The Routledge Handbook of Social Work Theory

The Routledge Handbook of Social Work Theory provides an interdisciplinary and international introduction to social work theory. It presents an analytical review of the wide array of theoretical ideas that influence social work on a global scale. It sets the agenda for future trends within social work theory.

Separated into four parts, this handbook examines important themes within the discourses on social work theory, as well as offering a critical evaluation of how theoretical ideas influence social work as a profession and in practice. It includes a diverse range of interdisciplinary topics, covering the aims and nature of social work, social work values and ethics, social work practice theories and the use of theory in different fields of practice. The contributors show how and why theory is so important to social work and analyze the impact these concepts have made on social intervention.

Bringing together an international team of leading academics within the social work field and newer contributors close to practice, this handbook is essential reading for all those studying social work, as well as practitioners, policymakers and those involved in the associated fields of health and social care.

Malcolm Payne is Emeritus Professor, Manchester Metropolitan University and has worked in probation, local government social services, the local and national voluntary sector and in a hospice in the UK. He is the author of many books including *Modern Social Work Theory, Older Citizens and End-of-life Care,* and *Humanistic Social Work.*

Emma Reith-Hall is a senior social work lecturer at Nottingham Trent University and a PhD student at the University of Birmingham. She remains involved in child and adolescent mental health practice.

The Routledge Handbook of Social Work Theory

Edited by Malcolm Payne and Emma Reith-Hall

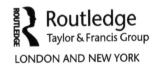

Routledge
Taylor & Francis Group

LONDON AND NEW YORK

First published 2019
by Routledge
2 Park Square, Milton Park, Abingdon, Oxon OX14 4RN

and by Routledge
605 Third Avenue, New York, NY 10017

First issued in paperback 2021

Routledge is an imprint of the Taylor & Francis Group, an informa business

British Library Cataloguing-in-Publication Data
A catalogue record for this book is available from the British Library

Library of Congress Cataloging-in-Publication Data
A catalog record for this book has been requested

Typeset in Bembo
by Apex CoVantage, LLC

ISBN 13: 978-0-367-78384-6 (pbk)
ISBN 13: 978-0-415-79343-8 (hbk)

To Margaret, wife and mother, who enriches our lives and social work, and without whom this book would not exist

Contents

Contents

Figures

Tables

Contributors

Peter Benbow is a senior lecturer in social work at Nottingham Trent University. His background is in adult mental health, and his academic interests include mental health practice and legislation.

Kyle Bennett is a doctoral student in the School of Social Work, University of Illinois at Urbana-Champaign, USA.

Professor Christine Bigby is Director, Living with Disability Research Centre, and Chair, Academic Board, at the School of Allied Health, La Trobe University, Australia.

Paul Blakeman is a senior lecturer in social work and course lead for the masters programme at Nottingham Trent University.

Robert Blundo is Professor Emeritus at the School of Social Work at the University of North Carolina Wilmington. He has spent his career writing and teaching social work students about the fundamentals of the strengths perspective and solution-focused practice.

Kristin W. Bolton is Associate Professor in the School of Social Work at the University of North Carolina Wilmington. She specializes in resilience and the evidence base of solution-focused brief therapy.

Beverley Burke is a senior lecturer in social work at Liverpool John Moores University, UK. She has practised as a youth and community worker and as a social worker and has published widely in the areas of anti-oppressive practice, values and ethics. Beverley is co-editor of the practice section of the international peer-reviewed journal *Ethics and Social Welfare*.

Alice K. Butterfield is a professor at the University of Illinois at Chicago, Jane Addams College of Social Work. Her international experience includes Romania, Ethiopia and India. Her work has focused on the development of MSW and PhD programmes, university-to-university and community partnerships and social development in impoverished communities.

Malcolm Carey is Professor of Social Work at the University of Chester. He previously taught at the Universities of Manchester and Liverpool following many years working as a social worker with older and disabled adults. His research interests include ageing and care, disability, applied ethics and professional identities and deviance.

C. M. Cassady is a doctoral student in social work and anthropology at Wayne State University in Detroit. Previously, she worked as a clinical social worker applying cognitive behavioural concepts in medical and hospice social work settings. Her research follows her clinical experience focusing on end-of-life choices and healthcare.

Simon Cauvain is Acting Head of Department, School of Social Sciences, Nottingham Trent University, UK, responsible for strategic and operational leadership and management. He oversees the social work teaching team, curriculum developments and student experience. Simon's main research interests include social worker experiences and associated feelings about practice, and the connection between research and professional practice and in the role of the university in qualifying social work education. Simon also supports the development of social work in Malawi, Africa.

Cecilia L. W. Chan is Chair Professor in the Department of Social Work and Social Administration of the University of Hong Kong. She is renowned for her integrated east–west mind–body theories in clinical practice that can empower people with special needs such as persons with stroke, cancer, divorce, bereavement, trauma and loss. Besides improving quality of life and subjective self-report, her Integrative Body-Mind-Spirit Social Work (IBMS) Intervention can also bring about improvements on physiological markers on stress, anti-aging and immune system.

John Coates is Professor Emeritus in Social Work at St. Thomas University, Fredericton, New Brunswick, Canada. He is a founding member of the Canadian Society for Spirituality and Social Work, and has long been an advocate of attending to the physical environment in social work. He has published widely on issues related to the environment and social work, the indigenization of social work, and spirituality and social work. His most recent books include *Decolonizing Social Work* (with Gray, Hetherington, & Yellow Bird, Routledge, 2013) and *Environmental Social Work* (with Gray & Hetherington, Routledge, 2013).

Polly Cowan is a doctoral student at the University of Edinburgh. Her research is on adoption disruption in Scotland. Polly is a social worker, working in the third sector, having previously worked in statutory settings (children and families) in England and Scotland.

Viviene E. Cree is Professor of Social Work Studies at the University of Edinburgh. She previously worked with children and families in voluntary and statutory settings and has researched and published widely on social work. Her most recent research, with Morrison and others, was on social workers' communication with children.

Beth R. Crisp is a professor and discipline leader for social work at Deakin University in Australia, and the editor of the *Routledge Handbook of Religion, Spirituality and Social Work*. She has degrees in social work, theology and political science and has written extensively about spirituality for both secular and religious audiences.

Jane Dalrymple is a freelance trainer and consultant and associate lecturer at the University of the West of England. She is an accredited Dementia Care Matters Trainer and as such is part of a group of trainers who seek to be leading edge to improve dementia care. She practised as a social worker for many years and has published widely in the areas of anti-oppressive practice and advocacy.

Lesley Deacon is Senior Lecturer in Applied Social Studies and Social Work; Programme Leader MSc Practice Development at the University of Sunderland and co-author with Stephen J. Macdonald of Social Work Theory and Practice (Sage, 2017). Her PhD and post-doctoral research primarily focus on how generic social work practice can effectively respond to individuals with specific, complex needs; by listening to, and advocating for, the service user voice.

Lori L. Egizio is Visiting Clinical Trainer of Social Work, University of Illinois at Urbana-Champaign, USA.

Iain Ferguson is Honorary Professor of Social Work and Social Policy at the University of the West of Scotland. His books include *Radical Social Work in Practice* (with Rona Woodward, Policy Press, 2009), *Global Social Work in a Political Context: Radical Perspectives* (with Lavalette and Ioakimidis, Policy Press, 2018), and *Politics of the Mind: Marxism and Mental Distress* (Bookmarks, 2017). He is Advisory Editor for the international journal *Critical and Radical Social Work* and a founder-member of the Social Work Action Network (SWAN) (www.socialworkfuture.org).

Michael D. Fine is Honorary Professor in the Department of Sociology at Macquarie University, Sydney, Editor of the *International Journal of Care and Caring* and Principal Researcher on an Australian Research Council (ARC) project concerning the development of an Australian Measure of Outcomes in Community Care (ACCOM). His book, *A Caring Society?*, was published by Palgrave Macmillan in 2007.

Candy H. C. Fong, Ph.D. was Senior Education Officer of the Jockey Club End-of-life Community Care Project of the University of Hong Kong. She has contributed to research and training for persons with cancer, patients at their end-of-life and community rehabilitation.

Y. L. Fung is Post-Doctoral Fellow in the Department of Social Work and Social Administration, University of Hong Kong. He is now managing a large number of practice-research projects on Integrative Body-Mind-Spirit Intervention for various target groups such as children with eczema, family members of cancer patients and children whose parents are in prison.

A. Antonio Gonzalez-Prendes, PhD, is Associate Professor at Wayne State University's School of Social Work, where he serves as lead teacher of the Cognitive Behavioural Theory track for advanced-year MSW students. He has over 25 years of clinical experience in the treatment of mental health and substance use disorders.

Mel Gray is Professor Emeritus, Social Work, at the University of Newcastle, New South Wales, Australia. With John Coates, she published the first edited book on *Environmental Social Work* (Routledge, 2013) and has authored numerous journal articles and book chapters on social work engagement with the environment.

Tom Grimwood is Senior Research Fellow and Academic Lead of the Health and Social Care Evaluations (HASCE) research centre at the University of Cumbria. His books include *Key Debates in Social Work and Philosophy* (2015) and *Irony, Misogyny and Interpretation* (2012).

Michael Anthony Hart, PhD, MSW, is a citizen of Fisher River Cree Nation in central Canada and is the Vice Provost (Indigenous Engagement) at the University of Calgary, Alberta, Canada.

He was the Canada Research Chair in Indigenous Knowledges and Social Work at the University of Manitoba from 2012 to 1018 where he also spearheaded the development and implementation of the Master of Social Work program based in Indigenous Knowledges. His research focuses on Indigenous practices and the incorporation of Indigenous knowledge, experiences and perspectives into social work.

Stan Houston commenced his career as a social worker and worked in various child-care settings in Belfast for around 20 years. He then moved to higher education, and worked in Queen's University Belfast for a further 20 years. He recently retired but decided to return to employment by taking up an academic post in Trinity College Dublin. His main academic interests lie in the application of critical social theory to social work.

David Howe is Emeritus Professor at the University of East Anglia, Norwich. Before that he was a teacher, child-care officer, and social worker. His research and writing interests include child and family social work, attachment and social work theory. He is the author of 21 books and more than 100 peer-reviewed papers and book chapters.

Christopher G. Hudson is a professor in the MSW Program at Salem State University, Massachusetts, USA, and is best known for his research in mental health policy and services and psychiatric epidemiology. His publications include *Dimensions of State Mental Health Policy* (Praeger, 1991), *An Interdependency Model of Homelessness* (Mellen, 1999), and *Complex Systems and Human Behavior* (Lyceum, 2010). Recent research includes theoretical reviews on complex systems theory and testing theories of psychiatric disparities. This research led to new methodologies for estimating local rates of psychiatric disability, which have been validated in Israel, New Zealand, and the United States. Dr. Hudson was awarded the William J. Fulbright Award for research, in Hong Kong (2002–2003) and in the Czech Republic (2017–2018). Recently, he served as elected president of the Massachusetts Chapter of the (US) National Association of Social Workers.

Vladimír Labath is a Professor of Social Work, with a PhD on educational psychology. After training in group psychotherapy, he worked as a therapist and counsellor and remains an active practitioner. In 1991, he established the first university social work department in Slovakia at Comenius University in Bratislava. He has also been involved in civil society development programmes and took part in projects in ten countries worldwide. His research focus is youth, delinquency and group work. At present he is a member of the Department of Social Work at the Catholic University in Ruzomberok, Slovakia.

Peter Lehmann is a professor in the School of Social Work at the University of Texas at Arlington. His clinical and research interests include teaching and using strengths and competency-based approaches with youth and adult offender populations as well as in the treatment of children and families.

Hilda Loughran is Associate Professor in the University College Dublin School of Social Policy, Social Work and Social Justice. Prior to taking up that position, she worked as a social worker and addiction counsellor in an addiction treatment service. She has written on social work counselling skills and brief interventions. She works with service users in substance use settings, building on their expertise to improve the social work curriculum. She has also engaged with service users around social justice issues, disadvantage and substance use.

Stephen J. Macdonald is a reader in Social Science at the University of Sunderland and co-author with Lesley Deacon of *Social Work Theory and Practice* (Sage, 2017). His published research has employed both qualitative and quantitative research methods to analyze disabled people's experiences of structural barriers.

Kenneth McLaughlin is a senior lecturer at Manchester Metropolitan University, where he teaches modules on sociology, social policy and mental health. Prior to this, he worked as a social worker in a social services mental health team and as a support worker with homeless families. His research is concerned with the way wider social and political concerns are reflected within social policy in general and social work in particular. His previous work has highlighted the implications of a risk-averse culture and the process of psychologization on contemporary social work theory and practice.

Kathleen Manion is Associate Professor and Program Head, BA Justice Studies, Royal Roads University, Victoria, British Columbia, Canada. With 25 years' experience in social and community services and academic institutions, her research interests include supporting children to thrive; bridging the gap between practitioner experiential knowledge, theory and policy and international social work. Her projects have explored child protection, homelessness, childhood development, environmental intersections, family violence and youth justice.

Ewa Marynowicz-Hetka is a social pedagogue; Professor of the Humanities, Full Professor and Director of the Department of Social Pedagogy at the University of Łódź, DHC of the University of Ostrava (Czech Republic); member of the Pedagogy Sciences Committee of the Polish Academy of Sciences (2003–2011), President of the Polish Association of Schools of Social Work (1991–2011) and President of the European Research Resource Centre for Social Work.

Fiona Morrison is a lecturer at the Centre for Child Wellbeing and Protection at the University of Stirling. She worked in the third sector in children and families' settings. Her most recent research, with Cree and others, was a UK-wide study of the 'everyday' encounters between children and social workers.

David P. Moxley serves as director and professor in the University of Alaska, Anchorage School of Social Work. Previously, he served on the faculties of the University of Oklahoma and Wayne State University. His interests span social work and social action, and his practice has taken him to high-need communities across the globe.

Pavel Navrátil is Associate Professor in the Department of Social Policy and Social Work, Masaryk University, Brno, Czech Republic.

Carolyn Noble, PhD, is Associate Dean (Social Work) at NPI ACAP Sydney as well as Professor Emerita at Victoria University, Melbourne. Her research interests include social work philosophy and ethics, work-based learning and professional supervision and critical theory and practice development in social work. Further areas of research include gender democracy and equal employment opportunity for women in higher education and human services. She has published widely in her areas of research and continues to present her work nationally and internationally.

Elena Ondrušková psychologist, lecturer and consultant in social work practice, worked as a lecturer and researcher at the Social Work Department at Comenius University, Bratislava,

Slovakia. She is associated with critical theories, empowerment, gender-sensitive ideas and feminist theory in social work. In her research she focused on examining relationships in families at risk and exploring women's strategies to manage violence in close relationships. She is an author of six books, manuals on practice with families and many scholarly and popular articles.

Malcolm Payne is Emeritus Professor, Manchester Metropolitan University and worked in probation, local government social services, the local and national voluntary sector and in a hospice in the UK. He is author of many books including *Modern Social Work Theory* (Palgrave Macmillan, 4th ed., 2014), *Older Citizens and End-of-life Care* (Routledge, 2017) and *Humanistic Social Work* (Lyceum, 2011).

Michael Reisch is Distinguished Professor of Social Justice at the University of Maryland and a former Woodrow Wilson Fellow and Fulbright Scholar. His most recent books include *Macro Social Work Practice in a Multicultural Society*; *Social Policy and Social Justice: Meeting the Challenges of a Diverse Society*; *Social Work Practice and Social Justice: Concepts, Challenges, and Strategies*; *The Routledge International Handbook of Social Justice*; and *The Handbook of Community Practice*. In January 2017, he became a Fellow of the American Academy of Social Work and Social Welfare.

Emma Reith-Hall is a senior social work lecturer, Nottingham Trent University and PhD student at the University of Birmingham. She remains involved in child and adolescent mental health practice.

Karen Roscoe is a senior lecturer in social work, University of Wolverhampton. Karen is published in a variety of academic journals including the *British Journal of Social Work*. Her work captures the narratives of service users who have encountered domestic violence in rural Wales and social workers applying the concepts of reflective letters in integrated family services, drawing on new models for intervention. Karen's research draws on transdisciplinary methodologies using critical discourse analysis to enhance creatively innovative and productive theory formation.

David Shemmings, OBE, PhD, is Professor of Child Protection Research and co-director of the International Centre for Child Protection, University of Kent and Visiting Professor, Royal Holloway, University of London.

Yvonne Shemmings, MA (by research), is Continuing Professional Development specialist and an honorary lecturer at the International Centre for Child Protection, University of Kent.

Guy Shennan is a social worker who works as an independent consultant, specializing in solution-focused approaches, having pioneered their use within statutory social work with children and families in the UK. From 2014–18, he was chair of the British Association of Social Workers.

Abiot Simeon is Assistant Professor in the College of Social Science and Humanities, Debre Berhan University. He received his PhD in Social Work and Social Development from Addis Ababa University. His dissertation examined the Mission for Community Development Program, a local NGO, as a locality-based social development organization in Ethiopia.

Douglas C. Smith is Associate Professor of Social Work, University of Illinois at Urbana-Champaign, USA.

Paul Stepney is Adjunct Professor of Social Work at the University of Tampere, Finland and visiting professor at one other Finnish university. Prior to this he taught at four UK universities and worked as a hospital social worker. Paul's research interests are in critical practice and prevention, and he is co-author of three books. His latest book is with Neil Thompson: *Social Work Theory and Methods: The Essentials* (Routledge, 2017).

Stéphanie Wahab is Professor of Social Work, Portland State University, USA.

Penelope Welbourne worked as a residential social worker, child and family social worker and social work manager prior to beginning work as an academic at Plymouth University. Her teaching and research interests are centred on work with children and families, especially the intersection between law and the family.

Sarah Wendt is Professor of Social Work, College of Education, Psychology and Social Work, Flinders University, South Australia.

Tom Wilks is a lecturer in Social Work at the University of Winchester. He worked for many years as a social worker and service manager, primarily in mental health and in drug and alcohol services. His academic interests are in social work ethics, service user involvement in social work education and advocacy. He is the author of *Advocacy and Social Work Practice* (Open University Press, 2012).

Karen Winter is a senior lecturer in social work at Queens' University Belfast, having practised as a qualified social worker for more than 16 years, working with children and families. Her research and teaching focuses on young children on the edge of care and in care. She has an interest in their rights, relationships and outcomes. She is chair of the Advisory Committee for Fostering Network NI and non-executive member of the Board of the Northern Ireland Guardian *ad Litem* Agency.

Yuk-Lin Renita Wong is a professor in the School of Social Work at York University, Canada. Her scholarship and teaching aim at deconstructing power relations in the knowledge production and discursive practices of social work; as well as re-centring marginalized voices and ways of knowing and being. She brings contemplative pedagogy into social work education and takes up mindfulness as a pedagogy of decolonization and as critical reflective practice that nurtures awareness and wholeness in social justice work. She has been a mindfulness practitioner since 1998 and has been leading meditation and mindfulness training since 2007.

Introduction

Malcolm Payne and Emma Reith-Hall

In this Introduction, we set out the structure of this Handbook and explain how it is organized and some of the reasoning behind our editorial decisions.

The aim of the Handbook is to survey and review current theoretical analysis and debate within the discipline and profession of social work, making it available to scholars and practitioners to inform their own specialized research and scholarship. Managers of social work services, practitioners and students may also find the content useful as a guide to current theoretical analysis and debate.

Theory in social work

We have taken a very broad view of what constitutes theory in social work.

First, we recognized that social work and its theory is partly national. It depends on the culture, law, policy and traditions of each country and its region. But it is also international, because there is worldwide distribution of literature and global interaction among ideas. What is important in theory varies across the world, depending on the political, social and social science discourses present in any particular society, but it also reflects an international consensus about what is currently important in social work. This is highlighted in several chapters, but we chose to place early in the book, at Chapter 2, Labath and Ondrušková's account of the development of social work ideas in the political and social science context of Slovakia since revolutionary changes in 1989. We can see in their account the influence of international theoretical literature and the impact of debates among disciplines close to social work as a new profession and its theory emerged. The struggles to create a relevant theoretical consensus from these influences illustrate the processes of theoretical development that continuously inspire, stimulate and frustrate social workers everywhere.

Second, we have tried to balance coverage of ideas about social work's aims, its nature and the values that inform it (in Parts 1 and 2) with varying theoretical visions about how to practise it (in Part 3). We argue in Chapter 1 that all these issues interact in any application of theory. A practice theory considered in Part 3, for example, is not applied separately from social and political aims considered in Part 1, values issues (Part 2) or knowledge about particular client groups or services (Part 4).

Third, we recognize that sources of social science knowledge about the issues and problems that social workers face as they work with their clients are important to many social workers. We include, therefore, in Part 4, a selection of accounts of practice with client groups and social issues that practitioners and social care services work with. These show how ideas about the aims, values and practice of social work come together in the service of particular groups. These chapters allow readers to triangulate general ideas about power, stigma and oppression with practice approaches and how these make their impact on the individuals, groups, communities and social structures that practitioners seek to influence and change.

We sought contributions from writers in a wide range of countries and intellectual traditions. A balance of contributions from well-established writers and younger contributors from different countries sometimes gives us a new perspective on ideas that we thought familiar and introduces us to a local literature which is paralleled in other countries; Chapters 4 on epistemic discourses on assessment and 24 on social pedagogy are examples. Inevitably, though, a Handbook written in the English language must rely mainly on contributions from writers confident in being able to express their ideas in that language. Therefore, among nearly 60 authors, about a third are from the UK; a third from the US and Canada and about a third from Africa, Asia, Australia and mainland Europe.

Structure

The Handbook is divided into four parts.

Part 1 The aims and nature of social work

Conceptions of an activity such as social work and its social organization influence how it is carried out and its contribution to social relations and political and social debate. Chapters in this part of the book critically review ideas about the nature of social work and its objectives. They look at ideas and debates around different perspectives and positions about what social work is.

Part 2 Theory about social work values

The nature of social work reflects resolutions of value conflicts inherent in making social interventions within the economic, political and social structures in society. How social work resolves these issues creates some of the characteristics of the discipline and profession and its thinking. Chapters in this part of the book critically review ideas that have influenced social work values, considering important value positions that affect the practice actions, professional judgements and the governance and regulation of social workers.

Part 3 Theories of social work practice

Chapters in this part of the book critically review theories that propose ways of practising social work. They debate the intellectual sources, knowledge and evidence base, value and impact of these practice theories. The aim of these chapters is to promote an understanding of a practice theory's contribution to, and limitations within, the constellation of ideas available to social work practice and to appraise the value of the theory as a contribution to social work. These chapters do not provide enough detail for someone to practise according to any theory. By including these chapters, we aim to provide an informative account of what practitioners concerned with these theories are currently achieving.

Part 4 Theory in practice

Chapters in this part of the book explore that theoretical ideas in social work particularly influence practice with a client group or social issue. They cover theoretical ideas from related academic and professional areas as well as from within social work thinking. The aim of these chapters reflects the reality that practice actions are influenced by an interacting complex of conceptualizations, of social work practice and of social science knowledge. These chapters show how, in social work, theory must offer more than stimulating visions of the world. It must also contribute to practitioners' impact on the social situations that they face.

To conclude

We are grateful for the trouble contributors have taken to offer stimulating and interesting presentations of the issues that we asked them to consider and often to present us with the unexpected. One of the strengths of a big multi-contributor book such as this one is that each author addresses the topic in their own way, which really suits the variety and diversity of the social work profession.

Part 1

The aims and nature of social work

Social work theory, knowledge and practice

Malcolm Payne and Emma Reith-Hall

Introduction: social work theories as stories and knowledge management

Theory tells stories about social work. Each set of theoretical ideas expresses how we may represent some of the aims and practices of important aspects of social work. No one theory represents all social work; rather, each theory is brought together around important facets selected from the whole. In the first part of this Handbook, discussions of theoretical thinking are constructed around important areas of social knowledge that influence ideas about the nature of social work, such as biomedicine, culture, psychology and the social. Theoretical thinking in the second part coalesces around important value concepts that influence social work ideals, such as caring, autonomy and human rights. The third part explores a series of discrete formulations that theorize important ways of doing social work in practice. And in the fourth part, theoretical ideas formed around some selected human groups and services important in social work disclose another reconstruction of concepts explored elsewhere in the Handbook. In every part there would have been other perspectives, theorizations or analyses that could have been included, but we have tried to present a wide and representative range of ideas current in social work debate.

Theory is constructed in stories because the connections between different facets of social work cannot be defined only in one way; rather the stories show how they are linked and perceived in many ways. Some theoretical constructions may be of sequences. Examples are a story about how the ideas of social work as eclectic or integrated changed in a central European country over 25 years (Chapter 2), stories about the development of psychology as an influence in social work (Chapter 3) or about developments in critical thinking (Chapter 26). Other theoretical constructions are less linear and more complex, as befits accounts of human life and action, where there are constant intersections of knowledge from many different sources.

The stories that theories offer therefore show us encounters between ideas. Theories and the writings about them challenge, intertwine with and elude each other. Interconnected theories form groups that share many ideas and approach social work similarly. Examples of such groups are approaches based on positive psychologies (chapters 18–22) and critical approaches to social work (chapters 26–31). But each theoretical position within such groups elaborates the shared perspectives in different directions. In the positive psychologies group, strengths perspectives focus on positive contributions from peoples' social networks and relationships, solution-focused practice on positive thinking, motivational interviewing on developing positive energy and narrative practice on exploration in peoples' experiences. In the critical theory group, critical perspectives focus on ways of contesting the 'taken for granted'; macro perspectives on interventions working with social groups; empowerment engages with how people may take up and use the power available to them; anti-discrimination practice is about how to surmount social barriers and advocacy theory is concerned with helping people find ways of strengthening their influence and voice to make progress in their lives.

Theory groups that confront each other take genuinely different views of intervention in human lives but within the same framework of thought. Examples are the cognitive sciences (Chapters 16–17) and the positive psychologies (Chapters 18–22) as a basis for practices. Sometimes, these opposing theories speak past each other, not clashing but irrelevant to each other's concerns. They are operating at different levels or in different contexts of thinking. If we examine Chapters 15 and 16 on systems and cognitive behavioural therapy in social work, for example, we can see different ways of thinking about social work compared with Chapter 27's account of macro practice. The social work that each discusses is of a very different nature, and these ideas do not engage with each other.

Social work abounds in theoretical variety. This is because the array of possibilities offered by theoretically diverse stories assists its practitioners and scholars in knowledge management. Doing social work, teaching it and researching it means drawing information from the people engaged in the human situations that we are dealing with and evaluating and organizing that information. How does a practitioner choose what questions to ask of an applicant for service or what things to say to a resident of a care home? How does a social work educator decide what is most useful and appropriate for helping students learn to practice social work? How does a researcher decide important areas of the social work world to investigate and explain? Their choices reflect different theoretical positions and tendencies.

Healy (2014), noting that theory constantly evolves, identifies three important discourses that shape theoretical positions:

- Dominant discourses in services providing for health and well-being: medicine, law, economics and new public management. Healy neglects education, which is significant in some national systems of social work and in some social work theories.
- Behavioural and social science discourses that are important to social workers but are less significant than the dominant discourses: psychological and sociological ideas.
- Alternative discourses that are available but that she claims are not yet influential on the dominant discourses: citizens' rights, religion and spirituality and environmental and green perspectives.

How do we position alternative perspectives as part of the whole panoply of social work? This depends on where we come from and where we are aiming. For example, ecological systems theory was conceived as a more social form of practice than preexisting relationship-based practice. Coates and Gray argue, however, in Chapter 14, that it does not adequately represent environmental and green perspectives that are now important in social thought. Their contribution thus becomes part of the interaction between discourses. It asks questions. What are our 'social' objectives in ecological or green practice? How has that changed as theory has developed? And we may ask, looking at other chapters' stories about theory, do they adequately conceptualize the ecological: the macro focus on the political, for example, in Chapter 27? Hudson in Chapter 15 documents changes in systems thinking which also demonstrate limitations in social work's ecological systems theory. It is inadequate in the context of current systems thinking. And while social pedagogy (Chapter 24) and local social development practice (Chapter 25) are both represented as macro practices, Ferguson's account of macro practice in Chapter 27 would place them more at the mezzo level. Again, while Ferguson's conceptualization of macro practice and Wendt's account of feminist practice in Chapter 31 are clearly within the bounds of critical theory (Chapter 26), Ferguson (Chapter 27) expresses concerns about the limitations of identity politics as a foundation for macro practice. Differences of focus throughout Chapters 26–31 on critical theory suggest there is a complex of interacting connections, dissenting voices and confounding issues among these broadly consonant sets of ideas.

Social work knowledge in practice, discipline and profession

Social workers therefore have many sets of theoretical ideas to choose from and many nuances to apply. Why is this? We suggest that it is because social workers in practice are always generalists in a complex world. Social work educators and researchers, therefore, draw from a broad range of human sciences to inform and stimulate their practice. Pawson, Boaz, Grayson, Long and Barnes (2003), in an important research study, identified five knowledge sources that social workers use:

- Organizational knowledge, from the agency.
- Practitioner knowledge, from their practice experience.
- Policy community knowledge, about legal and policy information.
- Research knowledge, from systematic research.
- User and carer knowledge, gained from the experience and views of service users.

Social workers have to organize knowledge from all of these sources to carry out any act in their practice. The profession and discipline of social work must also bring together wide ranges of knowledge to organize and facilitate their use in professional actions.

A profession is an identifiable occupational group carrying out widely recognized social responsibilities by implementing practices that build on understanding derived from its discipline. A profession such as social work must therefore formulate those responsibilities into a recognizable and recognized system of practice that social workers are able to carry out in their daily practice activity. Theory informs the systemization of a profession's practice and facilitates practitioners in implementing practice appropriate to the profession.

Healy's (2000) valuable distinction between social work practice and practices points to the difference between the profession's system of practice and the social worker's practice activity. Practice, to Healy, is what social workers do when they interact with clients on behalf of and as part of social work agencies. Meeting a member of the public to 'do an assessment' or to 'safeguard a child', a social worker must perceive and collect complex practical information about many different issues and ally it to human understanding. They work in the context of public policy and as part of an organization, alongside colleagues from their own and other professions. To do all this, they must manage many different sources of knowledge and package their findings into clear decisions about intervention in human and social situations. They must then take action that requires collective engagement of carers, clients and colleagues. Social work educators and researchers must similarly incorporate into academic discourses a whole range of these complexities, co-producing with practitioners and clients the stories that will construct social work practice and theory.

Practices are the social processes that social work engages in through that practice and those agencies. Among other things, Healy refers to emancipation, creating and representing social identities, influence, power and social regulation. Discussing theorizing in social work, Thompson (2017) notes that one helpful aspect of theory is how it may help us to make sense of, understand and connect the practice with the practices. Thus, in practising with individuals, families and communities, social workers deal in people's social identities as gendered individuals with ethnic identities. These identities affect the identities conferred by their membership in family and community. But, unlike journalists, policymakers or politicians, social workers are not managing ideas of gender and ethnicity or of family and community at the level of policy, but in the impact of those ideas as they affect individuals and groups in their daily lives. The social work profession is one of several professions that practise within services that care for and help people within a social sphere that includes professions such as the church, clinical psychology, counselling, law, medicine, nursing and teaching. Social work's professional identity and its practice overlap with aspects of these professions and with community and youth work. Similarly, the services within which social workers practice interact with education, health, housing, social security and other services in the public sphere and with social institutions such as churches and religious organizations, the courts and criminal justice organizations and government and political structures.

Consequently, social work actions are 'distributed'. That is, they are carried out in networks of relationships in people's homes and communities and in networks with other organizations and professions. Social work actions are not part of an institution such as a centralized bureaucracy paying social benefits, a hospital or a school in which practitioners are enveloped in and protected by conformity to an established authority deriving from legal requirements (Orlikowski, 2002). Because what they do always involves discretionary action in an uncertain social world, social workers must, using theory from their profession, manage complex knowledge to achieve organized activity among a collective of people who may have differing aims and roles. They must negotiate dilemmas among a variety of participants. Their theory and the education and research that develops that theory must in turn enable them to explore and use the knowledge that contributes to discretionary action in an uncertain and complex world.

Having a range of ideas available through social work's theoretical stories therefore helps practitioners to manage information and decisions, disentangling competing interests and concerns. And research and education in such a field must reflect and respond to the complexity that practitioners must deal with. If the stories offered by theory allow social workers to manage the diversity of the knowledge as they practice and take part in social practices, social work's disciplinary discourse and their professional organization must also deal in that range. A discipline is a branch of knowledge and understanding, created through debate and critical analysis founded on empirical observation and research. The scholarship involved in theory and theorizing contributes to that discipline, since it shows ways of bringing together and using theory.

A professional discipline is not like an academic discipline: its disciplinary knowledge and understanding are created to be used in carrying out its practice, providing the services that meet the social responsibilities that fall within its sphere of concern. Social work practice and services therefore interact with and influence the discipline, which in its turn informs and structures the practice and services. They are nothing without each other. Disciplinary knowledge and understanding are only worthwhile if they usefully inform practice, but to be professional, practice must implement the discipline because a profession only exists where it is informed by a discipline.

But professional practice in the social sphere is not wholly defined by its discipline because practice also involves artistry and craft. This is because social work objectives and scholarship do not generate just 'do this-do that' actions. Instead, they require practitioners to use empathy and judgement to produce results that are experienced positively by the people involved. Artistry is about using imagination to create an outcome that people experience as worthwhile, emotionally and socially right. Craft focuses on practitioners' capacities to bring together different skills to achieve the results they and their clients want. Social work often involves making an application, following a procedure or carrying out some administrative action, but it is never only that. It also involves finding a satisfying and worthwhile outcome to these procedures and actions for practitioners' clients. 'Satisfying' implies achieving a positive emotional response to both the work's outcome and the processes pursued to achieve that outcome. 'Worthwhile' implies a value judgement about the personal and social outcomes of the work. The profession, discipline and practice are not only judged by clients and the people who surround them and by practitioners themselves. They are also evaluated by their community, political and social institutions that commission the profession and its practice and the other professionals and participants in the society that surrounds the practice.

Theory as ideas

Theory is about ideas, and exploring theory helps us understand the ideas that influence social work as a discipline, a profession and the practice that derives from that discipline and profession. Theories are both sets of ideas used to explain something and sets of principles that inform practitioners about how an activity is undertaken. Social work theories are used to help social workers understand the people, communities and societies they work with and to inform decisions about which methods, models and interventions will help effect change, achieve tasks and fulfil goals. Theory is not the (possibly fleeting) impact of stray ideas. As part of a discipline and profession, it implies systematic thinking applied to the social phenomena and structures of social work and in identifying and codifying its practices.

Ideas may also be important because of their heuristic character: that is, they stimulate and help us learn things about ourselves and the world around us. Houston, in Chapter 5, for example, discusses Bourdieu's conceptions of different forms of 'capital', and Marynowicz-Hetka in Chapter 26 and Benbow and Blakeman in Chapter 36 discuss other contributions to social work by Bourdieu. Ideas about capital alert us to the different ways in which people may accumulate opportunities to exercise power and control over their lives and the society around them. Social capital, in particular, is the extent to which individuals, families and communities build networks of relationships to support and develop their lives. This concept has influenced thinking about how people may be empowered in important ways that limit or alter the impact of coercion through economic, class or political power. The idea has influenced healthcare professions in rethinking possibilities of generating social means of health improvement (Morgan & Swann, 2004). It can also help social work find ways of understanding how empowerment might be relevant to social work and how it may be achieved in practice. People are empowered if we can increase their social as well as other forms of capital in living their lives.

Sociological research offers evidence for practitioners to use about important elements in social relations, such as families, communities and organizations. Increasingly, social theory focuses on ideas about society, to be applied in thinking about how social relations among human beings are influenced by movements and structures in society. Thorpe (2018), for example, explores ideas such as phenomenology, symbolic interactionism, the social self, Bourdieu's ideas about symbolic violence, feminist ideas and globalization. Some of the same ideas make their appearance in relevant chapters (see Chapters 5, 26, and 28) in this Handbook. Parrott with Maguinness (2017), while covering some of the same territory, focus on sociological ideas about interpersonal social relations of practical concern to practitioners, such as stigma, risk and poverty, and broad social issues of direct political concern to them, such as economic markets, managerialism and again globalization.

Analyzing theory

An important role of social work theory, therefore, is to assist both analysts within the discipline and professionals to resolve conflicts that are central to debate within and understanding of it. Connecting with Marynowicz-Hetka's ideas of social work as an action science (Chapter 24) and Navrátil's distinction between explanation and understanding (Chapter 4), Musson (2017) makes a useful distinction between theories of:

- Explanation, whose aim is to provide explanations of the behaviour and social conditions that practitioners work with.
- Application, whose aim is to construct how practitioners should think about society and approach the situations they deal with.

Beckett and Horner's (2016) approach is to accept elements of both as part of social work theory. This is because any practice that emerges from theoretical analysis in social work requires understanding of how to apply the explanations.

Deacon and Macdonald (2017) classify theories according to their disciplinary or intellectual source, and this is similar to the analysis by Pawson et al. (2003) of sources of social work knowledge:

- Psychological theories.
- Sociological theories.
- Ethics and moral philosophies.
- Political theories and ideologies.
- Organizational theories.

Analyses such as Healy's (2014) show us that the theory influencing the discipline and profession of social work is contested. Because social work relies heavily on theoretical sources from elsewhere and is practised in various organizational contexts trends, in those disciplines and organizations inevitably affect social work. We can see this in several chapters in this Handbook. Carey (Chapter 6) for example draws attention to how biomedical knowledge, one of Healy's dominant discourses, influences social work thinking.

If it is to achieve artistry and craft, social work must have theory that also helps practitioners respect and respond to the complexities of social relations in general as they affect practice in particular instances. The issues include:

- Social work roles in political and social change and interpersonal change.
- Social work's position in relation to other professions, to policy and law and to organizations within which it operates.
- Social work's position in relation to political and cultural issues in current social debate.

Connolly and Harms (2015) classify social work theories into five somewhat ironically named groups:

- Ecosystems theories, which they regard as central, particularly work involving risk and protection, because they enable the exploration of multiple factors in people's lives.
- Onion-peeling theories, which offer ideas to enable practitioners to explore layers of experience in people's lives.

- Faulty-engine theories, which focus on unhelpful aspects of behaviour and thinking in people's lives.
- Story-telling theories, which seek to help people understand events and attitudes that have occurred in their lives.
- Mountain-moving theories, which focus on collective solutions in economic, political and social aspects of society that will benefit people's lives.

They argue that practitioners can see the practice solutions proposed by any of these theories according to a lens: that is, a way of looking at social situations. Lenses that practitioners use may be:

- relational: that is, focusing on human relationships among people and within societies.
- social justice, concerned with achieving different conceptions of fairness.
- change, concerned with achieving individual and social change.
- reflective, exploring cultural and social interpretations and understandings of social situations.

These different lenses generate alternative approaches to the social objectives set by different types of theory. They do so both by their interactions with each type of theory and by the diversity of ways each lens might be relevant. Practitioners might have a job that focuses on criminal behaviour: for example, using faulty-engine theories such as cognitive behavioural theory (CBT; Chapter 16) or motivational interviewing (MI; Chapter 20), but they can do so by exploring ideas offered by any or all of the lenses. At different times they might be more concerned with their clients' relationships, achieving social justice, individual or social change or inducing their clients to be more reflective, or they might aim their CBT or MI at relationship improvements for social work clients, while for others it might be more about being more reflective in understanding how they react to people with a different background or culture.

Social work theory and practice

We have argued that social work as a discipline and profession must deal with social complexity and uncertainty; therefore, discretion and thoughtful application of ideas must also be inherent in its practice. Practice demands that practitioners create a new story from their theoretical resources for each client, social issue and social group that they engage with. Such individual stories must also draw on the situation, issue or group that is presented to the practitioner. Putting together different perceptions of the real-world situation and the theoretical story makes social work's practice interesting and rewarding, and this stimulates commitment among practitioners to using the sets of ideas that theory offers them. Yet that commitment enforces engagement with the complexity and uncertainty of the social world, making social work a challenging and anxiety-provoking profession. The plethora of causes and contributory factors associated with all the different modes of human and social disadvantage and distress have generated a wide range of interventions and practices employed at the micro, meso or mezzo and macro levels of intervention. In turn, these demand attention to a varied array of continually expanding knowledge, values and skills. For social work practitioners, and for students in particular, adapting to the possibilities and learning what to think about, what to do, how to do it, why and with whom, can be a daunting and overwhelming prospect.

In Part 4 of this book, the chapters begin to explore how social work theories help us to make sense of the circumstances and predicaments we encounter in practice. Without this analysis of theory in practice, we could find ourselves floundering in unfathomable situations, with little recourse to understand or intervene in the lives of individuals, groups, communities and societies. Each chapter in Part 4 brings together knowledge about an important social work client group or social issue with the discrete practice theories examined in Part 3, to demonstrate how social work responds to social issues and needs. The practice theories in Part 3 provide direction, giving students and practitioners insight into sets of ideas which facilitate the understanding that might move people closer to their aspirations and goals. Using theories prevents each practitioner and student from having to start from scratch every time they work with a new client, social group or social issue. This does not mean an existing formula or off-the-shelf manual can be applied case after case, issue after issue, but it gives the student or practitioner an indication of what might work with a particular client group or in a specific setting, a set of ideas to inform practice, which can then be adapted to suit clients' needs and preferences.

Practitioners in the course of their work and students in social work education often struggle with theory because its generality makes it hard to use in the specificity of practice; there is a theory-practice gap. We have argued that the complexity of real human and social lives is hard to account for in a cogent theory. Our aim in Part 4 is to help practitioners and students explore how particular theories inform specific areas of practice. As they do so, their understanding and confidence in using theory to illuminate how to practise in particular situations grows. To be used effectively in social work practice, theory must be applied, and knowledge must be managed; Part 4 is concerned with developing accounts of how that application occurs. In addition to practitioners and students learning and reading about different theories, the role of managers, practice educators, supervisors, mentors and social work colleagues is to help practitioners and students cross theory-practice gaps. It is in the practice context, after all, that social work theories come to life and that their relevance and utility can be fully realized and tested out. It is also in the practice context where the nuanced individual facets of people's lives become apparent, for which a combination of theories is required to achieve appropriate understanding and intervention. Eclecticism, bringing together disparate theoretical sources to inform an episode of practice, represents a challenge for practitioners and students as they endeavour to draw on and apply different theories in a coherent and synthesized way; see Chapter 2 for further discussion.

In turn, practice informs theory. Many of the theories included in this book, particularly some of the theories that guide interventions, have their origins in practice. Social workers and allied professionals have, through their own work with people, developed ideas about human behaviour and strategies for promoting change, which they have formulated, tested out and shared, producing new theories for social work practice. Principles underpinning person-centred and solution-focused theories were developed through observing what works with real people in practice. Practice also allows theories to evolve, shaping and refining them so that they remain useful and appropriate to the changing contexts and landscapes in which social work operates. The demise of the decisional balance activity in exploring ambivalence discussed in Chapter 20 provides a very clear example of how revisions have been made to the theory underpinning MI.

Research plays a crucial role in both generating and testing theories, adding to the knowledge base and contributing to evidence-informed practice. In some areas, as Chapter 35 on child and adolescent mental health considers, the evidence base is underdeveloped. Similarly, as new challenges emerge in the social world, it is research, along with practitioner, service user and carer expertise, that will contribute to ways that social work theories can inform new areas of social work practice.

Social work theory: contextual or universal

The difficulty of using theory to respond to complex practice situations raises questions about whether research can helpfully inform practice or theory in this way. If social work theory is concerned with the whole of social relations, society and the social at a high level of generality, does that mean that it is universal in its application? Arguments for evidence-based or evidence-aware theory propose that this must be the aim of a theory capable of use in practice. The assumption is that a general theory, like those reviewed in this Handbook, must be universal, capable of application everywhere. Yet Labath and Ondrušková (Chapter 2) show how political and social change generates different patterns in the use of theory; Houston (Chapter 5) and Crisp (Chapter 11) show how social and cultural variation must be understood in relation to their cultural and social contexts. Hart, discussing indigenist social work (Chapter 23), shows how theories must emerge from the social and cultural milieux in which they operate. Practice theory must be contextual, therefore. Part of the process of responding to complex social situations requires the adaptation of the theoretical formulations of practice contained in practice theory. This is part of the flexibility and discretion involved in competent practice and part of the theoretical competence required of students and supported by their mentors in social work education and practice.

The social and cultural contexts generated across the globe must, therefore, provide options for the use of different theories in a practice situation. We argued, discussing the theoretical analysis of theory, that different lenses can help us adapt theory to play its part in a variety of situations. We proposed, therefore, that the critical realism approach to social science research is the most appropriate to examining social work theory. This proposes that studies of interventions with similar social issues in different milieux allow for the accumulation of findings about the circumstances in which various interventions are worthwhile. The choices that practitioners must make, therefore, can be informed by an awareness of how the options for intervention have played out in different contexts. In turn, this permits adaptation of models of practice to meet the present circumstances, based on an understanding of their effectiveness in previous similar and dissimilar environments. Claims that research can identify universally relevant interventions to be applied without adaptation must, therefore, be rejected. Moreover, since much research on social provision is funded by governments with the aim of informing service provision rather than professional practice, it does not address issues of the effectiveness of practice theory. Governments and social science researchers do not necessarily want to ask the questions that social workers want to ask about social work practice, about how it might be done and done better. Rather, they want to ask about policy objectives and achievements.

The future of social work theory

Many of the more concrete forms of analysis of social work theory based on positivist assumptions that empirical research can support universal application of particular practice theories have, therefore, felt increasingly unsatisfactory in the social work discipline: hence attempts like that of Connolly and Harms (2015) to recognize the complexity of the interaction of different aspects of theory. Writers on theory increasingly deal with the social conditions that bear on practice issues, rather than seeking to differentiate practice theories. Hodgson and Watts's (2017) introductory text, for example, covers issues such as risk, power, poverty and disadvantage, difference, respect and dignity, social justice and fairness, human rights, spirituality and hope, organizational contexts for practice, empathy, professional judgement and decision-making, assessment and critical reflection. Gray and Webb's (2013) edited collection focuses on the impact of ideas drawn from different social scientists and from current social science debate, including ways of examining and understanding social concerns. Thus, this kind of theory explores practice implications of ideas rather than formulations of practice prescriptions.

An important development of the 21st century has been the shift from problem-based practice towards the positive psychology of strengths and solution perspectives. This is an example of one of the shifts in emphasis in social work theory that take place from time to time. The shift from practical and moral persuasion toward policy innovation to create active social provision and psychological understanding to inform it, for example, took place in the early 20th century. A further move from a mainly psychodynamic theory base to acceptance of a more diverse set of social science influences was a characteristic of the 1970s. The tension between social democratic theory focused on the person and individual, group and community change and radical and critical appraisals of social work and its role in the major social changes of the last half century also emerged strongly in that more diverse social work theory universe. Another important movement has institutionalized an emphasis on the role of empirical research of different kinds, to inform evidence-based, evidence-aware or evidence-informed practice. The fact that these different emphases on the role of evidence exist suggests that its contribution is widely accepted but still unclear and insufficient. As we have suggested, empirical research has not helped resolve practice dilemmas, though it may help improve service structures.

It is striking that none of these changes in theoretical focus within social work have displaced others. They are more a rebalancing of the direction of travel of practitioners and their profession. Such rebalancing is inevitably connected to the policy and political debates that inform it and that are, in turn, influenced by the reconstructions of theoretical relationships in social work thinking. The structure of this book, then, does not create divisions between social work's aims and nature, its values, its practice theory and the knowledge and theory about the needs of social groups. We argue that practitioners call on all these areas of knowledge in interaction. We cannot work with any aim, any value orientation, any practice prescription, any group of clients without at times integrating all these aspects of theory in our thinking. See, for example, in Chapter 34, how child safeguarding links theory, values and the social as important elements of theory combining in practice. That is why social work practice is complex and demanding of practitioners.

The shift from problem-based to positive psychologies chimes with the current commitment of many social workers to respect the people they work with and the promotion of the value of respect for their person and their personal and social identity (see Chapter 9). More broadly, for a profession whose gaze is directed to the social, wider social objectives demand a focus on social justice (see Chapter 10) in the face of social inequalities and the social determinants of ill health and pressures on social well-being (see Chapters 10, 36–40). Social work has always emphasized its responsibility for working with the outsiders, the powerless and the weak trampled on by the insiders, powerful and strong in every society (see Chapters 28–31). Although it is part of the state and an accepted professional response to social difficulty, and wants to be in this position so that it can help its clients and respond to the social pressures on them, social work also wants to be the outsider profession. The tension between these aims is painful for its practitioners and tough for its theory-writers.

One question for theory therefore frequently emerges in debates about theoretical analysis of social work and its practice. It is this: the detailed analysis of and attention to helping the person and modifying their behaviour or developing strengths is in tension with the social objectives of social work, to change society by seeking social justice in the face of important inequalities and oppressions. But does concern for one invalidate commitment to the other? Proponents of onion-peeling and faulty-engine theories are often impatient with the blue-sky gaze of those proposing to move mountains by social or political intervention (returning to the usage of Connolly & Harms, 2015). Does active focus on persons, groups and communities mean that we evade responsibility for the broader implications of the social forces affecting social workers' clients and the policymakers who set their agency's mandate? Does activism on the social damage the capacity of the discipline and profession to grapple with the personal?

Practitioners and social work theory have never resolved this tension in practice. It is always present, a tension inherent in our understanding of the profession of social work and the disciplines that inform it. This book seeks to review the present state of the theory that informs that professional discipline and that universal and timeless tension.

References

Beckett, C., & Horner, N. (2016). *Essential theory for social work practice* (2nd ed.). London: Sage.

Connolly, M., & Harms, L. (2015). *Social work: From theory to practice* (2nd ed.). Cambridge, UK: Cambridge University Press.

Deacon, L., & Macdonald, S. J. (2017). *Social work theory and practice*. London: Sage.

Gray, M., & Webb, S. (Eds.). (2013). *Social work theories and methods* (2nd ed.). London: Sage.

Healy, K. (2000). *Social work practices: Contemporary perspectives on change*. London: Sage.

Healy, K. (2014). *Social work theories in context: Creating frameworks for practice* (2nd ed.). Basingstoke: Palgrave Macmillan.

Hodgson, D., & Watts, L. (2017). *Key concepts and theory in social work*. London: Palgrave Macmillan.

Morgan, A., & Swann, C. (Eds.). (2004). *Social capital for health: Issues of definition, measurement and links to health*. London: Health Development Agency.

Musson, P. (2017). *Making sense of theory and its application to social work practice*. St Albans: Critical Publishing.

Orlikowski, W. J. (2002). Knowing in practice: Enacting a collective capability in distributed organizing. *Organization Science, 13*(3), 249–273.

Parrott, L., with Maguinness, N. (2017). *Social work in context: Theory and concepts*. London: Sage.

Pawson, R., Boaz, A., Grayson, L., Long, A., & Barnes, C. (2003). *Types and quality of knowledge in social care* (Knowledge Review 3). London: Social Care Institute for Excellence.

Thompson, N. (2017). *Theorizing practice* (2nd ed.). Basingstoke: Palgrave Macmillan.

Thorpe, C. (2018). *Social theory for social work: Ideas and applications*. London: Routledge.

2

Theoretical aspects of social work – from eclecticism to integration

Vladimír Labath and Elena Ondrušková

Social work education's rich tradition in the former Czechoslovakia was forcibly interrupted by a totalitarian communist regime in the early 1950s. After revolutionary changes in 1989 and a return to a democratic system, the Comenius University Pedagogical Faculty, Bratislava, established in 1991 the first department of social work in the territory that became Slovakia. The department's approach was created through a discourse among academics in group psychotherapy, psychological counselling, therapeutic pedagogy and resocialization. In the first academic year, teachers and students specializing in social work met, and none had qualifications in social work. The solution to the lack of qualification was twofold: study and inspiration from abroad and compensating for theoretical gaps by applying theories from other disciplines.

Alongside transition from a totalitarian, communist regime to a democratic, pluralist society, from a state-governed economy to a regulated market economy, scientific knowledge about the resolution of individual and social problems was reconstructed. In a society becoming more open, such reconstruction confronted existing knowledge in other areas of the scientific world, and that included social work.

Theory and knowledge in social work

We understand a theory to be an organized generalized system of claims and explanations of the nature of certain facts: in social work, social phenomena and social problems. Focusing on social work theories, we are going to consider general theories of social work, the theories of context-based social and humanistic sciences and specific, or 'small', theories connected to social work practice. These are generally concerned with methods to move towards chosen goals.

Two general attitudes towards theories in social work may be identified (Payne, 2014). One is where practitioners prefer frameworks, models and scientific interpretations to explain and justify their actions. They consider it inappropriate for their own ideas, values and preferences to influence their professional conduct. Instead, neutral action is more effective for achieving clients' needs and agencies' goals. In this view, professional action is about a 'technology' of procedures. On the other hand, some professionals view social work as a human, interpersonal process, in which it is appropriate to consider the human dimension, people's thinking and judgement, achieving higher efficiency than just by applying a technological procedure.

Professional discourse on reconstructing social work theories and using them in practice in our regime transition reflected a discourse between these two approaches.

Like Healy (2005) and others, we consider social work to be a highly contextualized activity, varying considerably in different contexts of practice. This creates opportunities for theories to develop directly 'on the ground'. According to her, social work theories do not determine what social workers will pay attention to or what procedures they use in practice. Healy examines how social work theories construct and reinforce discourses on services, especially from ideas in psychology and sociology, which construct understandings of clients' needs and frame the direction of practice.

Seeing theory and practice development in social work as context dependent, we identified several factors in the social transformation in our society which influenced this process. These comprised primarily the development of civil society, political and economic goals, the changing emphasis on certain values and the discontinuity of scientific knowledge. All these factors related to every aspect of the transformation of a totalitarian society into a democratic regime. We use the term 'democratic society' to refer to economic situation, the state of civil society, and issues such as attitudes towards human rights. Concepts are likely to have different connotations in socially and economically developed societies as compared with transition economies. Going through the process of transition itself affects thinking, the preferences for specific theories and human behaviour.

Regardless of how we understand the nature of theory, Payne (2014) and other authors propose that theories are '. . . socially constructed in interactions between clients and practitioners in their agencies and in wider political, social and cultural arenas' (Payne, 2014, p. 3). If we accept the concept of the social construction of theories then we can say that at least 'practical' theories are variable and applied in several ways, and their abuse cannot be ruled out. The goal of theory in this context then is to legitimize the practical procedures that serve to assess and fulfil clients' needs. Therefore, we see theories as frameworks that define the three basic objectives of social work – empowerment, social change and resolution of social problems.

Musil (2010) considers the identity of social work as a key issue in theoretical discourse. He denotes it as a 'non-crystallization' of social work. He analyzes the process of constructing or shaping the identity of social work in the Czech Republic through 'domestic' theories. These focus on the question of what perspectives are applied in describing the characteristics of the institutionalization of social work. He states that essentially three perspectives are applied, not necessarily explicitly by writers: critical modernity, conservative modernity and late modernity or postmodernism. Each perspective identifies, understands and defines the institution of social work in distinctive ways. Similar discourses took place in Slovakia, which has been long connected to Czech tradition culturally, historically and politically.

Wider political themes, phenomena and problems are reflected in the reality of agencies and influence preferences for specific approaches. Watson and West (2006, p. 13), as well as other authors, point out that politics and policy goals are necessarily reflected in agencies' governance, resulting in direct pressure on the form and manner of social workers' practice. It is never possible to exclude some form of monitoring that may serve political objectives. They write that 'every social worker must personally, individually evaluate how he will respond to political pressure, which may be of a different nature – more or less subtle'. It is then up to each worker's individual reflection and the subsequent decision to consider whether to reflect such pressures when they apply particular social work perspectives. The development of social work is changing. In the past, psychosocial casework was the fundamental method (Payne, 2005). Currently, evaluation processes are of the highest importance in social work, especially the evaluation of outcomes, while methods are less important. Pragmatic solutions are important, which is also a reflection of policy goals.

Indisputably, values, meaning and function are important factors in the development of knowledge. The question of how the personal and professional values of social workers are understood or defined plays a significant role in how they approach practice (see Part 2). Banks (2001) argues that one crucial feature of social work practice is the constant inspection of one's own values and their potential in relation to the service provided. Watson and West (2006) suggest that there are only two competing paradigms of procedures that aim to change the social structure: managerialism and anti-oppression. Whichever is adopted then affects how values are reflected both in the initial assertions of social work theories and especially in the way in which social work is carried out.

Thus, developing theories of social work as well as building a system of social assistance and support in post-communist countries, as in other democratic societies, is sensitive to the social and ideological context. The specificity of post-communist countries is the difficult-to-define discontinuity and the controversial nature of the development of knowledge, especially social and human sciences. In Slovakia, in the process of transition from communist to democratic society, reconstruction of content has taken place, related to theories, practice and the concept of education in social work.

Changes during the period of societal transformation

The need for a critical assessment of theories of social work has grown as social problems have grown and the welfare state has been developed and reconstructed. This chapter explores how knowledge, university development and practice in the field of social work have been represented as a totalitarian society changes into a liberal democracy. We divide this period – in terms of pragmatics, and theoretical and research development – into three consecutive stages.

Confrontation with the ideologization of knowledge

From previous practice, the view dominated that social work is a professional process with which to solve individuals' social problems. Musil (2010) describes how these distorted ideas about goals and practices of social work under socialism. In the first phase of the development of theories (especially those concerning practice procedures), most approaches and theories used relied on working with individuals even if the source of the problems was not primarily attributed to them. Subsequently, influenced by empowerment-based ideas of social work practice, some discourse emerged about structural sources of particular social problems. Yet this shift was reflected particularly in the thinking about social problems that had previously not been acknowledged or addressed, such as violence against women, poverty and social exclusion of some groups of people, such as homeless people and substance abusers.

Confrontation with the ideologization of knowledge about individuals and society during socialism happened in many scientific fields but was probably strongest in pedagogy, sociology and psychology. Discourses emerged that critically evaluated the goals or findings of research that had been conducted in the context of the ideologization of scientific research. At the same time, research in social and human sciences continued without a critical re-evaluation of past scientific practice. Creators of the knowledge of social theories, especially Keller (1993, 2006), came up with their own interpretation of current social problems, with an acknowledged leftist or socialist perspective. Specific issues arising in Slovakia included how socialism characterized previously unacknowledged poverty, unemployment and, in particular, the social problems of marginalized Roma communities.

In this period, theoretical discourse came to ignore the conception of such issues as the acute consequences of the limited ability of poor or disadvantaged individuals to sustain by themselves a reasonable quality of life. Consequently, seeing such issues, as views within the international social work discourse might, as concerning the interaction between individuals and society requiring work with social structures or social environments was not perceived as problematic in post-communist societies. As a result, they were not a subject of theoretical research in the early period during which social work was being restored.

Education in social work (leaving aside organizational and administrative issues) was taking place in the context of social transformations around the liberalization of the economic environment and legitimation of civil society. It also felt the impact of changes in the social system, including transition from a concept of total social security towards the creation of social assistance and social service provisions. It meant that key concepts of social work were being continuously redefined and reconstructed. The themes of the functioning of the welfare state and social policies and the system of social services were dominant in these contemporaneous processes, with discourse about individuals being weaker.

Expert and theoretical discourse took place against a backdrop of diverse processes. The main aims were to depoliticize and de-ideologize education, knowledge and practice. Depoliticization concerned the removal of state power structures from the education system. De-ideologization involved opening communication channels, building information systems and stimulating diversity in thinking, knowledge and creativity. It meant liberation from the omnipotent universally applied dogma of Marxist-Leninist philosophy and materialistic interpretation of social reality. Part of this process were efforts to make helping professions less paternalistic and form the profession of social work, departing from administrative-legal practice and moving towards a biomedical paradigm. This process was followed by the differentiation and development of social services, changes in the role of social policy in society and building and legitimating civil society.

In that period, the study programme was modular, providing teaching on personality, social environment, helping professions, man in society, social pathology and development of social competencies. The starting point was positivist theories with a microsocial focus, inspired by different psychotherapeutic traditions. Since university-level social work education did not exist, social work conceptualizations emerged as parallel theories within several disciplines – psychology, sociology, psychotherapy and counselling, law and philosophy. Knowledge was multidisciplinary, and an eclectic approach prevailed in practice. The aim was to synthesize information, knowledge, concepts and approaches selected from different approaches and resources to create understandable and practically applicable logical systems of knowledge. Relationships among individual knowledge systems were purely pragmatic. The ambition was to select models that reflected reality, had a wide application and might be modified to different social (sociopsychological, socio-legal, socio-economic and socio-political) phenomena. The eclectic nature of knowledge was evident mainly in the effort to provide a wide range of insights and knowledge that could be universally applicable. On the other hand, the intention was to point out alternative ways of thinking and open paths for theoretical and practical specialization. The order of the day was to search for context and interconnections within knowledge.

Theory vs. application dilemmas

The second phase of the development of thinking and knowledge in social work in Slovakia relied on the first experience of new phenomena such as unemployment, a sharp rise in the abuse of hard drugs, homelessness, poverty and other social issues alongside the emergence of a range of new institutions and specialized services in connection with theory, history, research and trends in social work. During this period, writings by Payne (1997, 2014), Healy (2005), Gray and Webb (2013), Mullaly (1997) and others, played a major role in the cultural land-scape of our country, in particular the translations of works and publications of Matousek's team (2001). A feature of this phase was the selection of new knowledge, the tendency to look for connections, especially between theory and practice. In this spirit, the scope of theoretical knowledge was extended even further. Identity, profession, specialization and the legislative defi-nition of social work dominated research topics. On the other hand, theoreticians also sought detailed understanding of the field with scientific thought. Issues of terminology, research and conceptualization of the subject came to the fore.

Theoretical discourse developed at three levels during this phase. The first was the penetra-tion of social work theories with an increased interest in macro social issues of social phenom-ena, demography and social policy. The second level concerned sensitization to important issues within society, as well as with experts and theoreticians, using empowerment theories; anti-discrimination and anti-oppression concepts, orientated to cultural, gender, sexual and gender equality; inclusive approaches and the promotion of diversity. Knowledge was stimulated by good quality outcomes in mobilizing the non-profit sector and the massive development of civil society. A strong need to standardize social work processes emerged. The third area was the research sphere where, alongside the quantitative methodology typical of the first developmental phase, interest in qualitative research strategies began to develop. The theoretical definition of social work also became a topic of research.

During this period, it became clear that it was essential to connect separate cognitive spheres, seeking out interrelated themes and promoting their interaction. The integrating element among various theories was the client. There was an effort to perceive different theoretical sources as aspects of one process, the process of giving assistance. With some degree of toler-ance, we could rely on the model of systematic selection by Epstein (in Matousek et al., 2001). Theoretical debates were dominated by the topics of assistance, individual theories, concepts and interpretations focused on the knowledge and development of helping activities. Theories focused on the client, and they intersected at the point of giving assistance, aiming for self-help. Selecting theoretical aspects is the task of a theoretician, the aim being provision of relevant theories. Research served more to verify knowledge and claims than to create new knowledge. Its task was to provide a sufficient theoretical basis for effective application in practice. At this stage, it was not possible to speak about full integration, but rather about partial integration with the intention of stimulating and meeting the needs of practice. The integrative element was mainly present in the reciprocal linking of theory and practice.

The opening of information channels by removing barriers to the communication of infor-mation in society and the availability of publications brought polarization of opinions, per-spectives and confrontation among supporters of individual concepts. New findings brought unexpected dilemmas of objectification and relativization, sociologizing and psychologizing opinions, positivist positions and discourse considerations. Elementary topics were overshad-owed by 'small' areas of interest specifically linked to national local needs and issues. The overall picture of knowledge in social work was frequently overtaken by concepts of local character and particular circumstances, attributing potential for universal application to them. The period of enthusiastic acceptance of innovation was gradually replaced by the phase of matter-of-fact assessment, the selection of essential resources and the redirection of attention to the Slovak potential of knowledge.

Development of local scientific discourse

Emancipated local research in social work can be illustrated by feminist activism and the development of feminist thinking. Bosa (2013), through her own research and interpretation of the history of social work in a global context, has offered in our context a unique feminist interpretation of the history of social work. She opened the way for understanding feminist thinking in social work, especially for students because they gained a scientifically sound and positive scientific text in a concentrated and attractive form. Her later publication *Feminizmy v sociálnej práci* (Bosa, 2014) influenced the quality of education with its focus on understanding the values, principles and methods of feminist social work. Feminist theory became linked to research into social work that reflects the domestic context, whereas it previously focused on historical research (Bosa, 2014).

The identity of social work (Levicka et al., 2015) is also a subject of research. Levicka J. and Levická K. (in Levicka et al., 2015) distinguish three historical phases in the professionalization of social work in Slovakia. In the first phase, various associations focused on 'social assistance' with social issues important at the time of their activity. The second phase began with the professionalization of voluntary activity through formal social work education, referred to as 'social care' in the Higher School of Social Welfare in Prague, 1918–19. The third phase reproduced the second some time later but focused on the activities of professional associations and the creation of codes of practice. These activities were limited by social events that shaped the definition of social problems and the application of procedures for giving assistance.

The professionalization of social work practice took place as national discourses on social work theory emerged. This also resulted in the development of ethical standards and practice guidance for different areas of practice. Some of them directly followed the standards of international social work organizations (BASW, IFSW) and built on the same values and principles. They were, importantly, about social work's role in mitigating social exclusion and ensuring access to social resources for individuals, groups and communities. An example is the standards for field social work in marginalized Roma communities (Ondrušková, Pruzinska, & Rusnakova, 2015). Standards for field social work aim to ensure high-quality professional work meeting theoretical and practical requirements for expertise in this area of practice as well as broader professional demands. They are also a basis for enhancing the quality of field social work performance. Ideologically, the standards are built on the values of civil society and participatory democracy. That means that respect for human and civil rights, and for dignity and human potential, are priorities in all areas of performance and in field social work processes. Field social work aims to make available to citizens whatever their social circumstances existing social resources, enabling them to participate in decision-making processes in society and to promote opportunities for living a good quality dignified life.

In creating and building theoretical knowledge, the discourse seeks both reflexivity and contextuality. In recent years, qualitative research strategies and differentiation of research across the country have dominated. With the wide-ranging 'big' theories, we may identify tendencies towards discourse models of reasoning.

Knowledge – from eclecticism to integration

Our analysis proposes that the theoretical discourse over these twenty-five years moved through a process of evolution from eclecticism to integration, a transition from multidisciplinary to interdisciplinary approaches. In the first phase theories were extracted mainly from psychological counselling, psychotherapy and resocialization without making deeper interconnections and interactions. This is an example of eclecticism, but with no deeper connection between theoretical models of thinking and knowledge. The breakthrough in knowledge came as theoretical insights were taken into social work environments. This inspired further conceptualizations and their practice consequences. It shifted the models of reasoning taken from other helping and mental health professions to develop a different quality. As local theories of social work emerged, building on the knowledge and experience of the earlier phases of development, combinations and connections were achieved not only in practical applications but also and especially in the fields of knowledge and thinking. Interactions among theories then brought about the integration of knowledge of different sources, which was characterized by an interdisciplinary approach. Theories do not exist separately, side by side, but become sources of mutual inspiration, stimulation and development.

Social work differs from other helping professions not in its methods, but above all in its perception of reality, its thinking, and its reasoning. Therefore, we agree with Mullaly (1997) that it is necessary to systematize social work knowledge; it is not enough to provide an overview of individual approaches, theories and effective practical models. But this does not mean creating a unified, universal conceptualization. Rather, it should be about searching for principles, patterns, categories and missions for social work that could sufficiently generalize and differentiate knowledge and experience into a coherent theoretical and scientific system.

The mission of an integrative model is not, then, to define the content of education, the subject of social work, or to unify frameworks of social reality. It seeks to describe the social work way of thinking when analyzing the selection of theoretical sources and, above all, to identify the process of expert, theoretical and scientific discourse. We were originally inspired by ideas about integrative processes in psychotherapy (Knobloch & Knoblochova, 1999; Prochaska & Norcross, 1999), and we tried to compensate for the ignorance of theories and prescriptions of social work practice within other sources. At present, we see our model of integrating different levels of knowledge as the optimal form of discourse, where interaction between several levels and areas of knowledge are mutually enriching. Thus, we can talk about social work's way of thinking and reasoning. The content of the various parts of the model has changed over the years, but the way of thinking appears to be fundamental.

The essence of our integrative model of social work is the interconnection of three sources of theoretical knowledge.

On the first level, we see knowledge from a reflected, conceptualized and generalized practice – best practice. 'Small' theories, those about methods of intervention (Watson & West, 2006), provide theoretical background and practical structure for the work processes. Over the past 20 years, short-term models have been preferred, emphasizing service efficiency. This first level should retroactively include evidence-based practice, drawing on broader disciplinary fields. In this period, the shift has been from paternalism, state centralization of services, an administrative-legal focus and 'objectivism', through eclecticism and experimentation to liberalism, participation, subsidiarity, solidarity, responsibility, contextuality and reflexivity.

The second level consists of applied disciplines, helping theory. Analyzing 'help' in this context is unnecessary; we use it as an umbrella concept for all forms of helping activities, including self-help. These concepts speak of possibilities and limitations in helping individuals, couples, families or other groups. Here we can distinguish two sources of knowledge:

- The authentic, original theories of social work, and
- Concepts originating in other areas applied in the practice of social work.

While the early 1990s were dominated by psychotherapeutic knowledge and consultancy theories, authentic social work concepts of thinking and interpretation of reality now prevail, with the aim of perceiving the connections in practice and, above all, in knowledge.

Our category of 'referential idea concepts' includes the sum of knowledge and theory from other disciplines – psychology, sociology, law, philosophy and other important thought streams, research projects and concepts. Here, there have been significant shifts from positivistic understanding of reality towards constructivist and critical models of reasoning (Berger & Luckman, 1971; Healy, 2005; Fook, 2002). These shifts constitute an important theme in the development of knowledge for social work.

Figure 2.1 shows these components of our model, connected with double arrows expressing their interconnection and interaction. We see mutual interaction not only as exchanges of knowledge, but as never-ending discourses of reciprocal inspiration, stimulation and influence. The circle consequently shows the new quality of knowledge achieved in social work. The uninterrupted line expresses the permeability and openness of the cognitive system.

The integrative model has a generic character – it describes the discursive interaction between specific theories, models and concepts that lead to social work's special interpretation of social reality. The content of the integrative model, unlike its form, is unique. The key factor of an integrative approach is the two-way interaction of three levels of knowledge. The subject of cognition is social, socio-psychological, socio-political, socio-economic and social-legal phenomena (not only problems), which may only be interpreted within particular cultural and political environments and specific historical periods.

Integration may be defined as unification and/or connection. Theory and practice interconnecting may achieve integration at the level of practice through eclecticism. Integration is also an opportunity to grasp and define the theoretical framework, specifically of social work. Van Hasselt (cited by van der Laan, 1998, p. 150) '. . . defines integration as a transition from ideological versatility to unity. The final unit is more than the sum of its parts, but it is still possible

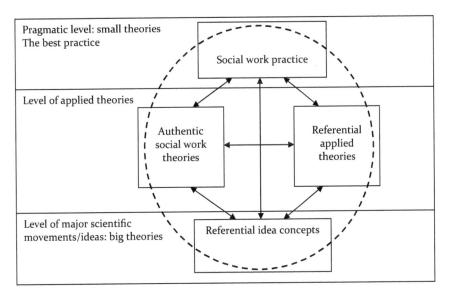

Figure 2.1 An integrative model of social work

to distinguish individual parts within the final unification'. The author suggests the wealth of knowledge resulting from the integration of theories, experience and facts. Payne (2011) explores integration, generalization and the specific conditions of particular cultures, countries and legal systems. He emphasizes the contextuality of helping theory and practice; universal systems of theories of social work cannot be considered real.

In this spirit, Payne (2014) distinguishes three levels of and limits to an integrated approach:

- The pluralistic availability of different theories of social work is beneficial, respected and real. The particularities of theories are tolerated depending on the conditions.
- The choice of theories among individual authors is within a wide range of theoretical considerations. The attempt to select theories always leads to a degree of narrowing and cannot cover the whole sphere of knowledge.
- Selective focus on underlying values is a necessary starting point for incorporating a wider framework of ideas into one thought system.

Our integrative approach is an attempt to seek common values, principles, patterns and categories of social phenomena in the helping theory and to create a distinctive framework for the interpretation of particular social realities.

Conclusion

Our integrative model of social work:

- Combines ideas, knowledge, concepts, theories and scientific disciplines in seeking a specific interpretative framework. By mutual interaction of theories, it creates a new quality of knowledge.
- Integrates various authentic theories created in the sphere of social work and referential theories, referential scientific knowledge, thought streams and positive experience from practice. It conceptualizes social work referring to cultural specifics in practice, theory and research.
- Perceives individuals (both clients and social workers) as integrated beings, viewing them as complex bio-psycho-socio-spiritual unities and as a dynamically evolving system that exists in a unique social context and time.
- Aims to strike a balance between support (relationship, cooperation), development (of potential) and correction (intentional change) as help is provided, with these elements being mutually complementary.

This integrative approach is determined by uniqueness in any culture, history, social structure and social issue; and in any preferred theoretical interpretation and conceptualization of social phenomena and the process of change. Interacting views, ideas, concepts and theories influence each other and create a new quality, an interdisciplinary dimension. This stimulates discourse among different sources of a given approach.

The integrative model has an interdisciplinary background. Unlike multidisciplinary thinking, interdisciplinarity seeks to overcome the mechanistic summation of theories and knowledge. Deeper theoretical and methodological linking of theories and their mutual interaction is essential and leads to a higher quality of knowledge. The integrative approach is a way of thinking not seeking to create universal content, which may be varied. It is dynamic, accepting and presupposing continuous theoretical and scientific development, and rejecting the creation of unified, universally valid theory.

In summary, the integrative concept of social work is characterized by its interdisciplinarity. The interaction among different theoretical sources has the potential to create a new quality of knowledge, which captures the fundamental goal of integration. Interdisciplinarity requires dynamic interconnection. The scientific space of social work arises at the intersection of interactions of referential resources, application level and practice. Our model does not seek universal adoption; it represents the development and method of the theoretical thinking of one group of university teachers.

References

Banks, S. (2001). *Ethics and values in social work.* Basingstoke: Palgrave Macmillan.

Berger, P. L., & Luckmann, T. (1971). *The social construction of reality.* Harmondsworth: Penguin.

Bosa, M. (2013). *Feministicke korene socialnej práce.* Presov: Filozoficka fakulta Presovskej University.

Bosa, M. (2014). *Feminizmy v socialnej praci.* Presov: Filozoficka fakulta Presovskej University.

Fook, J. (2002). *Social work: Critical theory and practice.* London: Sage.

Gray, M., & Webb, S. A. (2013). *Social work: Theories and methods* (2nd ed.). London: Sage.

Healy, K. (2005). *Social work theories in context: A critical introduction.* Basingstoke: Palgrave Macmillan.

Keller, J. (1993). *Az na dno blahobytu.* Brno: Hnutí DUHA.

Keller, J. (2006). *Soumrak socialniho statu.* Praha: Sociologicke nakladatelstvi SLON.

Knobloch, F., & Knoblochova, J. (1999). *Integrovana psychoterapie v praxi.* Praha: Grada Publishing.

Levicka, J., Levicka, K., Kovalcikova, N., Kallay, A., & Slana, M. (2015). *Identita slovenskej socialnej prace.* Trnava: Typi Universitatis Tyrnaviensis spolocne pracovisko TU v Trnave a VEDY, vydavatelstva SAV.

Matousek, O., Kodymova, P., Kovarik, J., Macek, Z., Musil, L., Navrátil, P., . . . Tomes, I. (2001). *Základy sociálni prace.* Praha: Portál.

Mullaly, R. P. (1997). *Structural social work: Ideology, theory, and practice.* Don Mills, Ont: Oxford University Press.

Musil, L. (2010). Tri pohledy na budoucnost socialni prace. In M. Smutek, F. W. Seibel, & Z. Truhlarová (Eds.), *Rizika socialni prace: Sbornik z konference VII. Hradecke dny socialni práce.* Hradec Kralove: Gaudeamus.

Ondrušková, E., Pruzinska, J., & Rusnakova, J. (2015). *Standardy terennej socialnej prace a terennej prace v socialne vylucenych komunitach.* 1. vyd. Bratislava: IA MPSVR SR.

Payne, M. (1997). *Modern social work theory* (2nd ed.). Basingstoke: Palgrave Macmillan.

Payne, M. (2005). *Modern social work theory* (3rd ed.). Basingstoke: Palgrave Macmillan.

Payne, M. (2011). Social work: vision and reality. In E. Ondrušková & Z. Koscurová (Eds.), *Realita a Vízia Sociálnej Práce* (pp. 8–18). Bratislava: Univerzita Komenského.

Payne, M. (2014). *Modern social work theory* (4th ed.). Basingstoke: Palgrave Macmillan.

Prochaska, J. O., & Norcross, J. C. (1999). *Psychoterapeuticke systemy: Prurez teoriemi.* Praha: Grada Publishing.

van der Laan, G. (1998). *Otázky legitimace sociální práce.* Ostrava: Albert.

Watson, D., & West, J. (2006). *Social work: Process and practice.* Basingstoke: Palgrave Macmillan.

3

Psychological and counselling theory in social work

A critical overview

Carolyn Noble

This chapter discusses how psychology and counselling have informed and influenced social work's theory and practice from its earliest beginnings. I do this by presenting psychological and counselling theories pertaining to individual change in historical order and identifying their adaptation and uses for social work's developing practice. In conclusion, I identify how the more contemporary theoretical developments in counselling and psychology and social work, which focuses on social justice issues, can link individual change with a structural analysis to address increasingly complex personal and social problems.

Introduction

Social work has been influenced by many theories from the social sciences and the humanities as it is practised at the meeting point between the individual and society. Like psychology and counselling, social work is characterized by its focus on face-to-face interactions and helping individuals and families with their personal and social problems. While psychology and counselling see themselves as distinct and separate professions, both claim that theories and practices such as psychoanalysis, psychodynamics, behaviourism, cognition, existentialism, person-centred counselling and narrative and strength-based therapy underpin their historical development, their philosophical and theoretical understandings and their current practice base, despite their different professional and training schemas (see Gilliland & James, 2003, pp. 4–5; Richards, 2008).

From the many theories influencing social work, the disciplines of psychology and counselling have been most influential in helping strengthen its early theoretical development and subsequent psychosocial assessment tools and relational skills, despite social work also developing its own distinct identity, epistemology, professional standing and training pathways (Payne, 2014; Healy, 2005; Dominelli, 2004). More latterly, though, social work has branched out to develop theories and skills in community work, social planning and research, advocacy and social change. Its emphasis on an anti-oppressive approach to practice highlights its commitment to including the wider social, political and cultural arenas in its analysis (Gray & Webb, 2013; Connolly & Harms, 2012).

Most commentators agree, however, that the influence of psychology and counselling still holds sway in informing the more traditional approach to social work practice. For social workers working in therapeutic settings, an understanding of the importance of personality development, social learning, lifespan and ego development, attachment and the impact of loss, grief and trauma on individuals, families and groups (Harms, 2010) has been beneficial. The advantages of using psychodynamic perspectives, cognitive behavioural therapy, social learning theory, ego-psychology, family therapy and the strengths-based and narrative approach have provided social workers with a strong professional practice base (Turner, 2017; Payne, 2014; Chenoweth & McAuliffe, 2015; Connolly & Harms, 2012). Psychology's and counselling's interpersonal helping and communication skills and the importance of a therapeutic alliance have also been successfully and importantly adapted into its practice base (Seden, 2005).

Psychodynamic theories

In the 1920s when psychology, particularly its psychodynamic theory, was becoming quite widespread as a therapeutic practice, early social workers were, at the same time, looking to strengthen their theoretical underpinnings. It was no surprise, therefore, to see that this popular approach was quickly incorporated into social work's developing narrative (see Chapter 12). Psychotherapists such as Freud (1901, 1920) Adler (1921), and Jung (1921, 1933, 2006) provided emerging social work with a ready-made practice model that aimed to change behaviour. Through reflection and insight, individuals could change their problematic behaviour by working with a therapist who would get them to focus on uncovering the layers of psychological responses; emotions, both conscious and unconscious and feelings built up from many varied experiences encountered during life's journey, encouraging them to reflect on how these psychological reactions impacted their emotional development. Mary Richmond (1917, 1922) adapted psychodynamic theories into the emerging psychosocial casework. This was given further credence by Hollis (1964) and then further refined by Turner (1978). Of course, psychodynamic practice is vast and complicated, but I will select a few of its key concepts that were and remain influential in the development of social work by way of illustration.

Psychodynamic practice

Freud's case studies were analyzed and presented to show how his theory of the conscious and unconscious emotions that are internal to individuals' early childhood development and outside their control can impact on individuals' intrapsychic development. Consequently, they may have lasting effects on how individuals deal with anxiety, trauma, loss, grief, separation, conflict and relationships. And Freud's descriptions of defence mechanisms, such as denial, projection, repression and rationalization, were presented as unconscious mechanisms to reduce anxiety and protect individuals from becoming overwhelmed by unacceptable impulses and threats. This helped social workers understand the way people react to their social environment and opened the inner world of social work's clients for scrutiny and change (Payne, 2014). Adler's (1921, 1958) suggestion that being in the world involved reflection on the environment, others and importantly on oneself to find authenticity in living and Jung's (1933) work on the role of the unconsciousness in relation to personality development which suggested that behaviour and personality problems are set in early childhood: these provided psychosocial casework with *prêt-à-porter* theories and suggestions about how to work with individuals who are psychologically distressed and unable to function normally. Drawing on these schemas, psychosocial casework believed that the challenge in therapeutic work was to find an equilibrium with the inner and outer world, which would reduce the individual's psychic pain and enable normal adult functioning.

Classical psychotherapeutic knowledge adapted from Freud and his fellow travellers, such as the value of tools like 'ventilation', 'resistance' and 'transference' and the function of 'defence mechanisms', provided social work practitioners with the psychosocial knowledge required to explore and understand the richness and the complexities of the inner world. These could hold clues for comprehending (ab)normal adult functioning by providing explanations for both clients' difficulties and obvious distress in maintaining psychic stability and well-being and those presenting with problems in developing and maintaining stable and functioning relationships. Such tools and strategies were adapted to help social workers deal effectively both with the emotional distress of their clients and with the strength of their emotional responses and psychological defences that seem to marginalize and isolate them from their community and larger social membership. They also help them work with their clients towards making positive behavioural changes in their lives. As a consequence, the generic base of social casework practice had begun its journey to explore theories and practices in its work with individuals so as to make sense of what is in reality a complex human world (Connolly & Harms, 2012).

Rollo May (1953) and Carl Rogers (1950, 1956), as early contributors to developing and refining (non-directive) communicative practices as distinct from the more directed focus of psychotherapy, developed concepts that were also readily adapted by early social workers and were and still are important developments for social casework. Examples include May's (1953) concepts of the search for human autonomy, life's meaning and self-realization and the belief that the whole person could determine their own destiny and Rogers's (1950, 1956) belief that individuals can only achieve authenticity and self-actualization (or a truth) in their lives if they experience such things as congruence, empathy, support and unconditional regard from significant relationships. Accepting the individual's uniqueness and helping the person obtain a balance between thoughts, feelings and experiences is presented as the very core of social work activity that enables people to find a congruence in their lives and solutions to their distress, anxiety and problems. Concepts by Hollis (1964) that were adapted from May's and Rogers's work are still a prominent feature of current traditional social work practice (Connolly & Harms, 2012). These include ideas such as acceptance, empathy, listening, reassurance, encouragement, self-determination, environmental manipulation, consideration of clients' inner and outer needs, the importance of talking and listening in treatment and encouraging the expression of feelings. Also drawn from these sources is incorporating the consideration of external factors such as cultural influences and economic pressures when working with individuals, couples and families. Some of Rogers's key qualities are now recognized as central to culturally safe practice where, for example, the exploration of full identity expression forms a part of this emerging practice (Connolly & Harms, 2012, p. 94).

Ego-psychology and life stage development

Ego-psychology (Erikson, 1959; Freud, 1968) extended psychotherapeutic practice away from exploring just the inner world to include the 'average acceptable environment', such as incorporating family, friends and groups into the psychodynamic perspective. Ego-psychology focused on strengthening the ego or individuals' sense of importance. This is because, according to these psychotherapists, optimal ego development results in the mastery of stage-specific psychosocial developmental events, associated tasks and the psychological crises attached to each stage.

Psychologists Erikson (1959), Winnicott (1968) and Piaget (Gruber & Vonèche, 1995) posited that all individuals are continually developing emotional maturity through their entire lives, and this development passes through specific life stages that have particular psychological crises to resolve in order to progress to the next stage. These stages can be described broadly as childhood, adolescence, adulthood (including childbearing and parenting), old age and on to ultimate death. Each stage presents the individual with an opportunity to balance biological forces with specific sociocultural influences. Normalizing these developmental theories can raise issues when applied to those who develop outside the norm or where cultural influences can engender different crises and different emotions and social and cultural responses. Nevertheless, having a broad understanding of human development can help social workers anticipate and respond appropriately to their clients. By supporting individuals to exercise rational control over life events, they can help them achieve an emotional maturity by dealing positively with the psychosocial challenge linked to each stage (Turner, 2017).

For example, because statutory work has responsibilities to protect and ensure the physical and emotional safety of children, adolescents, adults and older people, being well-informed about the complexities of moving through life stages helps social workers make care plans and policymakers design policies and programmes to protect, safeguard and resource clients if they are made vulnerable at any stage of their lives. Knowing that individuals and families have huge emotional investments in and attachment to each part of their life and to those people sharing it with them helps social workers deal with clients' experiences of loss and grief associated with these transitions (Harms, 2010).

Further psychological research into lifespan development has identified other important factors relating to and impacting the child/adult/old age/death progression. Exposure to a range of factors can alter how individuals, families and groups adjust (or don't) to life stages (Turner, 2017; Harms, 2010). These include toxic substances, stress, abuse, separation, neglect, inadequate nutrition and other social determinants such as educational opportunities and changes in health and cognitive ability, family and relationship breakdown, social isolation and deprivation or loss of work, physical strength, breaking down of cultural influences and religious and spiritual beliefs. Knowing about or looking for the possible impact of these events can provide social workers with additional information on how cultural and social pressures impact people's mental well-being and ability to deal with stress and anxiety while searching for practical and resourceful options for the challenges these transitions bring.

Attachment theory

Another aspect of life course development theory that made a valuable contribution to social workers' practice is Bowlby's attachment theory (see Chapter 13). I have singled this theory out for special attention because it had and still has to some extent influenced social workers' roles in child protection politics and practices as well as work with young people and families. Briefly, attachment theory is a spatial theory, both literally and metaphorically (Holmes, 2014, p. 47). Like Erikson (1959) and Winnicott (1968), Bowlby (1984) agreed that the external world has significant impact on the development of our inner worlds, particularly in the early years of infancy. In brief, Bowlby emphasized that the infant child develops a sense of self because of a quality relationship with their caregiver (Holmes, 2014). The pattern of holding, mirroring, responding to, attuning with and ultimately letting go or being released from this early infant attachment forms the schematic map of Bowlby's theory. That is, when I am close to my loved one, I am happy and secure, and conversely when I am apart, I am anxious, sad and lonely.

The vulnerability of a child who is separated from the attachment figure (usually the mother) or does not have the experience of a secure emotional base will suffer from attachment distress which can colour present and future relationships (Holmes, 2014). When early relationships are secure, then future relationships will be perceived as desirable, safe and containing a flexible level of support and tolerance for separation. From the security of this attachment, individuals can get on with living, forming secure relationships, undertaking projects and exploring their community and the world out there.

Conversely, when these early relationships are inconsistent, absent, interrupted or abusive, difficulties in future adult relationships can emerge as unsatisfactory relationships will generate defences against fears of possible abandonment, neglect and/or abuse linked to their earlier experiences (Miller, 2012, p. 65). That is, broken attachments can have long-term impact on children's ability to form lasting relationships. Knowing about the importance of secure attachments can help social workers working in child protection, particularly with the long-term impact on children who are separated from their first caregiver when taken into care, incarcerated in juvenile justice institutions or moved from one caregiver to another (Butler & Hickman, 2011). Children who experience broken attachments can also experience difficulties in parenting as parenthood can re-awaken their own attachment history (Holmes, 2014). Bowlby (1984) also suggested that secure attachments follow life cycles from infancy to adulthood. As individuals move across the lifespan, attachments begin to accumulate and deepen, and so their loss due to separation, divorce, or death can engender further emotional and psyche toll. In this place of loss, people can experience deep depression, disappointment and bereavement.

Attachment theory can also be applied to the worker-client relationship. When social workers form relationships with clients, the quality of the relationship and its helping value will be affected by the quality of the client's internal model of relationship. Social workers can gain a sense of how easy or difficult it is for clients to engage in a helping relationship and how they might handle the gaps between visits and the loss of significant worker relationships. This might arise because of foreseen or unforeseen circumstances, such as staff changes, resignations, internal promotion or transfer. The social worker may also experience such loss at the death of a client or the abrupt cancelling of the working relationship.

Cognitive behavioural therapies (CBT)

It was not until the 1950s and 1960s that learning theory or cognitive behavioural therapy (CBT) became a competitor to existing psychodynamic-oriented therapies and was quick to find favour with social workers who began to express an interest in exploring the immediacy of the problems being presented and helping clients learn new social skills as a way of assisting change. The slowness and complexity of psychodynamic therapies were seen as too cumbersome, time consuming and less suited to the type of clients social workers were working with. Emerging from the integration of cognitive and behavioural therapies, CBT was seen to have something of relevance to offer social work practice as it had the strongest evidence-based support for its effectiveness. By focusing on the 'here and now' and finding immediate solutions that would motivate individuals to change their behaviour in ways that would make life easier for them, CBT gradually replaced psychodynamic approaches. Moving away from self and retrospective analysis and focusing on specific issues that clients want to change, individuals map out a plan of addressing the behaviours by developing new adaptive learning experiences as a way of modifying the stresses caused by their current behaviour (Dobson & Dobson, 2009). CBT is time limited and seeks to teach clients to become their own therapists as they confront their fears, anxieties and avoidances by changing their cognitive schemata. It avoids blaming individuals by looking for strengths, competencies, capabilities and good attributes to motivate individuals to achieve measurable and realistic goals. This approach sits well with social work practice that is respectful of clients' own objectives and acknowledges the need to engage individuals 'in making their own changes and incorporating their own objectives into wider social outcomes' (Payne, 2014, p. 152).

The change process follows certain steps. The first is to identify the problem and the underlying core beliefs and assumptions, including its history and its impact. This is followed by a process of self-monitoring to identify its triggers and observing reactions including the physiological, behavioural and subjective responses. Once the physiological, psychological and social distress are identified, the process of changing unhelpful thoughts, re-attributing blame, and desensitizing events or emotions that cause distress is introduced. Then new behaviour changes are observed and assessed as useful or not. The underlying assumption is that, by changing pre-existing thought patterns, individuals can change behaviours that are unhelpful, cause anxiety and depression and impede adult functioning. Demanding the active participation of the client in identifying the problem and in implementing and monitoring agreed-upon behavioural changes to limit the stress, reduce the phobias or general anti-social behaviours gives the client the necessary knowledge and skills to adapt to other behaviours that cause distress and/or anxiety. Skills such as challenging existing beliefs and assumptions, using Socratic questioning, and observing problematic behaviours that cause depression or anxiety can help individuals untangle overpowering emotions and consequences that are impacting their lives (Neenan & Dryden, 2014). Social learning or re-learning can also take place by observing others' behaviour and the situation in which this behaviour is taking place, thereby picking up skills through modelling. Links with past behaviour and its consequences also can be transferred to new experiences. While not addressing broader environmental and societal influences such as poverty, deprivation, racism, sexism and homophobia, CBT can provide social workers with awareness of how individual equilibrium can be compromised by anxiety, phobias and depression and provide them with new learning strategies to reduce the impact of these debilitating emotions linked to both the internal and external worlds (Neenan & Dryden, 2014; Dobson & Dobson, 2009).

Problem and task-centred approaches

Helen Harris Perlman's (1957) book *Social casework: A problem-solving process* accepted the learning theory as a model for helping individuals change their behaviour. Perlman viewed problematic behaviour as learned behaviour, so she argued that to change behaviour based on learning principles was a good place to start. Current social workers will be familiar with Pearlman's four *P*s essential to working with clients – person, problem, place and process – and the learning theories linked to this approach. The process involves committed use of the worker-client relationship to undertake the problem-solving stages effectively. Motivation is garnered if the clients genuinely see the set goals as alleviating the problem (Payne, 2014).

One of the most enduring and influential frameworks to emerge from the CBT heritage was Reid and Epstein's (1972) 'task-centred casework' (see Chapter 17). Their approach to making the problem-solving approach more explicit and task focused helped bring the problem-solving strategies into daily practice. Focusing on short-term achievable goals mobilized the client's energy and reduced dependency on the worker as well. The fact that the clients determine their goals and see these goals achieved can contribute to their assuming control over what happens in their lives. In this approach, the social worker is active and direct, like a counsellor, guiding the client toward the implementation of the tasks designed to achieve the set goals. The social worker and the client together assess if the desired outcomes have been achieved (Payne, 2014). The theory behind these cognitive behavioural approaches is that a subsidiary goal of social work is to change behaviour, and that change can be achieved by setting objectives and specific outcomes and making plans as a means of resolving social problems that affect them. It was Turner (1978) who extended direct-practice casework to make use of community resources and noted the liberating effect on clients when such resources were made available. These perspectives are still valued concepts and skills in social work today and much appreciated by service users as well (Seden, 2005, p. 15).

Humanistic psychology and existentialism

The final theory from counselling and psychology (with a little help from philosophy!) that I want to include here that has had influence on social work's counselling practice is concepts from humanistic and existential approaches. The significance to social work is the way these approaches include the arts and spirituality and the value of shared experiences as an important aspect of the human experience. While their influence waxes and wanes, overall their belief in the power of the individual to undertake self-exploration and the personal meaning they attach to their awakening and how this awareness feeds into their perception of the world supports social casework's belief that human beings have the capacity to reason, make choices and act freely in their own interests (Payne, 2014, p. 277; Chenoweth & McAuliffe, 2015).

Humanistic perspectives strongly resonate with social work values and practice standards such as cherishing the integrity of the individual, seeing and valuing the humanity in all human beings as equal and affording human rights and that this equality also extends to seeking parity between and across different social groups. Valuing and showing respect for the whole person, humanistic ideas empathize a commitment to self-determination, social equity and belief in and advocacy of democratic human rights for all.

Existentialism is grouped with humanistic principles as this theory, too, values freedom and responsibility and believes in peoples' capacity to control their lives and change their ideas about how they should live. Change is directed by the person, and it is their responsibility and choice to effect positive change in their lives and to govern how they should live (Chenoweth & McAuliffe, 2015, p. 136). This still has resonance in direct social work practice.

Helping relationship – worker-client relationship

The significance of the therapeutic relationship underpins both Perlman's and Hollis's early work and is regarded as key to establishing a working alliance with the clients as a safe and secure environment to explore the emotions and solutions to their problems. According to John and Trevithick (2012, p. 65), social work was the first profession to highlight the importance of the relationships that are created with clients and other significant others (see also Biestek, 1961). The emphasis of the helping relationship provided social work with an important theoretical orientation, and the importance of the 'working relationship' remains central to current social work texts and as a key foundation for all client work.

Communication and interpersonal skills

Current social work skills emphasize the importance of both basic and advanced communication and interpersonal skills for practice which have been built up from these various helping approaches (Miller, 2012; Seden, 2005). Such skills are valuable for working towards a solution for the issues at hand. They include goal-setting, active listening, non-critical acceptance, reflection and checking, empathic understanding, observance of body language and the use of self and self-reflection, boundary awareness, avoidance of judgemental and moralistic responses and the ability to offer constructive feedback and skills for managing tensions and hostility (Miller, 2012; Seden, 2005). These practice skills underpin all social work's practice methods. Being listened to, being understood and having the ability to make meaningful connections with clients is still a much-valued professional attribute (Miller, 2012). The ability to hear, listen and respond with empathy and respect can contribute to good social work practice; failure in this regard can be a contributor when misunderstandings and gaps in practice emerge. Counselling skills and other interpersonal skills help significantly when trying to negotiate the legal and bureaucratic task-centred aspects of statutory social work or the complexity of working in teams, organization-ally and in research partnerships and community settings (Seden, 2005). As Seden (2005, pp. 6, 11) argues, it is almost impossible for social workers not to be competent in communicating as work with individuals and with other settings demands attention to what is being said, how it is said and how it is understood. Seden (2005) also argues that effective communication skills are appreciated by clients and their families as well as students; this is an area where students would have liked more training.

Strengths-based and narrative therapy

More recent influences of psychology and counselling can be seen in the growth of strengths-based approaches to practice. Strengths-based approaches (see Chapters 18 and 19) have a strong interconnection with psychology's learning theory as well as ego-psychology. The fundamental belief in strengths-based approaches is in the individual's ability to find their own strength and motivation to change behaviours towards their well-being and optimal functioning rather than 'being daunted and overwhelmed by the size of the problem' (Greene & Lee, 2011; Connolly & Harms, 2012, p. 125). Not being able to find solutions to their problems with the available resources, individuals can, by using a strengths-based perspective, find new solutions to old problems. For this reason, this approach has significantly influenced social work in recent dec-ades. What is attractive about this approach is the focus on empowerment, belief in individual resilience and the capacity of individuals to heal themselves and overcome adversity. Distress, abuse, isolation and depression are seen as challenges to face and overcome. This belief provides clients and workers with a powerful antidote to feelings of alienation, oppression, discrimination and isolation and the seemingly insurmountability of their daily problems.

The helping relationship stays centre stage as it acts as a conduit for dialogue and collabora-tion as social worker and client work together to overcome the adversity in the client's life. The focus moves from victimhood to strengths-based approaches and the belief in the restorative capacity of the human spirit to know what is best for themselves and their future. Its links with CBT can be seen in the belief that individuals will be motivated to change if they set their own goals and thus discover or rediscover their sense of self, purpose and power in their successful completion (Connolly & Harms, 2012, p. 126). As with CBT, the role of the social worker is to facilitate the development of client-determined goals and to link the client to available resources and community networks. As with CBT, its approach focuses on the short term and on solving the immediate problem. As with ego-psychology, the individual is strengthened and supported to seek positive solutions to the difficulties they are experiencing and the opportunities that might spring from them (Payne, 2014).

One particular addition to strengths-based approaches that has its genesis in Australian social work is narrative therapy (White, 2007; see Chapter 21). Narrative therapy sees people as sepa-rate from the problem and believes that individuals have the capacity to address the problem and its influence on their lives. It borrows concepts from personal construct theory, which proposes that each individual manages their behaviour according to constructs or the picture of the situ-ation in their minds and the shared social expectations about how to behave in certain social situations (White, 2007). If these constructs of reality are shared with family and with groups, then these pictures become a reality. When these constructs are not shared by all groups, and when some of these constructs place certain individuals and groups as outsiders relegating them to a marginal position in the dominant culture, then a narrative approach can help reorder the pictures by exploring new stories. Presenting an alternative story to the dominant one immediately challenges the status quo, undermining the legitimacy of the particular personal or societal construct.

By helping people think in alternative ways and extending the strengths approach to incorporate storytelling, clients can rewrite and re-author their stories in any way that facilitates their strengths and leads to re-imagining a different, more positive perspective. This, in turn, can lay the groundwork for a more hopeful future (White, 2007). Re-authoring stories into new empowering stories can help victims experience a cathartic release from guilt, shame or sadness (Connolly & Harms, 2012, pp. 135, 142) or indeed right a terrible wrong. This may especially be so when the dominant stories are unhelpful, create distress or perpetuate injustices or are false and misleading rewrites of history such as the stories of Australia's or the UK's colonial past. Narrative therapy helps individuals think differently about their experiences, and by constructing alternative ways to examine their experiences, individuals can transform themselves and their surroundings (Greene & Lee, 2011), especially their past perceptions and beliefs. Reworking dominant stories and identifying alternative constructions of events coming from the family, community or society can be transformational or an empowering experience for those whose identities, histories or experiences were subjugated within the dominant culture and their own family history. Its value to social work is the belief that social arrangements are not set in stone and can be challenged and changed. According to Greene and Lee (2011), clients do better when there are strong expectations of success.

Critical reflection

Historically, critical thinking has its genesis in John Dewey's pedagogical emphasis on reflection as the foundation for experimental learning. Psychologist Schön's (1983) notion of a reflective practitioner was one who, by engaging in critical reflection, could explore the gaps between factual knowledge and the emotionally intuitive knowledge gained from practice. Briefly, critical reflection involves looking at ideas and assumptions from as many perspectives as possible, where divergent ideas about the issues are vigorously sought and the affective disposition of open-mindedness regarding divergent views of the world are used when confronted with the messy complexities of daily practice (Noble, Gray, & Johnston, 2016; Morley, 2016).

Social workers, counsellors and psychologists see the same value in engaging in inquisitiveness and critically questioning assumptions, beliefs, decisions and actions in order to be fully informed about what is going on and how to intervene effectively in a positive and influential way. The process of reflection is a key strategy for use in supervision, as workers critically review and reflect upon their work, the consequences of their intervention and what might have been different with this new knowledge (Noble et al., 2016, pp. 201–215). The use of critical reflection has been adopted by each of these disciplines. Critical reflection is useful when informed by critical theory (see Chapter 26) and its commitment to social justice work and as a strategy to challenge structural power relations (Morley, 2016; Smith, 2008). It is to the influence of these ideas that I now turn.

Social work, psychology and counselling – social justice

The idea that counsellors and psychologists have for many years been concerned with the relationship between individuals' mental well-being and the social milieux in which people live, especially in marginalized populations, has in recent years resulted in calls to incorporate social justice and advocacy in their practice (see Chapters 10 and 30). Reisch (2014) posits that private troubles are only important at the individual level, while public issues have structural implications for society. To understand individual problems in their many facets needs a wider lens in order to comprehend the complexity of social influences, the political and cultural structures of modern life and their impact on individuals' functioning, sense of well-being and social advantage and privilege (Arthur & Collins, 2014).

Individual struggles are more often created or aggravated by oppressive systems such as age, gender, class, ethnicity or spiritual beliefs, sexual preferences and membership in either dominant or non-dominant groups (see Chapter 29). There is growing recognition in counselling and psychological scholarship that people's health and well-being is impacted positively or negatively by economic, social, political, and cultural structures as well as educational and organizational systems (Arthur & Collins, 2014). For example, domestic violence, racial and gender discrimination, poverty, social inequities and disproportionate privilege, unemployment, educational advantage, environmental health concerns and unequal social, political and economic access all have a human toll. The multifaceted problems involving losses, crises, trauma, personal difficulties and long-standing disadvantages stemming from conditions of poverty, unemployment, discrimination, socialization, and abuse are not just overwhelming, but to keep working within these complexities with an individual lens can seem indifferent to and at some level ignorant about the many structural injustices that form risk factors for mental health concerns.

In fact, current literature in both counselling and psychology (Arthur & Collins, 2010, 2014; Lee, 2007) would suggest there is more than a growing awareness that focusing solely on individual change is limiting, given increasing awareness of the impact of social structures. Many approaches presented in this chapter, such as person-centred and cognitive behavioural approaches, include some notions of empowerment. Also, strengths-based and narrative approaches can disrupt dominant understandings and structures by re-authoring and re-storying dominant narratives. In many psychological approaches, however, individuals and their context remain the focus, leaving the broader social structures in place. By concentrating on remediation of psychological issues located in the individual client, attention has been drawn away from the structures that lead to psychological distress and mental ill health (Arthur & Collins, 2010, 2014). Active involvement in resource advocacy, community outreach and public policy making are examples of interventions that can promote attention to social justice issues among counsellors and psychologists. Self-reflection on how therapist privilege might inadvertently replicate experiences of injustice and challenging therapeutic interventions practices that appear inappropriate or exploitative are other competencies for social justice work (Lee, 2007).

Here once again, there is a symmetry between this development within counselling and psychology and social work, with one key difference. The more progressive school of social work has always looked for theories and perspectives that seek to eliminate disadvantage outside the individual and their immediate social world. From Jane Addams's pioneering attempts in the early 20th century at social reforms and her and others' attempts to change social structures to help individuals, to the influence of conflict theory and then, from the late 1960s, the influence of a structural and feminist analysis (Baines, 2017; Mullaly, 2007; Dominelli, 2004; see Chapters 27 and 31), social work began to incorporate a social justice focus in working with clients a little ahead of counselling and psychology. Integrating key concepts such as the interrelatedness of the personal and the political with a socio-political framework towards emancipatory social justice and human rights goals provided social workers with a critical perspective that contrasted sharply with the person-centred approaches such as casework and its individualized treatment approaches, especially those that focused purely on the individual. How practitioners support

personal growth and human potential while addressing social inequality and injustice and acting as social advocates can be seen in feminist theory and its application in practice. Feminist
counselling has been embraced by all three discipline groups and has sequentially influenced the
growth of multicultural work (Arthur & Collins, 2010, 2014).

Feminist counselling and psychology

Feminist analysis has introduced a profound critique of traditional approaches to therapy, resisting the historically and culturally determined traditional roles prescribed for women 'such as
mother, carer and home-maker and being typed more problematically as "emotional", "irrational", more submissive, less independent, less reliable, less objective, more neurotic and less
well-adjusted than adult men' (Noble & Day, 2016, p. 17). These stereotypes have been seen to
exclude women from public life, relegating them to the private, mostly invisible sphere and, again
more problematically, objectifying them for the male sexual gaze. Traditional psychotherapists
were critiqued for their intrinsically male-centric focus on personality development, intrapsychic distress, diagnosis and symptomatology in relation to women and girl clients (Noble & Day,
2016). Not only were women clients subject to this sexist discourse, women psychotherapists,
such as Klein, Horney and Irigaray, who critiqued the founding fathers, were ignored, and their
theories received less attention than those of the men with whom they worked (McLeod, 2013).

As experts in their own lives, women are encouraged to take both individual and collective action to achieve change that empowers their social, cultural, sexual and political position
and reduces their isolation and marginalization (Noble & Day, 2016, p. 20). Feminist therapists
address issues such as marriage and partner relations, intimate partner violence, reproduction,
child care, career options, emotions (especially taboo ones like rage or jealousy), body image,
gender stereotypes, gender and trauma, self-esteem and individual and structural discrimination.
These are just some of the key influences impacting women's well-being and personal safety.

The therapist strives for an egalitarian relationship through transparency and relational self-
reflectivity and by being aware of the power imbalance in the professional relationship and
actively working to minimize its impact on client/therapist work by working towards establishing an egalitarian relationship (op cit, p. 21). Overall, the aim of feminist practice is to exercise
a commitment to the transformation of the socio-politico-economic and cultural relations and
power structures that limit women's agency. A significant aspect of feminist practice is to place
each woman at the centre of the helping process and together work to change women's lives for
the better (Brown, 2010; Dominelli, 2002).

Conclusion

This chapter has considered the major influences that counselling and psychology have had on
the development of social work. Social work practice has been enriched by the psychodynamic,
relational and cognitive behaviourist understandings of the individual and their theories of
human development, motivation and personal change. Drawing heavily from counselling and
psychology in its formative stage, social work was able to build its primary base for direct practice and an intellectually stimulating base for social work to grow its practice with individuals to
include children, families and then groups (Healy, 2005). Even today, social work continues to
be aligned with counselling and psychology in the shared use of interpersonal, communicative
and relational skills, especially the importance of a healthy relationship characterized by empathy,
authenticity and mutual regard (Healy, 2005, p. 53). A key contribution is in providing distress
and trauma with a human dimension and providing skills and knowledge for social workers

working in direct practice and in the mental health field. Latterly, counselling and psychology have paid increased attention to social justice and advocacy and how the realities of social justice and socio-political inequalities impact on individuals' well-being links with social work's progressive practice. This affects where people have access not only to the help and resources that better their lives but also to an advocacy and experience of empowerment that facilitates self-determination. This redirection of focus provides these disciplines with skills to challenge inequality and discrimination wherever it is found.

Further reading

Miller, L. (2012). *Counselling skills for social work* (2nd ed.). London: Sage.
Noble, C., & Day, E. (Eds.). (2016). *Psychotherapy and counselling: Reflections on practice*. S. Melbourne: Oxford University Press.
Payne, M. (2014). *Modern social work theory* (4th ed.). Basingstoke: Palgrave Macmillan.

References

Adler, A. (1921[2001]). *The neurotic constitution: Outline of a comparative individual psychology*. New York: Routledge.
Adler, A. (1958[2011]). *The education of the individual*. Eastford, CT: Martino.
Arthur, N., & Collins, S. (2010). Social justice and culture-infused counselling. In N. Arthur & S. Collins (Eds.), *Culture-infused counselling* (2nd ed.). Calgary, AB: Counselling Concepts.
Arthur, N., & Collins, S. (2014). Counsellors, counselling, and social justice: The professional is political. *Canadian Journal of Counselling and Psychology, 48*(3), 171–185.
Baines, D. (2017). *Doing anti-oppressive practice: Social justice social work* (3rd ed.). Halifax & Winnipeg: Fernwood Publishing.
Beistek, F. (1961). *The casework relationship*. London: George Allen & Unwin.
Bowlby, J. (1984). *Attachment (Attachment and Loss, Vol. 1)* (2nd ed.). Harmondsworth: Penguin.
Brown, L. S. (2010). *Feminist therapy*. Washington, DC: American Psychological Association.
Butler, I., & Hickman, C. (2011). *Social work with children and families: Getting into practice*. London: Jessica Kingsley.
Chenoweth, L., & McAuliffe, D. (2015). *The road to social work and human service practice.* (4th ed.). S. Melbourne: Cengage.
Connolly, M., & Harms, L. (2012). *Social work from theory to practice* (2nd ed.). Port Melbourne: Cambridge University Press.
Dobson, D., & Dobson, K. (2009). *Evidence-based practice of cognitive-behavioral therapy*. New York: Guilford.
Dominelli, L. (2002). *Feminist social work theory and practice*. Basingstoke: Palgrave Macmillan.
Dominelli, L. (2004). *Social work: Theory and practice in a changing profession*. Cambridge, UK: Polity.
Erikson, E. (1959). *Identity and the life cycle*. New York: Norton.
Freud, S. (1901). *The psychopathology of everyday life*. New York: Dover.
Freud, S. (1920). *A general introduction to psycho-analysis*. New York: Boni and Liveright.
Freud, A. (1968[1937]). *The ego and the mechanisms of defence* (Rev. ed.). London: Hogarth.
Gilliland, G., & James, R. (2003). *Theories and strategies in counselling and psychotherapy* (5th ed.). Boston, MA: Allyn & Bacon.
Gray, M., & Webb, S. (2013). *The new politics of social work* (2nd ed.). Basingstoke: Palgrave Macmillan.
Greene, J., & Lee, M. Y. (2011). *Solution-orientated social work practice: An integrative approach*. New York: Oxford University Press.
Harms, L. (2010). *Understanding human development: A multidimensional approach*. S. Melbourne: Oxford University Press.
Healy, K. (2005). *Social work theories in context: Creating frameworks for practice*. Basingstoke: Palgrave Macmillan.
Hollis, F. (1964). *Casework: A psychosocial therapy*. New York: Random House.
Holmes, J. (2014). *John Bowlby and attachment theory* (2nd ed.). New York: Routledge.
John, M., & Trevithick, P. (2012). Psychodynamic thinking in social work practice. In P. Stepney & D. Ford (Eds.), *Social work models, methods and theories* (2nd ed.). Lyme Regis: Russell House.
Jung, C. G. (1921 [2017]). *Psychological types*. Abingdon: Routledge Classics.

Jung, C. G. (1933[2001]). *Modern man in search of a soul*. London: Routledge.

Jung, C. G. (2006). *The undiscovered self*. New York: Signet.

Lee, C. C. (Ed.). (2007). *Counselling for social justice* (2nd ed.). Alexandria, VA: ACA.

May, R. (1953). *Man's search for himself: Signposts for living and personal fulfillment*. New York: Condor Books.

McLeod, J. (2013). *An introduction to counselling* (5th Ed.). New York: Open University Press.

Miller, L. (2012). *Counselling skills for social work* (2nd Ed.). London: Sage.

Morley, C. (2016). Critical reflection and critical social work. In B. Pease., S. Goldingay, N. Hosken, & S. Niperess (Eds.), *Doing critical social work: Transformative practices for social justice* (pp. 25–38). Sydney: Allen & Unwin.

Mullaly, B. (2007). *The new structural social work*. Don Mills, Ont: Oxford University Press.

Neenan, M., & Dryden, W. (2014). *Cognitive behavior therapy: 100 key points & techniques*. (2nd ed.). London: Routledge.

Noble, C., & Day, E. (Eds.). (2016). *Psychotherapy and counselling: Reflections on practice*. S. Melbourne: Oxford University Press.

Noble, C., Gray, M., & Johnston, L. (2016). *Critical supervision for the human services: A social model to promote learning and value-based practice*. London: Jessica Kingsley.

Payne, M. (2014). *Modern social work theory* (4th ed.). Basingstoke: Palgrave Macmillan.

Perlman, H. (1957). *Social casework: A problem solving process*. Chicago: University of Chicago Press.

Gruber, H. E., & Vonèche, J. J. (Eds.). (1995). *The essential Piaget*. Lanham, MD: Aronson.

Richards, G. (2008). *Psychology*. London: Routledge.

Richmond, M. (1917). *Social diagnosis*. New York: Russell Sage Foundation.

Richmond, M. (1922). *What is social case work?* New York: Russell Sage Foundation.

Reid, W., & Epstein, L. (1972). *Task centered casework*. New York: Columbia University Press.

Reisch, M. (2014). *Social policy and social justice*. Los Angeles: Sage.

Rogers, C. R. (1950). Client-centered therapy: A helping process. *University of Chicago Round Table, 698,* 12–21.

Rogers, C. R. (1956). A counseling approach to human problems. *American Journal of Nursing, 56,* 994–997.

Schön, D. (1983). *The reflective practitioner: How professionals think in action*. New York: Basic Books.

Seden, J. (2005). *Counselling skills and social work practice* (2nd ed.). Maidenhead: Open University Press.

Smith, S. (2008). *Applying theory and policy in practice: Issues for critical reflection*. Farnham: Ashgate.

Turner, F. J. (1978). *Psychosocial therapy*. New York: Free Press.

Turner, F. J. (Ed.). (2017). *Social work treatment: Interlocking theoretical approaches*. Oxford: Oxford University Press.

White, M. (2007). *Maps of narrative practice*. New York: Norton.

Winnicott, D. (1968). *The family and individual development*. London: Tavistock.

4

Epistemic discourses of 'explanation' and 'understanding' in assessment models

Pavel Navrátil

Introduction

Holland (2010) and Czech writers Glumbíková, Gojová and Grundělová (2018) note that social work assessments are strongly influenced by practitioners' own values and personal expectations, more so than their investigations of their clients' social realities. It is not necessarily a problem that social work is affected by personal values and beliefs, though these need to be articulated and systematically studied (Hubíková & Havlíková, 2017); perspectivism is a prominent and accepted epistemic viewpoint in the philosophy of social science. It is, however, a serious issue that social work practice with clients does not strongly reflect clients' social realities and perceptions. It is not that social workers are following the principles of perspectivism, but rather that they are epistemologically blind; they are unaware of the ways in which they acquire and use knowledge in their practice. If we want to return epistemological sight to social workers, it is important to raise and analyze the use of knowledge in social work. Since assessment is a crucial knowledge collection task in all social work, it is a useful focus for thinking about these issues.

In this chapter, I use two key epistemic discourses, 'explanation' and 'understanding', to analyze important models used in social work to assess living situations. The aim of this analysis is to contribute to the debate about and premises for building knowledge in social work as an academic discipline and practice profession, as the International Federation of Social Workers (IFSW) defined it in the current definition of social work. I chose discourse on explanation and understanding because these are among key epistemological strategies in the social sciences, which are often presented not only as very different but also as sometimes contradictory. In some ways, these epistemological strategies delimit the terrain for epistemology. Therefore, it is reasonable to assume that the dichotomy between explanation and understanding should be a useful tool for grasping the diversity of our epistemological models, or understandings, of social work. I focus on assessment because this is a crucial aspect of all social work, and a number of different models of assessment may be clearly identified.

Assessing clients' living situations is basic to the social work task (Dyke, 2016), but how this is done influences the quality of the performance of social work as a whole. Assessments in social work are carried out in a variety of contexts, similarly with a variety of purposes. Social work is a diverse profession, which intersects with the complexities of social life from various angles. Social workers work in distinct contexts (Van Ewijk, 2018) and for distinct reasons (Coulshed & Orme, 2012). Social work's contexts are determined by the network of social institutions and organizations within which it is carried out and by the nature of the target group and the specific knowledge and skills required by a situation (Baláž, 2012; Svein & Katya Nogales, 2017). For example, when clients contact a social services organization for the first time, a decision needs to be made about which services are to be offered while, in other cases, the agency needs to assess risks that the client is exposed to, such as by determining the extent of addiction (Navrátil, 2007). The assessment may be at the client's request or by referral from another organization, such as the courts. Assessments are also carried out throughout the phases of intervention. While we usually think of assessments as undertaken in the context of the beginning of collaboration with clients, they may also be carried out to decide what services should be provided, when contact with clients should be terminated, or, during an intervention, when social work interventions should be adapted as clients' needs change or develop (Turney, Platt, Selwyn & Farmer, 2012).

There are several models of assessment which not only react to social work's diversity in the variability of their forms, but also reflect diverse epistemic viewpoints. Epistemic premises are fundamental building blocks for any field striving to solidify its position in academic discourse, but how social work tackles constructing its epistemology is insufficiently studied. This is not only an academic question: epistemic premises directly apply to the methods used in social work (Lorente-Molina & Luxardo, 2018). It is important, therefore, not to avoid thinking about the prerequisites for creating and using social work's epistemology. Furthermore, epistemology and its premises are present and relevant when practitioners are assessing living conditions and situations. This is because assessing clients' living conditions is about understanding and learning from the significant characteristics of those living situations and deciding on aims and plans for intervention.

Explain or understand?

The social work process includes a series of decisions affecting clients' lives. The assessment process plays out as a specific domain of social work from the first moment a social worker initiates contact with a client. Social workers aim to reach conclusions and evaluations of clients' situations quickly because of the expectation that they will provide help and support in a timely fashion. During this time, social workers face several diverse questions, such as *Who is this person? What do they want and need? What can I do for them? How does the person view their situation? What resources do they have?* Two basic epistemological methods exist for trying to answer these questions; these *assessment strategies* differ from each other in their view of the parameters of assessment. The first is an *objectifying strategy*; the second is about *subjectivity and interpretation*.

In introducing consideration of assessment models in social work, I distinguish two extreme viewpoints that reflect these strategies. Barker's (2013) view is close to the objectifying perspective, the aim of which is to grasp the client's situation as an objective set of facts that can be described and explained. He describes assessment as a task in which a social worker aims to understand the nature, cause and development of a problem and, potentially, also a prognosis. To these ends, the characteristics of both the person and the situation, both related to the problem, are being analytically evaluated. Understanding the problem's cause makes it possible to design an effective intervention. Using the second assessment strategy, social work also offers an alternative, different image of the notion of assessment. It sees the goal of assessment as finding an in-depth understanding of the client's situation, which may help identify and consensually approve potential changes to the client's life (Milner & O'Byrne, 2004). Social workers using this discourse view aspects of the problem and the client's situation through the lens of various interpretations. This leads them to gather alternative viewpoints, with the aim of agreeing with the participants on the one that will seem the most useful. The first approach is an *explanation discourse*. This is often seen as a notion that appears in the natural sciences but is less adequate in social contexts, such as social work. The second approach is a *discourse of understanding*, which social work often prefers to explanation. These two discourses (see Table 4.1) are extremes; they do not provide an exhaustive description of all possible discourse strategies that are available in argumentation and conceptualization of processes. However, in many respects, they are present in all debates about approaches to assessing situations in any context.

Is social work an objectified science or (only) based on intuitive understanding? This question is central to professional identity (Schön, 1983) and to discussion about how to approach the epistemological process. This aspect of debate about the nature of social work appears extensively in early literature (Levická, 2002; Lorenz, 2016; Munro, 2008; Reamer, 1995; Richmond, 1899, 1917; Thyer & Pignotti, 2015), contemporary debates surrounding evidence-based social work (Webb, 2001, 2002, 2017) and the identity of social work (Otava, 2016). There are significant parallels with questions about how to approach epistemology. The argument in both discussions follows a similar logic. Proponents of objectivity emphasize the scientific nature of social work, while those who support subjectivity and interpretation prefer to view social work as a form of art.

Social work is sometimes viewed as an artform because practising it requires a wide range of personal prerequisites and talents, developed through experience over time. In this approach to social work, Parker (2017) argues, assessments cannot be strictly and exhaustively defined. The intuitive nature of the work means that practitioners cannot reach outcomes exclusively using

Table 4.1 The discourses of explanation and understanding in assessments

Characteristics	Discourse of explanation	Discourse of understanding
Discourse origin	Natural sciences	Social sciences
Epoch	Modernity	Postmodernity
Nature of social reality	Objective (social facts)	Constructed (social constructs)
Epistemological goal	Creation of a formal theory	In-depth understanding of individual facts
Epistemological category	Cause	Meaning
Approach to practice	Preparation and application of a single 'correct' model that explains how things happen and how interventions should be carried out	Searching for various perspectives, interpretations and paths towards a solution
Purpose of reflection	Technically understanding and improving practice	Cultivation of personalities, expansion of knowledge of influences and impacts that affect ongoing processes
Timing	Before commencing work with a client	While working with a client
Method for argumentation of practical steps	Justification of the procedure based on research and theory (objectivized with evidence), a gold standard in the field	Justification of the procedure based on consensus, the best possible outcome, tradition, cultural interpretation and experience

Source: adapted from Holland (2010)

predefined questionnaires and checklists. Consequently, assessment depends on practitioners' ability to improvise, developed through practice and personal experience. Nevertheless, Parker (2017) draws attention to issues with viewing assessments as an art. In particular, clients are left at the 'mercy' of their social workers' qualities, approach and premises. Such assessments do not provide a systemic approach to the process, and their quality is correlated with the personal qualities of the practitioner or team performing the assessment.

Social work, however, has some attributes of science, because it has access to and devises theories that explain how problems arising in individuals, groups and communities are created and resolved (Navrátilová & Navrátil, 2016). Taking a scientific perspective, assessment is an exact measurement and may be carried out through steps described in social work methodology. This means that all social workers should reach the same assessment conclusions in given situations. A scientific assessment allows for the proposal of a standardized procedure for intervention. Parker (2017) comments that this model often reduces the complexity of clients' situations and does not capture the diversity of clients' circumstances, the impact of available facilities and services, cultural backgrounds and interpretations.

Both approaches to social work – viewing it as a science (explanation) or an artform (understanding) – offer a range of stimulating ideas about appropriate qualities of social workers and their work. Social workers' personal abilities, their talents and their creativity form a fundamental baseline, paralleling an artist's talent for their art. Social workers nevertheless cannot perform well without education and cultivation of their talent. Complicated social situations require state-of-the-art professional training. Practitioners not only need the right knowledge, but they also need to know how to work with information and apply learned skills creatively. Consequently, I believe assessment in social work has a specific property: both viewpoints may be used simultaneously. A good social worker must be capable of both understanding and explaining clients' situations. For instance, practitioners must be able to explain the stages of alcohol addiction and the characteristics of each stage, but must also understand the specific difficulties that the person needs help with.

Some important assessment models

In this section, I analyze assessment models considered representative of social work practice by a variety of authors (Holland, 2010; Horwath & Platt, 2018; Milner, Myers, & O'Byrne, 2015; Navrátil, 2014; Parker, 2017). Although most emphasize either objectivity (explanation) or subjectivity (understanding), many also strive to connect both viewpoints and bring them together in various ways.

Diagnostic model: where did the problem arise?

Richmond (1917) is an important source for a diagnostic model of assessment. She saw a diagnostic model as an anchor for social work as a systematic scientific method, putting social work on a level similar to medicine and psychiatry as an emerging 'big profession' (Lovelock, Lyons, & Powell, 2016). She understood the assessment process as rigorous:

> In social diagnosis there is the attempt to arrive at as exact a definition as possible of the social situation and personality of a given client. Investigation, of the gathering of evidence, begins the process, the critical examination and comparison of evidence follow, and last come its interpretation and the definition of the social difficulty.
>
> *(Richmond, 1917, p. 51)*

The diagnostic discourse in social work was supported by parallel processes which took place in medicine and psychiatry, culminating, for example, in the standardized formulations of mental disorders in the diagnostic and statistical manuals (DSM) of the American Psychiatric Association (2013; see Chapter 36). The impact of psychodynamic approaches to social work meant that diagnostic approaches to assessment remained prominent in the US as late as the 1970s. Diagnosis played an important role in problem-solving, which could be achieved by psychotherapy or social service provision. Prominent works of the period include Perlman (1957) and Hollis (1964). Both emphasized proper diagnosis of the client's problem, with plans for social intervention then based on this diagnosis.

Social work emphasized the need for diagnosis to pay attention not only to individuals but also to the family and its problems. Krakešová-Došková (1946) first introduced the notion of social diagnosis in Czech social work, pioneering in the way her work tackled social-educational work (Krakešová, 1973a, 1973b). While her approach was developed in the 1940s, political restrictions meant it remained unpublished until the 1970s.

The diagnostic trend remained influential and dominant until the 1970s (Řezníček, 1994). For example, Kempe et al.'s (1962) introduction of the notion of 'child abuse' understood child abuse as a syndrome, a disease with specific causes requiring diagnosis and treatment. Until the 1960s, social work practice betrayed no prominent doubts that this was the correct approach to assessment. Since then, the diagnostic discourse has been the target of critical analysis (Adams, Dominelli, & Payne, 2009; Fook, 2016; Janebová & Truhlářová, 2017), calling attention to the potential threat of pathologization of clients, misuse of power and lack of ability to perceive and deal with the wider social context of clients' problems.

Diagnostic thought crystalizes an objectivist, modernist view, believing correspondingly in truth and realistic ontology. It is clearly situated in the logic governing natural sciences and strives to analyze clients' situations and often their personalities with an emphasis on objectivity and the neutrality of the assessor. The goal of diagnostic assessment is to determine a theory for the given problem, which can subsequently be used to solve it via a formally described standard procedure.

Diagnostic thought is today applied mainly in areas of social work that are close to disciplines for which a diagnosis is the foundation for further work, typically psychiatry, medicine and pedagogy for intellectual disabilities. It is also important where rapid assessment of serious risks is needed, such as in social-legal interventions with children (Hyun & Adams, 2016; Turner, 2005). And yet, terms such as 'diagnosis' and 'diagnostics' remain controversial in European social work and are often replaced by more general terms, such as 'assessment' (Navrátil & Janebová, 2010).

Risk assessment model: when will the situation break down?

In the 1970s, predictive discourses developed within diagnostic models. As science's ability to predict future phenomena in other fields grew, social work interest also increased in finding predictive factors for risks. The ability to predict was considered to be an attribute of a fully fledged profession based on scientific methodology (Schön, 1983). It was logical that social work saw the creation of risk assessment systems.

The protection of children was a prominent target (Garbarino, 1976; Garbarino & Gilliam, 1980; see Chapter 34). Researchers tried to identify risk factors which would allow for the timely identification of high-risk families even before a dangerous situation arose. The characteristics of discourses on risk assessment do not diverge significantly from diagnostic discourses; their origin also lies in natural and technical sciences. Explanation plays a prominent role in predicting high-risk situations, operating with an epistemology of causes and consequences.

Risk can only be assessed or predicted by assuming that facts are objective, identifiable entities that cause risk.

Based on this predictive model, practice goals are to prevent high-risk situations, such as a neglected child, broken family or drug addiction. For the risk prediction process to be meaningful, practitioners must predict risks early, whereas predictions are mostly based on statistics verified with a formal theory. This may be unrealistic, adding additional problems to social work in practice (Littlechild, 2008).

Research on prediction is well justified by the goal of prevention and may expand understanding of families where, for example, children are neglected, but this approach has its weaknesses. Some studies on identifying risk factors did not operationalize the concepts used. Some predictive factors were commonplace rather than distinguishing high-risk families: for example, that the parents experienced unhappy childhoods or bad health or that the child experienced poor health. May-Chahal, and Coleman (2003) concluded that the factors identified as high risk are usually too general to be useful for predicting high-risk families in practice. Examples such as single parenthood, poverty, problematic relations with a partner, isolation and weak social networks, personal immaturity or the parent having themselves experienced abuse and neglect in childhood were too non-specific. Punová (2012) points out that protective factors present need to be taken into account alongside risk factors. Even though work on creating predictive tools continues, therefore, it is accepted that they cannot be 'infallible' and may not even be 'sufficient' to perform a complex assessment or unambiguous identification of high-risk situations (Watson & West, 2006).

Nevertheless, where social work takes place in areas of high risk to the psychological and corporal integrity of clients, a search for tools allowing for timely identification of risk continues to be important, and inspiration from other fields may be helpful (Calder, 2016).

Decision-making models: which decision is best?

As interest in predictive models in social work grew, decision-making theory began to be applied in social work. Models of rational decision-making were described earlier – for example, by Max Weber and Henri Fayol – but the pioneering work of Allison (1971) on the Cuban missile crisis of the 1960s was influential in the 1970s. He analyzed implicit decision-making models in human activities. The *rational model*, which expects that individuals (or groups) analyze available possibilities to reach their goal, was a starting point. Rational behaviour, however, requires access to relevant information. In Allison's model, people chose paths which led to their goal with minimum 'cost'. He also proposed two alternative models which might facilitate decision-making analyses. The *organizational-process model* emphasizes the variety of factors which apply when decision-making is carried out within an organizational context. Factors such as routine, organizational procedures, regulation of information, avoiding personal risk and how problems are defined have important impacts. The *policy management model* analyzes decision-making procedures in the context of governance and bureaucracy.

The discourse origins of this approach to assessment lie mostly in natural science, cybernetics and management. It is based not only on the assumption of an objective reality, but also on a model that rational human behaviour maximizes personal gain. It is also based on other discourse characteristics, such as a causal model of cause and consequence, and assumes behavioural models that decision makers will seek rationally to enhance performance. It assumes that the timing of assessment and decisions about it are focused on the beginning of work with clients, but, as I have already argued, assessment may be required at a later stage. A positive contribution of decision-making theory is the attempt to understand the meaning and significance of various alternatives in the problem situation and their consequences from clients' perspectives. While general decision-making seeks efficient solutions, therefore, applied in social work this approach must be understood in a more flexible light, balancing rational efficiency with clients' engagement and participation.

In social work, the rational decision-making discourse was applied especially in approaches which include, notably, the goal-oriented approach (Reid & Epstein, 1972; see Chapters 17 and 19) and in problem-solving ideas (Egan, 2014; Tolson, Reid, & Garvin, 2003). Critics of the rational decision-making discourse, however, claim that it cannot be applied on its own; this is because it does not take into account values, emotionality or social and cultural contexts and fails to consider the possible development of situations when new and additional information will be needed (Winkler, 2002). All these factors are relevant in social work (O'Sullivan, 2010). In the Czech Republic, Musil (2004) inspired a promising research direction targeting decision-making dilemmas (Janebová, Hudečková, Zapadlová, & Musilová, 2013; Nečasová & Musil, 2006; Otava, 2016).

Assessment in the critical perspective: what caused the problem?

The diagnostic approach to assessment and its derivatives were criticized as pathologizing clients, individualizing problems and preventing strategies directed towards social reform. Rather than narrowly placing the core of the problem in clients, a wider social standpoint contributed to a new perspective influenced by critiques from social theories, especially (neo)Marxism and feminism (see Chapters 26–28). Clients' problems were seen to lie in social failings, in the context of social networks, communities or the social order. Proponents of this approach emphasize social rather than psychological circumstances and stress oppression as a key social issue (Dominelli, 2018; Fook, 2016; Glumbíková, Gojová, & Grundělová, 2018; Janebová & Celá, 2016).

Assessments in the social context are discursively based on social sciences. Perceptions of social reality are, nevertheless, objectivistic, since they examine the social world from the perspective of its order and laws and strive to arrive at generalizable interpretations. Critical theory is, consequently, still based on the connections between causes and consequences, rather than on the individualized significance of a person's life (McNeill & Nicholas, 2017). Clients' satisfaction with their own social situations may be understood as stemming from a lack of information or a culture of silence requiring social action and liberation (Freire, 1972; Mullaly & Dupré, 2018).

Social work assessment in the critical perspective needs to take into account factors such as age, disability, ethnicity, family, sexual orientation and the role of these characteristics in the client's situation. For instance, Thompson's (2016) P-C-S analysis assesses the structural dimension of clients' situations as a way of understanding the role of discrimination and inequalities in the issues that they face. It focuses on the understanding of and interactions among the personal (P), cultural (C) and structural (S) dimensions of their lives. This offers a tool to analyze and understand clients' situations in relation to the general conditions in society.

A more specialized, less structural emphasis on assessing clients' situations in wider social contexts emerged in the UK during the 1980s. This was related to the deaths of children caused by neglect and abuse by parents and foster carers, many already known to social agencies and social workers (Corby, 2000). Reviews of these cases showed that coordination of information on the lives of these families from the various agencies responsible for their care and supervision was insufficient. As new events arose, practitioners did not use all relevant information about the family history, preventing them from getting a general picture. Criticism was also directed at the absence of a single comprehensive framework or system for their assessments. Studies also showed that social workers did not succeed in evaluating the needs of families as a whole and either focused on the needs of the parents or the children (Barber & Delfabbro, 2000; Holland, 2010). The outcome of these debates was the proposal of a framework for assessing children in need and their families, which later also inspired Czech methodology for assessing families where child protection concerns were raised (Navrátil, 2007).

Bureaucratic model of assessment: which decision cannot be attacked by anyone?

Bureaucratic or proceduralization trends, by increasing managerial prescription and scrutiny of assessment, are legitimized by claims that they help to eliminate risk and protect clients, but the consequences are problematic both for clients and for social workers (Harlow, Berg, Barry, & Chandler, 2013). Professional tools with the capacity to respond to complexity are often replaced by mechanized management measures which are driven by efforts to develop simple, unambiguous and cheap solutions (Tsui & Cheung, 2004).

Bureaucratization of social work processes is often linked with the so-called managerialism or new public management in public administration at the end of the 20th century, which extended to the social services. Musil (2004) explains that applying this approach in social services is on the one hand an endeavour to make social services processes closer to those of market economies and, on the other hand, the vision that, to make this market-based ideal a reality, social workers must be prevented from deciding the targets of services, instead offering 'products' which are predefined activities and services. This necessarily limits the ability of social workers to assess clients' situations comprehensively. Managerialism and bureaucratization of assessment processes leads to neglect of professional skills and competences of social workers and to the transfer of decision-making authority regarding services and resources to managers (Watson & West, 2006). Baláž and Musil (2016) also identified these trends as a factor which prevents social work from achieving its professional goals.

Trends towards bureaucratization are inspired by objectivistic discourses of explanation, but only loosely. Bureaucratic models of assessment create their own epistemic logic, centred around the principle of 'administrative correctness': that is, compliance with procedures. Since this principle is not linked to an epistemic reflection of reality, its application in the context of assessment goes completely against the purpose of this activity.

A moral panic around the abuse of children in the UK in the 1980s led to both bureaucratic forms of assessment and a shift of intervention from complex family support towards a more narrow focus on children protection (Musil, 2004; Parton, 2014). This shift reacted to both social workers' uncertainties and the need for greater public trust in the operation of social service systems. Bureaucratic assessment models are based on completing lists and check boxes, allowing social workers to verify whether the client is authorized to receive an agency's services. In this model, the expert is the person who created the forms, with the social worker's task being to collect information through the assessment process. This may be criticized for not fully respecting the client's personality, nor paying attention to their needs and positions. The social worker becomes a tool of the organization and its systems, performing predefined operations. Procedural models were created to standardize and regulate assessment processes to meet the administrative needs.

Some bureaucratic assessment tools were developed through research findings that legitimated them as practice improvement, remedying theoretical and practice deficiencies and securing consistent approaches to identifying and meeting clients' needs. Nevertheless, using procedural models of assessment means that social workers perform assessments through predefined questions and scales, rather than being able to assess situations flexibly, using their professional skills and values.

Coulshed and Orme (2012) argued that such systems are often rigid and require many forms to be completed during assessments. Increasingly, data are entered into computers to facilitate documenting and processing information. One result is that collecting data is sometimes so demanding that it restricts other activities of social workers. Assessment then becomes unidirectional, led by the needs of social workers and their agencies, and the outcome of the assessment may then lack engagement with and positive impact on clients.

Assessments in the participative model: what will the client think about that?

The participative assessment model appeared during the 1990s, reflecting interest in postmodern approaches in this period. It aims to democratize social work processes (Adams, 2008). Here, I focus on two postmodern assessment models: the exchange and narrative models. In both, the client's participation is of crucial importance.

In the exchange model (Smale, Tuson, Biehal, & Marsh, 1993), clients are perceived as experts in their own needs, and so they participate to the maximum in the whole assessment process. The relationship between the social worker and the client should allow clients to identify their own strengths, limitations and sources of understanding. Consequently, clients are enabled to assume control over the assessment process as well as over working on the issues which led them to the agency. An exchange assessment process is not 'only' about the open sharing of information between clients and practitioners. Assessment is seen as a full collaboration between two equal 'colleagues'. Social workers' competences lie in their knowledge of problem-solving processes, while clients are expert in their own problems. Exchange assessment aims to ensure the participation of all involved parties in the search for the understanding of needs and methods for responding to them. Social workers do not 'create' assessments but control the process and negotiate agreement about who should do what and for whom. The social worker also strives to target assessment on the *social situation* rather than on the *personalities* of the people involved, acknowledging that people seek out social services because other supporting systems are unavailable. Ideally, all individuals in clients' social networks should be included in the assessment, since each has their own perspective on the problem and its solution. Also, there are no sharp boundaries between assessment and management of social care. They form a continuous process, carried out in ways that emancipate the participants. Thus, Smale et al. (1993, p. 45) define the primary task of social workers in exchange model assessment as:

- Supporting full involvement by all participants in decision-making
- Creating a comprehensive assessment of the social situation, not just of the individual referred
- Helping establish and maintain the social networks which will be the foundation for the required care
- Facilitating negotiations about needs and possibilities
- Strengthening mutual trust
- Making responses to the situation flexible, when required

Coulshed and Orme (2012) proposed a narrative assessment model, different from the exchange model in two ways. The narrative approach acknowledges the social worker's expertise in offering knowledge about the processes of problem-solving while clients maintain influence in their interactions with the social worker. The narrative assessment model emphasizes that clients are also equipped with many useful skills and have key responsibilities in decision- making while also contributing their interpretations of the assessment. Another crucial component of narrative assessment is that information is not simply exchanged between clients and practitioners, but both engage in a process of jointly narrating or co-producing a story (Fook, 2016). Practitioner and client need not reach agreement in the end, since creating the narrative enables the possibility of debating and exchanging opinions. Fook's account of methodologies favours interviewing as the basis for narrative assessments. She recommends avoiding questions: for example, by the practitioner asking the client to 'talk about their experiences'. This helps immerse clients in the interview, treating it as an open discussion rather than as a formal interview or a questioning. Parton and O'Byrne (2000), however, do not exclude the use of questions and even propose the use of so-called 'scaling sheets' for various situations. Scaling sheets should not, however, be used merely to calculate a numerical score, but rather should aid the social worker in creating a narrative and allowing reflection on it. The narrative provided by the client allows the social worker to glimpse the client's life in the way the client sees it. The narrative draws the social worker into a conversation which is not controlled by theory. The conversation itself becomes part of the story.

To allow clients to participate fully in assessment processes, practitioners may usefully attend to the conditions which have an impact on clients' collaboration with practitioners (Navrátil, 2015). Clients may, for instance, require time to think about their situations, and attention needs to be paid to the intelligibility of the information on which decisions are made. It is also necessary to ensure that the structure and management of the agency make it possible for clients to influence decision-making. While clients need not be experts in individual matters, therefore, the participative model emphasizes that they should be equally involved participants in the assessment process, respecting decisions they make as it progresses.

Participative assessment models are within the discourse of understanding, which is based in social sciences. Social work agencies and their practices, rules and norms are social constructs which vary culturally, geographically and historically. The epistemic categories are interpretations and narratives. The purpose of reflection in practice is rather to expand one's understanding of both desirable and undesirable impacts on a problem and its solution. These models are mainly based on openness to possibilities which form the subject of negotiations. Assessments are understood as a permanent, cyclical process, in principle open to new findings, viewpoints or experiences; there is an emphasis on agreement. One potential risk of these models is a lack of boundaries for the process, offering the expert role to clients where practitioners should take over control. Also, outcomes may be inadequately defined.

Conclusion

In conclusion, I argue that social work needs to have a situational, open and complex approach to assessments and to the professional choice of which assessment model to use. This chapter sought to analyze the role of two key epistemic discourses, 'explanation' and 'understanding', within prominent social work assessment models during the last hundred years. The six assessment models considered were diagnostic, risk assessment, decision-making, critical, bureaucratic and participative models.

The first three models – diagnostic, risk assessment and decision-making – emphasize the objectifying position of *explanation*, while participative models, both exchange and narrative models, accentuate constructivist *understanding*, viewing social work as an artform. The critical model lies between these extremes. In some aspects, it is closer to the explanatory perspective while in others it has the traits of the understanding perspective (see Figure 4.1). The bureaucratic model inclines to the objectifying logic of the discourse of explanation, but analysis

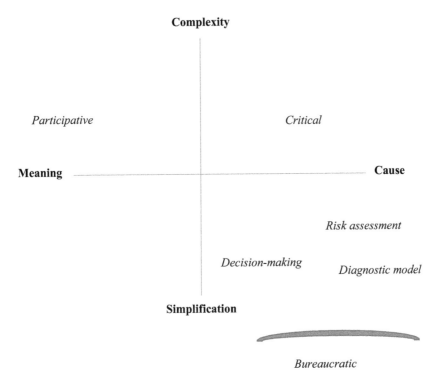

Figure 4.1 Assessment models with respect to their complexity and epistemological aims

suggests that it does not apply to either discourse. Its method is to create a system of understanding in which truth is given by directive. Though it endeavours to manage administratively limitations in the outcomes of assessment, this standpoint does not provide a professional tool of epistemology, and therefore it contravenes social work ethical standards. It does so by imposing the authority of the agency on how information is constructed. Consequently, it displays neither discourses of explanation nor understanding based on engagement between practitioners and clients with knowledge generated by the practitioners' investigation of the clients' situation.

A strong point of explanatory models of assessment is the ability to see the unique situation that clients are facing and to identify patterns and probabilities in comparison with many other similar situations known to practitioners. However, assessment models tending towards the extreme of the explanatory discourse do not help the people affected by the situation understand its meaning to them. Similarly, explanatory models over-simplify complex human and social data and consequently do little to manage the impact of social workers' biased expectations and professional and agency assumptions. Such models also emphasize the practitioner's expert role, while a strong point of models based on understanding is emphasis on respecting clients and their perceptions. They do this by visibly incorporating clients' experience and understanding and accepting the significance of their personal interpretations. Assessment models based on understanding accentuate the process rather than the outcome of the assessment and suppress the expert role of the social worker. As they strive to accommodate several viewpoints, they are closer to the ideal of achieving greater complexity.

The advantages and disadvantages of assessment models based on explanation and understanding suggest that only their active combination can lead to an appropriately complex approach to assessments. None of these polarities will suffice on its own. The objectifying approach is systematic, and the constructivist viewpoint opens the path towards quality and deeper understanding.

Parker (2017) supports an integrated approach, where assessments take advantage of the benefits of the social work of both science and art, also including parameters such as experience, wisdom, skills and acknowledging diversity as being among the prerequisites of high-quality assessments. If social work wants to be a profession that emphasizes solidarity, it must be able to generate and apply approaches to assessment and knowledge use more widely in order to understand human and social complexity if it is to assess client situations and social contexts adequately. Social workers cannot accept the dictatorship of administrators but should strive to win the trust of clients and the general public in their professional skills through active re-professionalization (Healy, 2017; Healy & Meagher, 2004).

References

Adams, R. (2008). *Empowerment, participation and social work* (4th ed.). Basingstoke: Palgrave Macmillan.

Adams, R., Dominelli, L., & Payne, M. (Eds.). (2009). *Critical practice in social work* (2nd ed.). Basingstoke: Palgrave Macmillan.

Allison, G. (1971). *Essence of decision: Explaining the Cuban missile crisis.* Boston, MA: Little, Brown & Co.

Baláž, R. (2012). Společenské kontexty sociální práce a jejich vliv na práci s cizinci. *Sociální práce/Sociálna práca, 12*(4), 134–149.

Baláž, R., & Musil, L. (2016). Faktory bránící dosahování oborových zájmů sociální práce. *Sociální práce/Sociálna práca, 16*(5), 52–71.

Barber, J. G., & Delfabbro, P. (2000). The assessment of parenting in child protection cases. *Research on Social Work Practice, 10*(2), 243–256.

Barker, R. L. (2013). *The social work dictionary* (6th ed.). Washington, DC: NASW Press.

Calder, M. C. (2016). *Risk in child protection: Assessment challenges and frameworks for practice.* London: Jessica Kingsley.

Coulshed, V., & Orme, J. (2012). *Social work practice* (5th ed.). Basingstoke: Palgrave Macmillan.

Corby, B. (2000). *Child abuse: Towards a knowledge base* (2nd ed.). Buckingham: Open University Press.

Dominelli, L. (2018). *Anti-racist social work* (4th ed.). London: Palgrave Macmillan.

Dyke, C. (2019). *Writing analytical assessments in social work* (2nd ed.). St. Albans: Critical Publishing.

Egan, G. (2014). *The skilled helper: A problem-management and opportunity-development approach to helping* (10th ed.). Belmont, CA: Thomson/Brooks Cole.

Van Ewijk, H. (2018). *Complexity and social work.* Abingdon: Routledge.

Fook, J. (2016). *Social work: A critical approach to practice* (3rd ed.). London: Sage.

Freire, P. (1972). *Pedagogy of the oppressed.* Harmondsworth: Penguin.

Garbarino, J. (1976). A preliminary study of some ecological correlates of child abuse: The impact of socio-economic stress on mothers. *Child Development, 47*(1), 178–185.

Garbarino, J., & Gilliam, G. (Eds.). (1980). *Understanding abusive families.* Lexington, MA: Lexington Books.

Glumbíková, K., Gojová, A., & Gřundělová, B. (2018). Critical reflection of the reintegration process through the lens of gender oppression: The case of social work with mothers in shelters. *European Journal of Social Work*, Online. Retrieved from https://doi.org/10.1080/13691457.2018.1441132

Harlow, E., Berg, E., Barry, J., & Chandler, J. (2013). Neoliberalism, managerialism and the reconfiguring of social work in Sweden and the United Kingdom. *Organization, 20*, 534–550.

Healy, K. (2017). Becoming a trustworthy profession: Doing better than doing good. *Australian Social Work, 70*, 7–16.

Healy, K., & Meagher, G. (2004). The reprofessionalization of social work: Collaborative approaches for achieving professional recognition. *British Journal of Social Work, 34*(2), 243–260.

Holland, S. (2010). *Child and family assessment in social work practice* (2nd ed.). London: Sage.

Hollis, F. (1964). *Casework: A psychosocial therapy.* New York: Random House.

Horwath, J., & Platt, D. (2018). *The child's world: The essential guide to assessing vulnerable children, young people and their families* (3rd ed.). London: Jessica Kingsley.

Hubíková, O., & Havlíková, J. (2017). Reflektivní praxe v sociální práci: Diskuse na příkladu sociální práce s lidmi v hmotné nouzi. *Sociální práce/Sociálna práca, 17*(2), 42–57.

Hyun, J., & Adams, S. R. (2016). A comparative study of child abuse risk assessment in the United States and Korea. *Asian Social Work & Policy Review, 10*(2), 210–224.

Janebová, R., & Celá, B. (2016). Kritická praxe mezi 'jinou' sociální prací a aktivismem. *Sociální práce/ Sociálna práca, 16*(2), 22–38.

Janebová, R., Hudečková, M., Zapadlová, R., & Musilová, J. (2013). Příběhy sociálních pracovnic a pracovníku, kteří nemlčeli – popis prožívaných dilemat. *Sociální práce/Sociálna práca, 13*(4), 66–83.

Janebová, R., & Truhlářová, Z. (2017). Janusova tvář sociální práce: Tři pohledy na pojetí kontroly v sociální práci. *Sociální práce/Sociálna práca, 17*(6), 116–130.

Krakešová, M. (1973a). *Výchovná sociální terapie 1. Díl.* Praha: Organizační a tiskové oddělení Ministerstva práce a sociálních věcí ČSR.

Krakešová, M. (1973b). *Výchovná sociální terapie 2. Díl.* Praha: Organizační a tiskové oddělení Ministerstva práce a sociálních věcí ČSR.

Krakešová-Došková, M. (1946). *Psychogenese sociálních případů. O vzniku sociální úchylnosti.* Praha: Nová Osvěta.

Levická, J. (2002). *Teoretické aspekty sociálnej práce.* Trnava: Trnavská univerzita v Trnavě.

Littlechild, B. (2008). Child protection social work: Risks of fears and fears of risks – Impossible tasks from impossible goals? *Social Policy & Administration, 42*(6), 662–675.

Lorente-Molina, B., & Luxardo, N. (2018). Towards a science of social work: Epistemologies, subalternity and feminization. *Cinta de Moebio, 61,* 95–109.

Lorenz, W. (2016). Research as an element in social work's ongoing search for identity. In R. Lovelock, K. Lyons, & J. Powell (Eds.), *Reflecting on social work: Discipline and profession* (pp. 145–160). Aldershot: Ashgate.

Lovelock, R., Lyons, K., & Powell, J. (2016). *Reflecting on social work – Discipline and profession.* New York: Routledge.

May-Chahal, C., & Coleman, S. (2003). *Safeguarding children and young people.* London: Routledge.

McNeill, T., & Nicholas, D. B. (2017). Creating and applying knowledge for critical social work practice: Reflections on epistemology, research, and evidence-based practice. *Journal of Ethnic and Cultural Diversity in Social Work,* Online. Retrieved from https://doi.org/10.1080/15313204.2017.1384945

Milner, J., Myers, S., & O'Byrne, P. (2015). *Assessment in social work.* London: Palgrave Macmillan.

Milner, J., & O'Byrne, P. (2004). *Assessment in counselling: Theory, process, and decision-making.* Basingstoke: Palgrave Macmillan.

Mullaly, R. P., & Dupré, M. (2018). *The new structural social work: Ideology, theory, and practice.* Ontario: Oxford University Press.

Munro, E. (2008). *Effective child protection* (2nd ed.). London: Sage.

Musil, L. (2004). *'Ráda bych vám pomohla, ale': Dilemata práce s klienty v organizacích.* Brno: Marek Zeman.

Navrátil, P. (2007). Posouzení životní situace: Úvod do problematiky. *Sociální práce/Sociálna práca, 2007*(1), 72–86.

Navrátil, P. (2014). *Reflexivní posouzení v sociální práci s rodinami.* Brno: Masarykova univerzita.

Navrátil, P. (2015). How to develop and manage a participative organization in social services with children and youth? In M. Pech (Ed.), *The international scientific conference INPROFORUM 2015* (pp. 87–92). České Budějovice: University of South Bohemia.

Navrátil, P., & Janebová, R. (2010). *Reflexivita v posuzování životní situace klientek a klientů sociální práce.* Hradec Králové: Gaudeamus.

Navrátilová, J., & Navrátil, P. (2016). Educational discourses in social work. *Social Education, 4*(1), 38.

Nečasová, M., & Musil, L. (2006). Pracovní podmínky a dilemata pomáhajících pracovníků: Poznatky z výzkumu charitní pečovatelské a ošetřovatelské služby. *Sociální práce/Sociálna práca, 2006*(3), 57–71.

O'Sullivan, T. (2010). *Decision-making in social work* (2nd ed.). Basingstoke: Palgrave Macmillan.

Otava, L. (2016). Institucionalizace sociální práce a sebezkušenost sociálních pracovnic. *Sociální práce/ Sociálna práca, 16*(3), 105–116.

Parker, J. (2017). *Social work practice: Assessment, planning, intervention and review* (5th ed.). London: Sage.

Parton, N. (2014). *The politics of child protection: Contemporary developments and future directions.* Basingstoke: Palgrave Macmillan.

Parton, N., & O'Byrne, P. (2000). *Constructive social work.* Basingstoke: Palgrave Macmillan.

Perlman, H. H. (1957). *Social casework: A problem-solving process.* Chicago: University of Chicago Press.

Punová, M. (2012). Konceptuální vymezení resilienční sociální práce s mládeží. *Sociální práce/Sociálna práca, 12*(4), 67–75.

Reamer, G. (1995). *The philosophical foundations of social work.* New York: Columbia University Press.

Reid, W. J., & Epstein, L. (1972). *Task-centered casework.* New York: Columbia University Press.

Řezníček, I. (1994). *Metody sociální práce: Podklady ke stážím studentů a ke kazuistickým seminářům.* Sociologické nakladatelství.

Richmond, M. E. (1899). *Friendly visiting among the poor: A handbook for charity workers.* New York: Macmillan.

Richmond, M. E. (1917). *Social diagnosis.* New York: Russell Sage Foundation.

Schön, D. A. (1983). *The reflective practitioner: How professionals think in action.* New York: Basic Books.

Smale, G., Tuson, G., Biehal, N., & Marsh, P. D. V. (1993). *Empowerment, assessment, care management and the skilled worker.* London: HMSO.

Svein, T., & Katya Nogales, C. (2017). A matter of politics: The effects of the political context on social work in Norway and Bolivia. *Journal of Comparative Social Work, 12*(1), 1–27.

Thompson, N. (2016). *Anti-discriminatory practice: Equality, diversity and social justice* (6th ed.). London: Palgrave Macmillan.

Thyer, B. A., & Pignotti, M. (2015). *Science and pseudoscience in social work practice.* New York: Springer.

Tolson, E. R., Reid, W. J., & Garvin, C. D. (2003). *Generalist practice: A task centered approach.* New York: Columbia University Press.

Tsui, M-S., & Cheung, F. C. H. (2004). Gone with the wind: The impacts of managerialism on human services. *British Journal of Social Work, 34*(3), 437–442.

Turner, F. J. (2005). *Social work diagnosis in contemporary practice.* New York: Oxford University Press.

Turney, D., Platt, D., Selwyn, J. & Farmer, E. (2012). *Improving child and family assessments: Turning research into practice.* London: Jessica Kingsley.

Watson, D., & West, J. (2006). *Social work: Process and practice.* Basingstoke: Palgrave Macmillan.

Webb, S. (2001). Some considerations on the validity of evidence-based practice in social work. *British Journal of Social Work, 31*(1), 57–80.

Webb, S. (2002). Evidence-based practice and decision analysis in social work: An implementation model. *Journal of Social Work, 2*(1), 45–63.

Webb, S. (2017). *Professional identity and social work.* Abingdon: Routledge.

Winkler, J. (2002). *Implementace: Institucionální hledisko analýzy veřejných programů.* Brno: Masarykova univerzita.

5

Theorizing social work in the domains of culture, politics and society

Stan Houston

Introduction

It is axiomatic that social work is deeply immersed in society. It aspires to advocate for the most vulnerable members of the social order and thereby challenges oppression. Societal institutions, by way of contrast, seek to define, enable and limit the nature of social work through legislative and social policy instruments. Put another way, social work is 'caught in the middle' between the politico-economic state and civil society, seeking to interpret personal problems within a context of public issues. Into this challenging zone can be added a burgeoning identity politics that makes culture not simply the domain of benign, symbolic meaning but, tellingly, the sphere of contested, intra- and intergroup relations.

It could be argued that this zone takes on a further resonance when the ever-changing nature of modern politics and economics is additionally considered. When Fukuyama (1992) declared, boldly, that we had reached the endpoint of political ideology, as a consequence of the universalization of liberal democracy, he neglected to consider the evanescent nature of geopolitical affairs. Far from signalling the apogee of humanity's evolution, we have seen liberal democracy overtaken in some nation-states by the rise of a nascent, authoritarian populism centring on a fortress mentality that reawakens fears of the outsider or stranger. Moreover, despite threats of much greater fiscal protectionism, the continuance of neoliberal economics and politics has led to ever-widening cleavages between the economically advantaged and disadvantaged in society (Davies, 2014; Wilkinson & Pickett, 2009). The consequences of such discrepancies are typified in a raft of biopsychosocial indications of well-being including educational attainment, rates of mortality, statistics on crime, and the incidence of mental ill health, to name a few areas.

In this chapter, I expand on these themes by examining how the domains of society, culture and politics not only shape social work practice, but also afford opportunities for the profession to intervene in these spheres to implement anti-oppressive interventions. However, to understand fully the deep-seated nature of these intersecting social constellations, and how they affect social work, we need to embrace relevant metatheory (Ritzer, 1991). At this juncture, it is important to define what is meant by this type of theory in the social sciences. Furthermore, we need to consider how it differs from the more customary usage of explanatory theory in social work: theory that draws mainly from the disciplines of psychology, sociology and social anthropology. Basically, metatheory is *theory* about theory. It seeks to provide a much deeper understanding of concepts and schemas in the social sciences that are commonly used to explain human action in the real, social world.

By offering a penetrating analysis of explanatory theory, metatheory excavates the philosophical precepts, or elemental foundations, underpinning observations about human action and society. It therefore makes plain often unarticulated, higher-order presuppositions about explanatory concepts. Gaps in the latter can then be debated and tested. Not only that, a metatheoretical inquiry can lead to an overarching, systematic perspective on the interrelationship between human agency and social structure; the interplay between 'micro' and 'macro' social processes (see Chapters 15 and 27); and the vexed question of whether the social sciences should focus on the attributes of individuals as part of a project of methodological individualism (for example, the nature of individual minds) or methodological wholes (for instance, the nature of social structure, social institutions and society, more generally).

Delving into metatheoretical inquiry is not only necessary when examining the highly complex, differentiated focus of this chapter; it must, correspondingly, have a wider relevance within social work theory *per se* if the nature of suffering, power and oppression is to be more fully apprehended. My contention, here, is that social work thinkers could draw, more fully, on the philosophy of social science (as a central, metatheoretical source) to illuminate such themes, broadening their focus beyond explanatory schemas deriving, for example, from attachment theory; or expository models, such as systems theory; or what Merton (1968) referred to as 'middle-range' theory: that is, concepts drawn from observation in empirical research. Such an argument in no way downgrades these latter types of theory; it merely reinstates the need for a wide paradigm of understanding in social work.

In this chapter, I explore social work's position within society, culture and politics by drawing on the metatheoretical work of the French social theorist Pierre Bourdieu (1977, 1980, 1990; see also Chapters 24, 27 and 36). Having set out Bourdieu's main ideas on these areas, I explore their implications for two critical dimensions of social work: the first aiming for cultural sensitivity and the second, political awareness. Bourdieu's theory has been chosen because of his international acclaim in providing penetrating, erudite insights into the nature of modern life, power, oppression, disadvantage and social division, social reproduction, the political state, culture, human perception and consciousness, ideology and threats to social welfare (Jenkins, 2002). In short, Bourdieu connects the individual with the domains of the social, cultural and political. With the pre-eminence of the 'cultural turn' in modern thought, Bourdieu's ideas on social class unite the domains of culture and the economy (Flemmen, 2013). What makes his work so important is that it helps explain a raft of social phenomena including the rise of new forms of individualism in neoliberal society, putting such orientations within a context of power, the resources available to people and the social arenas in which action takes place.

If ever there was a metatheorist qualified to provide insights into the areas explored in this chapter, it is Bourdieu. For him, metatheorizing is a form of *socio-analysis* where the social theorist is to the social unconscious of society as the psychoanalyst is to the patient's unconscious mind. Both approaches foster insight into not only the blind spots of human experience, but also the possibility of human betterment. More stridently, socio-analysis enables the social theorist to 'avoid being the toy of social forces' (Bourdieu & Wacquant, 1992, p. 183). Once the social theorist comprehends the nature of such forces, they will be in a much better position to control them.

Bourdieu's sociocultural theory

Bourdieu's metatheoretical work on the sociocultural domain relies profoundly on a cache of interlinked explanatory concepts. The first of these is denoted by the term 'habitus'. Bourdieu

(1989, p. 18) views habitus as 'internalised, embodied social structures'. Elsewhere (p. 76), he defines habitus as our 'cultural unconscious' or 'mental habits' or '. . . master dispositions' which lead to particular perceptions and actions that are durable in character. Implicit within the concept, then, is an acknowledgement that social structure and culture are deeply ingrained within us, that our ways of interpreting the social world are influenced by our social and cultural milieu. However pervasive this influence may be, though, Bourdieu reminds us that we are not automatons or mindless vehicles of our governing habitus. Rather, habitus acts as a very loose set of guidelines permitting us to strategize, adapt, improvise or innovate in response to situations as they arise. This type of action is not typically premeditated, but more often works in a pre-reflective manner as part of an inner set of dispositions that result in 'a feel for the game' (Jenkins, 2002, p. 65). Moreover, habitus is both a product and (re)producer of the social world and cultural experience: 'on the one hand, habitus is a structuring structure; that is, it is a structure that structures the social world. On the other hand, it is a structured structure; that is, it is a structure which is moulded by the social world' (Ritzer, 1996, p. 541). Put differently, action is a dialectical process whereby we internalize the external world but also externalize the internal world.

Through continuing socialization, an individual's habitus will come to mirror social divisions within his or her surrounding culture. More specifically, it will reflect class and material differences and cultural preferences: 'habitus, then, represents a sort of deep-structuring cultural matrix that generates self-fulfilling prophecies according to different class opportunities' (Swartz, 1997, p. 104). Structural disadvantages which may be present, for example, within the educational system, are internalized within children as they mature, leading to particular ways of viewing the world and enacting cultural norms. According to Bourdieu, fundamental life chances are determined by our habitus because it becomes embodied in the way we speak and our preferred cultural tastes, proclivities and deportment. Others react to us on the basis of these class markers to reinforce existing perceptions of our place in the stratified social world.

Bourdieu evinces a second conceptual tool related to habitus to add to the cache. This is referred to as the 'field'. For Bourdieu and Wacquant (1992, p. 97), the field represents a:

> . . . network, or configuration, of objective relations between positions. These positions are objectively defined, in their existence and in the determinations they impose upon their occupants, agents or institutions, by their present and potential situation in the structure of the distribution of species of power (or capital) whose possession commands access to the specific profits that are at stake in the field, as well as by their objective relation to other positions (domination, subordination, homology, etc.).

We can therefore think of fields as arenas of social relationship that are characterized by power differentials amongst the actors who make them up. Thus, they are better described as *force fields*. There are a number of these fields within modern neoliberal society that have a determinative effect on individuals and their habitus, including the economic sphere, the world of art, academia, sports and so on. To reiterate an earlier point, they are not founded on consensus. Rather, Bourdieu presents the field as a battleground where interests, power and prestige all vie for influence. Thus, domination and subordination lie at the heart of cultural experience. So, instead of being socialized into consensual arrangements, actors are thrust into a 'zero-sum' game where the 'curators of culture' (those with established power) and the 'creators of culture' (those seeking power) struggle for tactical advantage (Swartz, 2013).

Bourdieu suggests that the education system is a field of noted significance for it is here that social inequality is most evident. Children from working-class backgrounds will enter the school environment with a habitus that reflects particular assumptions about the role and value of education. For them, education is often seen as a means of acquiring practical skills. Teachers within the school may also work on the basis of pre-conceived views about what children from different classes or cultural groups (for example, travellers) can or should achieve. Indeed, basic markers of class (the way the child talks) or cultural deportment (the way the child gesticulates) lead to different expectations and approaches from those in authority.

Bourdieu's conceptual cache is made complete by a third and final heuristic: that of *capital*. Earlier, it was suggested that the field was characterized by struggle. For Bourdieu, the outcome of the struggle will be determined by the amount of capital (or resources) possessed by competing actors within a given field. He delineates four types of capital: namely, economic, cultural, social and symbolic. Economic capital refers to wealth defined in monetary terms; cultural capital involves a person's or institution's possession of recognized knowledge; social capital is constituted by social ties; and symbolic capital refers to one's status, honour, rank or prestige.

Our position in the social hierarchy will be determined by the amount and type of capital possessed. Dominant classes within society are invariably endowed with large amounts of capital, whereas subjugated or subaltern classes struggle hard to supplement their meagre assets. But even within the dominant classes there are discernible cleavages. On the one hand, there are those with large amounts of economic capital but few cultural resources (for instance, those in business); on the other, there are those who mainly possess cultural capital (that is, the intelligentsia or cognoscente). Regardless of how capital is configured, though, it will be utilized to attain strategic ground. This may necessitate converting or transmuting one form of capital into another. For example, cultural capital attained through recognized academic qualifications can be used in the employment field to increase one's economic capital. Hence, those possessing higher education qualifications may gain greater access to the employment market, improve their situation and avail themselves of new cultural pursuits.

The interrelationship between habitus, field and capital helps explain how culture impacts on people and how they socially reproduce their taken-for-granted worlds: worlds that are arbitrarily moulded and *naturalized*, yet misrecognized. Bourdieu elaborates on this process of naturalization (1980). He introduces the term 'doxa' to make the case in a compelling manner. Doxa shapes what can be thought and said at any one time within the field. Certain thoughts and words are permissible and others dismissed because they do not fit normatively with the group's way of being or form of expression. Consequently, doxa enforces parameters on social mobility and cultural expression within fields. Certain cultural artefacts will become 'out of bounds' and policed by an internal voice: 'this is not for us'.

Bourdieu proceeds to illuminate the interrelationship between culture, power and social reproduction. A central pillar of his theoretical edifice relates to the question of how social systems reproduce hierarchy and domination in culture without mass opposition arising. The answer to this question can be found in Bourdieu's view that at the heart of culture lies vested interests and struggles to attain symbolic and material advantage over others. Inherent within all forms of action, then, is power and a drive to attain the 'upper hand' through sometimes deliberate, but more often habitual or tacit, strategizing. The analogy of a chess game is relevant here. So, within the different arenas of social life, actors are socialized to plan the best move to accumulate prestige, kudos or wealth. In turn, they unwittingly reproduce existing divisions, social hierarchies, stratification profiles and class formations.

These essential premises about culture are reflected in Bourdieu's celebrated work on aesthetics entitled *Distinction* (1980). In this work, he charts how class influences everyday lifestyle and taste: the food we eat, our preferred newspaper, whether we are interested in so-called 'high' culture or its opposite, the world of the so called 'hoi polloi'. Accordingly, taste serves to differentiate people, to situate them in specific social groupings: 'taste is first and foremost the distaste of the tastes of others' (Wacquant, 1998, p. 223). More to the point, the higher classes are able to indulge their tastes freely because they have the resources to do so, whereas their working-class counterparts have limited means to achieve their aspirations in the chess game of social progression. Freed from the exigencies of material subsistence, the new bourgeoisie focus their attention on ways of accumulating prestige and wealth.

The cache of concepts used by Bourdieu to make sense of society and culture also has a formative bearing on his elucidation of the domain of politics. The next section elaborates on this theme, showing how Bourdieu's political theorizing has relevance for an understanding of power, the state, the political field and the impact of neo-liberalism on citizens' well-being.

Bourdieu's political theory

It is wrong to limit Bourdieu's corpus by branding it merely as a sociology of culture and education. In rejecting this myopic stance, Swartz (2013, p. 1) opines adroitly that Bourdieu 'offers not only a sociology of politics but also a politics of sociology'. In other words, the sociologist ought to be a social scientist uncovering the nature of existing political relations, including relations of power and domination. Yet, more than that, they must surpass the 'fact-value' antimony and engage in political activism. So, according to Bourdieu, sociology is not just a science; it is a decisive form of political engagement that debunks anti-humanist, globalizing forces. However, to do justice to this Janus-faced political endeavour, the right metatheoretical tools must be established to unearth the political terrain with dexterity. For Bourdieu, these tools are synonymous with the following concepts: (i) symbolic power, symbolic violence and symbolic capital; and (ii) the political State, neo-liberalism and globalization. Let us briefly consider what Bourdieu has to say on these themes.

Symbolic power, symbolic violence and symbolic capital

At the heart of Bourdieu's political sociology lie the intermeshed concepts of symbolic power, symbolic violence and symbolic capital (Schinkel, 2003). Collectively, they perpetuate social hierarchy, stratification and inequality in society and are pivotal in political processes of domination. Symbolic power, to examine the first notion, is a chief plank in the political infrastructure. In particular, it is used as a force for legitimation.

What makes the concept of symbolic power matchless, however, is that it links politics to the construction and maintenance of social identities, bodily expression and the perception of social reality. Symbolic power ensures, through a governing political doxa and habitus (see earlier references to these constructs), that dominated subjects internalize their conditions of domination from childhood onwards. Accordingly, they see them as *natural* and, in doing so, *misrecognize* their arbitrary character. In concrete terms, inequality and social divisions are viewed as 'the way things are' as subjects ease themselves into the social hierarchy and find their given niche without protest. Accordingly, symbolic power is used to impose classifications of meaning upon subjects – through the education system, cultural sphere and familial socialization – making them legitimate and, consequently, aiding their reproduction over time. Symbolic power is an inimitable form of political influence in that it is discrete, diffuse, subtle, invisible, imposed, constitutive and impalpable. It generates self-regulation through foisting 'the cop in one's head'.

The effects of symbolic power on the person are viewed by Bourdieu as tantamount to acts of symbolic violence. To reiterate, such violence has a demonstrative bearing on bodily activity, comportment, cognition and emotion. It leads to a kind of false consciousness. Subjects believe that they are responsible for their own suffering: a stance reinforced by the dominant framework of neo-liberalism and societal tendencies such as psychological reductionism and individualism. Yet self-blame masks the role of society as a primary causative agent of personal travail. Moreover, symbolic violence leads to a *dehistoricization* and *universalization* of political structure and cultural practice, both of which blind us to the true reality of lived experience. In terms of the former process, political and social structures are presented by the powerful as timeless, inviolable entities, whereas, in fact, we know on inspection that they are the product of contingent historical struggles (Marx, 2004). Likewise, although the latter process leads us to believe that the same political and social structures are present everywhere, regardless of time, context and place, we know this claim is problematic based on the findings of cultural studies (Huntington, 1996). Gender relations, for example, have changed dramatically throughout history because of political struggles, *contra* dehistoricization, and they are far from universal realities, *contra* universalization (de Beauvoir, 2011).

Symbolic power and symbolic violence are intimately linked with symbolic capital. Every person has some symbolic capital, but its social dispersal is very imbalanced. Simply put, symbolic capital provides governing members of society or political elites with the *resources* to dominate citizens. To wield symbolic power and exert symbolic violence, those individuals adopting positions of political power require the right kind of resources or capacity to influence the masses. Symbolic capital takes the form of rank, privilege, status, social position or the economic standing that makes one's position authoritative. Or it can be expressed through a charismatic personality exerting their political sway. A war veteran – the people's hero – returns from the battlefield and is immediately encouraged to stand for political office. Another way of saying this is that symbolic capital denotes socially acknowledged and permitted authority. Thus, for Bourdieu (1989, p. 23):

> As any form of performative discourse, symbolic power has to be based on the possession of symbolic capital. The power to impose upon other minds a vision, old or new, of social divisions depends on the social authority acquired in previous struggles. Symbolic capital is a credit: it is the power granted to those who have obtained sufficient recognition to be in a position to impose recognition.

Symbolic capital is effective because it is legitimated by society. It is perceived as making valid, fair-minded claims on others, commanding their respect, obedience and deference. At the same time, such claims can masquerade as political interests. Hence, a political leader of great standing possesses symbolic capital due to their social position in society, their educational qualifications, the esteem with which they are held, and the charisma that they exude. They make reasoned claims, advocating for necessary welfare cuts because of austerity management policies. Their claims have the ring of authority. A citizen might be forgiven for thinking that these claims are based on disinterested, rational assessments of the state of the economy. However, subterranean party and political interests might well be driving the politician's rhetorical flair.

The political state, neo-liberalism and globalization

Far from being a unitary phenomenon in the Western world, the political state, according to Bourdieu, is the amalgam of a set of overlapping bureaucratic fields that vie to control the social regulation of populations within society. Not only does it hold the monopoly on the means for physical violence; it also wields enormous symbolic power. Using and centralizing this latter form of power, the state legitimates social divisions by exercising the power of classification – or the authority to define what acceptable or unacceptable norms are in society. For instance, the state delineates which groups can be classified as legal or illegal immigrants. What is more, through the legal system and law-making channels, it determines which behaviours are permissible in civil society and the business world. The prospects for social mobility are shaped by its policies on education and how much funding is given over to this sector. In all of this, the state is not a detached reality; rather, it 'thinks through us', colonizing our habitus and doxa, directing us to make tacit judgements about what is acceptable politically or otherwise. Simply put, our state of mind is the mind of the state. Thoughts concerning the state are likely to be state-thought. This power to control the classificatory systems of meaning constitutes the ability to form and utilize ideology to promote social order and civic mindedness.

Bourdieu argues that the state has two primary functions: namely, to manage the economy, firstly, and to develop welfare entitlements, secondly. He claims that, in modern western societies, the former function has eclipsed the latter. This has resulted in large part from the rise of neo-liberalism: the practice of unfettered capitalism, free trade, speculative investment, the shrinkage of the state and its welfare arm, privatization and the deregulation of business. Bourdieu contends that neo-liberalism is part of a conservative revolution whose actors seek 'to sink and dissolve, in a cold water of calculation, all relationships and institutions of solidarity among people' (Mitrovic, 2005, p. 41), replacing the collective with the individual, the welfare state being one of those central collectives. While it foregrounds its mission in declarations of human rights and calls to liberty, in reality, it propagates the interests of big business and transnational corporations. Such trends are manifested in the European Union. In this geopolitical zone, contends Bourdieu, social democracy exists in tension with unencumbered capitalism, only to see the latter gain a turbo-charged momentum. More graphically, Bourdieu argues that the EU has now been prised apart, fragmented into two camps: the Europe of bankers and the Europe of workers.

For Bourdieu, the rise of big corporate business and the retrenchment of the welfare arm of the state have led to growing unemployment, economic cleavages of ludicrous proportions, the reduction of worker rights (zero-hour contracts being one example) and the social Darwinization of social life, where winners take all, greed is seen as good, the strong prevail over the weak and competition is valorized. In this movement, those who maximize their acquisition of various forms of capital, who excel in strategizing in the various fields in which they manoeuvre, are deemed to be the finest and fittest. By way of contrast, the poor (in capital and resources) are branded as incapable but nevertheless culpable for their own ineptitude. These are not only symbolic effects but material ones as well. Indeed, one analyst, Mitrovic (2005), refers to this economic model as killer capitalism because of the association between economic conditions and rates of mortality. Primarily, though, neo-liberalism reduces the person to a *homo economicus*, a rational actor concerned with maximizing his or her own gain and competitive advantage, materially and symbolically speaking.

Neo-liberalism thrusts outwards, Bourdieu contends, across the boundaries of the nation-state, becoming a global *force majeure*. Yet it continues to perpetuate the power and influence of a small number of leading countries over the entirety of other nations' stock exchanges and economic affairs. What exercises Bourdieu, though, is how globalization further erodes social democratic advances in welfare states, leading to inadequate housing, two-tier health systems, insufficient public transport, cuts to education and the dumbing down of the arts (which become commercialized and commodified by an ethos of profitability). Global, unelected and non-democratic economic bodies – the World Trade Organization, the International Monetary Fund and the World Bank – through their conditions of investment and loan management protocols affect the nature of work, promoting an ambient insecurity in the workplace, the emasculation of union power and the pursuit of short-term financial reward – all to keep investors happy. Coalitions of financial oligarchs, political bureaucrats, military elites and media interests strategize in their respective fields to accentuate such changes.

If this summary of Bourdieu's metatheory on the cultural and political domains has any credence, then power lies at the heart of all social life, as does the struggle for recognition in the various fields in which social actors are placed. Symbolic power, more specifically, creates and sustains the social hierarchies that form the substratum of political, societal and cultural experience. But what does this theorizing mean for social work? The next section addresses this central question.

Developing culturally sensitive and politically aware social work practice

Unless we acknowledge the unassailable link between culture, politics, social structure and social inequality, social work practice will at best prove to be ineffectual and at worst, may serve to reproduce unwittingly the divisions that it is attempting to challenge. For Bourdieu, there is a fundamental danger of misrecognizing how the domains of culture, politics and society cement individuals and groups into patterns of domination. Because we are immersed in these domains, they determine our thoughts and actions, often in subliminal ways. To make what is concealed overt, social workers must don the mantle of the engaged social scientist, become familiar with pertinent metatheory and apply it to their practice.

Taking these points to heart, there are three essential ways in which we can extrapolate Bourdieu's ideas to the practice domain: (i) enhancing professional reflexivity so that we can cogitate relentlessly on the impact of culture, politics and society on our taken-for-granted assumptions and actions and how these affect others; (ii) being sensitive to clients' experiences of the cultural, social and political fields, the meanings they have produced for them and their narratives about oppression; and (iii) developing practical strategies for empowering the excluded and marginalized: that is, those individuals whose capital in neoliberal society is very limited and who struggle in social fields to gain recognition.

Enhancing professional reflexivity

Unless we reflect on our personal and professional habitus and the professional field within which it is anchored, there is a danger of replicating biased notions that have been inculcated through professional training, managerial directives or experiences within embattled social work agencies. This awareness is gained through *reflexivity*. To summarize, then, reflexivity refers to the process whereby we continually reflect on how the assumptions underpinning our practice have been moulded by habitus, field, capital, doxa, symbolic power and the neoliberal order.

Bourdieu (1988) lays tremendous emphasis on this reflexive process but applies it mainly to the higher education field. Nonetheless, his ideas on the subject have relevance to the social work profession, which, like its educational counterparts, is concerned with human betterment. To take forward this imperative, Bourdieu recommends that we attend to two key areas. First, there is a need to reflect on our personal values, attitudes and perceptions and how they shape our actions. More specifically, the effects of socialization, education, gender relations and, importantly, social class need to be considered. Three important questions arise here. First, in what ways have our cultural identity and political attitudes been shaped by these factors? Second, can we identify any blind spots in our perceptions or areas enclosed by our professional doxa? Last, have we perpetuated symbolic violence on clients, even unintentionally, causing them shame and self-blame?

The effect of the field in which we operate is the second area of consideration. All professional groups are immersed in a governing field. This field will shape our professional view of the world. It therefore acts like the beam of a torch, illuminating certain parts of the path while leaving other parts in shadow. Accordingly, the field allows us to pose certain questions but excludes others. Alternatively, it acts as a censor to either allow or prohibit key ideas, according to the prescribed doxa. For Bourdieu, therefore, reflexivity promotes awareness of how the field distorts perceptions of reality. For social workers, the welfare or bureaucratic field will exact its own requirements and impose its own strictures, but what are they?

Peillon (1998) uses Bourdieu's notions of field, habitus and capital to explore the dynamics of the welfare field and address this question. He suggests that a key facet of this field is its normalizing tendencies: 'a wide range of highly personalized features of supervision and control have been set in place and the main normalising agents in the welfare field are doctors, teachers and social workers' (p. 218). Peillon is essentially saying that welfare agents act firstly to pacify discontent amongst the working classes or to avert a legitimation crisis within the neoliberal state. This effect is achieved through the provision of benefits and services which mollify welfare recipients' needs. Secondly, the role of social care professionals is primarily one of surveillance based on investigatory and classificatory practices. Thus, 'welfare agencies and welfare clients belong to a structure of domination' (p. 221). But it is a structure that is often misrecognized by both. For Bourdieu, misrecognition not only occurs within a particular field, but is also endemic to society as a whole. In short, it is a result of widespread *symbolic power*, *symbolic violence* and *symbolic capital* within the cultural and political domains. Social workers, as with any professional group, operate to perpetuate this symbolic violence but often unwittingly.

Hence, it is imperative for social workers to reflect relentlessly on these aspects of the welfare field and its impact on their professional habitus. However, although habitus has a determining effect on behaviour, it must be remembered that it is not a psychic prison. People, according to Bourdieu, exercise their agency: clients adopt resistant strategies to social work interventions (Peillon, 1998), and street-level bureaucrats can apply discretion when responding to administrative and controlling imperatives in their work (Lipsky, 2010). Indeed, the various types of capital mentioned above are often utilized in these counter-offensives. With this in mind, social workers ought to reflect on how they can dis-identify with the welfare field and their own personal habitus to expose practices founded on the application of symbolic power, symbolic violence and symbolic capital (Schirato & Webb, 2003).

The act of dis-identification entails adopting a *critical posture* towards social life. Here, social workers must avoid the risk of uncritically accepting official state classifications of meaning as orthodoxy, classifications often embedded in state policy and law. Reflexivity, here, demands that we maintain a critical distance from such classifications, posing a reflexive question: 'what if the state is only a human construction formed by power interests and elites'? Revealingly, the way social work has been classified by some commentators as a technocratic, scientific discipline has occluded the professional's emancipatory obligations to promote social justice (Garrett, 2007; Ferguson, 2008).

Developing cultural and political sensitivity

Cultural and political sensitivity may be equated with an affective empathy which seeks to remain open to others' experiences and resists defensive closure. Such attunement hinges, though, on an 'active and methodical listening as opposed to half-hearted understanding based on a distracted and routinized attention' (Garrett, 2013, p. 42). In this context, empathy is a process that involves accurate understanding of another person's cultural experience, emotions and behaviours and the doxa shaping them. Adopting this stance leads to several important areas of inquiry. First and foremost, what experiences has the client had within the various fields impacting on their life? In particular, what gains and losses have been accrued within the educational and welfare fields, and how have they been sculpted by the political field? Remember, these are the fields most associated with symbolic power, symbolic violence and symbolic capital. Second, how have life events, including childhood socialization, affected the client's taken-for-granted perceptions of self and others and the social world? This question relates to the nature and functioning of habitus, doxa and cultural identity. Third, how has the client experienced the material aspects of life under the stringent conditions of the neoliberal order: that is, work, economic livelihood and class relations? Last, have there been opportunities for the client to seek out new forms of capital or use the capital available to its best advantage in relevant fields? Conspicuously, a change in circumstances can occur during a period of crisis when there is a disparity between habitus and the social world, when doxa no longer fits with reality. At such moments, how can social workers help clients reflect on their circumstances to re-work constraining narratives?

In posing these questions, social workers should be attentive to an experience which Bourdieu refers to as 'hysteresis'. This occurs when a person is uprooted from one country and placed in another. It represents a profound disjuncture between habitus and field. The effect of hysteresis will be most pernicious when the two cultures and political arrangements differ radically in their social formation. Take, for example, a political refugee from an agrarian country who comes to live in a Western metropolis for the first time. Consider how this person's habitus will be thrown into complete disarray. Customs, social graces, deportment and basic meaning will all be problematized. What is more, the fields in the new culture will have different stakes and stakeholders. For the refugee in question, feeling like a 'fish out of water' is likely to lead to great mental uneasiness. Similar feelings could also be produced in ethnic minorities living in a society whose sensitivity to difference is limited by notions of liberal tolerance. On a lesser scale, hysteresis also operates whenever we are thrust out of our taken-for-granted social milieu. Thus, young people leaving home for the first time often experience bouts of homesickness.

These thoughts aside, culturally sensitive and politically active social work must also be attentive to the fundamental existential ground of being. In this context, Bourdieu points out that people are basically motivated by a need for recognition. Having a designated place in the social world, an acknowledged position, an acknowledged achievement or a particular skill serves to lessen the effects of existential repudiation, suggests Bourdieu. In this sense, our finitude is assuaged by the mark we make in life. However, for the culturally and politically excluded, misrecognition is often the defining experience. In existential terms, it is tantamount to an abnegation of self, an imprint of symbolic violence.

Such a depth of existential engagement can be heightened through social workers' adopting Bourdieu's notion of *relational analysis*: a process in which we bring not only our professional knowledge, but also our personal selves into the quest for accurate empathy with subjects and how they are positioned socially. This is to repudiate the call for professional objectivity at all times and to argue for a holistic form of identification: one that encourages the social worker to develop a deep understanding of and connection with the client and their social networks, using the worker's cognition and emotion to identify with the hurt of misrecognition.

Raising awareness and empowering

Social workers can assist clients to comprehend the effects of symbolic power and symbolic violence on their lives. This is similar to what has been termed as 'conscientization': 'conscientization requires helping oppressed people to gain a critical consciousness of the social structures that are implicated in their oppression . . . by this process, they become aware of their oppression rather than accepting it as inevitable' (Payne, 2014, pp. 332–33). But more than this, it involves *praxis*. Bourdieu's theory has particular purchase here because it explains how oppressive structures within the neoliberal order become part of our mental world. Furthermore, the idea of social fields helps us locate these structures spatially and fosters the idea that different recompenses (or interests) are being fought for within them.

To make conscientization a meaningful process, we need to assist the client to focus on areas where inequality has been most felt. We might, for example, facilitate insight into the workings of the educational field and how it has affected personal identity, social competence and educational achievement. Experiences related to social class also form an essential part of this analysis. However, this should not be a purely cognitive activity. For Bourdieu, habitus is literally embodied within physical presentation, movement and gesture. Finding ways to encourage bodily awareness of oppression is therefore a necessary if challenging facet of culturally sensitive social work.

In carrying out this work, social workers must challenge fatalistic ideas which assume that change is impossible because of structural barriers (Fram, 2004). It is important to remember that Bourdieu (1977) rejects the claim that his theory is overly deterministic and lacking in agency. Moreover, throughout the Western world there is evidence of the power of people in social movements (Tarrow, 2011). Where there is fatalism, it is often a result of labelling or pathologizing responses which become internalized within habitus. These negative dispositions – durable as they may be – should be challenged. One way of achieving this is to encourage the identification of a preferred habitus. The act of creating and reflecting on this idealized mind-set demonstrates the limitations of current dispositions. This technique is used to great effect by the Brazilian social pedagogue Augusto Boal (1979) in his 'theatre of the oppressed' stratagem.

Conscientization might also be fostered through helping clients analyze formative fields in their lives (Emirbayer & Williams, 2005). There are many critical questions fuelling this analysis: Who is in the field? What stakes or interests feature? What types of capital are being used and by whom? Are there any alliances? Where are the main divisions? Are there discernible contradictions between the various actors in the field, and how are they manifest? Young people leaving care might, for instance, scrutinize the employment field with these questions in mind. Their analysis might throw up a major contradiction between, on one hand, legislative requirements for specialized training schemes for care leavers and, on the other, the absence of this resource within the agency. The exposure of this contradiction might then result in a strategic alliance between the young people and a voluntary organization working in the field.

There is another way in which a Bourdieusian form of conscientization might unfold. This involves a strategic use of capital. With an increasing emphasis on citizenship and rights discourses (Ife, 2001), service users and their carers have gained symbolic capital in the sense that their power to influence services and practice standards within the social care field has never been greater. However, this type of capital must be used strategically and will be maximized when it is 'collectivized' or pooled. Thus, isolated individuals will make little inroad within a power-saturated field, and so alliances with other service users should be fostered. Mullender, Ward and Fleming's (2013) self-directed groupwork offers a useful template for collective action and welcomes the theorization of oppression. Collectivization might also mean drawing in specialist knowledge or, in Bourdieu's terms, cultural capital. Social work academics can offer so much in this domain provided they adhere to Gramsci's prescription of the 'organic intellectual' who openly identifies with an oppressed class.

Conclusion

It could be argued that metatheoretical sociology is too abstruse and far removed from the everyday practical realities faced by social workers and their clients. Even more critically, can Bourdieu's specific metatheory be adapted for the purposes of conscientization in social work, as has been argued? Surely, his notion of habitus indicates that only structural change is achievable. Are social workers equipped to engage oppression at this structural level?

I think the case for Boudieusian social work lies in the fact that the profession unassailably delves into the person-in-environment nexus (see Chapters 3 and 12). This is the bridge whereby we can assimilate Bourdieu's ideas into social work. Crucially, his notions of symbolic power, habitus, field and capital indicate how wider social, cultural and political systems colonize one's consciousness, affect one's attitudes and, subsequently, one's behaviour. This process of colonization through subtle power impacts not only the client, but also the social worker. Such insights ought to lead to a heightened empathy for the client and a much greater reflexive awareness within the social worker. This is the platform upon which conscientization can build. Despite various misapprehensions about his work, for Bourdieu, actors are not puppets. By engaging in struggle, they can disrupt entrenched social reproduction.

It is self-evident that we are living in a time of rapid societal, cultural and political change. Lenin's axiom that there are decades when nothing happens and then there are weeks when everything happens is most apposite when reflecting on today's world. To understand such changes, perspicaciously, and how they disturb everyday lives, we need to draw on pertinent metatheories. Without attending to the insights that they bring, there is a danger of falling prey to psychological reductionism with its attendant naming, shaming and blaming effects: effects that are germane to the scourge of neo-liberalism.

Further reading

Garrett, P. M. (2013). Pierre Bourdieu. In M. Gray & S. Webb (Eds.), *Social work theories and methods* (2nd ed., pp. 36–45). London: Sage.

Gray, M., & Webb, S. (2013). *The new politics of social work*. Basingstoke: Palgrave Macmillan.

Emirbayer, M., & Williams, E. (2005). Bourdieu and social work. *Social Service Review, 79*(4), 689–724.

References

Boal, A. (1979). *Theatre of the oppressed*. New York: Theatre Communications Group.

Bourdieu, P. (1977). *Outline of a theory of practice*. Cambridge: Cambridge University Press.

Bourdieu, P. (1980). *Distinction: A social critique of the judgement of taste*. London: Routledge & Kegan Paul.

Bourdieu, P. (1988). *Homo Academicus*. Cambridge, UK: Polity Press.

Bourdieu, P. (1989). Social space and symbolic power. *Sociological Theory, 7*(1), 14–25.

Bourdieu, P. (1990). *In other words: Essays toward a reflexive sociology*. Palo Alto: Stanford University Press.

Bourdieu, P., & Wacquant, L. (1992). *An introduction to reflexive sociology*. Cambridge, MA: Polity.

Davies, W. (2014). *The limits of neoliberalism: Authority, sovereignty and the logic of competition*. London: Sage.

De Beauvoir, S. (2011). *The Second Sex*. New York: Vintage Books.

Emirbayer, M., & Williams, E. M. (2005). Bourdieu and social work. *Social Service Review, 79*(4), 689–724.

Ferguson, I. (2008). *Reclaiming social work: Challenging neo-liberalism and promoting social justice*. Los Angeles, CA: Sage.

Flemmen, M. (2013). Putting Bourdieu to work for class analysis: Reflections on some recent contributions. *British Journal of Sociology, 64*(2), 325–342.

Fram, M. S. (2004). Research for progressive change: Bourdieu and social work. *Social Service Review, 78*(4), 553–576.

Fukuyama, F. (1992). *The end of history and the last man*. London: Free Press.

Garrett, P. M. (2007). Making social work more Bourdieusian: Why the social professions should critically engage with the work of Pierre Bourdieu. *European Journal of Social Work, 10*(2), 225–223.

Garrett, P. M. (2013). Pierre Bourdieu. In M. Gray & S. Webb (Eds.), *Social work theories and methods* (2nd ed., pp. 36–45). London: Sage.

Huntington, S. (1996). *The clash of civilizations and the remaking of the world order.* New York: Simon and Schuster.

Ife, J. (2001). *Human rights and social work: Towards rights-based practice.* Cambridge: University of Cambridge Press.

Jenkins, R. (2002). *Pierre Bourdieu.* London: Routledge.

Lipsky, M. (2010). *Street level bureaucracy: Dilemmas of the individual in public services.* New York: Russell Sage Foundation.

Marx, K. (2004). *Capital: A critique of political economy.* London: Penguin.

Merton, R. (1968). *Social theory and social structure.* London: Free Press.

Mitrovic, I. (2005). Bourdieu's criticism of the neoliberal philosophy of development, the myth of mondialization and the new Europe. *Philosophy, Sociology, and Psychology, 4*(1), 37–49.

Mullender, A., Ward, D., & Fleming, J. (2013). *Empowerment in action: Self-directed groupwork.* Basingstoke: Palgrave Macmillan.

Payne, M. (2014). *Modern social work theory* (4th ed.). Basingstoke: Palgrave Macmillan.

Peillon, M. (1998). Bourdieu's field and the sociology of welfare. *Journal of Social Policy, 27*(2), 213–229.

Ritzer, G. (1991). *Meta-theorizing in sociology.* Lexington, MA: Lexington.

Ritzer, G. (1996). *Sociological theory.* New York: McGraw-Hill.

Schinkel, W. (2003). Pierre Bourdieu's political turn? *Theory, Culture & Society, 20*(6), 69–93.

Schirato, T., & Webb, J. (2003). Bourdieu's concept of reflexivity as metaliteracy. *Cultural Studies, 17*(3–4), 539–553.

Swartz, D. (1997). *Culture and power: The sociology of Pierre Bourdieu.* Chicago: University of Chicago Press.

Swartz, D. (2013). *The political sociology of Pierre Bourdieu.* Chicago: University of Chicago Press.

Tarrow, S. (2011). *Power in movement: Social movements and contentious politics.* Cambridge: Cambridge University Press.

Wacquant, L. (1998). Pierre Bourdieu. In R. Stones (Ed.), *Key sociological thinkers* (pp. 261–277). Basingstoke: Palgrave Macmillan.

Wilkinson, R., & Pickett, K. (2009). *The spirit level: Why more equal societies almost always do better.* London: Allen Lane.

6

Paradigm shift? Biomedical science and social work thinking

Malcolm Carey

Introduction

Biomedicine is the study and practice of medical science and includes biology and the physical functioning of the human body. It has for more than a century endured as the principal belief system on which modern medicine and the clinical components of healthcare are built. Although often dynamic and sometimes capable of reform (or reinterpretation through active agency), biomedicine vigorously endeavours to remain objective and emotionally detached and historically has struggled to engage democratically with other theories, professional belief systems and models of practice (for example, Estes, Biggs, & Phillipson, 1996; Witz, 1992). Diagnosis, the use of evidence-based research and treatments to alleviate illness and the relative abstraction of human experiences all appear central to biomedical thought and praxis. Yet other priorities have been noted, including attempts to move beyond epidemiology and the treatment of the body's ills to enter the domains of politics, ethics, political governance and everyday life itself (Illich, 2010; Rose & AbiRached, 2013).

In recent years, social work education and practice have come under the increasingly direct influence of clinical healthcare and medicine, including many of the core political and cultural principles of biomedical science. For example, social policies and related legislation such as the Care Act 2014 in the United Kingdom (UK) remain indicative of government attempts to promote closer organizational and ideological ties between social work and healthcare. As I have argued elsewhere (for example, Carey, 2016a, 2016b), such policies reflect broader political agendas which link to ambitious neoliberal wishes to reduce state welfare to the basic provision of healthcare and education. Such an agenda is also tied to other reforms, such as the ongoing medicalization of 'social problems' such as mental health or ageing, privatization and the promotion of self-support for proactive citizens in 'communities' (Estes, Biggs, & Phillipson, 2003; Rose & AbiRached, 2013).

This chapter examines the relationship between biomedical science and social work thinking. It looks at the similarities and differences between two unique but increasingly closely associated 'helping professions'. As part of the discussion, the roles of paradigm, power and ideological disparities and distinct traditions are stressed, as well as the impact of ongoing policy-led reforms which continue to bring the professions closer together. Part of the general argument is that biomedicine is arguably becoming as influential as neo-liberalism in its capacity to directly influence and govern the role and purpose of social work. As we shall see, however, the ideological ties between biomedicine and social work thinking have a much longer history.

Paradigm, professional hegemony and discourse

Some clarification of definitions and concepts will help support the arguments set out in this chapter. These concepts have distinct traits but also relate closely to one another. First, a *paradigm* is not simply a theory but represents a whole system of thinking (and doing), complete with its own culture, rules and practices. The analogy of a 'map' is sometimes used to distinguish a paradigm from a theory as it can provide direction and guidance and tends to move beyond the hypothetical conjecture on which it rests (Carey, 2013). For example, biomedicine as paradigm contains theoretical elements that stress ideas such as objectivity and neutrality. Yet it integrates with these cultural and political traditions such as maintaining formal relations with patients alongside promoting professional expertise and patient autonomy and rational choice. Second, *hegemony* represents a subtle and typically manipulative expression of ideology that expresses the beliefs, values and enacted principles articulated by powerful groups to serve their own interests. Crucially, hegemony often seeks to compromise and entice to capture hearts and minds. For example, the medical profession may seek to emphasize positive traits such as care and the treatment of illness whilst concealing any intentions to dominate or control patient perspectives. Similarly, social work as professional hegemony may stress its positive roles in safeguarding and human rights and understate social control elements, such as those tied to its many legal responsibilities: for example, removing children or reducing the independence of older people.

Discourse represents the linguistic rules and structures which subtly or otherwise dictate how established traditions and beliefs form to produce 'versions of knowledge that then gain legitimacy' in a political, social, cultural and professional sense (D'Cruz & Jones, 2004, p. 156). Discourses emerge in all welfare professions including social work and medicine because they develop from knowledge production, aspiration and power to generate, say, a biomedical paradigm which becomes part of a wider medical discourse and subsequently elevates legitimacy, status and power. Like hegemony, discourses go on to establish what is acceptable or not to say and do, as well as strongly influencing how we understand and relate to people. Finally, biomedicine is recognized as a dominant paradigm and medicine as a master discourse because they each have significant powers and influence, due, not least, to their capacity to gain high levels of legitimacy and public support, which social work has struggled to consistently achieve (see, for example, Jones, 1983; Witz, 1992; Estes et al., 2003).

Shared traits and influence: Plato, positivism and the logos

A key Western belief system and core paradigm shared between biomedicine and social work is positivism. This encapsulates not merely an attempt to apply the laws of science to the study of society but, moreover, represents a powerful 'nineteenth-century post-Enlightenment ideology'. Indeed, the philosophical roots and ideals of positivism to be able to acquire 'absolute truth' through objective empirical investigation lie deep within Western culture and draw from core ideas initiated by Plato and other influential Western scholars. Crucially, Plato argued that citizens who were educated and knowledgeable remained superior to citizens who lacked the reliable insight gained from deep thought, self-reflection and a capacity to develop 'pure ideas' (Delanty, 2005, pp. 13–14). In Greek philosophy and tradition, the related principle of the *logos* (knowledge and insight) contrasts with common sense and spurious opinion (*doxa*) to represent a foundation upon which positivism – and the principal project of professionalism – draws influence. As Foucault (1992, p. 89) noted, the logos includes the art of persuasion and enlightenment based on evidence and careful reflection, alongside a sense of morality, self- restraint and a yearning for truth and 'the maintenance and reproduction of an ontological order'.

From the logos/doxa binary and later rational ideas embedded within Western analytic philosophy, we can locate where foundational and modern biomedical/social work doctrines and related processes originate. These include priority given to objectivity during diagnosis and assessment or evaluation, alongside the individualism and apparent emotional restraint of treatment or casework. This tradition is apparent within Fabianism and more recent and seemingly humanistic ideals such as empowerment, anti-oppression and participation, since each implicitly presumes the centrality of the dominant professional to enlighten or emancipate the service user or 'lay' expert. Thus, while the ideals of objectivity, expertise and logical truth persist as firmly embedded within biomedicine, they also carry significant influence within social work, especially in its ongoing search for public and trans-professional acceptance and legitimacy. Jones (1983), for example, argues that an organized form of 'scientific charity' social work has historically endeavoured to drape its practice and teaching in 'the cloak of science'. Motives include the use of science as hegemonic veil to conceal an underlying 'class based morality', alongside a low cost means by which to valorize 'professional' practices. Indeed, Jones draws attention to Eileen Younghusband's (1947) advocacy of the use of scientific discursive idioms to achieve more traditional ends in fields of practice:

> Social science and research make it respectable to talk about 'factors in social pathology' instead of the undeserving poor; 'community stimulation' instead of 'getting lonely people to the Settlement . . .' 'psychopathic personalities' instead of 'hopeless scroungers . . .' The essential rose remains unchanged by this change in names but, if anyone is helped thereby to see more clearly, to think more deeply, to diagnose more truly, and to treat more effectively, then this change and all others that succeed it are all to the good.
>
> *(cited in Jones, 1983, p. 91)*

More recently, Shaw (2016, pp. 27–28) has emphasized caution when he highlights two problems which over-reliance on elements of positivism may engender for social work. First, as a relatively crude instrument in dynamic social fields, it lacks a capacity to appreciate fully 'social wholes' or context. Both remain typically paramount in human relations and core social work activities such as assessments or evaluations. Second, as some critics of evidence-based practice have noted, the positivist tendency to measure and quantify objective 'variables' is a major challenge in dynamic social environments and (multi)cultural domains. For example, although measurement may be relatively straightforward when dealing with the human body within confined institutional settings such as the surgery or hospital, it is a very different proposition to quantify emotions or power, nurture, neglect, loneliness, discrimination or abuse. In addition to such critiques, concerns linger about how implicit positivist cultures of 'objectification' affect relations between the professional as 'expert' and patient or service user. Also, the underlying principle of experts disseminating truth and reason – or as being able to offer forms of emancipation – has been challenged, including (ironically) as being oppressive and ultimately maintaining established power relations (Carey & Foster, 2011).

Disembodied care and risk

A common criticism levelled at biomedical science remains the formal distance typically generated between medics and patients within discursive fields of praxis. Consequently, according to Twigg (2006, p. 83), medicine has become 'far removed from our everyday experiences of ourselves and others'. For example, in an eagerness to objectify patient needs scientifically during brief bouts of formal contact, subjective and embodied patient experiences will often be ignored. Indeed, under a medical gaze, the person 'becomes a body, an object, a site of physical and causal processes', whereas the patient's narrative is often presented as offering little more than 'a subjective and mistaken account'. Hodge's (2005, p. 164) ethnographic study of the attendance of service users with mental health needs at a healthcare forum in England illustrates this point. Through observation and the use of critical discourse analysis, Hodge articulates how, in meetings with medics and other healthcare staff, user views and personal experiences were carefully controlled and effectively dismissed by staff whose understandings appeared to be rigidly trapped in a medical discourse and biomedical paradigm. For example, common user perspectives regarding their experiences of poverty, structural disadvantage and numerous related mental health concerns were discouraged and removed from committee minutes and agendas. Related 'difficult' conversations were also politely yet effectively averted by the chair or non-participant attendees throughout meetings. Hodge concludes that proactive participant discussions initiated by users and which included tangible experiences or personal opinion were considered relevant 'only in so far as they [could] be incorporated instrumentally into [a dominant medical] discourse'. Such ideological rituals subsequently generated 'discursive inequality' between service users and officials, which 'mirrors and thus reinforces wider institutional power inequalities'.

In a detailed account which echoes similar concerns, Kitwood (1997) has argued that patients with dementia are commonly reconceptualized as being less than human within medical discourse following diagnosis. Indeed, personhood and many emotional needs can quickly disappear as priorities in favour of military-like treatment regimes or formal care, which effectively leads to a 'slow death'. Such attitudes have been recognized in response to other conditions in numerous reports of insincere care, neglect or even abuse within a variety of health and social care settings (see, for example, Goodley, 2013; Phillipson, 2013; Scull, 2015). Such political processes, attitudes and techniques of 'othering' and objectification have also lingered within social work and can include formal relations promoted with 'service users' who are care managed, probed or interrogated with intense questioning as part of bureaucratic assessments of need, restricted to briefly offering viewpoints within other formal meetings or routinely referred to or moved like objects between institutions. Their bodies might be mechanically processed as part of highly rationalized protocols and standardized services or entirely invisible and only briefly listened to by a nurse or 'social worker' asking scripted questions from one of many call centres (Dustin, 2007; Baines & van de Broek, 2017). A lack of meaningful contact between social workers and children has also been noted, including when vulnerable children are taken into care, with institutional priority instead being given to concerns about care commissioning, forensic investigations and collecting evidence during typically brief time frames (Bissell, 2012; Ferguson, 2011; Parton, 2014).

Modern-day attempts to use assessments of need to limit eligibility for support in adult care, ensure evidence-based objectivity or manage risk draw direct influence from medicine. Jones (1983, pp. 96–97), for example, argues that in Victorian London the Charity Organisation Society (COS), which gave birth to social work, had concrete ideas about how assessments should proceed, which appear remarkably like some components of modern-day practice:

> All COS visitors were supposed to do was to undertake a thorough enquiry into the claimant's life, asking for example landlords, neighbours, local shopkeepers, relatives and the parish priest, about the claimant's character and general moral state, and visiting the home

to assess cleanliness and order. They were then to report back to the local COS district committee with their assessment and, with the committee, determine whether the claimant was 'curable', and if so, what treatment strategy was required.

Importantly, social workers were to avoid becoming overemotional in their assessments or personally involved with clients. Too much sympathy might lead to political 'contamination' and questioning by the professional of the harshness or injustices of wider policies or acts of intervention. Despite recent claims that assessments are now more 'holistic' or 'person-centred', Webb (2006, p. 74) contests that such technologies of care increasingly seek to determine risk in target populations and complex social fields through a 'rational-linear model of reality'. Here, evidence-based hegemonic procedures and tools invariably narrow their focus through technologies such as structured questionnaires and cursory meetings, which generate 'fixed categories of meaning whilst filtering observed empirical reality' to grasp quantifiable 'needs'. Such methods also limit professional autonomy and detach the service user, who is disempowered, within neoliberal-inspired professional discourses and related assessment technologies, from a legion of structurally determined events and experiences. According to Baines & van de Broek (2017, p. 132), by enacting the policies of an austere state, many health and social care workers now regretfully 'act as conduits of control of scarce resources', while providing variable standards of fragmented care to 'increasingly frustrated and desperate service users'.

Iatrogenics, social control and resistance

Despite its strong influence, the biomedical paradigm has faced numerous challenges, which include some powerful critiques. Illich (2010), for example, argued that modern medicine and related expertise generate over-dependence and medically inflicted 'iatrogenic' harm and risks within society. Moreover, longer life and better standards of health are more often associated with factors outside direct biomedical control. McKeown (1976) reiterated the much wider positive impact of nutritional, environmental and personally motivated behavioural changes upon good health, including improved public water and sanitation systems, better education provision, public health, technologies, diets, exercise and so forth. These and other challenges posit most biomedical interventions as brief, superficial or counterproductive: for example over-relying upon prescribed drugs in treatment regimes which may have limited efficacy or cause as many side effects as they alleviate symptoms. The medical profession has also maintained strong ties to big business and new technologies, whilst regularly reinterpreting fundamental human experiences such as ageing as embodying decay or dependence. For example, Phillipson (2013, pp. 132–134) notes how physicians have been 'placed in charge of the definition and treatment of old age as a disease', ultimately neglecting cultural, political or social influence. Within biomedical discourse, alternative social models or cultural reinterpretations of ageing have been marginalized or dismissed, alongside patient opinions and lay knowledge bases. Nevertheless, the invisibility of ageing bodies can also be regularly expressed outside professional discourse, including at a personal and public level of engagement (Katz, 2010; Phillipson, 2013, pp. 132–134).

Related social iatrogenic criticisms have been levelled against the social work profession. Examples include the consistently poor 'life chances' and relative neglect experienced by many children placed into residential or foster care, the deterioration of health experienced by many older residents who receive increasingly fragmented residential or nursing care, and the fact that a significant majority of *effective* care is still provided in the home by families and relatives. So much formal professional social work and safeguarding of children, adults and families is now effectively authoritarian yet socially detached (Parton, 2014; Wrennall, 2013). Brown (1997) argued that 'clientization' is a delicate political process which encourages vulnerable people to be unnecessarily dependent on state bureaucrats, who subsequently hold a monopoly over power, information and other resources. These perspectives suggest that, in tandem with the biomedical model, modern social work fails to offer substantive longer-term preventative care and support to people most in need, limits meaningful engagement or co-production and at times increases disadvantage or neglect for service users. The key role of medicine, healthcare and social work in the collection and processing of personal information as part of complex state surveillance initiatives, alongside the wider dissemination of dominate norms to seemingly passive citizens, has also been emphasized. Such accounts often suggest that state social work remains more control focused, not least because services are forced onto clients rather than initiated through patient choice (Jones, 1983; Althusser, 1971[1989]; Cruickshank, 1999).

Although interesting and persuasive, such accounts may exaggerate the power or social control elements of professional interventions while understating the *potential* active role of users, patients or practitioners in circumventing or resisting 'negative' power. Many ongoing advances in the treatment of longer-term conditions within biomedicine and key support roles such as safeguarding within social care may again be understated or ignored. Despite deficits, within increasingly atomized societies and fragmented communities, the provision of effectively resourced health and social care might be more crucial than ever before, especially to many minority groups who otherwise would be left without any formal care.

Contested integration and biomedical dominance

Although the medical profession and biomedical ideas have always maintained some sway over social work's professional aspirations and cultures of praxis, such influence has recently begun to intensify. In particular, repeated government calls for greater levels of organizational and professional integration between health and social care and other sectors such as education or the police in many countries, including the UK, have begun to change the relationship between medicine, healthcare and social work. Previously, the Seebohm committee (1968) argued that social work should be independent from the National Health Service (NHS) in the UK, due to its understandable reservations that the medical profession would seek to control, limit and distort the activities of social workers. Such anxieties reflected the medical profession's long history of successfully controlling other female-dominated professions, such as midwifery, nursing and social work within healthcare domains (Webb & Wistow, 1986; Witz, 1992).

Subsequently, in England and Wales during the 1970s and 1980s, social work within local authorities gained relative independence from the NHS and was briefly freed from direct medical control. This structure began to change, however, with the implementation of the watershed NHS and Community Care Act in 1990 and other subsequent legislation such as the Care Act 2014. Since then, profound changes have included the demise of semi-independent local authority-based social service departments in England and the formation of integrated health and social care teams, alongside similar spatial and ideological moves in sectors such as higher education. Increasingly, social work has been encouraged to embrace biomedical and clinical healthcare paradigms and related discursive cultures of practice. Examples include the adoption of evidence-based practice and positivist, quantitative and grant-centred research cultures and specialist knowledge bases. These often privilege hard science, measurement, pathology and, as consequence, a more limited understanding of epidemiology, policy, social history and the crucial role of political and social context in the life chances of users, patients and carers (Rose & AbiRached, 2013, p. 196). In recent years the extent to which social work academics have embraced or resisted such ideological principles has often had a major bearing upon personal career development or promotion. This can breed a corrosive learning culture in which compliance and opportunism rather than omniscient insight, theory development, analysis, critique and innovation are rewarded (Furedi, 2006). Consequentially, a plethora of often uncouth rebranding exercises has taken place, with the emergence of seemingly newer forms of 'social work' which carry much closer hegemonic ties to a pervasive biomedical paradigm. Among other examples, these include the emergence of 'gerontological', 'palliative care' – and perhaps most revealing – 'clinical' and 'forensic' social work.

Despite often significant power disparities between welfare professions, policy documentation concerning health and social care integration has tended to ignore or understate any such differences. Advocates claim that integration will increase efficiencies, improve communication within more 'seamless services' and avoid unnecessary duplication of core work such as assessments (Gray & Birrell, 2013; Glynos, Speed, & West, 2014). Critics have offered different perspectives. For example, it has been proposed that keeping costs down and getting more input from fewer staff remain among the key motives for health and social care integration, an example of which has included the reduction of adult social workers in community settings (Poxton, 1999; Lilo, 2016). Integration policies have not offered further resources to already severely underfunded social care sectors in the UK, and rigid eligibility criteria to access support services endure or have increased (Age UK, 2014). Others identify integration as offering a versatile hegemonic construct through which further competition, outsourcing of public services and privatization can be justified (Estes et al., 2003; Glynos et al., 2014). Integration has also been recognized as offering another ideological means by which to focus the combined social control elements of health, social care and agencies such as the police, such as by providing more organized and effective levels of surveillance and early intervention, especially within child and adult protection services (see, for example, Wrennall, 2013).

Another ethical concern with integration for the social work profession remains the significant power disparities which are embedded within health and social care, including the tendency of biomedicine to discount perspectives which sit outside its paradigmatic comfort zone. Estes and Binney (1989, p. 588), for example, highlight biomedicine's tenacious capacity to 'seal itself off' from other perspectives, which often includes discrediting other paradigms or professional discourses (see also Witz, 1992; Illich, 2010). For example, attitudes towards social work within medicine have included apprehension regarding its various non-clinical, ambivalent or seemingly hazy activities which struggle to secure a clear evidence base, especially in the short term. Concerns also prevail about social work's apparent over-reliance upon an unsound knowledge base that includes the use of superfluous theory alongside seemingly unsound 'therapeutic' practices (see Bell, 1961; Brewer & Lait, 1980; Bywaters, 1986). In sum, when compared to the more meticulous or grounded clinical practices present within biomedicine, social work can appear a somewhat vague, if not strange, science. Whether such prejudices are unfair or not, they inevitably impact upon professional reputations, identity, status and role and can promote tensions or conflict within discursively contested multi-agency fields, in which different beliefs and practices sit alongside significant power and status disparities (Hudson, 2002; Carey, 2016b). In contrast, Lymbery (2006) has argued convincingly that effective collaboration and integration is heavily dependent upon the promotion of mutual respect and status. This remains, however, more an aspiration than a reality within health and social care. Numerous studies suggest that social workers are often little more than uninvited 'guests' under the 'benign control' of nursing and medicine within healthcare domains (for example, Beddoe, 2013; Bell, 1961; Bywaters, 1986).

Neuroscience, resilience and children

One area where biomedicine has established a strong influence within welfare, policy and social work is in studies of the developing brain, especially its purported impact on early childhood and later life. As prominent yet broad fields, neuroscience and neuropsychology have enjoyed a surge of interest in recent years, which has gradually been supported to varying degrees within professions such as education and social work, especially in America. This movement has included ongoing debate about the impact of the developing brain upon cognition, memory, emotions, skills, behaviour and later life chances. This has led some neuroscientists to insist that people 'are nothing but their brains' (Green, 2017, p. 61). Egan, Combs-Orme, and Neely-Barnes (2011, p. 270) argue that neuroscience can enrich social work's understanding of the 'transactional and ecological nature' of human development and inform interventions with service users, better support 'client systems' and facilitate practitioners' language and knowledge so as to enhance interdisciplinary practice. Again, no recognition of power disparities or consequences is provided. Whilst the rapid growth of neuroscience has spawned a variety of perspectives and applications from different disciplines, in recent years two politically diverging discourses have emerged.

First, closed-system perspectives within neuroscience (and neuropsychology) claim that the developing brains of children are almost set or 'hardwired' in their first four years of life. Indeed, emotional intelligence within the brain seemingly develops in the first 18 months and up to 80 percent of the brain develops in the first three years. Politically, this has led to calls for increased state intervention at an earlier age, including the removal of children from parents at a younger age before permanent and seemingly irreversible damage is inflicted. Scan images of children's brains have been used to emphasize a link between smaller 'walnut-shaped' brains and apparent neglect or poor parenting in earlier life. Such neuroscience-based evidence and arguments have become influential in American social policy and sections of the Coalition and Conservative Governments in the UK (Williams, 2014). Scull (2015, pp. 392–394) has detailed how during the 'decade of the brain' (during the 1990s and events beforehand) in America, crude psychiatric biological interpretations of the brain were used within psychiatry to recapture successfully the profession's previously lost legitimacy and power. Such a paradigm shift, however, has also been motivated by economic and related political factors, including supporting the pharmaceutical industry in generating new costly drugs to treat, with varying degrees of success, chronic mental health conditions such as schizophrenia and depression.

In contrast to this popular discourse, a more fluid set of arguments has remained, which include stronger emphasis placed on evidence that privileges the plasticity and resilience of the infant, adolescent and early adult brain, including a capacity to cope with adversity. This discourse can include recognition of the more durable impact of support systems leading to enhanced life chances upon children's and adults' well-being and longer-term health. This suggests that the strong biological emphasis placed upon early-years development has been grossly exaggerated. In the same way that concerns have been raised about the misuse of attachment theory as apparent 'evidence' for unfairly removing children, Wastell and White (2012, p. 409) question the increasingly prominent use of neuroscientific data in the UK to justify expanded programmes of statutory intervention, leading to the removal of children experiencing neglect or poor parenting. The authors claim that much biological 'evidence' has often been oversimplified or exaggerated, while moral debate is shut down in favour of simple and quick yet largely superficial policy-led solutions. The authors conclude with a call for practical help for families 'rather than moral panics about damaged brains' (Wastell & White (2012, p. 409). Recognition of the later limited life chances of most children brought into care is rarely a part of closed system–led debates or policy solutions.

Such research and debates are of interest for three reasons. First, they suggest ongoing ideological tensions and discursive disparities *within* biomedicine, which includes questioning about the validity and potential abuses of hard science, especially if used as evidence to support authoritarian policy initiatives. Second, they again reveal the tendency for some policymakers to selectively use medical 'evidence' to reify quick, appealing but often superficial policy-enacted solutions, rather than examining or responding meaningfully to the complexity or nuances of people's lives and forms of disadvantage. Finally, the promotion of neuroscience illustrates the potentially powerful hegemonic impact of crude elements of biomedicine upon social work practice. Green (2017, p. 63), for example, notes how some social workers have been persuaded by brief bouts of continuing professional development training in the UK to apply closed-system neuroscientific arguments and 'essentialist' research uncritically in practice. In addition, evidence has, at times, been routinely misunderstood and/or misused 'to over-biologize human behaviour, scaremonger, and blame parents in poverty', whilst misrepresenting working-class women as 'a threat to their child's developing infant brain' (Green, 2017, p. 63).

Bioethics, inequality and power

Alongside an influence upon parenting, education and interventions within professional social care, biomedicine has more recently enjoyed an enhanced role within welfare ethics, including in relation to social work research. Debates about the impact of utilizing professional codes of ethics have continued to generate debate. Advocates have emphasized the use of codes to offer moral guidance for practitioners, as well as establishing a coherent professional identity. Numerous critics, however, have stressed their individualizing and didactic nature and tendency to deal in broad universal concepts which may struggle to cope with human diversity and ever-changing societal norms or, indeed, shifting care-related domains of professional praxis (Carey & Green, 2013). Traditionally, professional social work has founded its ethical frameworks upon a bedrock of duty-based Kantian principles (which stress the rightness or wrongness of acts), alongside utilitarian-consequential frameworks that privilege moral outcomes. Nevertheless, one of social work's notable strengths in its adoption of ethics and theories to apply in practice has remained its relative openness to new perspectives. Its epistemological and ontological openness includes a tendency to embrace eclectic and often contrasting paradigms. This established tradition is often based on a rationale that diverse perspectives, including an ethic of care or virtue ethics (see Chapter 7), offer more flexibility in attempts to understand an ever-changing and diverse world, alongside the many different settings in which social work is practised (Congress, 2010; Carey & Green, 2013; Baines, 2013). As we have seen, however, biomedicine as paradigm operates as a much more closed system of ideas which focuses more upon utilizing rigorous science to attain certainty and 'truth'.

Since the 1970s, bioethics has established itself as the dominant paradigm attached to medicine and healthcare, but increasingly, this paradigm is having an influence within social work. Among other attributes, bioethics tends to use essentialist Kantian principles alongside 'ready-to-use kits of moral principles' (Zielinska, 2015, pp. 270–273), which can be applied to a raft of complex moral issues or social needs. Questions have been raised about the suitability of this paradigm, including its limited capacity to support all forms of care and research (Carey & Green, 2013). The close ideological links between bioethics, neo-liberalism and marketization indicate that they are far from politically neutral constructs. For example, within bioethics, strong emphasis tends to be placed on the decision-making capacities of patients, their autonomy and choice, alongside the promotion of a special one-to-one relationship built between medic as knowledge-rich 'expert' and patient as 'customer'. This model, however, ignores key differences in power between professional and patient or user, such as according to them any competing knowledge and status, alongside any acknowledgement of material or cultural forms of inequality. Indeed, as Estes et al. (2003, pp. 94–96) surmise, it is as if the person as customer loses their soul in the eyes of the knowledge-rich expert:

> [Within bioethics] the focus on individual autonomy and the responsibilities of health practitioners effectively obscures the underlying dynamics – economic, symbolic and interpersonal – which perpetuate health inequalities [whilst] . . . wider circumferences of policy and power relations are not addressed as it is assumed that the application of general moral principles rather than the interactive dialogue and legitimising discourses that shape relationships are sufficient to aid professional judgement . . . Interactions [can subsequently] take on a Buberian . . . I-it quality, whereby the humanity of the other is not seen, except as a thing like material, subject to manipulation and control.

As we have seen, social work, within the spirit of logos, also privileges the decision-making, sense of reason and expert power-base of the professional, and its associated ethical frameworks are often mired in over-generalized universal themes or aspirations to instil ontological order into the apparently chaotic life of the 'othered' client. There is a focus upon Western belief systems within core ethical frameworks utilized and a discounting of culturally rich indigenous moral traditions and ethics (see, for example, Brown & Strega, 2005). However, in contrast to morally rigid bioethical stances, social work's relative epistemological and ontological openness may endorse greater practitioner discretions or support better understanding, including possibly to appreciate and act upon power disparities, inequalities and the importance of political context.

Conclusions

The social work profession continues to gain closer ties to healthcare and medicine, for example as part of health and social care integration policies pursued in the UK since the 1990s. Such policy-based reforms are neither politically benign nor exclusively concerned with the provision of more focused care. Instead they have strong ties to political processes, which include the greater role of the market in the provision of care alongside biomedicalization within wider society (Estes et al., 2003, pp. 94–96; Rose & AbiRached, 2013; Scull, 2015). Although many such reforms are quite recent, the ties of influence between biomedical science as dominant paradigm and social work have a much longer history. There is indeed much in common between the professions, including a tendency to prioritize expertise and knowledge, objectivity and, to varying degrees, science-based interventions.

Despite such and other ties, social work contains unique traits which distinguish it from bio-medical science. Among other examples, these include a tendency to integrate more theoretical and ethical paradigms, especially in its teaching and some elements of practice. Social work is also not a clinical profession, and most of its disparate activities tend to be community based and are less likely to be housed in institutional settings.

There is a real danger, however, that many of social work's more positive and unique traits remain under continued threat. Not uncommonly, biomedicalization can lead to discursive and paradigmatic colonization, professional subjugation and the further objectification or exclusion of service users and carers (Carey, 2009). Indeed, many such outcomes have been established within inter-professional community mental health settings for many years now (Scull, 2015; see Chapter 36). As a political process, the impregnation of biomedical science into any social work discourse and related paradigms may go on to further restrict or even suffocate creative practices within fields such as education, such as by limiting, discrediting or opposing qualitative or critical research and teaching. As the dominant paradigm attached to a master medical discourse, it is likely to continue to seek to determine and restrict roles within integrated fields of practice (Carey, 2016b). Consequently, social work faces a moral and political challenge in attempts to generate viable resistance strategies to such hegemonic control. This ongoing paradigm shift is perhaps now on a par with any longer-term corrosive impacts generated by neo-liberalism.

Further reading

Illich, I. (2010). *Limits to medicine: Medical nemesis – The expropriation of health* (4th ed.). London: Marion Boyars.
A classic radical yet essentially libertarian critique of the often counterproductive impact of medical power and interventions, including beyond the hospital or clinic.

Twigg, J. (2006). *The body in health and social care.* Basingstoke: Palgrave Macmillan.
A detailed and theoretically adept exploration of the complex relationship between medicine, health and social care alongside the often objectified or discounted bodies of patients and service users alike.

Shaw, I. (2016). *Social work science.* Chichester: Columbia University Press.
Although regrettably lacking explicit engagement with political economy, this well-written book offers a thorough and intelligent exploration of the ongoing ties between social work and science.

References

Age UK. (2014). *Care in crisis: What next for social care?* London: Age UK.
Baines, D. (2013). Resistance in and outside the workplace: Ethical practice and managerialism in the voluntary sector. In M. Carey & L. Green (Eds.), *Social work ethics: Complex dilemmas within applied social care* (pp. 227–245). Farnham: Ashgate.
Baines, D., & van de Broek, D. (2017). Coercive care: Control and coercion in the restructured care workplace. *British Journal of Social Work, 47*(1), 125–142.
Beddoe, L. (2013). Health social work: Professional identity and knowledge. *Qualitative Social Work, 12*(1), 24–40.
Bell, E. M. (1961). *The story of hospital almoners.* London: Faber.
Bissell, G. (2012). *Organisational behaviour for social work.* Bristol: Policy Press.
Brewer, C., & Lait, J. (1980). *Can social work survive?* London: Temple Smith.
Brown, J. (1997). Circular questioning: An Introductory guide. *Journal of Family Therapy. 18*(2), 109–114.
Brown, L., & Strega, S. (Eds.). (2005). *Research as resistance: Critical, indigenous and anti-oppressive approaches.* Toronto: Canadian Scholar's Press.
Buber, M. (1958). *I and thou.* New York: Scribner.
Bywaters, P. (1986). Social work and the medical profession: Arguments against unconditional collaboration. *British Journal of Social Work, 16*, 661–677.
Carey, M. (2009). Happy shopper? The problem with service user and carer participation. *British Journal of Social Work, 39*(1), 179–188.
Carey, M. (2013). *The social work dissertation – Using small-scale qualitative methodology* (2nd ed.). Maidenhead, Open University Press.
Carey, M. (2016a). Journey's end? From residual service to newer forms of pathology, risk aversion and abandonment in social work with older people. *Journal of Social Work, 16*(3), 344–361.
Carey, M. (2016b, 28 June). Biomedical nemesis? Critical deliberations with regards health and social care integration for social work with older people. *International Social Work,* Online First.
Carey, M., & Foster, V. (2011). Introducing deviant social work: Contextualizing the limits of radical social work whilst understanding (fragmented) resistance in the state social work labour process. *British Journal of Social Work, 41*(3), 576–593.
Carey, M., & Green, L. (Eds.). (2013). *Practical social work ethics: Complex dilemmas within applied social care.* Farnham: Ashgate.
Congress, E. (2010). Codes of ethics. In M. Gray & S. Webb (Eds.), *Ethics and value perspectives in social work.* Basingstoke: Palgrave Macmillan.
Cruikshank, B. (1999). *The will to empower: Democratic citizens and other subjects.* Ithaca, NY: Cornell University Press.

Delanty, G. (2005). *Social science* (2nd ed.). Milton Keynes: Open University Press.

D'Cruz, H., & Jones, M. (2004). *Social work research – Ethical and political contexts.* London: Sage.

Dustin, D. (2007). *The McDonaldization of social work.* Farnham: Ashgate.

Egan, M., Combs-Orme, T., & Neely-Barnes, S. L. (2011). Integrating neuroscience knowledge into social work education: A case-based approach. *Journal of Social Work Education*, 47(2), 269–282.

Estes, C. L., Biggs, S., & Phillipson, C. (2003). *Social theory, social policy and ageing: A critical introduction.* Maidenhead: Open University Press.

Estes, C. L., & Binney, E. (1989). The biomedicalisation of ageing: Dangers and dilemmas. *The Gerontologist*, 29(5), 587–598.

Estes, C. L., Kelly, S. E., & Binney, E. (1996). Bioethics in a disposable society: Healthcare and the intergenerational state. In J. W. Walters (Ed.), *Ethics and ageing* (pp. 95–119). Chicago: University of Illinois.

Ferguson, H. (2011). *Child protection practice.* Basingstoke: Palgrave Macmillan.

Foucault, M. (1992). *The use of pleasure: The history of sexuality* (vol. 2). London: Penguin.

Furedi, F. (2006). *Where have all the intellectuals gone?* (2nd ed.). London: Continuum.

Glynos, J., Speed, E., & West, K. (2014). Logics of marginalisation in health and social care reform: Integration, choice, and provider-blind provision. *Critical Social Policy*, 35(1), 45–68.

Goodley, D. (2013). Why critical disability studies? In C. A. Ogden & S. Wakeman (Eds.), *Corporeality: The body and society.* Chester: University of Chester Press.

Gray, A. M., & Birrell, D. (2013). *Transforming adult social care: Contemporary policy and practice.* Bristol: Policy Press.

Green, L. (2017). *Understanding the life course: Sociological and psychological perspectives.* (2nd ed.). Cambridge, MA: Polity.

Hodge, S. (2005). Participation, discourse and power: A case study. *Critical Social Policy*, 25(2), 164–179.

Hudson, B. (2002). Interprofessionality in health and social care: the Achilles' heel of partnership? *Journal of Interprofessional Care.* 16(1), 7–17.

Illich, I. (2010). *Limits to medicine: Medical nemesis – The expropriation of health* (4th ed.). London: Marion Boyars.

Jones, C. (1983). *State social work and the working class.* Basingstoke: Palgrave Macmillan.

Katz, S. (2010). Sociocultural perspectives on ageing bodies. In D. Dannefer, & C. Phillipson (Eds.), *The Sage handbook of social gerontology* (pp. 357–366). London: Sage.

Lilo, E. (2016). *Mental health integration: Past, present and future.* Liverpool: Health Education North West.

Lymbery, M. (2006). *Social work with older people.* London: Sage.

McKeown, T. (1976). *The role of medicine: Dream, mirage or nemesis?* Oxford: Blackwell.

Parton, N. (2014.). Social work, child protection and politics: Some critical and constructive reflections. *British Journal of Social Work*, 44(7), 2042–2056.

Phillipson, C. (2013). *Ageing.* Cambridge, UK: Polity Press.

Poxton, R. (1999). Primary and community mental health and social care: Making a difference at the interface. *The Mental Health Review*, 4, 24–27.

Rose, N., & AbiRached, J. M. (2013). *Neuro: The new brain sciences and the management of the mind.* Princeton, NJ: Princeton University Press.

Scull, A. (2015). *Madness in civilisation.* London: Thames and Hudson.

Seebohm Report. (1968). *Report of the committee on local authority and allied personal social services.* Cmnd 3703. London: HMSO.

Shaw, I. (2016). *Social work science.* Chichester: Columbia University Press.

Twigg, J. (2006). *The body in health and social care.* Basingstoke: Palgrave Macmillan.

Wastell, D., & White, S. (2012). Blinded by neuroscience: Social policy, the family and the infant brain. *Families, Relationships and Society*, 1(3), 397–414.

Webb, S. A. (2006). *Social work in a risk society.* Basingstoke: Palgrave Macmillan.

Webb, A., & Wistow, G. (1986). *Planning, need and scarcity: Essays on the personal social services.* London: Allen & Unwin.

Williams, Z. (2014, 26 April). Is misused neuroscience defining early years and child protection policy? *The Guardian.*

Witz, A. (1992). *Professions and patriarchy.* London: Routledge.

Wrennall, L. (2013). Where did we go wrong? An analysis of conflicts of interest, perverse financial incentives and NOMBism. In M. Carey & L. Green (Eds) *Practical social work ethics: Complex dilemmas within applied social care* (pp. 171–98). Abingdon: Routledge.

Younghusband, E. L. (1947). *Report on the education and training of social workers.* London: Constable.

Zielinska, A. C. (2015). Moral principles and ethics committees: A case against bioethical theories. *Ethics and Social Welfare*, 9(3), 269–279.

Part 2
Theory about social work values

7

Care and caring

Michael D. Fine

After decades, if not centuries, of neglect, the concepts of care and caring have become central to contemporary social thought. While essential for human existence, approaches to providing care change over time. As the core concepts signify activities, ideals and phenomena that are inherently value based, their meaning and character remain contested, making them difficult to define and analyze. It is, nonetheless, increasingly vital to understand their meaning and significance as terms and, even more importantly, as forms of action and as relationships.

In the late middle ages and early enlightenment, the word 'care' generally referred to worries and concerns, a sense still recognized as 'cares and woes'. By the 19th century, the concept was increasingly used to refer to a responsibility for containing or confinement, as in the phrase 'in the care of her majesty' (Fine, 2007a, pp. 23–39). Today, while the subtleties of its meaning and the ownership of the concept are often contested, the word is used in a much more positive and active sense.

Leaving aside their widespread popularity in marketing, where they are attached to everything from vehicle maintenance and beauty products to food preparation and real estate management, the terms 'care' and 'caring' are used in contemporary language to refer to closely related aspects of social behaviour. From this, it is possible to identify three core components of meaning.

First, care is a mental disposition (to care *about* someone) that involves a concern for the wellbeing of self and others. Second, it can refer to activities that are a form of work (to care *for* someone). This work involves both physical and emotional forms of labour concerned with providing nurturance, personal maintenance, assistance or support or involving the provision of attention. Competence is a key requirement if the activity is not to result in harm. Importantly, this work is often taken for granted, marginalized, undervalued or overlooked. Third, caring takes place within a relationship among specific individuals or groups: a caring relationship. While this is often an intimate or familial relationship, it may also be a professional or occupational relationship or extended beyond the interpersonal level to encompass a community, political entity or society (Rønning, 2002; Fine, 2007a; Rummery & Fine, 2012; Thelen, 2015).

Each of these three components may legitimately be considered on its own as a form of care. Yet, in the practice of care in the field of human service, we have come to expect that these aspects will be brought together, aligning in a holistic sense to the greatest degree possible.

Undertaking the work of providing personal support without a disposition to care about the person receiving care and in the absence of any relationship with the care recipient is often looked upon as a form of uncaring care (Ungerson, 2005).

Care is also more than each of these components. It is a value, an ideal and an ascribed responsibility or duty that is commonly subject to cultural and often legal enforcement as a 'duty of care'. The ideals of care may invoke feelings of warmth or of coldness, as Hochschild (1995) comments, and cover a range of distinct meanings and activities. Care may thus be understood by some as a term referring to traditional forms of maternal nurturance and to the treatment of people in large social institutions, while to others it invokes ideas of more contemporary clinical, professionalized, commercial or home-based types of service (Hochschild, 1995). Despite deeply held beliefs that responsibility for care belongs to a particular set of social actors, such as the family (Finch & Mason, 1990, 1993; Weicht, 2015), responsibility for providing care is also inherently fungible. How and when can different sources of care be substituted or brought together in some form of working harmony is an issue of central importance for social workers as well as policymakers and care advocates (Glucksmann, 2005; Ungerson & Yeandle, 2006; Fine, 2007b).

Care as a professional value

The 'caring professions', in particular nursing and social work, have sought to place care at the centre of their concerns. Nursing, according to Nelson, derives in many ways from Christianity and has historically been concerned with the pursuit of an ethic, 'a mode of conduct', which has been to live out the Christian command of love or *agape* (Nelson, 2000, p. 1). While the humanistic reformulation of the nursing profession that took place following the work of Florence Nightingale in the 19th century has masked an underlying continuity in nursing's approach to care, these continuities, she argues, are evident in contemporary nursing theory, with its emphasis on holistic care (Nelson, 2000).

Today, in social work as in nursing, care and caring are discussed both as core values and as specialized professional skills (Baines, Evans, & Neysmith, 1998). Care, in this sense, increasingly represents a key professional concept, a foundational component of attempts to lay claim to a unique body of knowledge and skills. For example, there are few if any of the many theories of nursing developed since the 1960s that do not attempt to outline at least some elements of a definition of care. This is often contrasted with the curative, interventionist, depersonalized approach taken by medicine. In the writings that emerged from the profession of nursing from the 1970s onwards, care was seen similarly in a focused and very gender-specific way (Watson, 1979; Benner, 1984; Leininger, 1988; Lawler, 1991). Nonetheless, recent changes in the understanding of care and the orientation of the profession are significant. In contrast to the personalized approach to care commonly advocated today, nurses and social workers trained before the 1970s report that they were warned during their training not to become 'too involved' with their patients or clients (Dunlop, 1994).

Within just a few years, however, the meaning of the professional value of care in nursing changed dramatically. In place of the depersonalized task-focused view that placed priority on the physical process of providing assistance, it has increasingly moved toward seeing care in psychosocial terms. Benner and Wrubel, for example, argue that caring is a way of being in the world. It even determines what a person finds stressful and how they can cope with stress.

Writing about the adoption of an ethic of care in social work, Lloyd (2006) similarly argues

> The arguments for an ethics of care have considerable potency and relevance for social
> work practice . . . a central point of the feminist ethics of care is to re-conceptualize care as

a fundamental aspect of all human experience and to reject the current perception that it is relevant only to the weak and needy 'other'. Williams (2001) takes up this point, arguing that social policies need to be developed that would enable us to prioritize opportunities to give and receive care.

(Lloyd, 2006, pp. 1182–1183)

Yet, as Twigg (2006) has sought to remind us, care cannot be conceptually confined to a matter of sentiment nor understood simply as an expression of moral disposition towards others, spirituality or religion. Care, in important ways, is also a particular form of work, one that both responds to the vulnerability of the body and in turn requires physical and emotional exertion for its performance. To understand how these elements have come to be in tension, it is necessary, I contend, to engage with several countervailing contemporary debates about care and caring which have emerged alongside and, in many ways, as a product of contemporary social movements, especially feminism and the disability movement, since the 1970s (see Chapters 31, 38 and 39).

The rise of feminist thinking about care and caring

Until recently, care remained a neglected concept in academic social research and in philosophical thought. The development of rich research and critical scholarship concerning care is closely linked to the rise of political activism for women to achieve full citizenship and be able to enter public life in equality with men. Their advocacy concerned the liberation of women, which included removing the shackles on women's roles, amongst which responsibility for providing care within the family was foremost (Beck-Gernsheim, 2002). Academic interest in care developed alongside and, in many ways, as a product of agitation by feminists from the mid-1970s. Initially most attention was focused on concerns about the unpaid work carried out by women within the family. As the political and broader social significance of what had earlier been seen as a domestic matter began to be explored, so care theory developed in scope, ambition and significance.

The starting point for the original feminist analysis of care was that of the social identity of the carer or, more broadly, the position of women in society (Thomas, 1993). Care, according to this perspective, was broadly defined as women's social role or duties, which were seen, critically, as focused on reproductive activities which confined females to the domestic sphere. These duties, which included 'caring for their children, their elderly or sick relatives and, of course, their husbands' according to Land (1978, p. 360), also extended to other forms of unpaid care such as care of older people and of children with disabilities (Finch & Groves, 1983). In this view, care came to be considered, in the title of Graham's deservedly famous book, as the 'labour of love' (Graham, 1983) provided at home, informally, by unpaid and recognized female relatives of the recipients, as caring was linked to female gender identity, the home and family.

An important finding of the empirical research that followed was that, although they remained a minority of all unpaid carers, a significant number of men also provided care at home (Arber, Gilbert, & Evandrou, 1988; Arber & Ginn, 1990; Pickard, Wittenberg, Comas-Herrera, Davies, & Darton, 2000; Pickard, 2013). Yet this finding serves to reinforce the focus on the 'burden of care' and the identification of those responsible for providing unpaid care as 'carers' and, in the US, 'caregivers', that has remained an enduring contribution of research derived from this approach. Studies in the UK, for example, documented the hours devoted to providing hands-on care, providing supervision, company and simply being available. The hidden 'costs of care', which included social isolation and psychological distress as well as lost earnings and careers (Nissel & Bonnerjea, 1982; Glendinning, 1989), also began to be documented. In the US, Brody's research on 'women in the middle', those who provided care in their middle years to both parents and children, extended this perspective (Brody, 1981). From this body of work grew a national and now international social movement to represent and support carers (Barnes, 2001; Marking, 2017).

As research on care extended to formal settings and new service initiatives in the home, it became increasingly clear that while care remained a gendered activity, it could not be understood as an activity confined to the family or informal sphere. Researchers such as Ungerson insisted that the concept of care includes formal services and policy interventions of various kinds as well as support provided in the domestic sphere and called for the abolition of the false dichotomy between formal and informal care, which had in any case become increasingly difficult to sustain. Like many others involved in research on care, Ungerson followed developments in policy such as the introduction of payments for caregiving (Ungerson, 1987, 1997, 2000) and the emergence of the 'social care mix'. These were the product of what British policymakers termed 'the mixed economy of welfare' that resulted from marketization and quasi-market reforms introduced in the UK from the 1990s (Baldock & Ungerson, 1996; Ungerson & Yeandle, 2006).

Receiving and transforming care

While debate on care over the past 40 years has increasingly sought to link informal and unpaid care with formal and paid care, rather than distinguish these forms from each other, an enduring feature of the debate on care to this point had been its focus on giving, rather than receiving, care. The experience of receiving care and its impact on the personal identity of the care recipients or dependents had been relatively neglected. Researchers who focused on this aspect of care systems, such as Parker (1981), focused on the poor quality of formal care services. Parker argued that the way publicly funded facilities operated meant that the assistance available to frail older adults, children with learning disabilities, chronically ill people or children in child care failed and needed to be rethought. In place of care and caring, he argued, what was provided was an impersonal 'tending', as in the word 'care attendant'. The physical work of providing support was prioritized but the interpersonal aspects neglected.

In focusing on the receipt of care, the objective of those who shared this perspective was to formulate appropriate social policies for the support of those reliant on such assistance. Disability advocates also sought to change the system of services and entitlement, seeking even more fundamental changes that would overthrow the still-patronizing way that care was conceptualized. Keith (1992) and Morris (1993), who each experienced disability, argued that like existing services, the new feminist conceptions of care which sought to highlight the sacrifice undertaken by women assumed the passive dependency of recipients. Drawing on principles articulated as part of the 'social model of disability' (Oliver & Barnes, 1998; see Chapters 36, and 28–40) as well as those of feminism, Morris argues that the problems with the then-prevailing feminist conceptions of care can be traced to a failure to examine the factors which underlie the need for assistance in the first place.

> By taking the need for care for granted and by assuming the dependency of older and disabled people, feminist research and carers as a pressure group have not only failed to address the interests of older and disabled people but they have, unwittingly, colluded with both the creation of dependency and the state's reluctance to tackle the social and economic factors which disable people.
>
> *(Morris, 1993, p. 49)*

Care, they pointed out, was portrayed as a one-way process in which concern for recipients was based on pity and assumptions of incompetence. Concern for carers, in turn, led to the recipients of assistance being portrayed as nothing more than a burden, a problem to be managed. In seeking to lift the cloak of invisibility from women carers, feminists claimed to have emancipatory ideals. Disability activists, in response, sought to employ a similar strategy, calling for recognition and empowerment of the recipients of care. Other writers from a disability perspective were even harsher. Oliver and Barnes (1998, p. 8), for example, argued that the discovery of the 'carer' had not helped disabled people gain their independence nor freed family members from responsibility for caring.

Dependency, help and interdependency

The social model of disability makes a conceptual distinction between impairment (a bodily deficit) and disability (a socially constructed limitation) in a manner similar to the feminist distinction between sex and gender. Disability and the need for care are seen as social constructions produced by the social and economic structures and culture of capitalist society (Lloyd, 2001; Corker & Shakespeare, 2002). Importantly, this suggests useful ways in which the need for care can be reduced: for example, by appropriate use of technology and the principles of good design and by making buildings wheelchair accessible, removing the need for a wheelchair user to rely on carers to provide access. Other social causes, such as discrimination in employment, need to be removed through legislation or similar provision. Providing those reliant on assistance with access to their own resources might also enable them to take charge of the labour required for their ongoing care rather than remaining dependent on those who provide it.

While more radical solutions for dealing with social causes of dependency and exclusion can also be imagined, Shakespeare (2000a, 2000b) sought to articulate what might be considered a more conciliatory position. Instead of assuming relations of care based on an active caregiver and a dependent recipient, it is necessary to acknowledge the significance of 'interdependence'. Drawing on a well-established line of thinking in social work (Keith-Lucas, 1972; Jordan, 1979), what was required, suggested Shakespeare, was a simpler solution based on help.

A different voice: the values of care as an ethical virtue

Interdependence is also a core theme in a second feminist approach to care and caring that developed from the field of moral philosophy. In place of seeing care as a burden, it began by portraying it as a necessity and a virtue. The ethics of the care debate developed initially as an unanticipated by-product of the work of the psychologist Gilligan (1982) on the moral development of children. Undertaking research with the cognitive developmental psychologist Lawrence Kohlberg, Gilligan noted that girls typically seemed more concerned with preserving relationships and scored less well than boys of the same age on Kohlberg's moral development scale, which measured the emergence of a moral orientation towards justice. Gilligan undertook her own study amongst a group of women to explore these insights. Their responses suggested that many of the young women emphasized the responsibility they felt to maintain and strengthen personal ties between people, rather than seeking to impose the impersonal and abstract legalistic principles of justice. She termed this concern for sustaining personal relationships an 'ethic of care', noting that

> ... the logic of an ethic of care is a psychological logic of relationships ... The ideal of care is thus an activity of relationships, of seeing and responding to need, taking care of the world by sustaining the web of connection so that no one is left alone.
>
> *(Gilligan, 1982, p. 73)*

While Gilligan appears to have had doubts about whether an ethic of care was exclusively feminine and simply different from, or even equivalent to, an ethic of justice, Noddings (1984) and a number of others expressed no such doubt. At the time, many feminists had also argued that advancement for women required freeing women from domestic duties, replacing the burden of responsibility for domestic care with opportunities for employment and participation in public life outside the home. Noddings argued that the achievement of social, economic and political recognition by women should not mean abandoning the ideals of care, but its opposite, embracing the ethic of care as a public virtue. By seeking acknowledgement and greater recognition of the significance of care and caring activities, the goal was not to become honorary men but to transform the public sector to become more caring.

Following the early work of Gilligan and Noddings, other feminists sought to develop the approach. Tronto (1993), for example, proposed the following definition:

> On the most general level, we suggest caring be viewed as a species activity that includes everything that we do to maintain, continue and repair our 'world' so that we can live in it as well as possible. That world includes our bodies, ourselves, and our environment, all of which we seek to interweave in a complex, life-sustaining web.
>
> *(Tronto, 1993, p. 103)*

Tronto's definition sought to universalize the concept of caring, extending it beyond personal support and intimate relationships. It was ambitious and bold, staking a claim that extended the concept of care into almost all aspects of human existence and perhaps much beyond that. The ideal was posited as a counter to the ideal of the autonomous, independent, calculating rational man that is central to liberal political and economic theory. Her intention in this and in more recent work (Tronto, 2013, 2017) has been to understand the political as well as ethical dimensions of the concept. Tronto thus argues for care to be acknowledged as a social virtue which stands in contrast to the ideal of self-interest. The 'life-sustaining web' she invokes is neither an excessive reliance on others for our maintenance nor excessive self-reliance but suggests an alternative to the dichotomy of either wholesale dependency or extreme autonomy.

Building on this, the Dutch political philosopher Sevenhuijsen (1993) and other European care researchers, sought to acknowledge the ethics of care alongside a care as part of more politicized model of citizenship rights in a way that would recognize the *receiving* as well as *giving* care. In the Netherlands, Knijn and Kremer (1997) formulated this as a right to receive care, a right to give care and the right to be able to care for ourselves. This was amplified by Williams (2001), who pointed to the emergence of a new political discourse based on concerns for work/life balance, in which women (and men) needed to find ways to combine the pursuit of careers and employment with opportunities to provide care. The approach also sought to break down the sense of care as a one-directional relationship in which an active caregiver provides assistance to a dependent and passive recipient. Their argument seeks to recognize the reciprocal and embodied character of care. Caring relationships are often complex, reciprocal and mutually supportive rather than simple binary relationships between an active carer and a passive and dependent care recipient (Morris, 2001; Fine & Glendinning, 2005). While subsequent research on care has placed greater emphasis on the agency and recognition of the care recipient (Lloyd, 2000, 2004; Rostgaard, 2006; Yeatman, Dowsett, Fine, & Guransky, 2009; Needham, 2011), there remains considerable scope for developments that will help assist with the development of deeper analyses of the political, economic and relational aspects of care.

Dependency and care

In a powerful and comprehensive review of care ethics, Collins (2015, p. 169, cited in Tronto, 2017, p. 37) argues that the central proposition of the ethics of care approach is that 'dependency relationships generate duties' (see Chapter 8, and Chapter 40 on older people). This insight owes much to the work of philosophers such as Martha Fineman and Eva Fedor Kittay. Each saw dependency as at times an arbitrary and pernicious social construction, such as when applied to the social condition of women, and at others as a fundamental and unavoidable aspect of the human life course, a condition encountered in frail old age and disability as well as in early childhood and at times of illness. When grounded in the biology of the body, these conditions are what Fineman (1995, 2002, pp. 161–164) called the 'inevitable dependencies' of the human life course. But dependency is also socially produced within the family and outside as those responsible for caregiving are in turn made dependent on a third party whom Kittay (1999, p. 27) terms 'the provider', by their commitment to provide care. Political, economic, cultural and moral conditions in different societies and at different points in history need to be identified as responsible for the social response to bodily dependencies (Kittay, 1999).

Kittay's analysis of care places dependency and considerations of power that arise from the relationship between caregivers and recipients at the centre of the analysis (Kittay, 1999, pp. 30–40). She identifies a paradigm form of care as 'dependency work', which she uses as an analytic device to explore its complexities. In the paradigm case, the well-being of the 'charge' or recipient is the responsibility and primary focus of the dependency worker. The vulnerability of care recipients, she notes, arise from their lack of physical or mental capacity. Care workers are also vulnerable. This arises not just from their economic and social dependency on others, but from their readiness to assist the charge, their identification with the well-being of the charge and by their inability to express annoyance or vent frustrations in interacting with the charge in ways that would normally be acceptable in human relationships between equals (Kittay, 1999; Fine, 2005). The recipient of care may thus, in certain cases, exert a 'certain tyranny' by advancing false needs, making exaggerated demands on the worker, or 'exploiting the worker's concern and need for the connection forged through the relationship'. Kittay notes how a care recipient may 'graft the substance of another to one's own', failing to recognize the integrity of the one who undertakes the work on their behalf. The special vulnerability of the caregiver, in this view, arises as a result of the ties formed through the recipient's dependence on them, through which they experience their substance grafted onto the other. In such a case, the caregiver has effectively become overidentified with the charge and is unable to assert an independent sense of self.

Drawing together Rawls' (1971, 1982) concepts of social citizenship and the work of Sen (1997) concerning human capabilities, Kittay argues that if we lack the capability to care for ourselves and therefore need support, we should be able to receive it without those who provide the assistance being penalized. Rather than presuming that everyone has the capacity for autonomy, a recognition of the inevitability of dependence at some stage of each of our lives, and of the need for care of those who are dependent, must involve an acknowledgement of human interdependencies. Such a concept is not an assertion of interdependency as an alternative or negation of dependency, but rather one based on the recognition of 'nested dependencies' which link those who need support with those who help them and, in turn, link the helpers to a set of broader supports.

> Just as we required care to survive and thrive, so we need to provide conditions that allow others – including those who do the work of caring – to receive the care they need to survive and thrive.
>
> *(Kittay, 1999, p. 133)*

By understanding the goal of care as the nurturing and development of the charge's capabilities by the dependency worker, Kittay shows how a recognition of the complex nature and character of power is essential to understand the dynamics of interpersonal interaction between carer and recipient and the injustice of the exploitation and dependency experienced by carers and – she is quite explicit on this point–by women more generally.

Care, for so long regarded as a private matter, an unseen exchange that occurred within the intimacy of the domestic sphere, is clearly now a global and corporate concern. With the rise of ageing populations, the increasing prevalence of disability and the increased reliance on formalized child care arrangements to support working mothers, it is increasingly important that what Kittay, Jennings, and Wasunna (2005, p. 443) have called 'a global ethic of long term care' be recognized (see also Deacon, 2007; Fine, 2007a). The movement of low-paid care workers from the third world to advanced wealthy countries (Ehrenreich & Hochschild, 2002), as much as the persistent inequalities within care relationships, are issues of vital concern for health sociologists, as they are for others concerned with issues of global equity. The recognition of the vital importance of care for human life as a response to dependency, which she has come to call 'the elephant in the room' (Kittay et al., 2005), provides Kittay with a rationale for public policy supporting care and, through it, the individuals who take responsibility by caring.

Conclusion

The rapid explosion of the rich body of theory and research on the topic of care and caring which this entry has sought to outline is indicative of the vitality and enduring importance of the field. Looking back over the past 40 years of theory and accompanying research, what is perhaps most striking is the ambition of those working in the field to establish the fundamental importance of the topic, the diversity of theory that has arisen as a result and the still unsettled, incomplete and conflicting range of positions that have been given voice over that time. There is a record of the achievement in a number of countries of gaining at least some level of recognition for the work of family carers and, in policy terms, of developing responses to the problems they experience (Yeandle, Kröger, & Cass, 2012). An impressive and continually extending body of empirical research has been undertaken and has led to the growth of a number of specialist journals, including the *International Journal on Care and Caring* (Yeandle, Chou, Fine, Larkin, & Milne, 2017). However, attempts to develop a unified theory of care that has widespread acceptance beyond those who share the position of the proponents remain at best elusive.

A common theme amongst contributors to the theoretical discussions has been a recognition of the significance of care and caring as essential preconditions for every individual's existence and as a fundamental pillar of social life. Alongside this, a clear acknowledgement of the feminist origins and inspiration for much of this work has been the recognition of the importance of gender in allocating responsibility for care in both the family and in public domains and the generally devalued position of those responsible for providing care. Yet tensions remain, reflecting not just the frustrations of a still-incomplete political project, but real differences in outlook amongst the different contending schools of thought. A key question lying at the heart of this is whether it is sufficient to understand the degraded position of care as arising from its association with women or the inverse, as Kittay (1999) has argued, that women have suffered because it is they who have taken responsibility for the provision of care.

A second urgent set of challenges that confront those who theorize about care arises from the economic, market and political pressures encountered in the 21st century. What are the implications for care of marketization and ongoing managerial restructuring of formal services and public initiatives? Can settings in which profit maximization is the key incentive provide conditions under which care can flourish? Addressing the issues surrounding these sorts of questions requires going beyond simple managerial assertions of the importance of the market for choice and quality of care provisions (Bode, 2007; Williams, 2009). What they reveal is the unavoidably political character of questions surrounding care and caring and the need for social workers and others from the caring professions, as well as researchers, citizens, consumers and policymakers, to confront the issues of power, need and inequality that lie at the heart of issues of care.

A third core challenge for theory is recognizing and reconciling the need to receive care and the need to give care. While much care theory has been concerned with the giving of care, far less has focused on its receipt (Saraceno, 2008; Yeatman et al., 2009; Tronto, 2017). Certainly a body of research has pointed to the significance of individual consumers and the importance of addressing this gulf, particularly in response to the move toward increasing individualization and personalization of care (Fyson, 2009; Needham, 2011; Fine, 2013). The understanding of care that the new approaches invite and elicit differs in important and, at times, radical ways from that initially advanced in the feminist debate on care. It is one that must be built on an acknowledgement of the individualization of high modernity and the reconfiguration of risk. These points are eloquently set out by Morris:

> We need to challenge the social construction of dependency, but we should not at the same time deny the experience of our bodies and the consequences for the provision of assistance. Vulnerability is created by one person having a greater need for physical assistance than the person who is in a position to provide it and by the nature of the assistance required. This is why a focus on human rights is so important in our challenge to the meaning of care . . .
>
> Whatever 'care' is – whether it is in the form of formal services, cash payments, or personal relationships – if it does not enable people to 'state an opinion', to 'participate in decisions which affect their lives' and to 'share fully in the social life of the community', then it will be unethical. . . . We need an ethics of care which, while starting from the position that everyone has the same human rights, also recognizes the additional requirements that some people have in order to access those human rights.
>
> *(Morris, 2001, pp. 14–15)*

Such an approach to care, based firmly on ideals of care as a human right, provides a clear direction for the caring professions as well as for others concerned with ethical choices for the future.

Further reading

Lloyd, L. (2006). A caring profession? The ethics of care and social work with older people. *British Journal of Social Work, 36*(7), 1171–1185.

Rummery, K., & Fine, M. (2012). Care: A critical review of theory, policy and practice. *Social Policy & Administration, 46*(3), 321–343.

Tronto, J. (2017). There is an alternative: Homo curans and the limits of neoliberalism. *International Journal of Care and Caring, 1*(1), 27–44

References

Arber, S., Gilbert, N., & Evandrou, M. (1988). Gender, household composition and receipt of domiciliary services by the elderly disabled. *Journal of Social Policy, 17*(2), 153–176.

Arber, S., & Ginn, J. (1990). The meaning of informal care: Gender and the contribution of elderly people. *Ageing & Society, 10*(4), 429–454.

Baines, C. T., Evans, P. M., & Neysmith, S. M. (Eds.). (1998). *Women's caring: Feminist perspectives on social welfare* (2nd ed.). Toronto: Oxford University Press.

Baldock, J., & Ungerson, C. (1996). Money, care and consumption: Families in the new mixed economy of social care. In H. Jones & J. Millar (Eds.), *The politics of the family* (pp. 167–187). Aldershot: Avebury.

Barnes, M. (2001). From private carer to public actor: The carers movement in England. In M. Daly (Ed.), *Care work: The quest for security* (pp. 195–210). Geneva: International Labour Office (ILO).

Beck-Gernsheim, E. (2002). From "living for others" to "a life of one's own": Individualization and women. In U. Beck & E. Beck-Gernsheim (Eds.), *Individualization* (pp. 54–84, original pub. in German 1983). London: Sage.

Benner, P. (1984). *From novice to expert: Excellence and power in clinical nursing.* Menlo Park, CA: Addison-Wesley.

Bode, I. (2007). New moral economies of welfare: The case of domiciliary elder care in Germany, France and Britain. *European Societies, 9*(2), 201–227.

Brody, E. (1981). Women in the middle and family help to older people. *Gerontologist, 26,* 373–381.

Collins, S. (2015). *The core of care ethics.* Basingstoke: Palgrave Macmillan.

Corker, M., & Shakespeare, T. (2002). Mapping the terrain. In M. Corker & T. Shakespeare (Eds.), *Disability/postmodernity: Embodying disability theory* (pp. 1–17). London: Continuum.

Deacon, A. (2007). Civic labour or doulia? Care, reciprocity and welfare. *Social Policy and Society, 6,* 481–490.

Dunlop, M. J. (1994). Is a science of caring possible? In P. Benner (Ed.), *Interpretive phenomenology: Embodiement, caring, and ethics in health and illness* (pp. 27–42). Thousand Oaks, CA: Sage.

Ehrenreich, B., & Hochschild, A. (Eds.). (2002). *Global women: Nannies, maids and sex workers in the new economy.* New York: Metropolitan.

Finch, J., & Groves, D. (Eds.). (1983). *A labour of love: Women, work, and caring.* London: Routledge & Kegan Paul.

Finch, J., & Mason, J. (1990). Filial obligations and kin support for elderly people. *Ageing and Society, 10,* 151–175.

Finch, J., & Mason, J. (1993). *Negotiating family responsibilities.* London: Routledge.

Fine, M. D. (2005). Dependency work: A critical exploration of Kittay's perspective on care as a relationship of power. *Health Sociology Review, 14*(2), 146–160.

Fine, M. D. (2007a). *A caring society? Care and the dilemmas of human service in the 21st century.* Basingstoke: Palgrave Macmillan.

Fine, M. D. (2007b). The social division of care. *Australian Journal of Social Issues, 42*(2), 137–149.

Fine, M. D. (2013). Individualising care: The transformation of personal support in old age. *Ageing and Society, 33*(3), 421–436.

Fine, M., & Glendinning, C. (2005). Dependence, independence or inter-dependence? Revisiting the concepts of 'care' and 'dependency'. *Ageing and Society, 25*(4), 601–621.

Fineman, M. A. (1995). *The neutered mother, the sexual family and other twentieth century tragedies.* New York: Routledge.

Fineman, M. A. (2002). Masking dependency: The political role of family rhetoric. In E. F. Kittay & E. K. Feder (Eds.), *The subject of care: Feminist perspectives on dependency.* Lantham, MD: Rowman and Littlefield.

Fyson, R. (2009). Co-production and personalisation in social care: Changing relationships in the provision of social care. *Critical Social Policy, 29*(4), 727–729.

Gilligan, C. (1982). *In a different voice.* Cambridge, MA: Harvard University Press.

Glendinning, C. (1989). *The costs of informal care: Looking inside the household.* London: HMSO.

Glucksmann, M. (2005). Shifting boundaries and interconnections: Extending the 'total social organisation of labour'. *Sociological Review, 53,* 19–36.

Graham, H. (1983). Caring: A labour of love. In J. Finch & D. Groves (Eds.), *A labour of love: Women, work and caring.* London: Routledge and Kegan Paul.

Hochschild, A. R. (1995). The culture of politics: Traditional, postmodern, cold-modern and warm-modern ideals of care. *Social Politics, 2*(3), 331–346.

Jordan, B. (1979). *Helping in social work.* London: Routledge and Kegan Paul.

Keith, L. (1992). Who cares wins? Women, caring and disability. *Disability and Society, 7*(2), 167–175.

Keith-Lucas, A. (1972). *Giving and taking help.* Chapel Hill: University of North Carolina Press.

Kittay, E. F. (1999). *Love's labor: Essays on women, equality, and dependency.* New York: Routledge.

Kittay, E. F., Jennings, B., & Wasunna, A. A. (2005). Dependency, difference and the global ethic of longterm care. *Journal of Political Philosophy, 13*(4), 443–469.

Knijn, T., & Kremer, M. (1997). Gender and the caring dimension of welfare states: Toward inclusive citizenship. *Social Politics, 4*(Fall), 328–361.

Land, H. (1978). Who cares for the family? *Journal of Social Policy*, *3*(7), 357–384.

Lawler, J. (1991). *Behind the scenes: Nursing, somology and the problem of the body.* Melbourne: Churchill Livingstone.

Leininger, M. M. (Ed.). (1988). *Care: The essence of nursing and health.* Detroit: Wayne State University Press.

Lloyd, L. (2000). Caring about carers: Only half the picture? *Critical Social Policy*, *20*(1), 136–150.

Lloyd, L. (2004). Mortality and morality: Ageing and the ethics of care. *Ageing & Society*, *24*(2), 235–256.

Lloyd, L. (2006). A caring profession? The ethics of care and social work with older people. *British Journal of Social Work*, *36*(7), 1171–1185.

Lloyd, M. (2001). The politics of disability and feminism: Discord or synthesis? *Sociology*, *35*(3), 715–728.

Marking, C. (2017). Enabling carers to care: Making the case for a European Union action plan on carers. *International Journal of Care and Caring*, *1*(2), 289–292.

Morris, J. (1993). *Independent lives? Community care and disabled people.* London: Palgrave Macmillan.

Morris, J. (2001). Impairment and disability: Constructing an ethics of care that promotes human rights. *Hypatia*, *16*(4), 1–16.

Needham, C. (2011). *Personalising public services: Understanding the personalisation narrative.* Bristol: Policy Press.

Nelson, S. (2000). *A genealogy of care of the sick: Nursing, holism and pious practice.* Southsea: Nursing Praxis Press.

Nissel, M., & Bonnerjea, L. (1982). *Family care of the handicapped elderly: Who pays?* London: Policy Studies Institute.

Noddings, N. (1984). *Caring: A feminist approach to ethics and moral education.* Berkeley: University of California Press.

Oliver, M., & Barnes, C. (1998). *Disabled people and social policy: From exclusion to inclusion.* London: Longman.

Parker, R. (1981). Tending and social policy. In E. M. Goldberg & S. Hatch (Eds.), *A new look at the personal social services.* London: Policy Studies Institute.

Pickard, L. (2013). A growing care gap? The supply of unpaid care for older people by their adult children in England to 2032. *Ageing & Society, FirstView*, 1–28. doi:10.1017/S0144686X13000512

Pickard, L., Wittenberg, R., Comas-Herrera, A., Davies, B., & Darton, R. (2000). Relying on informal care in the new century? Informal care for elderly people in England to 2031. *Ageing & Society*, *20*(6), 745–772.

Rawls, J. (1971). *A theory of justice.* Cambridge, MA: Harvard University Press.

Rawls, J. (1982). Justice as fairness. *Philosophy and Public Affairs*, *14*, 227–251.

Rønning, R. (2002). In defence of care: The importance of care as a positive concept. *Quality in Ageing – Policy, Practice and Research*, *3*(4), 34–43.

Rostgaard, T. (2006). Constructing the care consumer: Free choice of home care for the elderly in Denmark. *European Societies*, *8*(3), 443–463.

Rummery, K., & Fine, M. (2012). Care: A critical review of theory, policy and practice. *Social Policy & Administration*, *46*(3), 321–343. doi:10.1111/j.1467-9515.2012.00845.x

Saraceno, C. (2008). "Care" giving and "Care" receiving between individualization and re-familization. *Berliner Journal Für Soziologie*, *18*(2), 244–256.

Sen, A. K. (1997). *Choice, welfare and measurement.* Cambridge, MA: Harvard University Press.

Sevenhuijsen, S. (1993). Paradoxes of gender: Ethical and epistemological perspectives on care in feminist political theory. *Acta Politica*, *28*(2), 131–149.

Shakespeare, T. (2000a). *Help.* Birmingham: Venture Press.

Shakespeare, T. (2000b). The social relations of care. In G. Lewis, S. Gewiriz, & J. Clarke (Eds.), *Rethinking social policy* (pp. 52–65). London: Sage.

Thelen, T. (2015). Care as social organization: Creating, maintaining and dissolving significant relations. *Anthropological Theory*, *15*(4), 497–515.

Thomas, C. (1993). De-constructing concepts of care. *Sociology*, *27*(4), 649–670.

Tronto, J. (1993). *Moral boundaries: A political argument for an ethic of care.* London: Routledge.

Tronto, J. (2013). *Caring democracy: Markets, equality, and justice.* New York: New York University Press.

Tronto, J. (2017). There is an alternative: Homo curans and the limits of neoliberalism. *International Journal of Care and Caring*, *1*(1), 27–44.

Twigg, J. (2006). *The body in health and social care.* Basingstoke: Palgrave Macmillan.

Ungerson, C. (1987). *Policy is personal.* London: Tavistock.

Ungerson, C. (1997). Payment for caring – Mapping a territory. In C. Ungerson & M. Kember (Eds.), *Women and social policy: A reader* (2nd ed., pp. 369–379). Basingstoke: Palgrave Macmillan.

Ungerson, C. (2000). Thinking about the production and consumption of long-term care in Britain: Does gender still matter? *Journal of Social Policy*, *29*(4), 623–643.

Michael D. Fine

Ungerson, C. (2005). Care, work and feeling. *Sociological Review, 53*, 188–203.

Ungerson, C., & Yeandle, S. (Eds.). (2006). *Cash for care in developed welfare states*. Basingstoke: Palgrave Macmillan.

Watson, J. (1979). *Nursing: The philosophy and science of caring*. Boston, MA: Little, Brown & Co.

Weicht, B. (2015). *The meaning of care: The social construction of care for elderly people*. London: Palgrave Macmillan.

Williams, F. (2001). In and beyond new labour: Towards a new political ethics of care. *Critical Social Policy, 21*(4), 467–493.

Williams, F. (2009). *Claiming and framing in the making of care polices: The recognition and the redistribution of care*. Geneva. Retrieved from www.unrisd.org/unrisd/website/document.nsf/d2a23ad2d50cb2a280256 eb300385855/f0924ad817fe8620c125780f004e9bcd/$FILE/Williams.pdf

Yeandle, S., Chou, Y-C., Fine, M., Larkin, M., & Milne, A. (2017). Care and caring: Interdisciplinary perspectives on a societal issue of global significance. *International Journal of Care and Caring, 1*(1), 3–25. doi:10.1332/239788217X14866278171183

Yeandle, S., Kröger, T., & Cass, B. (2012). Voice and choice for users and carers? Developments in patterns of care for older people in Australia, England and Finland. *Journal of European Social Policy, 22*(4), 432–445.

Yeatman, A., Dowsett, G., Fine, M., & Guransky, D. (2009). *Individualization and the delivery of welfare services: Contestation and complexity*. Basingstoke: Palgrave Macmillan.

8

Autonomy and dependence

Tom Grimwood

What is autonomy?

The concept of autonomy, in the context of social work values, is constructed from several inter-linking aspects. Politically, to exercise autonomy is to claim authority over one's own actions; it is a right to self-determination and self-governance, rooted in the Greek *autos* (self) and *nomos* (laws). Physically, to exercise autonomy is the freedom to initiate one's own actions; an independence from the constraints or supports of others. Morally, autonomy is crucial to the capacity not only to act according to one's own reasoning and not under external influence, but also, in the Kantian tradition of moral philosophy, to follow rational, universal moral laws. Across all three, the key point is that autonomy does not simply describe particular actions, behaviours or choices made but rather a particular way in which the authority to act, behave and choose is exercised.

In some definitions (see Dworkin, 1989), autonomy is defined as 'self-rule', meaning the *independence of choice*, free from the manipulation of others, and the *capacity*, physically and mentally, *to rule oneself*. However, while all three of these aspects link autonomy with independence, autonomy and dependence are not diametric opposites. Technically, the opposite of autonomy is heteronomy (subjection to another), whereas the opposite of dependence is independence (which refers to a relationship of need). Arguably, the ambiguity over both these terms frequently blurs these differences in both social work practice and theory. How important or significant this blurring might be depends upon the context in which autonomy and dependence are invoked. The British Association of Social Workers (BASW) Code of Ethics, for example, situates the value of autonomy in terms of its relation to the service user:

> Social workers should support people to reach informed decisions about their lives and promote their autonomy and independence, provided this does not conflict with their safety or with the rights of others.
>
> *(BASW, 2012, p. 12)*

By running autonomy and independence together, this statement in fact utilizes two different concepts: positive freedom, the right to nurture and grow self-determination, and negative freedom, independence within the limits of encroaching on others' self-determination. While, as part of a code of ethics, the statement intends to be broad in scope, there is something instructive about the way in which 'informed decisions', 'autonomy', 'independence' and 'safety' are merged together, a merger which is reflected in some of the tensions which social work theory has long encountered when articulating the meaning of autonomy to practitioners. In contrast, the (American) National Association of Social Workers' Code of Ethics highlights 'self-determination', but does not reference autonomy. See www.socialworkers.org/pubs/code/code.asp.

Implicit in the BASW statement is a further use of autonomy, which reflects the social worker's ability to act on such values in the first place. Indeed, the importance of autonomy as a social work value emerges from the professional status of the role. For example, in Robison and Reeser's *Ethical Decision-Making and Social Work* (2000), autonomy appears as a kind of brokering skill between the social worker's duties to an employer (the state, the agency, etc.) and the duties to the service user, which may conflict in ways more pronounced than in other health professions (Carpenter, Schneider, Brandon, & Wooff, 2003). For Parrott, more generally 'professional autonomy remains important [. . .] as social workers have to apply and interpret policy in relation to individual cases' (2014, p. 46). In this context, it is perhaps no surprise that autonomy often figures in social work literature in discussions of supervision; both Munro (2011) and the Social Work Reform Board (2012) in the UK looked to professional supervision to protect the reflective space necessary for practitioners to assess their 'critical consciousness' (Bransford, 2011). This consciousness is built upon the fact that social work's origins have meant that practice is always dependent upon higher authorities for its resources (Dominelli, 1997), whether these were Victorian philanthropists, the state, or – increasingly so – the consumer market. Thus, the autonomy of decision-making is required, as well as enabled, by a range of dependencies.

In contrast, other views of autonomy explicitly challenge the association of autonomy with independence. Jordan, for example, argues that social work should not simply defend a service user's 'negative liberty', but should instead be based on the value of emancipation, which translates as 'increasing autonomy and opportunity'. But he clarifies:

> I take autonomy to include choice, and acknowledge that the choices most important for most agents in the present-day world are made in markets [. . .]. However, the notion of emancipation also includes collective action [. . .] and has no associations of rational egoism or possessive individualism.
>
> *(Jordan, 2004, p. 6)*

In this case, achieving the benefits of autonomy may well involve dependence on other people, groups or structures, in which case, treating autonomy and independence as similar would risk being short-sighted (see MacKenzie, 2014). Regardless, Jordan notes that this alignment of autonomy and dependence produces an irony for social work as an emancipatory project in the 21st century:

> In local authorities and other statutory agencies it is charged with motivating and cajoling [. . .] service users towards projects of autonomy and self-development, while controlling the deviant and destructive aspects of resistance strategies (crime, drugs, benefit fraud, self-harm, mental illness). It becomes both more demanding ('tough love'), more controlling, and more coercive. It focuses on the assessment of resources and risks, despite the rhetoric of empowerment and inclusion. It also, in the process, becomes more impersonal, arm's length and office-bound.
>
> *(Jordan, 2004, p. 10)*

This irony is important, as this quotation encapsulates the different levels at which particular tensions between autonomy and dependence emerge for social work today: a micro level around the autonomy of the service user (their rights as individuals, legally, socially and morally); a meso-level concerning the autonomy of the social worker in the field (the role of autonomy in the values, ethics and decision-making of practice, as well as the organizational and structural autonomy of the social worker's practice, which facilitates and mediates these); and a macro level regarding the autonomy of social work as a profession, embedded within society as a whole (see Chapter 27).

The reality is, alas, far less tidy than these three tiers initially suggest. In part, this is because autonomy often emerges as a presupposition of, rather than a theory within, social work practice. As such, the technical specificity of the concept itself can be difficult to articulate distinctly from the concepts it is so frequently aligned with, such as independence, freedom and determination. Furthermore, this specificity is frequently obscured in much of the current and past social work literature, which is enthusiastic to reference autonomy but reluctant to embed it within a clear *theoretical* context. For example, the narrative of increased managerialism and neoliberal marketization leading to a loss of professional autonomy is by now well established (Lavalette, 2011), and suggestions that moving away from state-controlled social work provides 'more autonomy' as a benefit (see, for example, Preece, 2012) can be carried without question. Or a different example: in their critique of the discourse of 'well-being' as a measure of service user need in contemporary English social work, Simpson and Murr argue that this 'continues to include autonomy and self-determination'; but that 'this is focused primarily upon the *narrower* concepts of independence and choice' (Simpson & Murr, 2014, p. 891, my emphasis). But if we find autonomy referenced alongside independence, self-determination, self-esteem, professional integrity, freedom of choice and so on, then what differentiates autonomy from these things in a social work context? If it's something broader than independence and choice, what then renders it specific enough to be still meaningful in practice?

The tensions that these questions raise require careful thinking through, if the use of the concept of autonomy is not to become, at best, a meaningless stock phrase of practice, or, at worst, actively complicit in the concealment of oppressive ideologies of practice. Surprisingly little work has been devoted to unpacking the limits and substance of both what autonomy 'is', and in what sense it is 'good': under what measures and in what context, to the extent that Murdach has argued that 'in contrast with other values such as social justice and confidentiality, there today appears to be little interest in the profession exploring the value of self-determination' (2011, p. 371). The risk in play here is precisely illustrated by the quotations from Jordan above, which highlight the way in which 'projects of autonomy' can find themselves uncomfortably and ironically twisting from discourses of emancipation into acts of control; similarly, there is a risk of conflating a model of autonomy as 'freedom of choice' with the narrow values of neoliberal consumerism (Cree, 2013, p. 155) or, indeed, a risk that teaching the values of autonomy to social work students falls short in the face of what Preston-Shoot (2012) describes as the 'secret curriculum' of social work education, whereby the cultural practices of organizations overrule the values and models of good practice taught on degree programmes. As I have argued elsewhere, 'the moment that an ethical basis or legal framework ceases to be questionable – either by virtue of becoming "just common sense", or by standing atop unassailable moral heights – is the same moment that we lose the ability to critically discern appropriate use from inappropriate' (Grimwood, 2016, p. 83).

The ethics of autonomy

Within the history of ideas, the concept of autonomy takes on a principal moral and political role in the European Enlightenment and the development of a secular humanist modernity which followed (see Payne, 2011, pp. 30–31). Whereas the notion of self-sufficiency is valued as far back as the Ancient Greeks (Aristotle notes the highest value in life is to need nothing but that this would *also* require a large amount of dependency on sustenance, friendships and other supporting goods), modern autonomy arises from a context where, as Marcuse describes, 'reason took the form of rational subjectivity. Man, the individual, was to examine and judge everything given by means of the power of his knowledge. [. . .] Self-sufficiency and independence from all that is other is the sole guarantee of the subject's freedom' (1992, pp. 6–7).

This principle of autonomy as self-sufficiency within modern moral philosophy is chiefly associated with the work of Immanuel Kant. For Kant, modernity required man [sic] to emerge from 'his self-incurred immaturity', which he defined as 'the inability to use one's own understanding without the guidance of another' (Kant, 1996, p. 11). Autonomy was, therefore, the key to understanding moral authority in the modern age, once the older structures and systems of moral authority, such as the feudal system and the influence of the Church, had dissipated. Freedom to choose, for Kant, was not simply the absence of restrictions (the 'negative liberty' espoused by utilitarian and liberal thinkers such as J. S. Mill), but rather the ability to reflect on and validate moral laws which individuals themselves arrived at rationally. In this way, Kant uses autonomy to mean 'self-sufficiency', independence from others, but specifically the self-sufficiency of reasoning:

> the good will is good not because of what it performs or effects, not by its aptness for the attainment of some proposed end, but simply by virtue of the volition – that is, it is good in itself and considered by itself is to be esteemed much higher than all that can be brought about by it in favour of any inclination.
>
> *(Kant, 1998, p. 279)*

Kant's focus on rationality is also key to his model of autonomy: we cannot, he argues, choose our 'inclinations', such as our emotions, our relationships or our social circumstances, and therefore should be wary of using them in our moral decision-making. We can, though, choose between following our inclinations and following our duties. Such duties are to moral laws: laws which are decided upon by the application of reason to moral dilemmas. Because these laws are fundamentally rational, and therefore universal, then our duty to them is absolute. In this sense, the moral autonomy he describes is both highly individualistic (we can only decide what is right and wrong for us to do) and overwhelmingly universal (if we follow rational principles, what Kant terms the categorical imperatives, then as individuals we will *all* arrive at the same outcome). Hence, the fundamental duty of Kant's moral system is to act only in respect of others' autonomy: treat other people as ends in themselves, never as means to an end. Autonomy, for Kant, is difficult to achieve and part of our development as individuals, but it is nevertheless the cornerstone of moral values.

There is a clear lineage between the kind of moral society envisaged by Kant that was, via the work of Fichte, subsequently applied to early social contexts. This is primarily seen in the work of British philosopher T. H. Green, and the work of the early forms of social work practice – most notably, the Charity Organization Society (COS) and the Settlement House Movement in the United Kingdom and the United States – who were heavily influenced by these ideas (see Pierson, 2011). But while Kantian ethics decreed that the moral actor 'utters moral commands only to himself' (MacIntyre, 2002, p. 147), the influence of social reform agendas, married with the moralistic hubris of idealism, led to a widening of the remit of autonomy as a tool for a specific form of 'emancipation'. As Harris notes, in these early forms of social work, 'poor people were not seen as at the mercy of [. . .] social and economic processes and were not regarded as requiring sympathetic intervention' (Harris, 2008, p. 664). Instead, they took Kant's view of a 'self-incurred immaturity' quite literally: 'caseworkers stressed the importance of isolating the causes of individual difficulties and locating people's problems within themselves in order to intervene more directly in their lives' (Harris, 2008, p. 666). This resulted in a discourse which merged 'individual help for the deserving, [. . .] with the Poor Law in an overarching welfare regime' which in turn refashioned people 'in accordance with the requirements of the new capitalist society' (Harris, 2008, p. 666).

From its very inception, then, the notion of autonomy has never been a tidy one within social work, even when the 'paternalist' strategies of the COS fell from fashion, at least for a time, during the 20th century. But while social work may not draw on Kant directly – tellingly, BASW replaced references to 'duty' with 'responsibility' in their 2011 revised code of ethics – there remains a widespread assumption across social work literature that more autonomy is a *good thing*. Furthermore, this normative value retains echoes of Kant's model: not only in the more overt uses – such as Biestock's assertion (1974) that client self-determination was a 'natural right' and the highest value of social work – but also in the implicit Kantian requirements of a developed sense of rational self-sufficiency. As Singh and Cowden note, 'historically' the notion of autonomy refers to the control social workers have over their own practice, in their role as 'experts' who are able to 'make independent judgements free of political interference', on the basis of 'an absolute commitment to ethics' (2013, p. 81). At the same time, the untidy nature by which autonomy translates into practice raises problems for the traditional Kantian model. The general concept of autonomy in social work today remains a complicated interweaving of the value of *emancipatory* autonomy (seen, for example, in the mantra of person-centred practice) with the material conditions of practice (both for the service user and social worker). It may be useful, therefore, to follow the theories which respond to the problems for Kant's thinking when considering how autonomy is articulated as a value in social work in the 21st century.

Autonomy and relationships

The alignment of autonomy with self-sufficiency raises a key question over the extent to which this overlooks the physical and emotional relationships already in existence around the exercise of autonomy and the ways in which these relationships are recognized and maintained. Does a commitment to autonomy as a social work value in fact run counter to what Lynn refers to as the 'person-in-the-situation' that social work is committed to (2006, p. 110) or Garrett describes as the 'fleshiness' (2013, p. 166) of working with others to address disadvantage?

One of the issues here is that, in general parlance, autonomy is frequently explained in terms of its political meaning, translating the 'self-rule' of the body politic into the freedom of choice for the body personal (see Murdach, 2011, p. 372). But as Gilligan (1993) argued in the classic feminist work *In a Different Voice*, an emphasis on the self as a representative of, or in relation to, the state is a poor analogy, as it overlooks the attachments to others that an individual has (which do not correlate to any relationship between states). Furthermore, it overlooks what Bourdieu has termed the 'symbolic violence' of the body politic itself in prescribing the 'practical schemes of perception, appreciation and action' which frame such relationships (2000, p. 175; see Chapter 5) and legitimize current structural social inequalities (Fineman, 2004). As such, one of the main criticisms of autonomy as a social work value is that it imposes a specifically gendered, classed and cultured view of the individual, modelled on the most politically powerful in society, which overlooks the tangible relations these are embedded within.

In the 1980s, Gilligan's work laid a significant foundation for criticizing Kantian accounts of personal development, notably Kohlberg's. His work suggested that rational and objective autonomy is the highest level of moral development. This account, Gilligan argued, reflects a gendered account which privileges what have been traditionally masculine characteristics and values. Relational aspects of identity, such as caring, have traditionally been viewed as secondary, or obstructive, to more 'male' aspects such as autonomy, objectivity and universality. Hence, while the Kantian model of autonomy remains the norm, Barnes notes that 'choice and control' for service users are typically framed as the ideal for interventions, with 'care and protection' only the 'booby prize' (Barnes, 2011, p. 160). Such views and their subsequent development in feminist ethical theory (for example, Noddings, 1984; Held, 2006) have thus formed the launching pad for a number of variations of a 'care ethics' within social work, which challenges the idea that autonomy equates to a substantive independence and suggests instead that mutually caring relations allow for genuine personal transformation and actions which address actual needs (see Hugman, 2005; Reamer, 2016; see Chapters 8 and 31).

This does not do away with the notion of autonomy altogether, however. When viewed in the context of relationships, rather than atomistic individuals, Gilligan herself suggests that autonomy can still be a worthy ideal, both practically and psychologically. Using the relational account of development employed by Loevinger and Wessler (1970), Gilligan argues that, while Kohlberg's account of development uses autonomy as a means to arrive at an 'objectively fair or just resolution to moral dilemmas upon which all rational persons could agree', relational autonomy 'focuses instead on the *limitations* of any particular resolution', as well as their conflicts (1993, pp. 21–22, my emphasis). Autonomy is thus redefined, somewhat poetically, as 'modulating an excessive sense of responsibility through the recognition that other people have responsibility for their own destiny' (Gilligan, 1993, p. 21). The subsequent development of this notion of relational autonomy has taken root in many health discourses, particularly around the topics of patient and service user empowerment (see, for example, Wardrope, 2015; Walker & Ross, 2014), as well as areas of social work (Banks, 2012, p. 93). It remains, however, a broad umbrella term, rather than a clearly defined theory of autonomy (MacKenzie & Stoljar, 2000, p. 4).

The persuasiveness, or usefulness, of relational autonomy as a guiding value for social work largely hinges on what role relationships play in autonomous acts. For example, some theorists, such as Nedelsky, suggest this is a *causal* relationship because 'if we ask ourselves what actually *enables* people to be autonomous, the answer is not isolation, but relationships – with parents, teachers, friends, loved ones', and, presumably, social workers and/or their clients (Nedelsky, 1989, p. 12, my emphasis). Conversely, the absence of such enabling relationships can prevent a person from asserting autonomy, whether personally, as in the case of domestic abuse, or at a broader social or historical level, as in the case of displaced persons. This also suggests, though, that the concept of autonomy can and should only be understood within *localized* causal contexts. This seems at odds with a far more prominent emphasis of references to autonomy within social work literature which is geared towards a more encompassing, universal definition. Indeed, if relationships are causally linked to autonomy, this still seems to require a more specific set of values to be ascribed to autonomy itself, what Singh and Cowden (2013, p. 81) saw as an 'absolute commitment to ethics', in order for social workers to separate its *normative* significance from any old act that arises from a relationship with, or responsibility to, others. In light of this criticism, other theories of relational autonomy suggest that for a person to be autonomous, they must not only act or decide on something themselves but include *within* this act or decision some kind of moral attitude towards themselves, such as self-worth, self-respect, or self-dignity (see, for example, McLeod & Sherwin, 2000). This model finds resonance with certain approaches to anti-oppressive practice (Dominelli, 2002) by combining a commitment to social justice with the promotion of human rights, acknowledging relational needs while insisting on a clear definition of self-rule. In this way, the level of autonomy one has, or doesn't have, can still be mapped in a developmental way.

Autonomy and ideology

Relational autonomy may provide a more promising foundation to many contemporary approaches to social work than Kantian self-sufficiency. But a question remains whether relational autonomy retains from Kant too much of a focus on the *individual's* development, at the expense of broader and far more complex *ideological* relations. Nowhere is this complexity more visible than in the rise of the 'personalization' agenda, which has been a key route to challenging the 'paternalism' of social work practice (Ellis, 2007).

Beginning in the late 1980s and 1990s, autonomy developed a specific value related to the rise of what Cannan described as 'enterprise culture' in the United Kingdom: embodied by 'a self characterised by autonomy, responsibility, initiative, self-reliance, independence and willingness to take risks, to "go for it"' (1994, p. 7). Alongside this was a shift in social care towards quasi-markets for personalized service user budgets, using the logic of neoliberal economics to counter the perceived 'dependency culture' of social security which '"produces" the poor' (Cree, 2013, p. 147).

Our focus here is not the merits of personalization but rather the question of what *model* of autonomy it invokes, particularly when, for example, Leece and Peace (2010) argue that service users in the United Kingdom have valued the extent to which personalization provides enhanced levels of 'independence' and 'autonomy'. Such a notion of autonomy is rooted in the liberal development of Kantian thought. Rather than attempt to map the content of autonomous acts, in the sense that theories of relational autonomy do, theorists such as Rawls developed Kant's model in the opposite direction, by theorizing a distinctly *procedural* account of autonomy in order to protect the basic freedoms of the individual (Besthorn, Koenig, Spano, & Warren, 2016, pp. 148–149). Rather than specify the moral norms which autonomy entailed, it concentrated on establishing the minimal conditions by which an individual's autonomy could be maintained. The liberal view begins from the idea of a self-interested individual, who must reconcile their own self-interested activities with that of other self-interested individuals through some kind of social contract (see Grimwood, 2016, pp. 40–46). As such, 'in a pluralistic society and even more clearly in a pluralistic world, we cannot agree on our visions of the good life [. . .] but we can hope to agree on the *minimal conditions* for justice, for coexistence within a framework allowing us to pursue our visions of the good life' (Held, 1999, p. 338, my emphasis). This model is present in the development of liberal economic visions for society by writers like Hayek and Friedman, for whom autonomy could be said to roughly equate to 'consumer-power', and the autonomy of the service user to their enablement as a 'citizen-consumer' (Clarke, Newman, Smith, Vidler, & Westmarland, 2007). Interference from the state can only be debilitating to an individual's autonomy; thus, dependency is a wrong to be corrected.

This model of autonomy is entrenched in tensions, however. Because the autonomy of personalization remains fundamentally focused on a 'floating self' which grounds liberalism and neo-liberalism, this procedural autonomy can overlook the importance of physical and relational dependencies. Lymbery argues that personalization 'exposes an enduring form of inequality: if we take into account the physical and cognitive frailties of many people in need of services, there are apparent limitations on their ability both to exercise choice and to have that choice turned into positive action' (2012, p. 788). This is problematic, given that social work values are premised on supporting 'people who have the lowest levels of capacity to act as self-actualising consumers' (Lymbery, 2012, p. 788). Jordan suggests that this procedural model of autonomy requires 'technologies of the self', driven by the state and aimed at the mainstream population to develop particular self-characteristics, such as motivation, self-esteem and entrepreneurship. But, Jordan notes, 'in relation to poor and disadvantaged people, they have to be motivated and instructed in how to get their projects of the self started' (2004, p. 9). This is problematic, Schram argues, because within the shift to 'personal responsibility' narratives (2000, p. 27) behind the delivery of social care:

> In the liberal contractual society that particularly valorizes choice, 'personal responsibility' is [. . .] especially paradoxical. It implies being willing to take responsibility for what the dominant culture has already assigned as one's responsibility, and on terms predetermined by the culture.
>
> *(Schram, 2000, p. 31)*

In part, these anachronistic categories arise from the shifts from the classical liberal model of autonomy found in writers like Rawls and the neoliberal policies which have dominated Western social policies: neo-liberalism requires a focus on economic self-determination to be 'directed, buttressed, and protected by law and policy as well as by the dissemination of social norms' (Brown, 2005, p. 41); as such, procedural accounts of autonomy are merged with substantive cultural assumptions. Fraser has termed this the 'Juridical-Administrative-Therapeutic apparatus' (Fraser, 1989, p. 154), whereby 'a form of bureaucratic "needs talk" [. . .] imputes to welfare recipient's personal deficiencies that need to be treated if they are to leave welfare for a life of "self-sufficiency"' (Schram, 2000, p. 72). In this sense, the concept of autonomy, far from liberating, can instead become a mode of cultural disciplining of the disempowered. Adding to the complexity of this is what Mead (1997) has described as a 'New Paternalism' arising within social policy. Here, traditional values are reasserted at the core of welfare directives – such as the need to work, the centrality of the nuclear family, and so on – *despite* these being arguably unsustainable in post-industrial society. In such cases, Estes suggests that a 'focus on rational problem resolution by technical experts serves to obfuscate the substance of class, gender, and racial/ethnicity', citing social policy around ageing as one context where 'the purportedly "gender neutral" policy [. . .] is biased toward the autonomous nuclear family' (Estes, 2001, p. 18). It is not simply the model of autonomy being utilized at issue here, but the relevance of autonomy *as a model* for the contemporary circumstances both social workers and service users practice within.

Autonomy and agency

It is perhaps not surprising that this tension underlies many of the discussions in contemporary social work around the relationship between a social worker's autonomy in the field and the management of risk accompanying this: a tension between the self-governance a social worker has over their own practice and the broader institutional and legal governance their practice sits within. It is of note that this complex sense of autonomy is largely articulated in terms of its loss. Fook, for example, argues that the 'autonomy of all professionals is challenged in the current context. Increased managerialism and changed funding arrangements effectively place more control of professional practice within the hands of managers or bureaucrats' (Fook, 2012, p. 28). Gray and Webb likewise align 'managerial control' and 'the undermining of practitioner discretion' with 'loss of professional autonomy' and criticize the 'surrender' of '"technical" and "ideological" autonomy within the rationalized care management process' (2012, pp. 12–13). For Lawler (2007), professional knowledge is undermined by 'management principles and practices [which have] trumped professional autonomy, knowledge and judgement'. The perceived 'objectivity' of 'management efficiency' is thus 'the main measure of effectiveness' (Lawler, 2012, pp. 102–103). Murdach (2011), too, suggests that the loss of self-determination as a value in social work is linked to the rise of 'verification' measures in practice. Conversely, Evans (2013) has argued that the imposition of more procedures and guidelines for practice may, in fact, *increase* the amount of discretion surrounding professional decision-making – for example, if practitioners find themselves working with contradictory guidelines or overly bureaucratic processes – and the fluidity this creates is not *necessarily* a good thing as it can lead to inconsistent service delivery.

In such arguments, the managerialism which obstructs social workers' autonomy is tied to the economically focused values of neo-liberalism, whereas 'practice autonomy' is aligned with the contextualized wisdom of the social worker. The complexity of this notion of autonomy is thus, in part, related to the debates around the validity of such practice wisdom. For example, Robison and Reeser argue that 'one of the marks of being a professional is having autonomy – the capacity, among other things, to make decisions about what is or is not in a client's best interests independent of the oversight of others' (2000, p. 128). But they also note that this autonomy 'means that most of our work is done with clients in such a way that others have few ways to judge whether we are competent or not' (Robison & Reeser, 2000, p. 128). In other words, the notion of autonomy as a form of contextual discretion is far removed from the Kantian universalist model, but it retains a sense of judgement and accountability that is rooted in the principle of autonomy *itself*, rather than more 'objective' measures.

But given the shrinking space for such autonomy to appear, negotiating these tensions regarding the critical relationship between practice and its institutional frameworks has in some cases led to a reformulation of autonomy as 'agency'. The primary theorists associated with agency are Foucault and Bauman. For both, there is a dissatisfaction with the modernist assumption that the self is either determined by its social context or separable from it. Foucault criticizes the notion of autonomy as straightforward self-rule by exploring the notion of 'governmentality': that is, the techniques and technologies which shape the way individuals govern themselves. In this way, *contra* the more deterministic views of Marxism, 'the subject constitutes itself in an active fashion through practices of the self', but 'these practices are nevertheless not something invented by the individual himself [sic]'. They are instead 'proposed, suggested, [and] imposed upon him by his culture, his society, and his social group' (Foucault, 2003a, p. 34). There can, then, be no self-sufficient autonomy, as the rationality this depends upon is itself a technique of governmentality. However, an individual does have agency. They are still concrete individuals in concrete social contexts, and while these contexts are created through various arrangements of power relationships, Foucault argues that governmentality is 'always a versatile equilibrium, with complementarity and conflicts between techniques which assure coercion and processes through which the self is constructed or modified by himself' (Foucault, 1993, pp. 203–204). He thus reframes autonomy as the 'permanent creation of ourselves' within our domains of practice (2003b, p. 52), which is not an isolated effort but rather created through 'the interplay of care of the self and the help of the other' which 'blends into preexisting relations, giving them a new coloration and greater warmth' (1986, p 53). Establishing one's own critical agency is thus an 'intensification of social relations' (Foucault, 1986, p. 53). Or, as Powell puts it, 'on the one hand, professional surveillance restricts practice while, on the other, complexity opens up the space for resistance and new formulations of power relations' (2013, p. 51).

Contrary to some critics' views, for example, Hugman (2003), this is not a re-articulation of the free-floating self of liberalism, but rather an awareness of the fragmented way in which autonomous practice appears. Similarly, Bauman has argued that the changes in material practices, modes of production and cultural fluency in late modernity have produced a 'habitat' where the relationship between individuals and organizations becomes more complex. For example, social work agencies have 'become seen as increasingly specialized, able to exercise authority over narrower and narrower domains. At points where different interests interact, therefore, there emerges a constant sense of "indeterminacy", where competing claims for legitimacy and authority are played out' (2008, p. 54). The notion of a dynamic 'habitat' for practice has thus grounded what Fook terms 'contextual practice' (2012, p. 161) as a specific response to the changes to the practical idea of social workers' autonomy, which is rooted in 'habitats in which autonomous agents act in an environment characterized by chronic indeterminacy, ambivalence and contingency' (Leonard, 1997, p. 108) rather than a transcendent or universal set of principles. For Bauman, 'autonomy means that agents are only partly, if at all, constrained in their pursuit of whatever they have institutionalized for their purpose' as there is no longer a single '"goal-setting" agency with overall managing and coordinating capacities' (1992, p. 192). The agency of the social worker is guided, not by the determination of protocols and procedures within the habitat, but rather by an 'unconditional' moral responsibility to the Other (Kendall, 2016, pp. 196–198), and in particular the need to work within a specific habitat to allow individuals to narrate their own agential development. On this view, autonomy takes a substantially different appearance to its modernist form: one that is less around self-sufficient decision-making or practice discretion and far more like the capacity – and the support of others' capacity – to claim authorship of a self-narrative through a complex of differing and often antagonistic social contexts.

Autonomy and universality

The problem with merging context dependency and autonomy in this way is, however, that if an individual's reason turns out to be only contingent upon their relationships or the reflection of a wider set of power discourses, relations or ideologies, then it cannot guarantee the universality and necessity of a moral principle. One route that social work theory has taken to overcome this problem, whilst maintaining the value of autonomy, is to turn to the thinking of Habermas (see Houston, 2013; Lovat & Gray, 2008). Unlike both theories of relational autonomy and Foucauldian critiques, Habermas retains the Kantian principle that rational autonomy is still a value to celebrate and heteronomy a threat to avoid. But he argues that this needs to be separated from a straightforward subject-object ontological distinction, which is found not only in Kant, but also in the structure-agency debates of 20th century sociology. Instead of seeing autonomy as being tied to the individual subject, Habermas locates it in the use of a particular form of reasoning, which is not monological but *dialogical* (Habermas, 1984). Both modern scientific and social knowledge has come to use almost exclusively a monological, 'instrumental' form of rationality, subservient to particular ideologies which shape our practices. This enforces a separation between individuals and the communities and relationships around them, and, subsequently, the value of autonomy becomes aligned with the value of the individual over and above their social context. The dominance of instrumental reason, bureaucratic, targets-driven managerialism, for example, is premised on monological strategies of ideology.

It is true, Habermas suggests, that a human being can only develop their reason, and therefore their autonomy, in dialogue with others. We are not born with a sense of autonomy but learn it throughout cultural upbringing. Hence, the oft-cited distinction between the value of autonomy in 'Western' and 'Eastern' cultures (even if the reality is perhaps more complicated – see, for example, Chirkov, 2004). As such, every genuine attempt to communicate involves an attempt to create consensus as this is the basis of any further conversation (Habermas, 1996). This suggests an 'ideal speech situation' which is created when such a consensus is fully realized. That is to say, communication should aim to create the conditions that allow for all interlocutors to both communicate and challenge one another, using only rationality and evidence, without the coercion of force or ideology. This suggests that 'the ideal speech situation creates the possibility of decisions not merely reflecting pre-held positions' (Spratt & Houston, 1999, p. 320) and thus reclaim the notion of autonomy. For Houston, this model of autonomy allows social work to address the broken and dysfunctional relations that it is often called to address. Social workers can accept that autonomy is not, in fact, possible for service users within particular regimes of disciplinary power: for example, benefits systems, social care bureaucracy and austerity measures. But, precisely *because* of this, they can also insist on the *ideal* of autonomy as the basis for effective intervention.

Summary

I have suggested here that, despite being a core social work value, the concept of autonomy within social work faces several questions to resolve. Some of these are rooted in the concept itself and the philosophical questions it raises, some in the specific contexts in which it emerges in 21st century social work practice, and some due to the lack of in-depth theorization it has received within such contexts. In this sense, the discussion in this chapter has attempted to describe the parameters of the concept in both its implicit and explicit uses. But the real theorization of autonomy and dependence in social work takes place, I think, by considering such questions specifically in terms of how one refers to and uses the term 'autonomy' within one's own practice: far more so than a recourse to an 'off-the-shelf' theory from philosophy, politics or psychology. The focus of these questions would be:

- Does autonomy enable contextualized decision-making or provide a universalist principle for decision-making?
- Does autonomy require specific rules, procedures or universals to govern self-determination? What kind of rules?
- Is service user autonomy a different concept to social worker autonomy or a variation on the same?
- To what extent does autonomy imply a specific type of individual – gendered, cultured or reflecting a particular physical or economic position?
- Is autonomy a byword for consumerism? In what way is the difference between the two made clear?
- If autonomy has been eroded, then what *is* it that has gone, and how did it go?

Further reading

Conly, S. (2013). *Against autonomy: Justifying coercive paternalism*. Cambridge: Cambridge University Press.
Fineman, M. (2004). *The autonomy myth: A theory of dependency*. New York: New Press.
    These books offer provocative critiques of the idea of autonomy in terms of contemporary social care.
Weinberg, M. (2016). *Paradoxes in social work practice: Mitigating ethical trespass*. London: Routledge.
    This book discusses many of the tensions in practice which surround the articulation of autonomy, particularly regarding the role of context and universals.

References

Barnes, M. (2011). Abandoning care? A critical perspective on personalisation from an ethic of care. *Ethics and Social Welfare, 5*(2), 153–167.
Bauman, Z. (1992). *Intimations of postmodernity*. London: Routledge.

Besthorn, F., Koenig, T., Spano, R., & Warren, S. (2016). A critical analysis of social and environmental justice: Reorienting social work to an ethic of ecological justice. In R. Hugman & J. Carter (Eds.), *Rethinking values and ethics in social work* (pp. 146–163). Basingstoke: Palgrave Macmillan.
Biestek, F. P. (1974). *The casework relationship*. London: Allen & Unwin.
Bourdieu, P. (2000). *Pascalian meditations*. Cambridge, MA: Polity.
Bransford, C. (2011). Integrating critical consciousness into direct social work practice: A pedagogical view. *Social Work Education, 30*(8), 932–947.
Brown, W. (2005). *Edgework: Critical essays on knowledge and politics*. Princeton, NJ: Princeton University Press.
Cannan, C. (1994). Enterprise culture, professional socialisation, and social work education in Britain. *Critical Social Policy, 14*(3), 7–26.
Carpenter, J., Schneider, J., Brandon, T., & Wooff, D. (2003). Working in multi-disciplinary community health teams: The impact on social workers and health professionals of integrated mental health care. *British Journal of Social Work, 3*, 1081–1083.
Chirkov, V. (2004). Culture, personal autonomy and individualism: Their relationships and implications for personal growth and well-being. In G. Zheng, K. Leung, & J. Adair (Eds.), *Perspectives and progress in contemporary cross-cultural psychology* (pp. 247–263). Beijing: China Light Industry Press.
Clarke, J., Newman, J., Smith, N., Vidler, E., & Westmarland, L. (2007). *Creating citizen-consumers: Changing publics and changing public services*. London: Sage.
Conly, S. (2013). *Against autonomy: Justifying coercive paternalism*. Cambridge: Cambridge University Press.
Cree, V. (2013). New practices of empowerment. In M. Gray & S. Webb (Eds.), *The new politics of social work* (pp. 145–155). Basingstoke: Palgrave Macmillan.
Dominelli, L. (1997). *Sociology for social work*. London: Macmillan.
Dominelli, L. (2002). *Anti-oppressive social work: Theory and practice*. Basingstoke: Palgrave Macmillan.
Dworkin, G. (1989). The concept of autonomy. In J. Christman (Ed.), *The inner citadel: Essays on individual autonomy* (pp. 54–62). Oxford: Oxford University Press.
Ellis, K. (2007). Direct payments and social work practice: The significance of 'street-level bureaucracy' in determining eligibility. *British Journal of Social Work, 37*, 405–422.
Estes, C. L. (2001). *Social policy and aging: A critical perspective*. London: Sage.
Evans, T. (2013). Organisational rules and discretion in adult social work. *British Journal of Social Work, 34*, 871–896.
Fook, J. (2012). *Social work: A critical approach to practice* (2nd ed.). London: Sage.
Foucault, M. (1986). *The history of sexuality, Vol. III: The care of the self* (R. Hurley. Trans.). New York: Vintage Books.
Foucault, M. (1993). About the beginning of the hermeneutics of the self. Transcription of two lectures at Dartmouth on 17 and 24 November 1980, ed. M. Blasius. *Political Theory, 21*, 198–227.
Foucault, M. (2003a). The ethics of the concern of the self as a practice of freedom. In P. Rabinow & N. Rose (Eds.), *The essential Foucault* (pp. 25–42). New York: New York University Press.
Foucault, M. (2003b). What is enlightenment? In P. Rabinow & N. Rose (Eds.), *The essential Foucault* (pp. 43–57). New York: New York University Press.
Fraser, N. (1989). *Unruly Practices: Power discourse and agenda in contemporary social theory*. Cambridge, UK: Polity.
Garrett, P. M. (2013). *Social work and social theory: Making connections*. Bristol: Policy Press.
Gilligan, C. (1993). *In a different voice*. Cambridge, MA: Harvard University Press.
Gray, M., & Webb, S. (2012). Towards a 'new politics' of social work. In M. Gray & S. Webb (Eds.), *The new politics of social work* (pp. 3–20). Basingstoke: Palgrave Macmillan.
Grimwood, T. (2016). *Key debates in social work and philosophy*. London: Routledge.
Habermas, J. (1984). *The theory of communicative action. Vol. I: Reason and the rationalization of society* (T. McCarthy. Trans.). Boston: Allyn & Beacon.
Habermas, J. (1996). *Between fact and norm*. Cambridge: Cambridge University Press.
Harris, J. (2008). State social work: Constructing the present from moments in the past. *British Journal of Social Work, 38*, 662–679.
Held, V. (1999). Feminist transformations of moral theory. In J. Sterba (ed.), *Ethics: The big questions* (pp. 331–345). Oxford: Blackwell.
Held, V. (2006). *The ethics of care*. Oxford: Oxford University Press.
Houston, S. (2013). Social work and the politics of recognition. In M. Gray & S. Webb (Eds.), *The new politics of social work* (pp. 63–76). Basingstoke: Palgrave Macmillan.
Hugman, R. (2003). Professional values and ethics in social work: Reconsidering postmodernism? *British Journal of Social Work, 33*, 1025–1041.

Hugman, R. (2005). *New approaches to ethics for the caring professions*. Basingstoke: Palgrave Macmillan.

Jordan, B. (2004). Emancipatory social work? opportunity or oxymoron. *British Journal of Social Work, 34*, 5–19.

Kant, I. (1996). An answer to the question: 'What is Enlightenment?' In M. J. Gregor (Ed.), *Immanuel Kant: Practical philosophy* (pp. 11–22). Cambridge, UK: Cambridge University Press.

Kant, I. (1998). Fundamental principles of the metaphysics of morals. In S. Cahn & P. Markie (Eds.), *Ethics history, theory and contemporary issues* (pp. 275–318). New York: Oxford University Press.

Kendall, S. (2016). Postmodern ethics for practice. In R. Hugman & J. Carter (Eds.), *Rethinking values and ethics in social work* (pp. 195–209). Basingstoke: Palgrave Macmillan.

Lavalette, M. (2011). *Radical social work today: Social work at the crossroads*. Bristol: Policy Press.

Lawler, J. (2007). Leadership in social work: A case of caveat emptor? *British Journal of Social Work, 37*, 123–141.

Lawler, J. (2012). Critical management. In M. Gray & S. Webb (Eds.), *The new politics of social work* (pp. 98–115). Basingstoke: Palgrave Macmillan.

Leece, J., & Peace, S. (2010). Developing new understandings of independence and autonomy in the personalised relationship. *British Journal of Social Work, 40*, 1847–1865.

Loevinger, J., & Wessler, R. (1970). *Measuring ego development*. San Francisco, CA: Jossey-Bass.

Lovat, T., & Gray, M. (2008). Towards a proportionist social work ethics: A Habermasian perspective. *British Journal of Social Work, 38*, 1100–1114.

Lymbery, M. (2012). Social work and personalisation. *British Journal of Social Work, 42*, 783–792.

Lynn, M. (2006). Discourses of community: Challenges for social work. *International Journal of Social Welfare, 15*(2), 110–120.

MacIntyre, A. (2002). *A short history of ethics*. London: Routledge.

Mackenzie, C. (2014). Three dimensions of autonomy: A relational analysis. In A. Veltman & M. Piper (Eds.), *Autonomy, oppression, and gender* (pp. 15–41). Oxford: Oxford University Press.

MacKenzie, C., & Stoljar, N. (2000). Refiguring autonomy. In C. MacKenzie & N. Stoljar (Eds.), *Relational autonomy: Feminist essays on autonomy, agency and social self* (pp. 3–33). Oxford: Oxford University Press.

Marcuse, H. (1992). Philosophy and critical theory. In D. Ingram & J. Simon-Ingram (Eds.), *Critical theory: The essential readings*. New York: Paragon House.

McDonald, C. (2006). *Challenging social work: The institutional context of practice*. Basingstoke: Palgrave Macmillan.

McLeod, C., & Sherwin, S. (2000). Relational autonomy, self-trust and health care for patients who are oppressed. In C. Mackenzie & N. Stoljar (Eds.), *Relational autonomy: Feminist essays on autonomy, agency and social self* (pp. 259–279). Oxford: Oxford University Press.

Mead, L. M. (Ed.) (1997). *The new paternalism: Supervisory approaches to poverty*. Washington, DC: Brookings Institution.

Munro, E. (2011). *The Munro review of child protection: A child-centred system*. London: Department for Education.

Nedelsky, J. (1989). Reconceiving autonomy: Sources, thoughts and possibilities. *Yale Journal of Law and Feminism, 1*, 7–36.

Noddings, N. (1984). *Caring: A feminine approach to ethics and moral education*. Berkeley, CA: University of California Press.

Payne, M. (2011). *Humanistic social work*. Basingstoke: Palgrave Macmillan.

Pierson, J. (2011). *Understanding social work: History and context*. Maidenhead: Open University Press.

Powell, J. (2013). Michel Foucault. In M. Gray & S. Webb (Eds.), *Social work theories and methods* (2nd ed., pp. 46–62). London: Sage.

Preece, H. (2012). *More client time and autonomy: Life in a social work practice*. Retrieved from www.communitycare.co.uk/2012/05/01/more-client-time-and-autonomy-life-in-a-social-work-practice/

Preston-Shoot, M. (2012). The secret curriculum. *Ethics and Social Welfare, 6*(1), 18–36.

Reamer, F. (2016). The ethics of care. *Social Work Today*. Retrieved from www.socialworktoday.com/news/eoe_0916.shtml

Robison, W., & Reeser, L. (2000). *Ethical decision making in social work*. Boston, MA: Allyn & Bacon.

Schram, S. (2000). *After welfare: The culture of postindustrial social policy*. New York: New York University Press.

Simpson, G., & Murr, A. (2014). Reconceptualising well-being: Social work, economics and choice. *Culture Unbound, 6*, 891–904.

Singh, G., & Cowden, S. (2013). The new radical social work professional? In J. Parker & M. Doel (Eds.), *Professional social work* (pp. 81–97). London: Sage.

Spratt, T., & Houston, S. (1999). Developing critical social work in theory and in practice: Child protection and communicative reason. *Child and Family Social Work, 4*, 315–324.

Walker, J. K., & Ross, L. F. (2014). Relational autonomy: Moving beyond the limits of isolated individualism. *Pediatrics, 133*(1), 16–23.

Wardrope, A. (2015). Relational autonomy and the ethics of health promotion. *Public Health Ethics, 8*(1), 50–62.

9

Empathy, respect and dignity in social work

David Howe

Introduction

Of the many human virtues that ethicists celebrate, curiosity and an interest in other people come high on the list. It might be also argued that they are prerequisites for empathy, respect and dignity.

Our lot in life is the human condition. We try to make the best of what we have and where we find ourselves. But life is often unfair. We have no control over the cards which fate deals us. Some hands are easier to play than others. If you are lucky enough to be born into a well-off family, benefit from a decent education and enjoy good health, the chances are that your mental health will be sound. Your levels of stress will be low. Your life prospects will be promising. It is easy to behave well when life runs smoothly.

In contrast, if you are raised in poverty by parents who suffer poor mental health, have problems with drug addictions, fail to have you immunized and neglect your safety, the chances are that life will throw more challenges your way. Indeed, one of life's mean tricks is that those who face the greatest number of challenges and the biggest stresses are often those least likely to have the resources – psychological, social, material – with which to handle them well. Risks are ridden best by the resilient. The vulnerable are more likely to stumble and fall.

All of which argues for a degree of understanding and humility when we work with those who are not coping well, in great need or behaving poorly. A well-worn adage, true, but we must remember that there for the grace of God go I. The more we know of the other person, their background, history, health, relationships, problems, circumstances, the more we can make sense of who they are and how they are, what they say and what they do. A compassionate interest in and caring curiosity about other people increase our understanding, and understanding is likely to increase our respect for the other and improve our ability to empathize. However, we must remember that respect and empathy do not mean that we necessarily condone the other's behaviour. There will be many things that other people say and do that are morally wrong, socially unacceptable, criminally bad and personally hurtful. But before we can work with people who are struggling with their feelings, their behaviour and other people, first we need to try and understand how they got to be in a position where they are being cast as either troubled or troublesome.

Most of us are less hostile towards those we feel are trying to understand us. We might not let our guard down immediately; after all, we have been hurt and caught out before, but if the other person seems as if they are trying to see things from our point of view, whether that view is right or wrong, then we might feel less wary, less defensive, less hostile.

Empathy

Many factors have been considered by evolutionary psychologists to account for our success as a species. These include diet, tool making, language, cooking and cooperation. Of these, our ability to cooperate appears as a key attribute. Our species, *homo sapiens*, has been around for the last 200,000 years. We are a group-living species, originally functioning in large kinship tribes of between 30 and 50 people. Cooperative behaviour allows the group to capitalize on the many and varied individual talents likely to be present in any large network. Some people will be good at either hunting, tracking, chasing, making or planning. Others might be good at caring, negotiating, managing or encouraging. However, before these different skills can be recognized and coordinated, individuals need to be in relationship with each other, and relationships don't work unless we can recognize and see how things look from the other's point of view. This allows collaboration.

'Mind reading,' therefore, became a primary skill in the business of human relationships. Without it, reading body language, gauging intentions, predicting behaviour and moderating one's own responses are difficult. So understanding the minds of others and their points of view makes cooperation possible. Cooperation allows the group to cohere and exploit the strengths of each individual to everyone's benefit. There is strength in numbers. And from an evolutionary perspective, there is safety in numbers too.

Seeing the world from other people's point of view, therefore, requires social intelligence. Other related psychological attributes also cluster around the concept of social intelligence. One of these is empathy. But whether we are talking about empathy or social intelligence, emotional literacy or mentalizing, each involves a complex set of reflexive psychological skills (Howe, 2008; Fonagy, Gergely, Jurist, & Target, 2002). The empathic, socially intelligent individual sees and senses how things might feel and look from different perspectives. The individual recognizes that, just as the other affects them, so they affect the other. And the way we are affected by the other influences what we think and feel, which in turn affects what we say and do. In other words, as an empathic, mentalizing, emotionally intelligent individual, I am able to recognize and monitor my own thoughts and feelings and how these affect what I say and do. I can recognize and understand that you have thoughts and feelings which affect what you say and do. I also understand that as I am trying to make sense of what you feel, think, say and do, you are trying to make sense of what I am feeling, thinking, saying and doing. And so together we create a dance of social interaction and psychological exchange in which there is endless scope for understanding and misunderstanding, pain and pleasure, hope and despair, cooperation and conflict.

Highly empathic people and those with good social intelligence generally enjoy more successful, less stressful relationships. They want to know what makes other people tick. They try to see things from the other person's point of view, given their history, background, worries, hopes, suspicions. And as they try to understand the other, they seek to *communicate that understanding*. The successful communication of what is recognized and understood is as important as the empathic understanding itself. Successful empathy, therefore, is an understanding of the other from the other's point of view *and* the communication of that understanding.

One of the major reasons clients give for believing that they are being helped by their social worker is that they feel their social worker is trying to *understand* them, understand where they are coming from, where they are at, what life is like for them, why they feel the way they do and why they do what they do (Howe, 1993). Not until the inner world of the other is grasped can that understanding be communicated. Not until it is communicated can the client feel understood. Not until the client feels understood can they engage with the worker. Not until they engage can they relate in a therapeutically useful way. Not until they relate can they feel safe, safe enough to stop, think, reflect, process, plan and move forward (Howe, 2012, 2014). None of this means that the social worker necessarily condones what the client says or does. It's just that the practitioner conveys that they are trying to 'get' the client and their story. They are trying to see things from their point of view, right or wrong.

Feeling understood by the other is often experienced as a moment of relief, a time of connection. Empathy, therefore, represents a way of being with the client. Every nuance of the other's body language, tone of voice and spoken word is observed and therefore felt. The empathic experience is visceral. The empathic, emotionally intelligent social worker senses that these resonating experiences are telling them important things about the other's thoughts, feelings, anxieties and beliefs. Empathy connects us with the other at the very moment when they are feeling sad, angry, frightened, anxious or happy. But unlike sympathy, empathy allows me to maintain the distinction between you and me, your feelings and my recognition of your feelings. Empathy puts me in *your* emotional shoes. Sympathy simply tells you that I've walked there too. Sympathy is me-oriented; empathy is you-oriented. Sympathy tells you that I've felt rejection too because my father also walked out on our family when I was a child. Empathy tells you that I can see that you still feel hurt and maybe even a little angry.

Psychologists recognize two types of empathy: emotional (affective) empathy and cognitive empathy. *Emotional empathy* is immediate. It's visceral; it's felt in the body. I see you hit your thumb with a hammer, and I take a sharp intake of breath, I wince and I might say 'Ouch!' Or you are free-climbing a sheer rock face. My muscles find themselves mimicking your body movements. My muscles tense. My hands grip. I have a look of anxious concentration on my face. By physically feeling the other's situation, we get to understand something of their world at that moment. More than any other component of empathy, the fact that we all share the same biology and the same senses means that we know at the physical, somatic level what it is to experience joy or jealousy, pain or pleasure. There are subtle physical resonances whenever we engage with another.

Cognitive empathy is more difficult, psychologically more demanding. It is based on seeing, imagining and actively thinking about the situation from the other person's point of view. It involves a more reflective process of trying to understand the other's state of mind. Some knowledge of the other's history, personality, circumstances and situation is necessary before we can set our minds to work imagining what it might be like to be them. Cognitive empathy requires you to watch, listen, concentrate and attend. For example, you might wonder: What must it feel like to be you, knowing that you have been fiercely independent all your life but now old age, a frail body and deteriorating health mean that you have to consider going into residential care? What must you be thinking and feeling?

When our empathy is at its best, both affective and cognitive empathy are involved. I am able to understand *and* feel your world while, at the same time, maintaining a clear sense of my own mental experience (Coplan, 2011, p. 5).

In summary, we might define empathy as (i) an affective reaction to the emotions of another, (ii) the cognitive act of adopting another's perspective, (iii) a cognitively based effort to understand the other person and their world and (iv) the successful communication of that understanding (Davis, 1994, p. 11; Howe, 2012).

If evolutionary psychologists have explored why empathy and social intelligence have played a key part in the success of our species, developmental psychologists have investigated how children develop empathy, social intelligence and mentalizing skills. Children need these skills if they are to become socially competent members of society. The ability to relate, take turns, share, care and cooperate depends on the child's ability to recognize that other people have minds with things going on in them different to their own. It is important to know what might be going on in those minds in order to relate well and behave in ways that are socially acceptable and culturally appropriate. Much of our behaviour that is regarded as moral and prosocial – that is, acting altruistically and selflessly on behalf of others – depends on our ability to be empathic, emotionally intelligent and socially competent. Our ability and willingness to care and show compassion, especially towards those who are weak, vulnerable and in need, is premised on the presence of empathy and good social understanding. In his modern retelling of Jane Austen's novel *Emma*, Alexander McCall Smith (2015) has Emma finally realize the unforgivable error of her small-minded prejudices and snobbish ways:

> …she had been able to make that sudden imaginative leap that lies at the heart of our moral lives: the ability to see, even for a brief moment, the world as seen by the other person. It is this understanding that lies behind all kindness to others, all attempts to ameliorate the situation of those who suffer, all those acts of charity by which we make our lives something more than the pursuit of the goals of the unruly ego.
>
> *(p. 358)*

Over the first few years of life, children gradually develop a 'theory of mind': that other people have minds and what goes on in them is different to what goes on in one's own. The infant brain is programmed to make sense of experience. The more the child is on the receiving end of experiences that credit them with an independent mind, one that is full of thoughts and feelings, the more the child can make sense of their own emotional, social and cognitive make-up. They can also begin to make sense of the emotional, social and psychological make-up of other people. This ability to reflect on the psychological state of the self and others allows children to begin to self-regulate their own aroused feelings. This is an important skill, one that helps children deal with their own as well as other people's emotions, stresses, behaviours and upsets.

Children cannot become empathic, socially intelligent beings, however, unless they have been in relationships with others who themselves are empathic and socially intelligent, with people who recognize and show an interest in the mental states of the children. The child's psychological, social and reflective self therefore forms as the child interacts with other self-reflecting, psychologically and socially complex selves. To be talked to in psychological terms helps children become good psychologists, able to make sense of the world socially and interpersonally (Meins et al., 2002; Fonagy & Target, 1997). Children who have not been in relationships with empathic and attuned parents, family and teachers fail to develop good levels of empathy, emotional intelligence and social understanding. Such deficits in the parent-child relationship, of course, are more likely to be found in children who suffer abuse, neglect and rejection. These children are often poor at social relationships. They are more at risk of mental health problems and dysfunctional behaviours (see Chapter 35). They don't deal well with stress. If these deficits continue into adult life, making sense of other people and regulating one's emotional responses remains difficult. This means that relationships are experienced as stressful, and stress is not something with which low empathy, non-mentalizing people deal well. They are also less likely to cope well with the stresses of poverty, poor housing and social disadvantage. Many clients therefore suffer a double blow. They experience higher levels of material and social stress, and they are psychologically less well equipped to deal with it, further compounding their stress.

Empathy and the social work relationship

It is more difficult to think straight when our emotions are running high. When we are anxious or angry, we become psychologically more defensive. Raised defences keep other people at bay. We don't hear what they say. Resistance increases. Cooperation evaporates. We cannot fully engage with another person until we feel safe. And not until we feel safe will we let down our psychological defences and allow our minds to think about and process our thoughts and feelings and those of other people.

Like attuned, empathic parents with a distressed child, relationship-based social workers know they have to tune into the distressed, suspicious, resistant client before any meaningful work can take place. The socially empathic worker needs the client to know that they are trying to see and understand things as the client sees and understands them. There is a shared struggle to make sense, to 'get it'. To feel recognized and understood by the social worker is an important first step in helping the client relax, collaborate, make decisions, and bring about changes in their life.

The simplest empathic responses generally take the form of 'You feel . . . because'. 'You feel angry because you think your mother doesn't believe you'. There is no evaluation. No moral judgement. Just a straightforward recognition of a feeling and the possible reasons for it. The empathic, attuned social worker might also say things like:

> I wonder if I'm right thinking that you might be feeling frightened about what the doctor might say when you visit her at the hospital tomorrow.
>
> My goodness, Sophie, are you sure that you couldn't care less whether Eddie goes or stays? You look furious to me!

In relationship with an empathic worker, the client can begin to 'down-regulate' their raised emotions. Having emotions recognized and named by the practitioner helps clients and service users feel less threatened, safer and more relaxed. When we feel less anxious, we are more able to think. When we drop our defences, our capacity to reflect and process thoughts increases. Social worker responses that are low on empathy generally lead to increases in client resistance. In contrast, high-empathy responses lead to reduced resistance (Miller & Rollnick, 2012). When resistance is low, there is a greater willingness to engage and cooperate. Low anxiety and increased trust mean that clients can begin to think, plan, decide and act more constructively and with less psychological distortion.

The argument so far is that if the psychological self forms in the context of close, empathic relationships with socially intelligent carers, then for the psychological self to *re-form* in healthy and emotionally literate ways, the self needs to get back into relationships with empathic, socially intelligent others including, in the case of clients, their social workers. As our selves form in the world of others, it is to that world of others that we must return if we are to change. The social formation of the self in childhood explains how we continue to be able to connect and communicate with others. It explains why we seek out empathically based relationships at times of need, distress and dysregulation. And it explains why such relationships and what takes place in them continue to have the power to change us, ontologically and psychologically, emotionally and behaviourally. Making sense is a shared, dynamic, reflexive business. Relationships in which it feels safe to talk hold the possibility of rethinking, re-feeling, redefining, and re-forming the self. This position echoes some of the ideas found in humanistic social work practices that seek 'human and social wellbeing by developing human capacities; personal growth; and social relationships of equality, freedom, and mutual responsibility through shared social experience' (Payne, 2011, p. 31).

Respect for persons and dignity

The principle of respect for persons has been a cornerstone in the ethical make-up of social work. At its most basic, the principle states that the individual person must be seen as a rational, self-determining being 'intrinsically worthy of respect simply because she or he is a person, regardless of whether we like the person, whether they are useful to us or whether they have behaved badly towards us' (Banks, 2012, p. 43). An individual is entitled to respect independent of any role he or she holds, any label which he or she is given, any legal category into which he or she is placed, any character trait he or she displays or any stereotype to which he or she is liable. Respect for persons is a reminder that we must be on our guard against 'objectifying' people, seeing them as a type such as 'schizophrenic', 'bed blocker' or 'alcoholic'.

Respect for persons requires us to acknowledge that other people have their own points of view about their choices, future and what's in their interest. We show a lack of respect when we override, ignore or dismiss the other person's agency and their right to have views about their own destiny and interests. Respect encourages other people to judge and choose things for themselves. We must listen to their claims and wishes and the reasons they give when they explain their intentions and justify their courses of action. The reasons they give may or may not be defensible, but they have the right to express them. However, by these same lights, they are also held responsible for the consequences of their actions. As with empathy, respect accepts the other person's right to be the author of their own thoughts and feelings and agent of their own actions, but it does not necessarily condone what is thought, said or done. The client must appreciate that actions have consequences, interpersonally, morally and legally.

There is an inevitable tension between respect for persons and our regulatory duties as social workers. Anxiety and discomfort increase our defensiveness and make us more likely to 'objectify' those who are making us feel anxious or uncomfortable. This can happen when we have to make difficult decisions such as removing a child or admitting someone into a psychiatric hospital. Describing a service user as 'a neglect case' or 'an aids and adaptations referral' not only objectifies the other, it distances us from the person and their humanity. Our practice risks becoming oppressive. A lack of respect denies the service user the chance to review and reflect on their situation. It blocks opportunities for them to explore their own point of view. It diminishes their right to be a self-reflecting, choice-making individual. It is undignified to be labelled, processed and explained. Many of these insights were anticipated by Ragg in 1977 when he titled his book *People Not Cases*.

The origins of the concept of respect for persons lie in the writings of the 18th-century German philosopher Immanuel Kant (see Chapter 10). Respect for persons has been the subject of much debate and discussion both in the philosophical and social work literature (for example, see Biestek, 1961; Banks, 2012; Downie & Telfer, 1969; Plant, 1970). Although this chapter is not the place to engage with these debates, we can take away from the principle the general idea that not only should people be presumed to be of intrinsic worth, no matter who they are or what they have done, but respecting the other is the only way to connect, communicate and relate meaningfully with our fellow human beings. Respect is achieved when the other person feels that we are trying to see and understand them from their point of view without prejudice, and such understanding is increased whenever we are being empathic and emotionally intelligent. We therefore find ourselves dealing with a set of concepts and ideas that are linked. Empathy, respect for persons, acceptance and understanding all appear as components of our ideas about morality and what it is to practise ethically. And it's in this ethical mix that we also find the idea of dignity and its promotion.

Loss of dignity is something that most of us have experienced at one time or another. It is often suffered when some aspect of our personality, performance or behaviour is made public when we would prefer it to have remained private. We feel the information revealed diminishes us in our own eyes if not those of others. You're drying yourself after a swim in the sea. A gust of wind blows away your towel, and there you are, naked for all to see. Or you are visiting the doctor's surgery when the receptionist pops into the waiting room and says in a voice for all to hear 'Can I check? Was your appointment for a prostate examination?' Loss of dignity can make us feel embarrassed, humiliated and devalued. When it takes place between people, the person inflicting the humiliation appears to be lacking empathy, whether the infliction was meant or not.

The risk of dignity being lost is reduced when workers show empathy, particularly cognitive empathy. You know how embarrassed 89-year-old Alice feels when she first realizes that she needs to ask for help to go to the toilet. Her request is best treated quietly, even matter-of-factly, as something ordinary and perfectly reasonable and that you are pleased to be able to help. Or you know that Rowanna feels ashamed. You've called round to see how she got on taking her two young children to their new nursery only to find her still in her pyjamas, clearly hungover. There is a smell of sick. She can't look you in the eyes. You know that she knows that you know she's let many people down, particularly her children, with her broken promises about not drinking, not disappointing the children, not 'screwing up' again. Rowanna's lost much of what little dignity she had, so there is no point in rubbing it in by saying the obvious. It's Rowanna's strengths that you have to salvage. She knows her weaknesses.

Our dignity is important (Social Care Institute for Excellence, 2008). It helps maintain our self-esteem, which in turn adds to our resilience. Resilience helps us recognize our strengths and supports the belief that with effort we can make a difference, bring about change. As social workers, we therefore need to respect people's rights to privacy, to choose, to be valued and heard and to be recognized as unique and individual. We need to respect people's choices and not make assumptions about the way they want to be treated, especially in matters of personal care. We need constantly to make that leap in which we try to imagine what it must be like to be 'you', to be frail and dependent, to be going to court with the distinct possibility that your children might be removed from your care, to be unable to gain access to a building because there is no signage to the ramp that grants wheelchair access.

Character and care

When clients and service users are asked what they want from social workers and what they value in the workers' attitude and behaviour, their answers have hardly changed over the years. Certainly, they want practical help, useful advice and effective interventions. But they also want services to be offered in ways that foster a relationship, maintain dignity and establish trust. There is much talk of appreciating social workers who come across as warm and friendly, who listen and who acknowledge and accept feelings, however ugly or uncomfortable. Clients and service users like to feel that the social worker is trying to understand them and that they are prepared to listen and see things from their point of view. If these elements are in place, there is an increased willingness by the service user to engage and form a relationship (Howe, 1993).

Much of what service users have to say about what makes a good social worker chimes with what virtue ethicists promote. Recently, a good deal of interest has been taken in what is known as *virtue ethics* or *relationship-based ethics* (Banks, 2012). This is a philosophical approach of great relevance for social workers. Virtue ethics pays attention to the qualities that workers possess as they engage with their clients (Houston, 2003; Clark, 2006). The *character* of the social worker matters. It is important what kind of person they are and are perceived to be (Houston, 2012). To practise ethically, and ultimately effectively, social workers need to possess one or more key virtues. These include such things as warmth, kindness, reliability, truthfulness, care, compassion, honesty, 'being straight with me', empathy, courage, integrity, impartiality and openness. Social workers who convey a sense of purpose and hope are generally viewed positively by service users. When we are asked to comment on the character of another person, we tend to evaluate them in terms of their virtues (and vices) (Beckett & Maynard, 2013). Indeed, observes Webb (2010, p. 119), if we are to develop good social workers, then along with many other things, we should also be promoting their moral education, cultivating their virtues and training their character.

However, there is a slight suspicion of cultural relativism in the promotion of particular virtues (Dracopoulou, 2015). It might be that what is regarded as virtuous in one culture or community might not be seen as such in another. It rules out notions of universal principles and rational touchstones by which to gauge the moral worth of an action. Even so, there is the broad feeling that, although particular virtues and their expression may be subject to cultural nuances, a compassionate nature and an empathic approach, by definition, should enable the worker to tune in to what is caring and appropriate in that practitioner's community of practice.

There is also another ethical position, one that suits social work particularly well. *Care ethics* is a form of relationship-based ethics (see Chapter 7). Care ethics recognizes and values the virtues present in close, caring, protective family relationships, particularly between mothers and their children. Care ethics differs from virtue ethics in the sense that it emphasizes what takes place in the caring relationship (Gray, 2010). It is only indirectly concerned with an individual's character and inherent virtues. 'Care is an activity *and* an attitude' (Featherstone & Morris, 2013, p. 348, emphasis original). It is when we feel fragile or vulnerable that we look for care and protection, acceptance and understanding, love and recognition. Recognizing and responding to other people's needs is the starting point for an ethics of care (Tronto, 1993; Noddings, 2003; Featherstone, 2010, p. 74). Caring relationships are ones in which relatedness, receptivity and responsiveness are present (Noddings, 2003; Featherstone, 2010; Featherstone & Morris, 2013).

Care, therefore, is an active ethic, involving feelings, thought and action. Behaviours which promote interdependence between people generally cement relationships and create a sense of belonging and well-being. They are life-sustaining, physically and emotionally. Care and mutuality are an integral part of citizenship and the idea of the civil society (Featherstone & Morris, 2013, p. 245). To give and receive care and offer compassion humanizes us. It makes us feel worthwhile. It makes us moral beings. It helps us feel that we belong. In fact, much of our moral development as children and our growing ability to care for others is the result of our being lovingly cared for throughout life (Hollway, 2006; Howe, 2012).

Empathy and structure

So far, we have given strong hints that skills such as empathy, virtues such as compassion and capacities such as care are not only good in themselves, but they are also key to the creation of successful relationships. There is a long-established research tradition which then goes on to argue that good quality relationships between clients and practitioners are more likely to lead to goal achievements and successful outcomes. Carl Rogers, a psychologist and counsellor, went so far as to say that the presence of *empathy*, *genuineness* and *warmth* in the professional relationship were not only necessary to bring about successful therapeutic outcomes, but they were often sufficient (Rogers, 1957; see Chapter 3). He referred to them as the 'core conditions' of the helpful relationship. They became basic to his idea of the therapeutic alliance and a person-centred practice.

Most research, however, suggests that although necessary, the 'core conditions' on their own are rarely sufficient. It seems that successful practices and effective interventions require both a good relationship *and* an evidence-based intervention, a strong working alliance *and* an effective technique, empathy *and* structure (Castonguay & Beutler, 2006).

Early last century, Sigmund Freud and Ernest Jones suggested that the best therapies and richest lives occur when there is a happy balance between love *and* work. Social work researchers and practitioners, too, have recognized the need for practice to be both responsive *and* systematic, to be relationship based *and* technically sound. Reid and Epstein (1972) say that a responsive worker is one whose discussions help clients feel understood, who expresses interest in what clients have to say about themselves and their lives, who listens attentively, who conveys appreciation and interest, who expresses warmth and goodwill and who accepts and does not judge. 'Perhaps the most critical component of responsiveness', they write, 'is the communication of empathic understanding' (Reid & Epstein, 1972, p. 129).

Bowlby (1988) pointed out that when feelings of anxiety are present, reflective thought, forward thinking and constructive action are difficult. If clients remain anxious, then thinking about problems and how to resolve them isn't easy. When our feelings are running high, we are more likely to behave defensively. It is the job of the social worker to try and bring down the emotional temperature by reducing feelings of stress whenever possible. Not until the practitioner has established a good working relationship will their client begin to feel that the encounter is a safe place in which to think about troublesome feelings, reflect on difficult memories, think positively and make plans for the future. Bowlby's position is therefore summed in the mantra *feel secure then explore*. You can't process thought and put your mind to work until your feelings have been regulated and anxiety levels are low. Good workers, therefore, try to act as a 'safe haven' for clients. And the more confident clients are in the presence and availability of the 'safe haven', the easier they find it to think about troublesome things and how they might be tackled.

Relationship-based practices in which empathy, care and compassion are present, although they have never gone away, are experiencing something of a revival in social work (Ruch, Turney, & Ward, 2010; Hennessey, 2011; Howe, 2014; Megele, 2015; McColgan, 2017). Most evidence-based and evidence-informed techniques also recognize that for an intervention to have any chance of success, the social worker needs to establish a good-enough working relationship. Cognitive-behaviour therapy, task-centred social work, brief solution–focused practices and strengths-based approaches (see Chapters 16–19) are unlikely to be effective unless the social worker can establish a relationship in which there is recognition, followed by acceptance, understanding, compassion, cooperation and finally collaboration with, in many cases, the prospect of hope. Most technical approaches only work when they rest on a bedrock of empathy, understanding and a good worker-client relationship (Howe, 2014).

Motivational interviewing (MI; see Chapter 20) offers a good example in which the twin elements of empathy and structure, feel secure and then explore and the need to be both responsive and systematic are present. The approach recognizes that clients first need to feel safe before they can go on to explore, problem-solve and change. In developing MI, Miller and Rollnick (2012) took a range of therapeutic insights from cognitive psychology, self-efficacy models and models of how we set about making changes and then married them with the more person-centred thinking of Carl Rogers (1957).

In collaboration with the client, the idea is to strengthen their motivation for, and commitment to change toward, a specific goal. 'Change talk' explores and picks up on the client's own ideas and arguments for change and then supports them. These ideas and arguments are drawn out of the client in the context of an empathic, collaborative relationship. Empathy facilitates change, and its absence frustrates it. A lack of empathy and the failure to create a caring relationship raise the client's anxiety. When clients are uncertain whether or not the social worker is interested in their feelings and point of view, they are likely to be more guarded. They begin to resist and become less inclined to cooperate. MI is a strengths-based approach that believes clients are capable of change if they really believe change is possible. Practitioners, therefore, focus on success, both past and present. Clients, of course, have to express a willingness and desire to change, even though they might be finding change difficult.

Conclusion

Baron-Cohen (2011) possibly went a little too far when he concluded that 'Empathy is like a universal solvent. Any problem immersed in empathy becomes soluble' (p. 127). There are certain situations when we need to put our empathy on hold, especially when we have to act quickly, be practical and not allow feelings to derail rational action. Surgeons in trauma units or social workers dealing with a physically abused toddler need to act quickly, rationally and practically. Empathic responses at such times need to be parked until the crisis is resolved.

At its best, though, empathy helps us to show compassion towards those who feel vulnerable and distressed. It underpins and supports our moral outlook. Some elements of empathy, however, particularly emotional empathy, do have a dark side. We tend to be most caring and empathic with people whom we are most alike. Empathy, particularly affective emotional empathy, tends to be easier between people of the same sex, age, class, ethnicity, race, ability or religion.

Lack of understanding is often greatest between people who are significantly different from one another. Lack of understanding can increase feelings of 'us' and 'them'. It can create in groups and out groups. When there are feelings of 'us' and 'them', there is a tendency to stereotype, homogenize and de-humanize those in the 'out group'. At times, we empathize with people we identify as being on the inside; we can be surprisingly harsh on others we deem alien and on the outside. Stereotyping other people denies them their individuality. It can deprive them of their humanity. It creates prejudice and can cloud moral judgement. It promotes *antipathy* and can lead to some of the worst, most violent and prejudiced behaviour.

More specifically, it is easiest to be empathic with an individual who presents us directly and immediately with their pain or sorrow, fear or outrage. We are much more likely to respond to human interest stories of individual cases than the general, abstract plight of whole communities. 'But the world', says Bloom (2017b), 'is not a simple place. One problem is that empathy is innumerate, favouring the one over the many'. Our heartstrings are tugged much more powerfully whenever we see the bleeding face of a war-wounded child or the haunted look of a grieving parent (Bloom, 2017a). It seems that the stronger our fellow feelings are for the individual in emotional pain, the more unfeeling, aggressive and punitive we feel towards those whom we believe caused the pain. Newspapers know all too well how to trigger our emotions when they picture the neglected child's sad face and report their tragic death. They also know that empathy for the one can lead to a profound lack of empathy for, and demonization of, the 'other' – the poverty-stressed, drug-using parents of the neglected child, the social workers who knew of the case, the health workers who failed to spot the broken bones and bruised arms (Jones, 2014; Shoesmith, 2016).

If these desensitizing tendencies are to be avoided, the social worker has to work hard at consciously promoting their own as well as other people's *cognitive* empathy and *social intelligence*. The more unlike the client is to them in terms of gender or race, age or religion, the more the social worker should try to see the world from the client's point of view. The social worker has to imagine what it must be like to be the client, to be in their shoes. Knowledge of the client's background, history, relationships and current circumstances should help the social worker think about what it might be like to be the other person: now, in this situation, with these people, under these pressures.

Clients who might not have had much experience of being on the receiving end of an empathic, emotionally intelligent relationship might find being empathic themselves difficult. They may not find it easy to see things from another person's point of view. This inability means that the 'give' and 'take' that normally facilitate a relationship tends to be erratic and unpredictable. The failure to moderate, adjust and take into account the other person's perspective can lead to behaviours that are defensive, hostile or withdrawn. Nevertheless, if the social worker can establish a relationship which offers the client a 'safe haven' and a 'secure base' it might be possible to help a defensive client begin to see the world from the other person's perspective, to think about their own as well as other people's state of mind.

Social intelligence might be increased by encouraging clients to 'wonder why'. Why do you think your elderly father seems to have lost interest in everything? You look so sad, as if you want to give up; are you thinking you've let your children down? There are also more formal techniques constructed to promote these reflective psychological skills. Mentalization-based therapies are designed to improve the social understanding and mentalizing skills of clients and patients so that they can recognize their own and other people's feelings, states of mind and intentions (Allen & Fonagy, 2006; Allen, Fonagy, & Bateman, 2008). And the idea of 'restorative justice' and 'truth and reconciliation' work is based on helping offenders, racists and prejudiced people see and understand how their crimes have affected those who have been victims of their anti-social, often violent behaviour.

As social workers we need to develop and maintain our social intelligence and rational compassion. Emotional intelligence and cognitive empathy sustain our willingness and ability to show care and be compassionate. We need to remain interested in and curious about other people and their lives. Books on psychology and sociology should not be left behind once our college days are over. Good quality fiction; engaging films; powerful drama, whether at the theatre or on television; stirring art and thoughtful poems can all feed our sensibilities. Case discussions with colleagues and reflective supervision are essential. If we are to remain professionally effective, it is important that we maintain interest in what goes on in our own and other people's heads and what takes place when the minds in those heads meet in the context of social, professional and everyday family relationships.

Recommended reading

Howe, D. (2012). *Empathy: What it is and why it matters*. Basingstoke: Palgrave Macmillan.
   Provides a general introduction to the concept and practice of empathy in the arts, sciences and helping professions, including social work.

Howe, D. (2014). *The compleat social worker*. Basingstoke: Palgrave Macmillan.
   Develops the argument that good social work is a combination of both social intelligence and evidence-informed practice, empathy and structure.

Payne, M. (2011), *Humanistic social work: Core principles in practice*. Basingstoke: Palgrave Macmillan.
   Promotes the idea that positive fulfilment in social relationships is a key aim of social work, one in which a fair and equal society might be promoted.

References

Allen, J., & Fonagy, P. (2006). *Handbook of mentalization-based treatment*. London: Wiley-Blackwell.
Allen, J., Fonagy, P., & Bateman, A. (2008). *Mentalizing in clinical practice*. Washington, DC: American Psychiatric Publishing.

David Howe

Banks, S. (2012). *Ethics and values in social work* (4th ed.). London: Palgrave Macmillan.

Baron-Cohen, S. (2011). *Zero degrees of empathy: A new theory of human cruelty.* London: Allen Lane.

Beckett, C., & Maynard, A. (2013). *Values and ethics in social work* (2nd ed.). London: Sage.

Biestek, F. (1961). *The casework relationship.* London: Allen & Unwin.

Bloom, P. (2017a). *Against empathy: The case for rational compassion.* London: Bodley Head.

Bloom, P. (2017b, 19 February). Think empathy makes the world a better place? Think again . . . *Observer*, p. 36.

Bowlby, J. (1988). *A secure base: Clinical applications of attachment theory.* London: Routledge.

Castonguay, L. G., & Beutler, L. E. (2006). Common and unique principles of therapeutic change: What do we know and what do we need to know? In L. G. Castonguay & L. E. Beutler (Eds.), *Principles of therapeutic change that work* (pp. 353–369). Oxford: Oxford University Press.

Clark, C. (2006). Moral character in social work. *British Journal of Social Work, 36*(1), 75–89.

Coplan, A. (2011). Understanding empathy: Its features and effects. In A. Coplan & P. Goldie (Eds.), *Empathy: Philosophical and psychological perspectives* (pp. 3–18). Oxford: Oxford University Press.

Davis, M. H. (1994). *Empathy: A social psychological approach.* Madison, WI: Brown and Benchmark.

Downie, R., & Telfer, E. (1969). *Respect for persons.* London: Routledge & Kegan Paul.

Dracopoulou, S. (2015). Major trends in applied ethics, including ethics in social work. In L. Bell & T. Hafford-Letchfield (Eds.), *Ethics, values and social work practice* (pp. 12–22). Maidenhead: Open University Press.

Featherstone, B. (2010). Ethic of care. In M. Gray & S. Webb (Eds.), *Ethics and value perspectives in social work* (pp. 73–84). Basingstoke: Palgrave Macmillan.

Featherstone, B., & Morris, K. (2013). Feminist ethics of care. In M. Gray, J. Midgely, & S. A. Webb (Eds.), *The Sage handbook of social work* (pp. 341–354). London: Sage.

Fonagy, P., Gergely, G., Jurist, E., & Target, M. (2002). *Affect regulation, mentalization, and the development of the psychological self.* New York: Other Press.

Fonagy, P., & Target, M. (1997). Perspectives on the recovered memory debate. In J. Sandler & P. Fonagy (Eds.), *Recovered memories of abuse: True or false?* (pp. 183–216). London: Karnac.

Gray, M. (2010). Moral sources and emergent ethical theories in social work. *British Journal of Social Work, 40*(6), 1794–1811.

Hennessey, R. (2011). *Relationship skills in social work.* London: Sage.

Hollway, W. (2006). *The capacity to care.* London: Routledge.

Houston, S. (2003). Establishing virtue in social work: A response to McBeath and Webb. *British Journal of Social Work, 33*(6), 819–824.

Howe, D. (1993). *On being a client: Understanding the process of counselling and psychotherapy.* London: Sage.

Howe, D. (2008). *The emotionally intelligent social worker.* Basingstoke: Palgrave Macmillan.

Howe, D. (2012). *Empathy: What it is and why it matters.* Basingstoke: Palgrave Macmillan.

Howe, D. (2014). *The compleat social worker.* Basingstoke: Palgrave Macmillan.

Jones, R. (2014). *The story of Baby P: Setting the record straight.* Bristol: Policy Press.

McCall Smith, A. (2015). *Emma: A modern retelling.* London: Borough Press.

McColgan, M. & McMullin, C. (Eds.) (2017). *Doing relationship-based social work.* London: Jessica Kingsley.

Megele, C. (2015). *Psychosocial and relationship-based practice.* St. Albans: Critical Publishing.

Meins, E., Fernyhough, C., Wainwright, R., Gupta, M., Fradley, E., & Tuckey, M. (2002). Maternal mind-mindedness and attachment security as predictors of theory of mind understanding. *Child Development, 73*(6), 1715–1726.

Miller, W. R., & Rollnick, S. (2012). *Motivational interviewing: Preparing people for change* (3rd ed.). New York: Guilford.

Noddings, N. (2003). *Caring: A feminine approach to ethics and moral education* (2nd ed.). Berkeley: University of California Press.

Payne, M. (2011). *Humanistic social work: Core principles in practice.* Basingstoke: Palgrave Macmillan.

Plant, R. (1970). *Social and moral theory in casework.* London: Routledge & Kegan Paul.

Ragg, N. (1977). *People not cases.* London: Routledge & Kegan Paul.

Reid, W., & Epstein, L. (1972). *Task-centred casework.* New York: Columbia University Press.

Rogers, C. (1957). The necessary and sufficient conditions of therapeutic personality change. *Journal of Consulting Psychology, 21*, 95–103.

Ruch, G., Turney, D., & Ward, A. (Eds.). (2010). *Relationship-based social work: Getting to the heart of practice.* London: Jessica Kingsley.

Shoesmith, S. (2016). *Learning from Baby P.* London: Jessica Kingsley.

Social Care Institute for Excellence. (2008). *SCIE practice guide 15: Dignity in care.* London: SCIE.

Tronto, J. (1993). *Moral boundaries.* London: Routledge.

Webb, S. (2010). Virtue ethics. In M. Gray & S. Webb (Eds.), *Ethics and value perspectives in social work* (pp. 108–119). Basingstoke: Palgrave Macmillan.

10

The interpretation of social justice, equality and inequality in social work

A view from the US

Michael Reisch

Introduction

Social justice has been a central normative component of social welfare and social work for over a century (Reamer, 2013). The *Code of Ethics* of the US National Association of Social Workers (NASW, 2017) explicitly states that the pursuit of social justice is an 'ethical imperative'. The International Federation of Social Workers (2014) makes a comparable assertion on its website: 'Principles of social justice, human rights, collective responsibility and respect for diversities are central to social work'. Yet the definition of this central tenet of practice is ambiguous, inconsistent and often in conflict with other goals, including social equality for excluded and marginalized populations (Reisch, 2008). To date, the profession has unsuccessfully attempted to resolve this conceptual and practical conflict despite repeated efforts by theorists from diverse ideological perspectives. This chapter explores the evolution of this conflict and its implications for contemporary social policies and social work practice.

Social justice, equality and social welfare: a brief history

Over several millennia, religious and secular views of social justice and equality throughout the world challenged, transformed or rationalized prevailing distributions of resources, power, status and opportunities. Although they all emphasized fairness, mutuality and loyalty, for the most part, they applied these values solely to people within the same community.

The 18th-century Enlightenment and the political revolutions of the 18th and 19th centuries expanded the meaning, if not the application, of these concepts. Subsequently, however, differences developed in the West between the Anglo-American emphasis on freedom and the continental emphasis on social solidarity. More recently, similar divisions emerged between the Western focus on universal, largely political rights and more culturally specific views of social justice and equality among developing nations. The diverse interpretation of these concepts reflects different assumptions about human nature, society and the state.

In the West, ideas about social justice and equality are closely associated with the concept of a social contract involving mutual rights and obligations that variously emphasize the preservation of individual liberty and property rights or the goal of social equality (Nozick, 1974; Tomasi, 2001). These distinctions have serious implications for modern social welfare systems (Roemer, 1996). Nevertheless, in the West a broad consensus exists that social justice involves a more equitable means of distributing societal goods (Miller, 1999). What constitutes 'fairness', whether it refers to individuals or groups and how it relates to the creation of a more egalitarian society remain subjects of considerable philosophical and practical contention (Nussbaum, 1999; O'Brien, 2011).

Contemporary perspectives on social justice and equality

Commentators usually frame debates over social justice and equality along a liberal-to-conservative spectrum, although contemporary interpretations of these concepts are complex. Over the past century, five major perspectives have framed Western discourse. Liberals focus on equal opportunity and the protection of political rights. Conservatives emphasize individual liberty, property rights and social stability. Communitarians stress social cooperation, trust and mutuality. Marxists or Social Democrats focus on socio-economic equality, the inevitability of change and the significance of culture. Postmodernists argue for the inclusion of marginalized groups and the development of socially just and egalitarian *processes*.

Sandel (2009) argues that three largely incompatible views of social justice currently exist: (1) utilitarianism, which seeks to maximize welfare to the greatest number of persons; (2) libertarianism, which prioritizes individual freedom; and (3) communitarianism, which focuses on virtue and the creation of the good life. In the practical realm, these philosophical approaches address two critical social functions, distribution and stability, and produce diverse views on the role of societal institutions in achieving social justice and equality. How to interpret and reconcile these concepts in increasingly diverse societies is, perhaps, the critical question for social workers in the decades ahead.

Philosophers have suggested several ways to resolve these differences. Rawls (1999, 2001) proposed a balance between equal individual and group rights and a more equitable distribution of opportunities and goods based on the principle of compensation. Conservatives would assign rights solely to individuals, not groups, and would limit these rights to the political sphere and the protection of property rights (Nozick, 1974). They also assert that social justice requires a balance between rights and responsibilities (Gilbert, 1995). Communitarians regard rampant individualism and the breakdown of community and morality as the major barriers to the attainment of social justice. Yet they have not specified how to apply this philosophy to practice (McNutt, 1997).

The 'capabilities approach' developed by Sen (2009) and Nussbaum (2011) represents an ambitious attempt to reconcile these conceptual conflicts by expanding Rawls's concept of distributive justice to include non-material 'goods' and the full participation of all individuals in key societal processes (Kim & Sherraden, 2014). In addition, Nussbaum highlights an issue both Rawls and Sen fail to address: that different individuals and groups in a society have different amounts of power. She argues that vulnerable populations cannot achieve their potential unless society corrects this power imbalance by enabling all people to acquire ten essential capabilities (Nussbaum, 2011). It would be challenging, however, to translate Nussbaum's ideas into policy or practice.

To date, most efforts to integrate these diverse perspectives into a coherent framework have not succeeded (Caputo, 2000). Similarly, little consensus exists about the balance between social justice (rights to social benefits) and equality (obligations to individuals or groups). There is general agreement nevertheless that justice and equality involve more than eliminating discriminatory laws to include provision for people's basic needs (Van Soest & Garcia, 2003).

To summarize, there are six current framings of these concepts:

1   Equal rights to intangibles such as freedom and equal opportunity to obtain social goods.
2   Equal distribution based on equal merit.
3   Equal distribution based on equal productivity.
4   Unequal distribution based on individual need.
5   Unequal distribution based on individual status.
6   Unequal distribution based on different 'contractual' arrangements.

Ryan (1981) simplified this list in two categories: approaches that emphasize 'fair play' versus those that stress 'fair shares'.

The welfare state and social justice

The emergence of the welfare state in the mid–20th century created a potential vehicle to advance social justice and equality through government intervention while strengthening social stability and the legitimacy of democratic institutions. For half a century, debates focused largely on how far to extend social rights and provide institutionalized compensation or redress (Titmuss, 1968). Since the 1970s, however, attacks on the welfare state have undermined its utility as an instrument for achieving social justice and equality.

Conservatives and neoliberals accused the welfare state of undermining freedom, personal choice, individual responsibility and motivation. Left-wing critics attacked the welfare state as an instrument of social control which primarily serves elite, corporate interests (Reisch, 2014a). Multiculturalists asserted that the welfare state ignored the specific needs of minorities and applied universal concepts of justice and equality without regard to different cultural norms (Banting & Kymlicka, 2006). Social workers must now consider the possibility that the goals of social justice and equality may not be compatible with the premises of the 20th-century welfare state.

European, North American and Australian social work scholars have addressed these issues to some extent (Hugman, 2008; Lorenz, 2014; Mullaly, 1997; Solas, 2008). They examined the effects of emerging paradigm shifts in policy and practice, the influence of market-oriented values on social services and changed meanings of professionalism. They have also analyzed the consequences of focusing on practice techniques instead of theoretical development and structural analysis.

Persistent questions further complicate this conceptual puzzle: How should societies achieve social justice and equality? Do these concepts apply to individuals or groups (Wakefield, 2014)? On what issues should they focus (Dominelli, 2012)? How can universal ideas about social justice and equality be reconciled with respect for cultural diversity (Reisch, Ife, & Weil, 2012)? Does the 'common good' even exist?

Social justice, equality and social work

Social workers in the US and UK first suggested social justice as a substitute for the traditional goals of charity at the turn of the 20th century. They proposed to replace hierarchical principles of charity with universal public standards of decency enforced by the state and rationalized by social scientific research (Addams, 1902; Wise, 1909). Their definition of social justice synthesized liberal, social democratic and moral principles (Holder, 1922). For most of the 20th century, this synthesis of individualistic and collectivist orientations formed the basis of Western social welfare (George & Wilding, 1994; Knight, 2005) and social work's dual focus on individual self-determination and social equity (Reisch, 2014a; Reynolds, 1951).

Yet, from the outset, the denial of citizenship rights to minority populations created obstacles to the translation of socially just and egalitarian principles into practice. Until recently, these frameworks largely excluded individuals who were not white heterosexual men. The profession's failure to overcome completely the influence of its hierarchical origins complicates its ability to work effectively with socially excluded groups (Kemp, 2014; Singer, 2014).

Several questionable assumptions compounded this difficulty. First, advocates for social justice and equality assumed that government-sponsored, modestly redistributive social provision would continue to reduce inequality by collectivizing the social costs of private enterprise. Second, they assumed that social workers' value-based goals required them to serve as benevolent instruments of the state without compromising their fundamental beliefs. Third, they assumed that social service 'commodities' differed from those produced by the for-profit system and, therefore, required different organizational structures and cultures. Until the late 1970s, these assumptions had some validity. Over the past four decades, however, economic globalization and major sociocultural changes have invalidated most of these assumptions with significant consequences for the foundations of social work practice.

From the origins of the profession, the failure of many social workers in the US to acknowledge the underlying contradictions of these assumptions produced several important developments. Socially excluded communities created services based on identity, not universal definitions of social justice and equality. In response to the profession's failure to recognize how 'universalist' rhetoric overlooked non-egalitarian concepts of race and gender (Drachsler, 1922), they emphasized mutual aid and self-help, concepts that mainstream social workers did not integrate into practice for decades (Beito, 2001; Chan, 1991; Iglehart & Becerra, 2013; Rivera, 1987).

Since the 1970s, many social workers have attempted to correct this historical omission by embracing the principle of distributive justice developed by Rawls (1999). Part of its appeal is its synthesis of two distinct philosophical traditions: the liberal tradition that emphasized self-determination and empowerment and the social democratic tradition, based on principles of mutuality and greater social equality (Lorenz, 2014). This synthesis appeared to be more open to alternative conceptions of need and helping and new criteria for evaluating the effectiveness of practice interventions (Green, 1999). More recently, social workers have sought to resolve this conceptual and practical dilemma through the incorporation of human rights into practice (Wronka, 2017).

Human rights, social justice and social work practice

The appeal of a human rights framework for a justice-oriented profession is obvious. Several social work scholars assert that a human rights framework complements the value of social justice because both emphasize the centrality of social cooperation, trust and mutuality (Flynn, 2013; Reichert, 2011). From this perspective, human rights offers a 'moral grounding for social work's more complex interpretations of social justice, equality, and empowerment' (Dewees & Roche, 2001, p. 137). Social work proponents of human rights also assert that they provide a comprehensive conceptual framework that addresses people's multidimensional needs (Healy, 2008) and promotes a focus on empowerment rather than individual pathology (Hawkins & San Marcos, 2009).

Although a human rights framework can be an effective bridging concept, some critics regard it as incompatible with social justice. Young (2011) argues that the pursuit of social justice requires more than universal rights that treat everyone identically. It requires basic changes in civil society and dominant cultural norms and values.

The most common criticisms of the human rights framework involve its Eurocentric bias (Reisch, 2014b) and its reflection of Western cultural and political hegemony (Akimoto, 2014; Thompson, 2014). Other criticism emerged within the West itself, based on perspectives as diverse as Marxism, postcolonial critiques of imperialism and postmodern arguments against the 'universalizing pretentions of Enlightenment thought' (Ignatieff, 2001, p. 105).

Some critics question the ability of the profession to apply this framework within established institutions (Murdach, 2011) or point out the distinction between rights and needs (Dewees & Roche, 2001). Others express concerns about opposition to rights-based tenets due to contested conceptual definitions (Reisch, 2002), the paucity of social work theories compatible with human rights (Payne, 2014), and the disjuncture between universalist human rights and the cultural relativism increasingly embodied in social work practice principles (Reisch, 2007).

While acknowledging the validity of these concerns, Wronka (2017) argues that the application of five human rights principles could resolve definitional ambiguities and clarify how to apply social justice principles to practice. These are: human dignity, non-discrimination; civil and political rights; economic, social and economic rights; and solidarity rights. Van Soest and Garcia (2003) assert that there is considerable compatibility between a focus on oppression and nine core human rights values: life; freedom and liberty, equality and non-discrimination, justice, solidarity, social responsibility, evolution, peace and non-violence, and reciprocal relations between humankind and nature (pp. 65–67). Ife (2010) proposed 'human rights from below' to resolve these dilemmas. His model preserves social work's long-standing commitment to ending injustices and inequalities yet avoids imposing hegemonic Western values by integrating local sources of knowledge and traditional cultural norms.

In sum, parallel discourses exist within social work. One focuses on the uncritical adoption of universal human rights principles, the other on group-specific inequalities rooted in social identity (Reisch, 2008). These differences emerged from the persistent conflict between universalist ideas about social justice and those that stress justice for specific oppressed groups (Kiehne, 2016). This conflict often puts the seemingly complementary values of social justice and equality in opposition to each other in nearly all areas of practice (McLaughlin, Gray, & Wilson, 2015).

Social justice vs. equality

During the early 20th century, the American conception of social justice expanded to include the reduction of social inequalities (Carson, 1990; Elshtain, 2002; Sklar, 1995). The patchwork social welfare system that emerged, however, reinforced gender and racial inequities, although it purported to advance the ideal of social justice (Abramovitz, 1999; Baynton, 2001; Schiele, 2013). Most social work leaders defined social justice in terms of political democracy and equality before the law, rather than equality of resources, status, opportunity or power. The isolation of most social workers from the populations with whom they worked prevented them from seriously considering concepts such as social equality (Lasch-Quinn, 1993).

Four distinct conflicts emerged: (1) between ideological homogeneity and heterogeneity, (2) between coerced assimilation and compulsory physical and social segregation, (3) between individual and group identity and rights and (4) over the meaning of citizenship (Carson, 1990; Johnson, 2001; Katz, 2001).

Most white social workers shared prevailing societal attitudes and could not embrace a vision of social justice that incorporated full social equality (Elshtain, 2002; Sklar, 1995). They failed to distinguish between the problems of European immigrants and those of African Americans or immigrants from Latin America or Asia (Stern & Axinn, 2013); they did not recognize that reducing social inequality required redistributive, non-egalitarian compensatory policies, not merely cultural assimilation (Lasch-Quinn, 1993; Salem, 1990; Hammond, 1920). The reforms the profession championed during the Progressive Era, around the turn of the century, and the New Deal, during the 1930s, therefore, had minimal impact on persons of colour and women. Only a few prominent leaders collaborated with African American scholars and activists, documented widespread discrimination against racial minorities and conducted research on the working conditions of women and girls (Reisch & Andrews, 2002).

In response, racial and ethnic minority groups consistently resisted coerced assimilation rationalized by social justice rhetoric because they feared it would destroy their cultural heritage. Wright (1920) argued that a socially just 'melting pot' was impossible without mutual respect, abolition of oppressive laws and institutions and establishment of equal rights and responsibilities. Perhaps the strongest argument for incorporating racial equality into universal conceptions of social justice in the 1920s appeared in the work of E. Franklin Frazier (1924). His ideas reflected a 'dual consciousness' regarding racial equality and social justice. It produced a 'dual agenda' among African Americans that distinguished their efforts to achieve social justice from those of their white allies (Hamilton & Hamilton, 1997).

Despite these efforts, the US took few steps towards racial or gender equality until the resurgence of the civil rights and feminist movements after World War II. These modest changes, however, focused primarily on eradicating discrimination, not on structural change (Valien, 1949, 1951). Social work researchers reinforced the tendency to view racial minorities and women through different lenses and to regard their 'deviance' from dominant cultural norms as distinct from class or religious differences (Barrabee, 1954). Consequently, policy advocacy focused more on 'fixing' these deficiencies than on addressing the structural roots of inequality.

Through the 1960s, most social service organizations largely ignored issues that affected racial and sexual minorities and women because of their physical and social segregation (Iglehart & Becerra, 2013). The first NASW *Code of Ethics* (1960) did not address racial equality and scant references to racism, sexism, sexual orientation and ability status appeared in social work literature until long after the decade's ferment subsided (Simon, 1994). It took NASW over a decade and a half after the modern civil rights movement emerged to take a forceful position against institutional racism and for social work scholars to address the practice implications of social justice ideals for women and people of colour. In fact, the emergence of so-called 'identity politics' produced increased tensions among social workers over goals and strategies and created a delicate problem to negotiate both intellectually and politically.

At the 1972 National Conference of Social Welfare, Dumpson (1972) proposed to shift the field's 'emphasis on individual pathology and rehabilitation' to 'the removal of socioeconomic and racial barriers to an equitable redistribution of the power, wealth, and income of the nation' (pp. 4–5). The movement for gender equality was particularly significant because for most of the 20th century the social work profession largely ignored issues of gender equality, particularly those of women of colour (Abramovitz, 1999). 'Selective' approaches to inequality and the resurgence of cultural and gender identity reinforced divisions within the profession (Chestang, 1970; De Anda, 1997; Morales, 1978). The shift Dumpson proposed never occurred.

The liberation movements of the 1960s, 1970s and 1980s, however, underlined the contradictions between the profession's social justice rhetoric and the focus of most practice on individual, family or community pathology, even when based on benign, if paternalistic, thinking.

The new social movements that appeared also altered the profession's vocabulary and practice focus (Lum, 2007; Devore & Schlesinger, 1996). Emerging theoretical frameworks analyzed issues through the lens of group rather than individual characteristics. They undermined efforts to establish a universal conceptual framework and obscured the relationship between social justice and equality (Gould, 1996). Few social workers could envision how an egalitarian, social justice–oriented conception of practice could emerge from this intellectual and cultural catharsis (Longres, 1997).

Nevertheless, mainstream theoretical constructs continued to presume the compatibility of social justice and equality (Caputo, 2000; Platt & Cooreman, 2001; Ramakrishnan & Balgopal, 1995). Yet an analysis of five contemporary theories of justice by Van Soest and Garcia (2003) identified only one that specifically addressed issues of race, ethnicity or culture. This distortion of social work theory continues to influence the education of practitioners (Bhuyan, Bejan, & Jeyapal, 2017). By contrast, alternative frameworks subsume a universal emphasis on social justice within the more immediate concerns created by group-specific inequalities and identity-based oppression, rather than broad structural analyses (De Anda, 1997; Goldberg, 2000).

Weaver (2014) takes this critique further. She asserts that while the injustices experienced by indigenous peoples are beyond dispute, the application of indigenous concepts of social justice to the goal of their liberation is somewhat ambiguous. She maintains that even well-intentioned efforts merely remediate these injustices and will never heal the damages caused by centuries of cultural domination, exploitation and genocide. This is why some social workers have called for the integration of indigenous concepts into contemporary views of justice (Calma & Priday, 2011; see Chapter 23).

Several unresolved issues complicate contemporary efforts to reconcile the concepts of social justice and equality in its theories and practice. One involves recognizing how the particular historical circumstances, needs and aspirations of marginalized groups shape their definitions of these concepts. A second is acknowledging how the professionalizing impulse has periodically fostered a search for universal theoretical frameworks that ignore the specific problems of minorities. A third issue is the persistent influence of cultural norms that stress individual responsibility and 'colour-blind' meritocratic principles (Young, 2011).

Social workers, therefore, must answer the following philosophical questions to develop practice models in which social justice and equality are complementary rather than conflicting goals: Are all inequalities equally unjust? How should we distinguish inequalities resulting from morally arbitrary contingencies from those produced by institutional discrimination? Should we measure equality in individual, group or societal terms? How can we balance respect for cultural differences with the creation of universal rights and greater equality? What types of interventions should we use to expand equality that do not compromise justice principles? (Fraser, 2012)

Implications for contemporary policy and practice

These conflicts have recently intensified in the social work field. The professional mainstream, influenced by neo-liberalism, continues to emphasize consensus approaches to social change, equality of opportunity not equity of outcomes and individual adjustment, now termed 'resilience' or problem amelioration ('evidence-based' interventions) instead of structural change (Reisch, 2013a). Although NASW recently embraced the concept of 'racial equity' (Kelly & Clark, 2009; NASW, 2013), it still endorses theoretical constructs that assume a benign relationship between individuals and the environment (Jani & Reisch, 2011).

In response, scholars from a broad range of ideological perspectives have increasingly criticized the theoretical foundations of practice (Potockey, 1997). Postmodernist critiques expand the concept of justice beyond a class-based perspective to include groups long denied the benefits of justice (Leonard, 1997). They stress the inclusion of excluded populations in socially just processes (Dominelli, 2010). Critical theorists like Fook (2014) and proponents of 'social justice feminism' have challenged the profession's cautious application of social justice (Gray, Agllias, & Davies, 2014).

Other social work scholars have criticized the positivist-empiricist and rationality-centred emphases of most contemporary social work research (Weick, 1999). Clinical social workers have connected the struggles for social justice and equality by integrating personal, political, professional and spiritual values and beliefs into their practice (Wakefield, 2014). Some argue that clinical social workers can engage in social justice work by eliminating oppressive practices in their agencies, developing client-centred programs and educating colleagues about social justice principles (Swenson, 1998).

Social workers in the macro arena have applied broadly defined concepts of social justice and equality to a variety of issues (Reisch, 2016; see Chapter 29). Some adopt a global perspective and connect social justice with opposition to economic globalization and militarism (Van Soest, 1994). Others emphasize the centrality of equality in the distribution of social goods to marginalized populations (Gibelman, 2000). Communitarians (McNutt, 1997) favour a balance between individual rights and responsibilities. Gal (2001) suggests that these different perspectives can be reconciled by using social policies to create horizontal equality in meeting needs while allowing the market to reward people for their efforts.

The combined effects of economic globalization, neo-liberalism and the profession's failure to overcome the influence of its quest for professional sanction and dominance further complicate the resolution of these differences (Dominelli, 2010; Fraser, 1995; George & Wilding, 2002). In different ways, the increase of involuntary clients, the expanded use of prescriptive individually oriented interventions, the narrow definition of 'evidence', the reluctance to become involved in politics or examine the effects of power and privilege on practice (Reisch & Garvin, 2016) and the persistence of inequalities even within qualitative research processes reflect these influences (Mikkonen, Laitinen, & Hill, 2016).

Conclusion

This overview of the struggle to clarify the meaning of social justice and equality for practice reveals several 'lessons' for the future. One is the tension between the application of social justice and equality in policy and practice and the acquisition of elite sanction. Perhaps more than any issue, the pursuit of enhanced occupational status continues to frustrate efforts to narrow the gap between the profession's rhetoric and practice realities (Wenocur & Reisch, 1989).

Another lesson is the need to incorporate selective policies and programs within a universal framework. A third is the importance of including marginalized populations as full and equal partners in *all phases* of policy and programme development and implementation and avoiding the reproduction of inequalities by using unjust means to achieve socially just goals (Gil, 2013). A fourth is that the translation of socially just ideals into practice is more likely to be realized when policies and programmes are guided by social democratic principles rather than market-oriented values (Marston, 2014). Fifth, the profession's greatest successes in implementing socially just and egalitarian values into practice have occurred when it incurred considerable professional and political risks. Finally, the most effective advocacy for social justice requires resisting the temptation to apply mono-cultural criteria to practice and recognizing its inherent political nature (Reisch & Jani, 2012).

Four significant obstacles to the attainment of these ideals, however, persist. The first involves the challenge of applying social justice and egalitarian principles in an institutional context based largely on the preservation of their opposites. The second concerns the difficulty of correcting injustices resulting from group membership through modes of intervention that focus primarily on individuals (Caputo, 2000; Katz, 2001; Prigoff, 2003). The third concerns the problem of translated contemporary concepts of justice and equality that include non-material resources and just participatory process into actual policy development and implementation. Finally, there is the growing need to overcome the reality – or perception – of resource scarcity produced by a combination of imposed fiscal austerity and the dominance of anti–social welfare, pseudo-populist ideology, often motivated by racial and nativist animus.

In the future, a socially just, egalitarian practice framework would include a re-emphasis on the structural analysis of society and its problems, with particular attention to the causes and consequences of inequality. It would include advocacy for programmes that diminish economic and physical insecurity and make vulnerable populations integral parts of society. It might even question the assumption that a universal idea of social justice exists (Witkin & Irving, 2014).

Practitioners and educators would acknowledge the significance of history, culture and context and the interconnectedness between domestic and international issues (Finn, 2015). They would integrate a critical perspective on the rationalizations for all forms of inequality and focus their practice on social transformation, not merely the amelioration of people's problems (Reisch, 2013b).

Despite these problems, there are hopeful signs throughout the world. Many social workers have reintroduced into their practice a broad social definition of health and an expanded awareness of the significance of the physical environment in well-being (Philip & Reisch, 2015). Using participatory action research, they have illuminated the structural origins of inequality and promoted expanded ideas of citizenship.

To take the risks involved in engaging in such activities, social workers have to confront several difficult truths. First, social justice and equality are complex, dynamic, conflict-laden and subjective concepts that look different in different contexts (Gasker & Fischer, 2014). Second, efforts to create a more just, egalitarian society can potentially reproduce injustice and inequality, albeit in different forms. Finally, the attainment of these long-standing goals will require sustained collective struggle particularly in the current inhospitable environment.

Further reading

The literature on social justice and equality is vast and ever growing. The following books explore the challenges involved in translating these ideals into policy and practice:

Finn, J. M. (2015). *Just practice: A social justice approach to social work* (3rd ed.). New York: Oxford University Press.
Reisch, M. (Ed.). (2014). *The Routledge international handbook of social justice*. London: Routledge. [Contains 36 annotated essays by international scholars from six continents.]
Reisch, M., & Garvin, C. (2016). *Social work practice and social justice: Concepts, challenges, and strategies*. New York: Oxford University Press.

References

Abramovitz, M. (1999). *Regulating the lives of women: U.S. social policy from colonial times to the present* (Rev. ed.). Boston: South End Press.
Addams, J. (1902). *Democracy and social ethics*. New York: Palgrave Macmillan.
Akimoto, T. (2014). Social justice in an era of globalization: Must and can it be the focus of social welfare policies? Japan as a case study. In M. Reisch (Ed.), *The Routledge international handbook of social justice* (pp. 48–60). London: Routledge.

Banting, K., & Kymlicka, W. (2006). *Multiculturalism and the welfare state: Recognition and redistribution in contemporary democracies*. New York: Oxford University Press.

Barrabee, P. (1954). How cultural factors affect family life. *Proceedings of the national conference on social welfare* (pp. 17–30). New York: Columbia University Press.

Baynton, D. C. (2001). Disability and the justification of inequality in American history. In P. K. Longmore & L. Umansky (Eds.), *The new disability history: American perspectives* (pp. 33–57). New York: New Press.

Beito, D. (2001). *From mutual aid to the welfare state: Fraternal societies and social services, 1890–1967*. Chapel Hill: University of North Carolina Press.

Bhuyan, R., Bejan, R., & Jeyapal, D. (2017). Social workers' perspectives on social justice in social work education: When mainstreaming social justice masks structural inequalities. *Social Work Education, 36*(4), 373–390.

Calma, T., & Priday, E. (2011). Putting indigenous human rights into social work practice. *Australian Social Work, 64*(2), 147–155.

Caputo, R. (2000). Multiculturalism and social justice: An attempt to reconcile the irreconcilable within a pragmatic liberal framework. *Race, Gender, and Class, 7*(4), 161–182.

Carson, M. J. (1990). *Settlement folk: Social thought and the American settlement movement, 1885–1930*. Chicago: University of Chicago Press.

Chan, S. (1991). *Asian Americans: An interpretive history*. Boston: Twayne.

Chestang, L. W. (1970). The issue of race in casework practice. *Social Work Practice* (pp. 14–26). New York: Columbia University Press.

De Anda, D. (Ed.). (1997). *Controversial issues in multiculturalism*. Needham Heights, MA: Allyn & Bacon.

Devore, W., & Schlesinger, E. G. (1996). *Ethnic-sensitive social work practice* (4th ed.). Boston: Allyn & Bacon.

Dewees, M., & Roche, S. E. (2001). Teaching about human rights in social work. *Journal of Teaching in Social Work, 21*(1/2), 137–155.

Dominelli, L. (2010). *Social work in a globalizing world*. Cambridge, MA: Polity.

Dominelli, L. (2012). *Green social work: From environmental crises to environmental justice*. Cambridge, MA: Polity.

Drachsler, J. (1922). Racial diversities and social progress. *Proceedings of the national conference on social work* (pp. 97–105). New York: National Conference.

Dumpson, J. (1972). Breaking the barriers to an open society. *Proceedings of the annual forum of the national conference on social welfare* (pp. 3–19). New York: Columbia University Press.

Elshtain, J. B. (2002). *Jane Addams and the dream of American democracy: A life*. New York: Basic Books.

Finn, J. M. (2015). *Just practice: A social justice approach to social work* (3rd ed.). New York: Oxford University Press.

Flynn, E. (2013). Making human rights meaningful for people with disabilities: Advocacy, access to justice and equality before the law. *International Journal of Human Rights, 17*(4), 491–510.

Fook, J. (2014). Social justice and critical theory. In M. Reisch (Ed.), *The Routledge international handbook of social justice* (pp. 160–172). London: Routledge.

Fraser, N. (1995). From redistribution to recognition? Dilemmas of justice in a post-socialist age. *New Left Review, 212*, 68–93.

Fraser, N. (2012, March–April). On justice. *New Left Review, 74*.

Frazier, E. F. (1924, April). Social work in race relations. *The Crisis, 27*.

Gal, J. (2001). The perils of compensation in social welfare policy. *Social Service Review, 75*(2), 225–244.

Gasker, J. A., & Fischer, A. C. (2014). Toward a context-specific definition of social justice for social work: In search of overlapping consensus. *Journal of Social Work Values and Ethics, 11*(1), 42–53.

George, V., & Wilding, P. (1994). *Ideology and social welfare*. New York: Palgrave Macmillan.

George, V., & Wilding, P. (2002). *Globalization and human welfare*. New York: Palgrave Macmillan.

Gibelman, M. (2000). Affirmative action at the crossroads: A social justice perspective. *Journal of Sociology and Social Welfare, 27*(1), 153–174.

Gil, D. G. (2013). *Confronting injustice and oppression: Concepts and strategies for social workers* (Updated ed.). New York: Columbia University Press.

Gilbert, N. (1995). *Welfare justice: Restoring social equity*. New Haven: Yale University Press.

Goldberg, M. (2000). Conflicting principles in multicultural social work. *Families in Society, 81*(1), 12–20.

Gould, K. H. (1996). The misconstruing of multiculturalism: The standard debate and social work. In P. L. Ewalt, E. M. Freeman, S. A. Kirk, & D. L. Poole (Eds.), *Multicultural issues in social work* (pp. 29–42). Washington, DC: NASW Press.

Michael Reisch

Gray, M., Agllias, K., & Davies, K. (2014). Social justice feminism. In M. Reisch (Ed.), *The Routledge international handbook of social justice* (pp. 173–187). London: Routledge.

Green, J. W. (1999). *Cultural awareness in the human services: A multi-cultural approach* (3rd ed.). Needham Heights, MA: Allyn and Bacon.

Hamilton, D. C., & Hamilton, C. V. (1997). *The dual agenda: The African American struggle for civil and economic equality*. New York: Columbia University Press.

Hammond, L. H. (1920). *Interracial cooperation: Helpful suggestions concerning relations of white and coloured citizens*. New York: National Board of the YWCA.

Hawkins, C., & San Marcos, T. X. (2009). Global citizenship: A model for teaching universal human rights in social work education. *Critical Social Work, 10*(1), Online. Retrieved from http://www1.uwindsor.ca/criticalsocialwork/global-citizenship-a-model-for-teaching-universal-human-rights-in-social-work-education

Healy, L. M. (2008). Exploring the history of social work as a human rights profession. *International Social Work, 51*(6), 735–748.

Hendricks, H. A. (1937). Social needs of Indian children. *Social Service Review, 11*(1), 52–65.

Holder, A. C. (1922). *The settlement idea: A vision of social justice*. New York: Macmillan.

Hugman, R. (2008). Social work values: Equity or equality: A response to Solas. *Australian Social Work, 61*(2), 141–145.

Ife, J. (2010). *Human rights from below: Achieving rights through community development*. New York: Cambridge University Press.

Iglehart, A., & Becerra, R. M. (2013). *Social services and the ethnic community* (2nd ed.). Boston: Allyn & Bacon.

Ignatieff, M. (2001). The attack on human rights. *Foreign Affairs, 80*(6), 102–116.

International Federation of Social Workers. (2014). *Global definition of social work*. Retrieved from http://ifsw.org/get-involved/global-definition-of-social-work/

Jani, J. S., & Reisch, M. (2011). Common human needs, uncommon solutions: Applying a critical framework to perspectives on human behavior. *Families in Society, 92*(1), 13–20.

Johnson, A. (2001). *Privilege, power, and difference*. Mountain View, CA: Mayfield.

Katz, M. B. (2001). *The price of citizenship: Redefining the American welfare state*. New York: Holt.

Kelly, J. J., & Clark, E. J. (Eds.). (2009). *Social work speaks: National association of social workers policy statements, 2009–2012*. Washington, DC: NASW Press.

Kemp, S. P. (2014). Social justice for children and youth. In M. Reisch (Ed.), *The Routledge international handbook of social justice* (pp. 286–299). London: Routledge.

Kiehne, E. (2016). Latino critical perspective in social work. *Social Work, 61*(2), 119–126.

Kim, S-M., & Sherraden, M. (2014). The capability approach and social justice. In M. Reisch (Ed.), *The Routledge international handbook of social justice* (pp. 202–215). London: Routledge.

Knight, L. W. (2005). *Citizen: Jane Addams and the struggle for democracy*. Chicago: University of Chicago Press.

Lasch-Quinn, E. (1993). *Black neighbors: Race and the limits of reform in the American settlement house movement, 1880–1945*. Chapel Hill: University of North Carolina Press.

Leonard, P. (1997). *Postmodern welfare: Reconstructing an emancipatory project*. Thousand Oaks, CA: Pine Forge.

Longres, J. (1997). The impact and implications of multiculturalism. In M. Reisch & E. Gambrill (Eds.), *Social work in the twenty-first century* (pp. 39–47). Thousand Oaks, CA: Pine Forge.

Lorenz, W. (2014). The emergence of social justice in the West. In M. Reisch (Ed.), *The Routledge international handbook of social justice* (pp. 14–26). London: Routledge.

Lum, D. (Ed.). (2007). *Culturally competent practice: A framework for understanding diverse groups and justice issues* (3rd ed.). Belmont, CA: Thompson/Brooks Cole.

Marston, G. (2014). Social justice and income support policies. In M. Reisch (Ed.), *The Routledge international handbook of social justice* (pp. 237–248). London: Routledge.

McLaughlin, A. M., Gray, E., & Wilson, M. (2015, December). Child welfare workers and social justice: Mending the disconnect. *Children and Youth Services Review, 59*, 177–183.

McNutt, J. (1997). New communitarian thought and the future of social policy. *Journal of Sociology and Social Welfare, 24*(4), 45–56.

Mikkonen, E., Laitinen, M., & Hill, C. (2016). Hierarchies of knowledge: Analyzing inequalities within the social work ethnographic research process as ethical notions in knowledge production. *Qualitative Social Work, 16*(4), 515–532.

Miller, D. (1999). *Principles of social justice*. Cambridge, MA: Harvard University Press.

Morales, A. (1978). Institutional racism in mental health and criminal justice. *Social Casework, 59*(7), 387–395.

Mullaly, R. (1997). *Structural social work: Ideology, theory, and practice* (2nd ed.). New York: Oxford University Press.

Murdach, A. D. (2011). Is social work a human rights profession? *Social Work, 56*(3), 281–283.

National Association of Social Workers. (1960). *Code of ethics*. Silver Spring, MD: Author.

National Association of Social Workers. (2013). *Achieving racial equity: Calling the profession to action*. Washington, DC: Author.

National Association of Social Workers. (2017). *Code of ethics* (Rev. ed.). Washington, DC: Author.

Nozick, R. (1974). *Anarchy, state, and utopia*. New York: Basic Books.

Nussbaum, M. C. (1999). *Sex and social justice*. New York: Oxford University Press.

O'Brien, M. (2011). Equality and fairness: Linking social justice and social work practice. *Journal of Social Work, 11*(2), 143–158.

Payne, M. (2014). *Modern social work theory* (4th ed.). Chicago: Lyceum Books.

Philip, D., & Reisch, M. (2015). Rethinking social work's interpretation of 'environmental justice': From local to global. *Social Work Education, 34*(5), 471–483.

Platt, A. M., & Cooreman, J. L. (2001). A multicultural chronology of welfare policy and social work in the United States. *Social Justice, 28*(1), 91–137.

Potockey, M. (1997). Multicultural social work in the United States: A review and critique. *International Social Work, 40*(1), 315–326.

Prigoff, A. W. (2003). Social justice framework. In J. Anderson & R. W. Carter (Eds.), *Diversity perspectives for social work practice* (pp. 113–120). Boston: Allyn & Bacon.

Ramakrishnan, K. R., & Balgopal, P. R. (1995). Role of social institutions in a multicultural society. *Journal of Sociology and Social Work, 22*(1), 11–28.

Rawls, J. (1999). *A theory of justice* (Rev. ed.). Cambridge, MA: Harvard University Press.

Rawls, J. (2001). *Justice as fairness: A restatement*. Cambridge, MA: The Belknap Press of Harvard University Press.

Reamer, F. G. (2013). *Social work values and ethics* (4th ed.). New York: Columbia University Press.

Reichert, E. D. (2011). *Social work and human rights: A foundation for policy and practice* (2nd ed.). New York: Columbia University Press.

Reisch, M. (2002). Defining social justice in a socially unjust world. *Families in Society, 83*(4), 343–354.

Reisch, M. (2007). Social justice and multiculturalism: Persistent tensions in the history of US social welfare and social work. *Studies in Social Justice, 1*(1), 67–92.

Reisch, M. (2008). From melting pot to multiculturalism: The impact of racial and ethnic diversity on social work and social justice in the U.S. *British Journal of Social Work, 38*(4), 788–804.

Reisch, M. (2013a). Social work education and the neoliberal challenge: The US response to increasing global inequality. *Social Work Education, 32*(6), 217–233.

Reisch, M. (2013b). What is the future of social work? *Critical and Radical Social Work, 1*(1), 67–85.

Reisch, M. (2014a). Social justice and liberalism. In M. Reisch (Ed.), *The Routledge international handbook of social justice* (pp. 132–146). London: Routledge.

Reisch, M. (2014b). The boundaries of justice: Addressing the conflict between human rights and multiculturalism in social work practice and education. In K. Libal, L. Healy, M. Berthold, & R. Thomas (Eds.), *Advancing human rights in social work education* (pp. 177–195). Alexandria, VA: Council on Social Work Education.

Reisch, M. (2016). Why macro practice matters. *Journal of Social Work Education, 52*(3), 1–11.

Reisch, M., & Andrews, J. L. (2002). *The road not taken: A history of radical social work in the United States*. Philadelphia: Brunner-Routledge.

Reisch, M., & Garvin, C. (2016). *Social work practice and social justice: Concepts, challenges, and strategies*. New York: Oxford University Press.

Reisch, M., Ife, J., & Weil, M. (2012). Social justice, human rights, values, and community practice. In M. Weil, M. Reisch, & M. Ohmer (Eds.), *Handbook of community practice* (2nd ed., pp. 73–103). Thousand Oaks, CA: Sage.

Reisch, M., & Jani, J. S. (2012). The new politics of social work practice: Understanding context to promote change. *British Journal of Social Work, 42*(6), 1132–1150.

Reynolds, B. C. (1951). *Social work and social living*. New York: Citadel Press.

Rivera, J. A. (1987). Self-help as mutual protection: The development of Hispanic fraternal benefit societies. *Journal of Applied Behavioral Science, 23*(3), 387–396.

Roemer, J. E. (1996). *Theories of distributive justice*. Cambridge, MA: Harvard University Press.

Ryan, W. (1981). *Equality*. New York: Pantheon.

Salem, D. (1990). *To better our world: Black women in organized reform, 1890–1920*. Brooklyn, NY: Carlson.

Sandel, M. J. (2009). *Justice: What's the right thing to do?* New York: Farrar, Straus and Giroux.

Schiele, J. H. (Ed.). (2013). *Social welfare policy: Regulation and resistance among people of color*. Los Angeles: Sage.

Sen, A. (2009). *The idea of justice*. Cambridge, MA: Belknap Press of Harvard University Press.

Simon, B. L. (1994). *The empowerment tradition in American social work*. New York: Columbia University Press.

Singer, J. (2014). Housing, homelessness, and social justice: Not fate but what we make. In M. Reisch (Ed.), *The Routledge international handbook of social justice* (pp. 300–318). Abingdon: Routledge.

Sklar, K. K. (1995). *Florence Kelley and the nation's work*. New Haven: Yale University Press.

Solas, J. (2008). Social work and social justice: What are we fighting for? *Australian Social Work, 61*(2), 124–136.

Stern, M., & Axinn, J. (2013). *Social work: A history of the American response to need* (8th ed.). Boston: Allyn & Bacon.

Swenson, C. R. (1998). Clinical social work's contribution to a social justice perspective. *Social Work, 43*(6), 527–537.

Titmuss, R. M. (1968). *Commitment to welfare*. Boston: Beacon.

Thompson, E. F. (2014). Social justice in the Middle East. In M. Reisch (Ed.), *The Routledge international handbook of social justice* (pp. 61–73). London: Routledge.

Tomasi, J. (2001). *Liberalism beyond justice: Citizens, society, and the boundaries of political theory*. Princeton, NJ: Princeton University Press.

Valien, P. (1949[1951]). Racial programs in social work. In M. B. Hodges (Ed.), *Social work year book, 1949, 1951*. Albany, NY: Boyd.

Van Soest, D. (1994). Strange bedfellows: A call for reordering national priorities from three social justice perspectives. *Social Work, 39*(6), 710–717.

Van Soest, D., & Garcia, B. (2003). *Diversity education for social justice: Mastering teaching skills*. Alexandria, VA: Council on Social Work Education.

Wakefield, J. C. (2014). Psychological justice: Distributive justice and psychiatric treatment of the non-disordered. In M. Reisch (Ed.), *The Routledge international handbook of social justice* (pp. 353–384). London: Routledge.

Weaver, H. N. (2014). Indigenous struggles for justice: Restoring balance within the context of Anglo settler societies. In M. Reisch (Ed.), *The Routledge international handbook of social justice* (pp. 111–122). London: Routledge.

Weick, A. (1999). Guilty knowledge. *Families in Society, 80*(4), 327–332.

Wenocur, S., & Reisch, M. (1989). *From charity to enterprise: The development of American social work in a market economy*. Urbana: University of Illinois Press.

Wise, S. S. (1909). The conference sermon: Charity versus justice. *Proceedings of the national conference of charities and corrections* (pp. 20–29). Fort Wayne, IN: Fort Wayne.

Witkin, S. L., & Irving, A. (2014). Post-modern perspectives on social justice. In M. Reisch (Ed.), *The Routledge international handbook of social justice* (pp. 188–201). London: Routledge.

Wright, R. R. (1920). What does the Negro want in our democracy? *Proceedings of the national conference of social work* (pp. 539–545). New York: National Conference.

Wronka, J. (2017). *Human rights and social justice: Social action and service for the helping and health professions* (2nd ed.). Thousand Oaks, CA: Sage.

Young, I. M. (2011). *Responsibility for justice*. New York: Oxford University Press.

11

Spirituality and secularity

Beth R. Crisp

Introduction

On matters associated with religion and spirituality, the question has been raised: 'Who tells social work's story?' (Vanderwoerd, 2011, p. 237). While the questioner argues that it should be social workers telling their own story rather than scholars from other disciplines, the experiences and perspectives of social workers on these issues are diverse and positionality may be critical in interpreting the stories which are told. Much of the social work literature on religion and spirituality has emerged from the UK and the US, but the concerns of social workers in these countries not only differ from those of their colleagues elsewhere, but also differ from each other (Crisp, 2017). Perspectives from social workers from former colonies differ from those of their colleagues in the UK (Stirling, Furman, Benson, Canda, & Grimwood, 2010), and even within the UK, the story varies for social workers in England, Scotland, Wales and Northern Ireland (Carlisle, 2016; Whiting, 2008).

This chapter seeks to provide a perspective on the impact of secularity and, more recently, postsecularity on social work as a profession, as well as considering the place of spirituality within social work practice, including that which occurs in faith-based organizations. Authored by an Australian social worker who identifies as Christian, this perspective, although contestable, may differ from but is arguably just as valid as any proposed by social workers from other countries or holding other religious beliefs. Prior to such discussions, it will first be necessary to discuss what is meant by 'secularity' and 'spirituality'.

What is secularity?

Secularity can be understood in different ways. At its most basic, the notion of secularity requires an understanding that there are realms or domains of life which are outside or separate to those which are perceived as being legitimately religious (Shook, 2010). In civil society, this is sometimes understood as the distinguishing of society into separate public and private spheres, with religion placed firmly in the latter (Taylor, 2007). Consequently, the existence of a secular state has come to be regarded as 'a necessary though not a sufficient condition for guaranteeing equal religious freedom for everybody' (Habermas, 2006, p. 4). Nevertheless, secularity does not imply hostility to religion although such assumptions are sometimes made (Modood, 2012).

In practice, it is less easy to divide the secular from the religious than it is in theory. Religious and secular values often coincide. What is proposed as secular often has a religious basis. For example, codes of human rights and legislation are typically secular guidelines for good conduct, but while the language is secular, the ideas are often rooted in religious values (Jivraj & Herman, 2009). Hence, 'it is undeniably true that in terms of vocabulary, concepts and institutional practices, each country in Western Europe is a secular state, but each has its own distinctive take on what this means' (Modood, 2012, p. 136). Whereas radical secularism demands absolute separation between the state and religion, moderate secularism allows for the accommodation of organized religion to serve the public good in cooperation with the state (Modood, 2013).

Another common understanding of secularity within a society is low levels of participation in formal religion (Taylor, 2007). Yet this must be balanced with the reality that five out of six people living on earth (84 percent) report identifying with one of the world's religions (Pew Research Center, 2012), although such affiliation may reflect cultural or other factors rather than religious beliefs (Crisp, 2010). Furthermore, expectations that religious sources of support should be accessible to all members of the community when they require it raises questions as to the extent religious participation is a relevant indicator of secularity (Collicutt, 2015). Davie's (1994) notion of 'believing without belonging', based on her finding that more than two-thirds of Britons were willing to claim a belief despite fewer than one in ten attending religious services, raises similar questions.

Secularity and social work

Professional social work in the English-speaking first world emerged as part of the broader secularization which occurred in the final decades of the 19th and early part of the 20th centuries. Until this time, welfare recipients were perceived as being morally deficient and in need of religious reform. Early social work rejected the notion that spiritual salvation was what those who were poor most needed. Consequently:

> . . . reducing charity to the pursuit of social rather than religious objectives, and in excising the evangelistic components . . . made possible the rational application of social scientific knowledge to the solution of social problems . . . A secular approach to charity produced a professional approach to social work.
>
> *(Bowpitt, 1998, p. 683)*

This professional approach was based on the premise that:

> Rational distancing from thoughts and emotions is used in cognitive – behavioural therapy to move towards fulfilment for the self. In the humanist view, spiritual or religious ideas are extraneous at best or pathological at worst.
>
> *(King & Leavey, 2010, p. 191)*

Such an approach sought to replace approaches underpinned by religious judgements with a form of professional practice which promoted respect for individuals and their resilience. This means, in the words of one respondent in a survey of UK social workers, 'there is no room for religion or spirituality or cooking tips in social work' (Furman, Benson, Grimwood, & Canda, 2004, p. 780). Hence, the generally accepted view among social workers for much of the 20th century was that:

> To fulfil its professional mission, social work must maintain itself as an essentially secular discipline. As a profession, social workers must strive to remain neutral toward any and all particular forms of religious and spiritual expression, even while recognizing the importance of such expression in human life.
>
> *(Liechty, 2013, p. 124)*

If the emergence of social work as a secular profession was intentional and didn't just happen by chance, so too were efforts to ensure secularity remained a professional hallmark such that it was lamented that 'the literature of the profession genially and serenely ignores religion' (Marty, 1980, p. 465). Social work practitioners have likewise tended to ignore or sidestep matters of religion, either having little knowledge or understanding of religious ideas and practices or not being equipped to address these issues within their professional practice (Cook, 2010).

Some authors have argued that this need to separate the profession from religion went as far as rewriting the history of social work by erasing any mention of its religious antecedents:

> According to the secularisation narrative, social work's Christian roots were anathema to its continued progress toward professionalization, and thus the histories that were told in the textbooks and journals of the emerging social work profession downplayed its Christian roots.
>
> *(Vanderwoerd, 2011, p. 238)*

Hence, the language of social work is decidedly secular, even when concurring with religious sentiments (Manthorpe, Harris, Samsi, & Moriarty, 2017). Religion is also conflated with ethnicity, such that matters of religion are treated as differences within a multicultural society rather than as being of theological significance (Jivraj & Herman, 2009). For individuals with a desire to work with what in religious language might be the 'poor and afflicted' but whose personal experiences of religion have been unfavourable, social work is the secular alternative to a religious vocation (Furman et al., 2004). Conversely, while there are many social workers whose decision to enter the profession has been influenced by their religious beliefs (Crisp, 2010), the religious social worker typically finds the workplace demands 'her theology is kept hidden and to all intents and purposes she is a practical atheist' (Whiting, 2008, p. 77). Social workers who identify as religious often accept the expectation that they never admit their religious beliefs and practices in the workplace (Elliott, 2017).

Hodge (2009) coined the phrase 'secular privilege' whereby secular identities, behaviours and practices are portrayed as normative, with religion to be unacknowledged or even deliberately obscured:

> Secular people . . . can expect their attempts to limit others' choices will be depicted favorably, that their legislative efforts will be depicted as a form of social justice. Conversely, identical efforts by people of faith to promote their perception of the common good are frequently labeled negatively . . .
>
> *(Hodge, 2009, p. 20)*

Not only do social workers who are religious perceive that they need to remain guarded about this aspect of themselves, but so too do many service users. This is particularly so in contexts where mental health has been associated with secularity and mental illness with religious beliefs and practices (Hodge, 2009) or with putting children at risk or in need of protection (Jivraj & Herman, 2009). While ensuring religion remains private may be protective for individual social workers and service users, the absence of religion in the public sphere may contribute to rein-forcing negative stereotypes being perpetuated (Cowden & Singh, 2017).

It is nevertheless recognized that individuals and organizations acting in the name of religion do at times challenge social cohesion and have provided additional rationales for secularism in social work (Cowden & Singh, 2017). For example, where religion has been integral to civil unrest, such as in Northern Ireland, the deep mistrust of anything associated with religion has prompted social workers to be perceived intentionally as neutral and non-sectarian. This has not just led to avoidance of matters associated with religion, even when directly pertinent to the experiences of service users (Carlisle, 2016).

Yet even in its most secular incarnations, social work has never entirely managed to displace religion. Where there are limited community resources, faith-based welfare providers may be perceived in terms of their capacity for charitable works and their religious faith overlooked (Jawad, 2012). Also, in some fields of practice, such as palliative care or foster care, at times of bereavement, social workers may be much more comfortable raising issues of religion and spir-ituality as a possible resource for service users, although the extent to which this occurs varies between countries (Stirling et al., 2010; see also Chapter 41).

From secularity to postsecularity

The 21st century has seen considerable rethinking about the applicability of the secularization agenda which sought to displace religion from public life. Whereas secularity embraced a desire to view religion as irrelevant, postsecularity is arguably a reality check:

> Today, public consciousness in Europe can be described in terms of a 'post-secular society' to the extent that at present it still has to 'adjust itself to the continued existence of religious communities in an increasingly secularized environment.' . . . The description of modern societies as 'post-secular' refers to a change in consciousness . . .
>
> *(Habermas, 2008, pp. 19–20)*

Postsecularity does not privilege either religious or secular viewpoints but recognizes both the merits and risks of both religious and secular thinking. Respect (see Chapter 9) rather than agreement with religious views denotes the postsecular (i.e. the need for tolerance and dialogue that nevertheless allows for religious beliefs to be considered as potentially either a cause or context of both liberation and oppression) (Fardella, 2017). This respect includes according indi-viduals and groups the right to use religious language in the public sphere to express sentiments which they cannot adequately express in secular language (Habermas, 2006).

In terms of welfare delivery, in a postsecular society, all religions are awarded the same privi-leges by the state (Gärde, 2015) and are not unfairly excluded from government funding or other opportunities (Jawad, 2012). In some countries the state has actively sought to partner with religious groups in service delivery (Gärde, 2015) as such partnerships may be crucial in providing services to 'hard-to-reach' communities. However, religious literacy by state authori-ties is often low, limiting both dialogue and the potential of any partnerships which are devel-oped (Jawad, 2012). Limited religious literacy has also resulted in 'multiculturalism' becoming rebranded as 'multifaithism' in public policy and practice (Cowden & Singh, 2017) although ethnicity and religion do not necessarily correlate.

Apart from providing legitimation for partnering with religious organizations, postsecularity also recognizes the integral place that spirituality has in the human experience (Hodge, 2012). Within professions such as social work, underpinned by the rise of science over religion and superstitions, rigid secularity has been found to be unduly simplistic because it negates the need for experiences of transcendence, ecstasy and mysticism (King & Leavey, 2010). At the same time, there has been a growing recognition, albeit strongly debated, that people who are not religious can be spiritual (Cook, 2010).

What is spirituality?

Spiritual traditions and practices present in both organized religion and movements concerned with the transcendental which occur outside religion, such as New Age (Hodge, 2012). Therefore, if it is not the same as religion, it is necessary to define spirituality. In doing so, it is necessary to acknowledge both that individuals who identify as 'spiritual' may also identify as 'religious' and that those who intentionally want to distance themselves from a religion may be wanting to do so from a religion other than Christianity:

> The 'spiritual-but-not-religious' discourse may speak well to the need of many people of Euro-Christian background to distance themselves from their Christian religion. As educators and practitioners, however, it is important that we do not make this stance the dominant and defining discourse of spirituality and religion in social work.
>
> *(Wong & Vinsky, 2009, p. 1356)*

Responding to such concerns, my working definition is as follows:

> Spirituality involves an awareness of the other, which may be God or other human or divine beings or something else, which provides the basis for us to establish our needs and desires for, understand our experiences of, and ask questions about, meaning, identity, connectedness, transformation and transcendence. While for some individuals these concerns will be integrally associated with their religious beliefs, and may only make sense within a specific religious framework, meaning, identity, connectedness, transformation and transcendence are intrinsic to the human experience, whether or not individuals regard these to be in the realm of spirituality.
>
> *(Crisp, 2010, p. 7)*

Being understood in terms of universal experiences such as needs for meaning, identity, connectedness, transformation and transcendence enables spirituality to be recognized as a normal part of human life rather than pathologized, as is the wont of secularism. While such an understanding is open to the criticism that spirituality has been reduced to be no more than a factor in individual psychological growth (Robertson, 2015), for many people their spirituality and religion are inseparable. In addition to being experienced within or outside a religious framework, spirituality can be understood at both individual and community levels (Perkins, 2015).

The emergence of spirituality in social work

Over the past two decades, there has been a growing interest in spirituality within the social work literature, suggesting a new legitimacy. To some extent this reflects broader changes in society and the emergence of postsecularity:

> . . . the rise of spirituality in social work . . . can also be linked to the failures of modernity and its depersonalising and alienating effects through the detraditionalisation and

secularisation of society, the rise of science, rationality, the professions, and industrial progress, and the decline in religion.

(Grey, 2008, p. 192)

Spirituality is now embraced by some social workers on the basis that holistic care cannot neglect the spiritual (Liechty, 2013). As such, it has been argued that attending to matters of spirituality is no more than good practice:

It comes down to good relationship-based practice. Social work touches at many points on the meaning we attach to our lives and it can be seen as a secular but spiritually attuned profession. Start where the client is, listen attentively with empathy, build relationships and be alert to narrative . . .

(Elliott, 2017, p. 97)

It is only in the 21st century that it has been acknowledged that newly qualified social workers require a basic understanding of religion and spirituality as part of their professional education (IASSW & IFSW, 2004). Legitimation by the state and other regulatory bodies that spirituality is important may encourage social workers to take this into account (Stirling et al., 2010). Other explanations which have been put forward for a renewed interest in spirituality among social workers include this being a response to the dehumanization and managerialism of social work (Garrett, 2014), increasing recognition of the need for and demands of environmental sustainability and the need to value and respect indigenous cultures in social work practice (Grey, 2008).

While recognition of the need for social workers to take into account spiritual matters has occurred in many countries, what this means in practice reflects the particular contexts including country or field of practice and the extent to which these are perceived as being imbued by secular or postsecular paradigms. For example, Stirling et al. (2010) note that while the British colonization of New Zealand resulted in considerable cultural similarities, the presence of the Maori people and their spirituality have resulted in differences in how social workers recognize and respond to spiritual issues. Similarly, variations can be found in comparing texts written during the same period by Holloway and Moss (2010) and Mathews (2009) in the UK, Canda and Furman (2010) from North America and Australian contributions by Crisp (2010) and Gardner (2011). The issues, demands and responses only vary further when considering perspectives from beyond first-world Anglophone countries (Crisp, 2017).

Despite a growing acceptance that in some circumstances it is legitimate to raise matters associated with religion and spirituality, many social workers are unwilling to do so (Furness & Gilligan, 2010). Even when this is far from their intentions, social workers fear any mention of religion or spirituality will be regarded as proselytizing and hence prefer that if such issues are to be raised, they are raised by service users (Furman et al., 2004). Consequently, 'if both service user and social worker are waiting for the other to give permission to raise this, then this is unlikely to occur' (Carlisle, 2016, p. 593).

Recognizing spiritual needs in service users is only part of the story. Social work is a stressful profession with high rates of burnout in some fields of practice (Crowder & Sears, 2017). It has been argued that the mandate of social workers in working for social justice (Hodge, 2012) and retaining their capacity for solidarity and compassion (Fardella, 2017) become impossible when their spiritual needs are neglected. Much of the work of social workers is emotionally taxing (Agger, Igreja, Kiehle, & Polatin, 2012), and even very experienced practitioners are not always able to cope with the distressing and traumatic experiences which their work may place them in (Farmer, 2015). With increasing recognition of the need for social workers to take active steps to prevent burnout (Sheridan, 2012), they are asserting that their own spiritual care practices are an essential aspect of, and not just an adjunct to, professional practice. For example, one social worker has written of her spiritual practice before or after seeing clients:

> In terms of cleansing processes, prayer and calling in the Divine, this was my practice for me, done before and after seeing each client, where I asked for the presence of God to guide my practice, or I used incense, oils or other methods to cleanse the room.
>
> *(Carrington, 2017, p. 297)*

While one might imagine such an approach may not be viable, or even perceived as desirable, by many social workers, the underpinning sentiments are perhaps ones which busy social workers can neglect: that the work we do with people is important and requires our respect. Even if only for a moment, taking time to reflect on our work is important. Other self-care techniques proposed by social workers include meditation techniques which promote mindfulness (Crowder & Sears, 2017) and yoga (Mensinga, 2011; see Chapters 22 and 41). Social workers' engagement in policy processes is arguably another way in which members of the profession can express their spirituality and meet their spiritual needs (Crisp, 2017).

While there is a growing recognition that social work practice can be enhanced by the appropriate incorporation of spirituality in the practice setting, there are some caveats. For example, despite spirituality having communal as well as individual expressions (Douek, 2015), it has been argued that the use of spirituality in social work has been to promote a highly individualistic view (Wong & Vinsky, 2009). There are also situations where spiritual beliefs or practices are neither beneficial nor benign and, unchallenged, can be harmful to individuals, families or communities (Sheridan, 2017). This includes use of mindfulness techniques, which can be misused to invoke violence and ruthless behaviours (Sun, 2014; see Chapter 22).

Spirituality as part of the social worker's toolkit

The secular imperative often results in social workers taking a less than holistic view of service users and their environments. Service users, even in times of crisis, can have a range of resources which can provide emotional and material support but may not consider these in difficult situations. These include religious or spiritual beliefs, practices and communities (Hodge, 2012). While there may be good reasons why service users might not want to take up such possibilities, such as fear of shame and stigma (Park, 2016) or because they have experienced the misuse of religion or spirituality (Sheridan, 2017), social workers who fail to consider religion and spirituality among the possible resources available to individuals and families may be doing a disservice to those they are working with (Liechty, 2013). This does not imply that religion or spirituality should be privileged, but it may be one of many community resources considered in an assessment process, along with schools, sporting groups, social clubs and so on, which individuals and families may or may not be part of. However, any mention of religion or spirituality needs to ensure that it is non-judgemental and not privileging any particular religion or spirituality (Puchalski, Ferrell, Virani, Otis-Green, & Baird, 2009).

Specific mention of religion and spirituality may not be appropriate in certain circumstances, and many social workers do not feel equipped to discuss such matters in a professional context (Perkins, 2015). However, there are other ways in which spirituality can be incorporated into social work practice which may feel more authentic for social workers, service users and the broader community. For example, while social workers have a long-standing commitment to the 'person-in-environment', this tends to be confined to the social environment (Crisp, 2017;

see Chapters 3 and 13). A more spiritual understanding of 'environment' (Zapf, 2008), has encouraged greater awareness among social workers as to the impacts of the built environment, climate change and natural disasters on the lives of those we work with (Crisp, 2017). Although such concerns might seem remote to many social workers, the definition quoted earlier in this paper – that spirituality involves concepts including meaning and connectedness – raises the importance of place as an issue, which frequently emerges in social work practice. Busy social workers may consider they have done their job by finding any place in a nursing home for a frail elderly person or housing for a homeless family, but when expediency or pressures result in such options not meeting other key needs of those service users, the placements may be at risk of failing (Crisp, 2010; Gardner, 2011).

Social workers can address the spiritual by facilitating service users' expressing the fundamentals of whom they understand themselves to be and their needs as they see them. Hence, narrative therapy has been proposed as one method which can

> ... address spirituality in practice, offering a respectful, non-judgemental and non-directive approach to working with issues related to spirituality and meaning-making. This provides a method for practitioners who would otherwise be uncomfortable with raising issues related to religion or spirituality to begin to open up spaces for people to speak about what gives them a sense of meaning and purpose.
>
> *(Béres, 2014, p. 112; see also Chapter 21)*

This requires an openness both to listening to the language and content of narratives and to recognizing that literal interpretations of these may preclude other explanations as to what is of critical importance in a situation (Gardner, 2011). As not everyone is good at expressing what is important in words, some social workers have utilized arts-based approaches to encourage individuals to express their feelings. Such work has involved children (Coholic & Eys, 2016), women (Coholic, 2006) older people and bereaved people (Renzenbrink, 2012) and individuals (Renzenbrink, 2012) as well as groups (Coholic, 2006):

> On the day before she died an 85-year-old woman who had been extremely anxious and in pain created what she called a 'bagel' out of soft white clay. She began to reminiscence about the first bagel she had ever tasted and the bagels she used to make for her family.
>
> *(Renzenbrink, 2012, p. 204)*

Other approaches including drawing and making collages (Renzenbrink, 2012) and writing (Coholic, 2006). Arts-based approaches may not only provide opportunities for participants to recollect past experiences, but can also be part of redressing oppression such as that experienced by indigenous communities (Coholic, Cote-Meek, & Recollet, 2012). Given that their marginalization has historically often been sanctioned by the state and welfare interventions have played a pivotal role (Briskman & Libesman, 2014), social work practice which ignores the spiritualities of indigenous communities will be unable to demonstrate its commitment to rectifying past injustices (Coates, Gray, & Hetherington, 2006).

Many social workers work in contexts in which the possibility of utilizing arts-based approaches is not viable in their direct client work. That does not mean that recognizing the importance of creativity has no place in their work. Rather, it is about acknowledging the creative element in everyone, which is often expressed in everyday tasks of living, including cooking, gardening, clothing and other adornments and creating a home (Crisp, 2010). Apart from reflecting something of their essential being, creativity can be a sign of the resourcefulness and resilience of those experiencing marginalization, oppression or other trauma; provide a means of commemorating or lamenting that which has occurred and be an expression of hope (Gero & Somerville, 2016). Despite there often being a fine line between adaptive creativity and signs of mental illness, a willingness to consider whether an action or object reflects resilience and not necessarily assume that it is a sign of pathology is another way in which social workers can enact their commitment to the spirituality of those they work with.

Recognizing the importance of rituals to individuals and communities is another way in which social workers can demonstrate their commitment to practice which takes account of the spiritual dimensions. As with creativity, ritual behaviours can be damaging to those involved or act as a sign of mental illness or other issues. Nevertheless, rituals can provide a structure for support in times of difficulty; opportunities to lament and share hopes and fears at times of transition and ways to celebrate. Some rituals have multiple functions. For example, in some cultures and families, the combination of funeral plus wake aims to provide not only spiritual consolation to mourners but also the opportunity to remember and celebrate a life and to commiserate with each other the ending of this (Crisp, 2010).

While some rituals are grand public affairs, others are relatively private. For many people, a cake lit with candles, the singing of a certain song and the receipt of a card are critical to any celebration of a birthday. They say to people that they are recognized above and beyond being a functionary (Crisp, 2010). Even very simple and solitary rituals can facilitate a sense of order, enriching our lives and even shaping our identities (Cooke & Macy, 2005). It is not the act itself but rather the symbolic value of an act which gives a ritual its meaning. Hence, what can be an important ritual for one person may have no such value for another person who ostensibly does the same things (Crisp, 2010). Good social work practice can involve facilitating rituals in partnership with service users (Crompton, 1998) or advocating on their behalf, particularly in institutional settings where there may be little understanding of how important a particular ritual is (Raman, 2007).

Whether it is professional self-care, creativity or rituals, the common component of these varying approaches to the incorporation of spirituality into social work practice is the recognition that human beings need to be regarded holistically, and effective work takes account of what is important to those we work with. Hence, people of differing abilities (Delich, 2014) or sexualities (Henrickson, 2007) or survivors of sexual abuse (Crisp, 2012) or couples dealing with infertility (Sewpaul, 1999) may be seen both as people with a specific issue or problem and also as being affected by spiritual implications related to their circumstances. The need for holistic care is also resulting in more social workers utilizing interventions such as yoga and tai chi, which seek to integrate mind, body and spirit, rather than regarding each as separate (Sun et al., 2013).

Spirituality and faith-based organizations

The imperative to do right is found in various religions, and a frequent expression of such beliefs is the provision of welfare services to disadvantaged members of the community. While this 'community' may be confined to members of a religious grouping, frequently services will be provided to members of the broader community irrespective of their religious beliefs. When funding is received from the state by faith-based organizations to provide services, it tends to come with the imperative for services to be secular at the point of delivery and available to all persons in the community irrespective of their religious beliefs (Crisp, 2014).

While such expectations are regarded as too much of a compromise by some welfare providers, others accept such restrictions on the basis that the needs of the community are more important than religious expression. Although the result has been that some faith-based organizations have become little different from their secular counterparts, others are exploring how they can express their spirituality without placing their funding at risk. Some of the ways this is happening include the setting of strategic directions and philosophies underpinning service delivery, staff recruitment and induction procedures and employment conditions which are congruent with the faith basis (Crisp, 2014), such that the experiences of social workers are frequently that 'faith-based organizations have a set of characteristics that distinguish them from their secular counterparts' (Clarke & Jennings, 2008, p. 15). Nevertheless, thinking about how organizations express their spirituality and respond to spiritual needs is far less advanced than it is for how individual social workers do this.

Conclusion

This chapter has provided a perspective on the dance which has emerged in recent years as the historical impact of secularity on social work practice has had to adapt to the influences of postsecularity and a growing recognition that holistic practice includes acknowledgement of the spirituality of both social workers and service users. This provides both opportunities and challenges to social workers and the organizations which employ them. Furthermore, many of the social work scholars who pioneered this work over the last two decades are now retiring, and there are new voices emerging who are both building on the work which has been done and taking it in new directions (Crisp, 2017). While this chapter has provided some insights, because of the rate of development in recent times, it cannot claim to be a comprehensive overview of spirituality and secularity in social work. Instead, this chapter has invited readers to reconsider their assumptions about religion and spirituality and to imagine ways in which these can appropriately be incorporated into professional social work practice.

Further reading

Crisp, B. R. (Ed.). (2017). *The Routledge handbook of religion, spirituality and social work.* London: Routledge.
   A recent international overview of the social work literature on religion and spirituality.
Fardella, J. A. (2017). Post-secular accommodation and Catholic health care: Corporate identity and the public good. *Ethics and Social Welfare, 11*, 47–61.
   An introduction to postsecularity and service delivery.
Hodge, D. R. (2009). Secular privilege: Deconstructing the invisible rose-tinted sunglasses. *Journal of Religion & Spirituality in Social Work, 28*, 8–34.
   More on the impact of secularity on social work.

References

Agger, I., Igreja, V., Kiehle, R., & Polatin, P. (2012). Testimony ceremonies in Asia: Integrating spirituality in testimonial therapy for torture survivors in India, Sri Lanka, Cambodia, and the Philippines. *Transcultural Psychiatry, 49*, 568–589.
Béres, L. (2014). *The narrative practitioner.* Basingstoke: Palgrave Macmillan.
Bowpitt, G. (1998). Evangelical Christianity, secular humanism, and the genesis of British Social Work. *British Journal of Social Work, 28*, 675–693.
Briskman, L., & Libesman, T. (2014). De-colonisation or re-colonisation? Contemporary social work and indigenous Australians. In S. Rice & A. Day (Eds.), *Social work in the shadow of the law* (4th ed., pp. 213–231). Annandale: Federation Press.
Canda, E. R., & Furman, D. L. (2010). *Spiritual diversity in social work practice: The heart of helping* (2nd ed.). New York: Oxford University Press.

Carlisle, P. (2016). Religion and spirituality as troublesome knowledge: The views and experiences of mental health social workers in Northern Ireland. *British Journal of Social Work*, *46*, 583–598.

Carrington, A. M. (2017). A spiritual approach to social work practice. In B. R. Crisp (Ed.), *Routledge Handbook of Religion, spirituality and social work* (pp. 291–299). London: Routledge.

Clarke, G., & Jennings, M. (2008). Introduction. In G. Clarke & M. Jennings (Eds.), *Development, civil society and faith-based organizations* (pp. 1–16). Basingstoke: Palgrave Macmillan.

Coates, J., Gray, M., & Hetherington, T. (2006). An 'ecospiritual' perspective: Finally a place for indigenous approaches. *British Journal of Social Work*, *36*, 381–399.

Coholic, D. (2006). Mindfulness meditation practice in spirituality influenced group work. *Arete*, *30*, 90–100.

Coholic, D., Cote-Meek, S., & Recollet, D. (2012). Exploring the acceptability and perceived benefits of arts-based group methods for aboriginal women living in an urban community within northeastern Ontario. *Canadian Social Work Review*, *29*, 149–168.

Coholic, D., & Eys, M. (2016). Benefits of an arts-based mindfulness group intervention for vulnerable children. *Child and Adolescent Social Work Journal*, *33*, 1–13.

Collicutt, J. (2015). Living in the end times: A short course addressing end of life issues for older people in an English parish church setting. *Working with Older People*, *19*, 140–149.

Cook, C. C. H. (2010). Spirituality, secularity and religion in psychiatric practice: Commentary on . . . Spirituality and religion in psychiatric practice. *The Psychiatrist*, *34*, 193–195.

Cooke, B., & Macy, G. (2005). *Christian symbol and ritual: An introduction*. Oxford: Oxford University Press.

Cowden, S., & Singh, G. (2017). Community cohesion, communitarianism and neoliberalism. *Critical Social Policy*, *37*, 268–286.

Crisp, B. R. (2010). *Spirituality and social work*. Farnham: Ashgate.

Crisp, B. R. (2012). The spiritual implications of sexual abuse: Not an issue only for religious women. *Feminist Theology*, *20*, 133–145.

Crisp, B. R. (2014). *Social work and faith-based organizations*. London: Routledge.

Crisp, B. R. (Ed.). (2017). *The Routledge handbook of religion, spirituality and social work*. London: Routledge.

Crompton, M. (1998). *Children, spirituality, religion and social work*. Aldershot: Ashgate.

Crowder, R., & Sears, A. (2017). Building resilience in social workers: An exploratory study on the impacts of a mindfulness-based intervention. *Australian Social Work*, *70*, 17–29.

Davie, G. (1994). *Religion in Britain since 1945: Believing without belonging*. Oxford: Blackwell Publishers.

Delich, N. A. M. (2014). Spiritual direction and deaf spirituality: Implications for social work practice. *Journal of Religion & Spirituality in Social Work*, *33*, 317–338.

Douek, S. (2015). Faith and spirituality in older people: A Jewish perspective. *Working with Older People*, *19*, 114–122.

Elliott, N. (2017). Faith, ethics and social work: Framework for an introductory lecture. *Ethics and Social Welfare*, *11*, 92–99.

Fardella, J. A. (2017). Post-secular accommodation and Catholic health care: Corporate identity and the public good. *Ethics and Social Welfare*, *11*, 47–61.

Farmer, B. (2015). *Walking together: A mental health therapist's guide to working with refugees*. Seattle: Lutheran Community Services Northwest. Retrieved from http://form.jotform.us/form/51666347065157

Furman, L. D., Benson, P. W., Grimwood, C., & Canda, E. (2004). Religion and spirituality in social work education and direct practice at the millennium: A survey of UK social workers. *British Journal of Social Work*, *34*, 767–792.

Furness, S., & Gilligan, P. (2010). *Religion, belief and social work: Making a difference*. Bristol: Policy Press.

Gärde, J. (2015). Shrinking religious communities and thriving interreligious social work in postsecular Sweden. *Journal of Religion & Spirituality in Social Work*, *34*, 1–23.

Gardner, F. (2011). *Critical spirituality: A holistic approach to contemporary practice*. Farnham: Ashgate.

Garrett, P. M. (2014). Re-enchanting social work? The emerging 'spirit' of social work in an age of economic crisis. *British Journal of Social Work*, *44*, 503–521.

Gero, A., & Somerville, K. (2016). *Making the Australian quilt: 1800–1950*. Melbourne: National Gallery of Victoria.

Grey, M. (2008). Viewing spirituality in social work through the lens of contemporary social theory. *British Journal of Social Work*, *38*, 175–196.

Habermas, J. (2006). Religion in the public sphere. *European Journal of Philosophy*, *14*, 1–25.

Habermas, J. (2008). Secularism's crisis of faith: Notes on post-secular society. *New Perspectives Quarterly*, *25*(4), 17–29.

Henrickson, M. (2007). Lavender faith: Religion, spirituality and identity in lesbian, gay and bisexual New Zealanders. *Journal of Religion & Spirituality in Social Work, 26,* 63–80.

Hodge, D. R. (2009). Secular privilege: Deconstructing the invisible rose-tinted sunglasses. *Journal of Religion & Spirituality in Social Work, 28,* 8–34.

Hodge, D. R. (2012). The conceptual and empirical relationship between spirituality and social justice: Exemplars from diverse faith traditions. *Journal of Religion & Spirituality in Social Work, 31,* 32–50.

Holloway, M., & Moss, B. (2010). *Spirituality and social work.* Basingstoke: Palgrave Macmillan.

International Association of Schools of Social Work (IASSW) & International Federation of Social Work (IFSW). (2004). *Global standards for the education and training of the social work profession.* Retrieved from www.ifsw.org/cm_data/GlobalSocialWorkStandards2005.pdf

Jawad, R. (2012). Serving the public or delivering public services? Religion and social welfare in the new British social policy landscape. *Journal of Poverty and Social Justice, 20,* 55–68.

Jivraj, S., & Herman, D. (2009). It's difficult for a white judge to understand: Orientalism, racialisation, and Christianity in English child welfare cases. *Child and Family Law Quarterly, 21,* 283–308.

King, M., & Leavey, G. (2010). Spirituality and religion in psychiatric practice: Why all the fuss? *The Psychiatrist, 34,* 190–193.

Liechty, D. (2013). Sacred content, secular context: A generative theory of religion and spirituality for social work. *Journal of Social Work in End-of-Life & Palliative Care, 9,* 123–143.

Manthorpe, J., Harris, J., Samsi, J., & Moriarty, J. (2017). Doing, being and becoming a valued care worker: User and family carer views. *Ethics and Social Welfare, 11,* 79–91.

Marty, M. (1980). Social service: Godly and godless. *Social Service Review, 54,* 463–481.

Mathews, I. (2009). *Social work and spirituality.* Exeter: Learning Matters.

Mensinga, J. (2011). The feeling of being a social worker: Including yoga as an embodied practice in social work education. *Social Work Education, 30,* 650–662.

Modood, T. (2012). 2011 Paul Hanly Furfey lecture: Is there a crisis of secularism in Western Europe?' *Sociology of Religion, 73,* 130–149.

Modood, T. (2013). Multiculturalism and religion: A three part debate. Part one Accommodating religions: Multiculturalism's new fault line. *Critical Social Policy, 34,* 121–137.

Park, C. J. (2016). Chronic shame: A perspective integrating religion and spirituality. *Journal of Religion & Spirituality in Social Work, 35,* 354–376.

Perkins, C. (2015). Promoting spiritual care for older people in New Zealand: The Selwyn Centre for Ageing and Spirituality. *Working with Older People, 19,* 107–113.

Pew Research Center. (2012). *The global religious landscape: A report on the size and distribution of the world's major religious groups as of 2010.* Washington, DC: Pew Research Center. Retrieved from www.pewforum.org/files/2014/01/global-religion-full.pdf

Puchalski, C., Ferrell, B., Virani, R., Otis-Green, S., & Baird, D. (2009). Improving the quality of spiritual care as a dimension of palliative care: The report of the consensus conference. *Journal of Palliative Medicine, 12,* 885–904.

Raman, S. (2007). Healing in Hinduism. In F. Gale, N. Bolzan, & D. McRae-McMahon (Eds.), *Spirited practices: Spirituality and the helping professions* (pp. 33–42). Crows Nest, NSW: Allen and Unwin.

Renzenbrink, I. (2012). Art therapy, healing and spiritual growth: A reflective essay. *Journal for the Study of Spirituality, 2,* 203–215.

Robertson, G. (2015). Spirituality and ageing: The role of mindfulness in supporting people with dementia to live well. *Working with Older People, 19,* 123–133.

Sewpaul, V. (1999). Culture, religion and infertility: A South African perspective. *British Journal of Social Work, 29,* 741–754.

Sheridan, M. J. (2012). Spiritual activism: Grounding ourselves in the spirit. *Journal of Religion & Spirituality in Social Work, 31,* 193–208.

Sheridan, M. J. (2017). Addressing spiritual bypassing: Issues and guidelines for spiritually sensitive practice. In B. R. Crisp (Ed.), *Routledge Handbook of Religion, spirituality and social work* (pp. 358–367). London: Routledge.

Shook, J. (2010). *Secularity and secularism explained.* Retrieved from www.centerforinquiry.net/blogs/entry/secularity_and_secularism_explained/

Stirling, B., Furman, L. D., Benson, P. W., Canda, E. R., & Grimwood, C. (2010). A comparative survey of Aotearoa New Zealand and UK social workers on the role of religion and spirituality in practice. *British Journal of Social Work, 40,* 602–621.

Sun, J. (2014). Mindfulness in context: A historical discourse analysis. *Contemporary Buddhism, 15,* 394–415.

Sun, J., Zhang, N., Buys, N., Zhou, Z-Y., Shen, S-Y., & Yuan, B-J. (2013). The role of Tai Chi, cultural dancing, playing a musical instrument and singing in the prevention of chronic disease in Chinese older adults: A mind-body meditative approach. *International Journal of Mental Health Promotion, 15*, 227–239.

Taylor, C. (2007). *A secular age*. Cambridge, MA: Belknap Press, Harvard University Press.

Vanderwoerd, J. R. (2011). Who tells social work's story? *Social Work & Christianity, 38*, 237–243.

Whiting, R. (2008). 'No room for religion or spirituality or cooking tips': Exploring practical atheism as an unspoken consensus in the development of social work values in England. *Ethics and Social Welfare, 2*, 67–83.

Wong, Y. L., & Vinsky, J. (2009). Speaking from the margins: A critical reflection on the spiritual-but-not-religious discourse in social work. *British Journal of Social Work, 39*, 1343–1359.

Zapf, M. K. (2008). Transforming social work's understanding of person and environment: Spirituality and the 'common ground'. *Journal of Religion & Spirituality in Social Work, 27*, 171–181.

Part 3

Theories of social work practice

12

Relational social work

Karen Winter

Introduction

Taking as the start point the internationally accepted definition of social work, most recently ratified by the International Federation of Social Workers [IFSW] (2014), social work is defined as 'a practice-based profession and an academic discipline that promotes social change and development, social cohesion, and the empowerment and liberation of people. Principles of social justice, human rights, collective responsibility and respect for diversities are central to social work. Underpinned by theories of social work, social sciences, humanities and indigenous knowledges, social work engages people and structures to address life challenges and enhance wellbeing'. Based on this definition, it is evident that relationships are core to social work practice, and relational social work is key to achieving its aims and objectives. There is a growing literature to support this view. That relationships are central is 'common sense' at one level, and yet, at another level, it is apparent that there are differences in definitions, conceptual and theoretical underpinnings and hoped-for outcomes.

Definitions of relational social work practice

An agreed definition of relational social work practice is hard to come by (Ruch, Turney, & Ward, 2010; Megele, 2015), but perhaps the best articulated is from Tosone (2004, p. 481) who states: 'relational social work is the practice of using the therapeutic relationship as the principal vehicle to effect change in the client's systemic functioning referring to the inherent interconnection of the intrapsychic, interpersonal and larger community systems'. The key characteristics of relational social work are threefold: first, the relationship is the mechanism through which change is achieved; second, the dyadic, potentially therapeutic, fluid and largely asymmetrical nature of the relationship between service user and social worker is key; third, the inextricable links between the interpersonal, intrapersonal and structural worlds of *both practitioner and service user* are central to the processes through which engagement, communication and collaboration to achieve desired outcomes take place. In considering definitional parameters, one of the emergent issues is whether 'relationship-based practice' is a set of principles or more of a conceptual, theoretical model or approach.

Relational social work as a set of practice principles

As a broad set of guiding principles that centre on the quality of professionals' relationships, it is no surprise to find that these resonate well with social workers because they reflect core professional values and our professional identities. These principles focus on being real, respectful, resourceful, reliable, accessible, flexible, truthful, genuinely interested, empathic, committed, responsive in thoughtful ways and also on being able to regulate one's own emotional responses and react responsibly to the emotions of others (see Chapters 8 and 9). A supporting body of research indicates that people involved with social services value professionals who demonstrate these qualities (Reimer, 2013). Often this is where discussion about relational social work begins and ends: a set of commonly agreed principles to which the profession can sign up. However, the literature on relational social work indicates several conceptual and theoretical frameworks that focus primarily on either the intrapersonal aspects of relational practice or its interpersonal social structural components. Importantly, it is understanding the processes by which social workers hold in tension the intrapersonal and interpersonal elements of relational encounters that is the focus of conceptual and theoretical frameworks of relational practice. As Bower (2003, p. 3) has argued, 'one of the uniquely valuable aspects of social work is the balance it holds between understanding and working with the internal and external realities of people's lives. The balance of course is an ideal, and in reality, workers may move between internal and external considerations and between action and reflection'.

Relational social work as conceptual and theoretical frameworks

Theoretical and conceptual frameworks focus on one of the following or a combination of themes from the perspective of the social worker or service user or both. These themes are the intrapersonal, the internal workings of the individual's mind and emotion; the interpersonal, the individual in their immediate context; the social structural positioning within society that takes account of stratifications and the discrete nature of these as well as their intersectionality. The relevant stratifications include class, gender, age, disability, race, religion, ethnicity, culture and political affiliation.

Intrapersonal

At the intrapersonal level, the psychodynamic approach, which houses many different theories including psychoanalysis, focuses primarily on individual psychology, personality and the individual's internal world, their internal reality. It provides both a theory of personality and an approach to practice. Often associated with clinical social work or psychiatric social work, the psychoanalytic approach was hugely influential historically. Goldstein (2009, p. 7) points out that in the 1920s, psychoanalysis contributed to the professionalization of social work and that: 'Social work practitioners, many of whom eagerly sought psychoanalytic treatment and supervision, began to use many psychoanalytic techniques with their clients'. Gaining further popularity in the 1940s onwards and associated with the work of Freud, Melanie Klein and Donald and Claire Winnicott, to name a few, within the parameters of a formal therapeutic relationship, the social worker and individual service user engage in a process that sought to explore, give expression to and resolve the internal, conscious and unconscious conflicts caused by the impact of adverse external events.

In the 1960s–70s onwards, the influence in social work of the psychoanalytic approach to understanding and addressing relationship dynamics fell by the wayside as a more sociological approach, with its emphasis on external, social structural processes and their impact, became increasingly influential (see Chapters 27–31). Mobilization around gender, race and poverty, which highlighted the impact of social structural issues as well as a growing antipathy towards the medical model, were contributing factors. Indeed, Hamilton (1958, p. 23), who advocated the psychoanalytic approach, argued that 'it was one of the aberrant features of the attempt to carry psychoanalytic principles and techniques into casework that treatment became so preoccupied with the inner life as almost to lose touch with outer reality and the social factors with which social workers were most familiar'.

Having said that, more recent work (Sudbery, 2002; Ruch et al., 2010; Megele, 2015) draws explicitly on psychodynamic theory. Sudbery (2002), for example, provides useful insights by explaining terms and their applicability. Of transference, Sudbery (2002, p. 153) states: 'Whatever its debatable characteristics, "transference" refers to the propensity of a helping relationship in the present to have echoes of the situation when the user of service was a child and needed assistance or care from their parent. "The patient sees in him[her] the return, the reincarnation, of some important figure out of his childhood or past, and consequently transfers on to him feelings and reactions which undoubtedly applied to this prototype"' (Freud, 1940/1949). On countertransference, Sudbery (2002) illustrates its use in helping the social worker identify how the person involved with social services makes them feel, stepping out of this and using the feelings to respond in a therapeutic way. Two points emerge from this of relevance to developments in individual psychology and social work. The first is that these concepts are equated with a medical model which is criticized because of its pathologizing tendencies, an over focus on the individual and their internal 'deficits'. The second is that knowledge of these terms and their applicability and relevance is seen to be the domain of specialist, therapeutically trained professionals and beyond the relevance of reach of the social work profession more generally. One exception to this is attachment theory, still used implicitly and explicitly to inform assessments and decision-making (see Chapter 13).

Interpersonal

As alluded to above, relationship-based practice involves an appreciation not just of the individual but of their social context, their positioning within it, their interaction with it and their daily lived experience of it. This conceptualization is captured in the social casework model and its iterations. Historically, the parameters of this approach were set out by Richmond (1922, pp. 98–99) in her work on social casework in which she states: 'Social casework consists of those processes which develop personality, through adjustments, consciously effected, individual by individual, between [people] and their social environment'. She identified four components to social casework: insight into individuality and personal characteristics; insight into resources, dangers and the influence of the social environment; direct action of mind upon mind; indirect action through the social environment (1922, pp. 101–102).

Effective relationships were built through casework which combined social investigation (gathering information), social diagnosis (identifying the main social issues), social relationships (cooperation with all sources of assistance) and social reinstatement (that is, the 'treatment' or restoration of an individual/family back to their former self and the (re)building of supportive relationships with extended family and community). In emphasizing the balance that should be given between the individual and the environment, she said that the social worker must be 'no more occupied with abnormalities in individual than in the environment . . . no more able to neglect one than the other' (Richmond, 1922, p. 98). In her summary, Richmond (1922, p. 255) noted that effective casework relationships depended on 'a knowledge of innate make-up and of the effects of environment upon an individual. The failure of a case worker to learn [their] client's social and personal background usually means failure to effect any permanent adjustment, but these diagnostic processes interplay with those of treatment [and that] action ranges from the humblest of services guided by affection, patience and personal sympathy, to such radical measures as complete change of environment, the organization of resources where none existed before, and the reknitting of ties long broken'.

This social casework framework that outlined the nature of relationships between social workers and the people they worked with has been taken forward and developed in different guises since that time. Its foundational pillars, 'person in their immediate and wider context' and the role of professional as intervening to effect change in the intrapersonal, interpersonal and wider social structural context, have remained untouched, but the ways this is understood have varied (Cornell, 2006). Cornell (2006) notes that from the 1940s, psychoanalytic concepts were incorporated into casework, with later additions drawn from systems theory.

Contemporary thinking regarding relational social work

In the most recent literature, Sudbery (2002), Ruch et al. (2010), Turney (2012) and Megele (2015) are agreed that following a period of declining popularity, relationship-based practice has seen something of a revival. They also agree that an effective model of relationship-based practice should be theoretically informed, practically relevant, accessible and applicable with all age groups, from diverse backgrounds and in any setting whether fieldwork, residential or therapeutic. Change for the better should be the goal and the outcome. Their contribution has built on an expanded knowledge in the intrapersonal, interpersonal and social structural elements of relational practice from the perspectives of both those at the receiving end of relational social work practice and the social workers engaged in relational work.

At the intrapersonal level, all writers explore the relevance to social work practice of key concepts associated with a broadly psychodynamic approach, attachment, transference, countertransference, defence, resistance and use of self. They note that there is an argument to say that where once there was a gap in social work knowledge regarding social structural issues and their impact on relational practice, the pendulum has swung the other way, and there is now a gap in basic understanding about individual psychology and its contribution to relational practice. Bower (2003) argues that given the issues, such as abuse, rejection, violence, neglect and trauma, experienced by people who come to the attention of social services, there is a need for social work professionals to be equipped with an understanding of the human mind, its conscious and unconscious workings and the role played by emotions. Not least, this understanding would enable social workers to make sense of why people respond to them in the ways they do through transference. It would also enable social workers to understand why different feelings, such as inadequacy, being overwhelmed, rage, sadness, confusion and untrustworthiness, are aroused in them when in contact with different people. And through countertransference they can appreciate how they can articulate and use these feelings to challenge and effect change in the people they work with. Focusing on intrapersonal elements to relational social work practice, Reimer's (2013) study explored parents' views of their relationships with social workers where child neglect had been an issue. Reimer noted that parental resistance, a common feature at the start of the relationship with the social worker, sometimes transformed into a trusting and collaborative relationship. This was especially so where the parents had 'tested out' the trustworthiness of the social worker and where a shared interest provided common ground from which to conduct their relationship. Understanding these relational dynamics in terms of transference and countertransference enhances the therapeutic potential of relationships between social workers who work in fieldwork and the families and individuals they are in contact with.

Combined with this, the interpersonal context that enables or hinders relational work for both social worker and those involved with social services has been further explored. People's willingness or unwillingness to engage with social workers has been explored; it may relate to family pressure, shame, fear and denial (Winter, 2015; Winter et al., 2017; Ruch et al., 2017). For social workers, greater recognition of the interpersonal context has led to research that focuses on work setting and organizational cultures (Ruch, 2005). Although representing attempts to re-align social casework or relationship-based practice to take better account of the social contexts in which people are positioned, one of the continued critiques of the psychosocial approach is whether it has been successful in achieving a balanced focus on both the individual and their social context (Turney, 2012). Whilst the interpersonal elements of models of relationship-based practice are well developed, articulations of the social context and social structural considerations remain less well developed.

To address gaps in thinking on the social structural context, Turney (2012) takes a different approach, using Honneth's (1995) work on recognition, respect and reciprocity to enhance our understanding of the social context in relationship-based practice. Applying this to social workers' statutory relationships with families, Turney (2012, p. 151) argues that 'an approach informed by recognition theory can support the development of a model of relationship-based practice that engages more effectively with both the social and the psychological'. She notes, however, that the critique of Honneth's work is its focus on micro interactions. A model that combines recognition (self, legal and social) and redistribution (goods and services), as outlined in Fraser's work (2003), for example, would allow for the development of a model of relationship-based practice where issues in the social context are more fully addressed through an explicit social justice approach. That said, Turney (2012) draws on Garrett's (2009) stance, arguing that Fraser's work has an underdeveloped conception of the state. This is an important consideration for social workers who both work for the state and who encounter individuals where the impact of social structural issues requires a state-level response.

Issues and challenges in relational social work

Social work as a field of practice is located within and shaped by several competing discourses that ultimately impact on the nature, purpose and anticipated outcomes of relational work. Prevailing discourses include managerialism, with its emphasis on the bureaucratic and technocratic elements of practice; risk adversity, with its emphasis on the identification and management of risk and accountability and value for money, with its emphasis on cost effectiveness, evidence of effectiveness and outcomes. Alongside that is the growing influence of counter discourses, including professional expertise in exercising judgement, intuition and creativity and on the value of meaningful relationships as the vehicle through which change is achieved. Each of these shapes relational social work in a different way.

At ground level, in working with people known to social services, social workers face the reality that there are contexts where elements of relationship-based practice remain aspirational rather than practicable because they cannot be all things to all people. The reality also is that some social workers may not like the people they encounter and vice versa. There are other contexts where the experience of a relationship with a social worker will be rated poorly by families, regardless of the existence of high-quality relationship-based aspects, because it is' what is it, a social worker relationship. Furthermore, there are contexts where relationship-based practice principles and real situations do not appear compatible. Social workers ask families to trust them and to engage in meaningful relationships. Yet at the same time they know that with staff turnover, staff sickness and the transfer of cases between teams, they are asking families to trust different social workers repeatedly. Social workers are tasked in their child protection work to retain a 'respectful uncertainty' and to 'think the unthinkable' about some of the information shared by families and the family issues to which they become privy, and it is obvious that this mind-set does not sit easily with the principle of establishing meaningful reciprocal relationships.

Beyond this, effective relational social work practice is related to emotional intelligence (see Chapter 9), the ability to work with uncertainty and the availability of good supervision and team working that incorporates space to reflect (see Chapter 34). It is known from research (Wastell, White, Broadhurst, Peckover, & Pithouse, 2010; Winter et al., 2017) that social workers' ability to 'put themselves out there' for the sake of relationships is compromised by pressures associated with organizational cultural norms where greater value is attributed to an 'objective, emotionally distant, detached' approach in executing roles and functions over and above a more 'subjective, close and relational' approach. This, in turn, limits opportunities to develop skills in emotional intelligence because these depend, in part, on the availability of safe space to reflect on and recognize the emotions of others, manage one's own emotions and manage the emotions of others. It is also known that, in a context of depleted resources and high caseload pressure, the potential of supervision is reduced to its managerial components only and its educative and supportive roles diminished. Lastly, with the growing emphasis on 'fluid workspace' (hot desking), teams are fragmented and the opportunity to derive support from colleagues reduced.

The workplace setting of the social worker in the statutory fieldwork sector, for example, in which most relationship-based social work practice, if we are honest, is instrumental and focused on the individual in their immediate context. Social workers are not engaged in relationships for relationships' sake. Nor do the people they work with engage in relationships with social workers for relationships' sake. Relationship-based practice is engaged in to achieve goals established as part of our professional and statutory duties. These, as Trevithick (2003) notes, could include gathering information for an assessment which will enable identification of where change might be best effected. Or a social worker might set out, under the guise of relationship-based practice, to gain insight into the views of a child for the purposes of a court report that will inform contact and living arrangements. This might be combined with applications to organizations to seek financial help or deal with housing issues and similar matters. In so doing, most of the work is aimed at enabling individuals to function better with the resources available to them rather than effecting fundamental change at the social structural level (Turney, 2012).

In a different workplace context – for example, the residential child-care sector – the meaning of relationship-based practice is somewhat different because the potentially therapeutic nature of the settings is more explicitly acknowledged, and the proximity and intensity of relationships is more evident. In residential child care, recent policy and practice developments have sought to embrace the value of therapeutic relationships and various models of care that stress this have been introduced into the sector (Winter, 2017). These include (Whittaker, del Valle, & Holmes, 2015): the attachment, self-regulation competence (ARC) model; the sanctuary model; the family teaching model (FTM); the social pedagogical approach; trauma systems therapy (TST); the children and residential experiences (CARE) model; promoting alternative thinking strategies (PATHS) and positive peer cultures (PPC). Common themes underpinning these approaches are a focus on the centrality of attachment relationships; the importance of trauma-informed practice (that is, understanding the impact on children of exposure to trauma); staff who are attuned, aligned and responsive to the circumstances and contexts of children and young people rather than reactive to their behaviour and an organizational context that supports staff and children. Research (Berridge, Biehal, Lutman, Henry, & Palomares, 2011; Macdonald,

Millen, McCann, Roscoe, & Ewart-Boyle, 2012) indicates that, while staff and young people value their relationships with each other where these models are in evidence, there are real challenges for workers in implementing elements of relationship-based practice, such as displays of emotion and intimacy, including holding, touching, comforting and showing acts of kindness. Such challenges are heightened in a context where discourses of managerialism and risk adversity dominate. The influence of these discourses is ever apparent given the recent media attention of appalling historical neglect and abuse in the sector (Brown, Winter, & Carr, in press).

In addition to these points is the question of how transformative relational social work is and can be. Or is it good enough that it is just instrumental? Looking critically at outcomes, effective relational social work practice could be measured in several ways. These include its intrapsychic impact, enabling people to develop an attachment and improve self-esteem, confidence and well-being and its interpersonal impact, helping people develop their strengths to better manage with what personal, social and economic resources they have and can gain access to. These outcomes in effect maintain the status quo. Alternative outcomes might include social structural impacts: for example, in empowering people to challenge the structural inequalities that have given rise to some of the needs in the first place and in lobbying on behalf of those in contact with social services so that the unacceptable never becomes acceptable. Research highlighting the views of service users indicates that in each of these aspects, they have found their relationships with social workers to have been transformative, either in how they felt about themselves, how the help they received helped them manage their circumstances or how they dealt with wider social structural issues. It is argued, however, that more needs to be done regarding positioning the profession as a 'political' enterprise in its broadest sense. That means not just engaging in relational work for instrumental reasons, but engaging in relational work to address and challenge the effects of inequality at all levels. This approach honours relationships in their totality, the individual, their immediate context and their positioning within wider social structures. It is also a way of honouring the true nature of the profession as defined at the start of this chapter. Featherstone, Gupta, Morris, and Warner (2016); Featherstone, Gupta, and Morris (2017) and Gupta (2017) reflect this in appealing to the social work profession to frame relationships with families within the context of a full understanding and appreciation of the impact of wider social structural disadvantages on them. Similarly, they propose a realignment of relational work away from its focus on 'intervention and problem-solving' concerned with intrapersonal and interpersonal characteristics to listening, challenging and supporting at a social structural level. The latter draws strongly on social workers' contribution to community development and on their broader advocacy role (see Chapters 25 and 30).

Going forward and doing things differently?

There have been developments with regards to relational work. At a conceptual and theoretical level, recent literature has focused on developing its social structural elements. Turney (2012) applies Fraser's conceptual framework to relational social work. With its core concern being social justice and its dual focus on recognition (personal, legal and social) and redistribution (resources and services), it emphasizes the importance of relational social work in a social structural context. Featherstone et al. (2016) and Gupta (2017) suggest a social model to the administration of child protection services based on Sen's (1985) capability approach (CA), again with its core focus on social justice obligations. Hence, both contributions remind us that relational work should fully take account of and engage with social structural inequalities.

At the levels of policy and practice, several developments have aimed to take forward more flexible approaches to relational social work that take account of wider social structural issues. In

England, in the Children's Social Care Innovation Programme (http://springconsortium.com), the government is investing £200 million to fund locally led innovative models of service delivery that generally have as one of their pillars the centrality of meaningful relationships.

At the level of social work training, Lefevre's (2015) work has made an important contribution to the social work curriculum regarding communication and relational skills. Such developments are having a noticeable impact on daily practice as evidenced in recent research (Smyth, 2017; Winter et al., 2017; Ruch et al., 2017).

To end, many of the contributions described above highlight three fundamental elements to relational social work practice: first, its central importance to all that we are as a profession and all that we seek to effect; second, that it is an endeavour that must encompass a combined, interrelated focus on the individual, immediate social context and wider social structural issues and third, to do this requires the profession to assert itself as a 'political' endeavour. In these sentiments there is nothing new; they reflect the thoughts of Richmond nearly 100 years ago. What is new is the current political, economic and social context that the social work profession finds itself in and how it organizes its priorities going forward.

Further reading

Folgheraiter, F. (2003). *Relational social work: Toward networking and societal practices*. London: Jessica Kingsley.

Tosone, C., & Gelman, C. R. (2017). Relational social work: A contemporary psychosocial perspective on practice. In F. J. Turner (Ed.), *Social work treatment: Interlocking theoretical approaches* (6th ed., pp. 420–27). New York: Oxford University Press.

References

Berridge, D., Biehal, N., Lutman, E., Henry, L., & Palomares, M. (2011). *Raising the bar? Evaluation of the social pedagogy pilot programme in residential children's homes*. London: Department for Education. Retrieved from http://dera.ioe.ac.uk/11857/1/DFE-RR148.pdf

Bower, M. (2003). Broken and twisted. *Journal of Social Work Practice, 17*, 143–153.

Brown, T., Winter, K., & Carr, N. (in press). Residential child care workers: Relationship based practice in a culture of fear. *Child and Family Social Work*.

Cornell, K. L. (2006). Person-in-situation: History, theory, and new directions for social work practice. *Praxis, 6*(4), 50–57.

Featherstone, B., Gupta, A., & Morris, K. (2017). Bringing back the social: The way forward for children's social work? *Journal of Children's Services, 12*(2–3), 190–196.

Featherstone, B., Gupta, A., Morris, K. M., & Warner, J. (2016). Let's stop feeding the risk monster: Towards a social model of 'child protection'. *Families, Relationships and Societies*. Retrieved from https://doi.org/10.1332/204674316X14552878034622

Freud, S. (1940/1949). *An outline of psychoanalysis*. New York: Norton.

Garrett, P. M. (2009). Recognizing the limitations of the political theory of recognition: Axel Honneth, Nancy Fraser and social work. *British Journal of Social Work, 40*(5), 1517–1533.

Goldstein, E. G. (2009). The relationship between social work and psychoanalysis: The future impact of social workers. *Clinical Social Work Journal, 37*(1), 7–13.

Gupta, A. (2017). *Relationship based practice in an unequal society*. Retrieved from www.healthcare.ac.uk/wp-content/uploads/2017/04/Anna-Gupta-Relationship-based-practice-in-an-unequal-society-190117.pdf

Hamilton, G. (1958). A theory of personality: Freud's contribution to social casework. In H. J. Parad (Ed.), *Ego psychology and dynamic casework* (pp. 11–37). New York: Family Service Association of America.

Honneth, A. (1995). *The struggle for recognition: The moral grammar of social conflicts*. Cambridge, UK: Polity Press.

International Federation of Social Workers. (2014). *Global definition of social work*. Retrieved from: https://www.ifsw.org/what-is-social-work/global-definition-of-social-work/.

Lefevre, M. (2015). Integrating the teaching, learning and assessment of communication with children within the qualifying social work curriculum. *Child & Family Social Work, 20*(2), 211–222.

Macdonald, G., Millen, S., McCann, M., Roscoe, H., & Ewart-Boyle, S. (2012). *Therapeutic approaches to social work in residential child care settings.* Belfast: Social Care Institute for Excellence.

Megele, C. (2015). *Psychosocial and relationship-based practice.* Northwich: Critical Publishing.

Reimer, E. C. (2013). Relationship-based practice with families where child neglect is an issue: Putting relationship development under the microscope. *Australian Social Work, 66*(3), 455–470.

Richmond, M. E. (1922). *What is social case work? an introductory description.* New York: Russell Sage Foundation.

Ruch, G. (2005). Relationship-based practice and reflective practice: Holistic approaches to contemporary child care social work. *Child & Family Social Work, 10*(2), 111–123.

Ruch, G., Turney, D., & Ward, A. (Eds.). (2010). *Relationship-based practice: Getting to the heart of practice.* London: Jessica Kingsley.

Ruch, G., Winter, K., Cree, V., Hallett, S., Morrison, F., & Hadfield, M. (2017). Making meaningful connections: Using insights from social pedagogy in statutory child and family social work practice. *Child & Family Social Work, 22*(2), 1015–1023.

Sen, A. (1985). *Commodities and capabilities.* Amsterdam: North-Holland.

Smyth, P. (2017). *Working with high-risk youth: A relationship-based practice framework.* Abingdon: Routledge Taylor & Francis Group.

Sudbery, J. (2002). Key features of therapeutic social work: The use of relationship. *Journal of Social Work Practice, 16*(2), 149–162.

Tosone, C. (2004). Relational social work: Honoring the tradition. *Smith College Studies in Social Work, 74*(3), 475–487.

Trevithick, P. (2003). Effective relationship-based practice: A theoretical exploration. *Journal of Social Work Practice, 17*(2), 163–176.

Turney, D. (2012). A relationship-based approach to engaging involuntary clients: The contribution of recognition theory. *Child & Family Social Work, 17*(2), 149–159.

Wastell, D., White, S., Broadhurst, K., Peckover, S., & Pithouse, A. (2010). Children's services in the iron cage of performance management: Street-level bureaucracy and the spectre of Švejkism. *International Journal of Social Welfare, 19*(3), 310–320.

Whittaker, J. K., del Valle, J. F., & Holmes, L. (2015). *Therapeutic residential care for children and youth: Developing evidence-based international practice.* London: Jessica Kingsley.

Winter, K. (2015). *Supporting positive relationships for children and young people who have experience of care.* Glasgow: Institute for Research and Innovation in Social Services.

Winter, K. (2017). *Systematic narrative review: Therapeutic model of intervention in respect of Children's House.* Belfast: Health and Social Care Board.

Winter, K., Cree, V., Hallett, S., Hadfield, M., Ruch, G., Morrison, F., & Holland, S. (2017). Exploring communication between social workers, children and young people. *British Journal of Social Work, 47*(5), 1427–1444.

13

Contemporary attachment theory

How can it inform social workers?

David Shemmings and Yvonne Shemmings

Introduction

In this chapter, we attempt to summarize the contribution attachment theory can make to social work practice. We argue that this contribution has been hampered by misunderstandings about what it does – and, more importantly, what it does *not* – say about close human relationships across the lifespan. Unfortunately, attachment theory and research have tended to be seen as more relevant to social workers working with children and families but less so with practitioners working with adult service users. Consider the attachment dynamics when a 60-year-old daughter provides personal care to her 80-year-old father if, when she was a teenager, he sexually abused her. In what follows, therefore, we will try to relate the growing compendium of research into attachment theory to all forms of social work practice.

We do not give an outline of attachment theory as such; there are many excellent summaries elsewhere that specifically refer to social work practice and topics (for example, Howe, 1995, 2011; Wilkins, Shemmings, & Shemmings, 2015). Instead, we offer a deepened and strengthened synthesis, firstly by identifying some key misconceptions and then by outlining four contemporary applications of attachment theory to social work practice.

Persistent misunderstandings

In 2011 Jennifer McIntosh edited an edition of *Family Court Review* devoted to 'Attachment'. With Eric and Siegfried Hesse, Mary Main, a key attachment researcher in developing Bowlby's theoretical insights – she was one of Mary Ainsworth's PhD students – contributed an article that should be read and digested by anyone teaching attachment to qualifying students (in any profession). In an important paper, Main, Hesse, and Hesse (2011) identify a worrying list of over 20 'misconceptions' about attachment, routinely applied inaccurately by a wide range of professionals. Here are three examples, to which we have added a short supplementary note of explanation:

1   *The 'window of opportunity' for the formation of a secure attachment endures only throughout the first three years of life'* (p. 439). If this were correct, professionals working with individuals over the age of three would be limited in what they could achieve. We should not unwittingly assume such

a deterministic stance. Individuals can and do change from an 'insecure' to a 'secure' internal working model of close relationships, although it is far less likely to occur the other way round, depending on who else they meet on their journey through life. (We return to this point later.)

2   'The amount of time spent with a child is the most important element in forming an enduring attachment relationship' (p. 439). The amount of time isn't the important dimension; it is the quality of the relationship that is far more influential and that in contemporary attachment research would now be referred to by terms such as 'parental sensitivity' or 'parental mind-mindedness' (i.e. 'caregivers' attunement to their infants' internal states') (Meins, 2013, p. 524).

3   'The great majority of parents, as well as infants, are secure' (p. 439). Many small- and large-scale surveys of attachment organization, including cross-cultural samples, routinely find that between 35 and 45 percent of individuals are 'insecurely attached', so it's scarcely true that this constitutes a 'great majority'. And attachment writers such as Crittenden (for example, Crittenden, 1995) argue that speaking of 'insecure' attachment, other than at its extremes, obscures its adaptive function – and can pathologize what clearly are very prevalent ways of relating to others. Another misconception we have also noticed is that many people assume that if an individual is securely attached then they are a 'nice' person, whereas insecurely attached individuals are not. Attachment organization ('styles' is a term that has almost disappeared from the lexicon) can reveal interesting things about how individuals process emotion within close relationships, but they are not a catch-all term to explain everything about human interaction. One of us (David) has consistently argued that the term 'attachment' is often better replaced by 'relationship' (Shemmings, 2016a): an *attachment* has four key components – the concept of a 'secure base' and 'safe haven', proximity-seeking behaviour and separation protest; hence, it should be distinguished from 'affectional bonds', 'love', 'affiliation' and other close relational constructs.

The need to keep abreast of research developments

It is good professional practice to stay up to date in one's area of interest and specialism; this is especially true in the field of attachment because so much research is undertaken. To give an illustration, we look briefly at the complex area of disorganized attachment (or 'D behaviour'). This is a set of behaviours seen in infants (i.e. 12–18 months) during an assessment technique, the strange situation procedure (SSP). They showed odd, conflicted, contradictory or fearful behaviour when reunited with a carer who had returned after a brief separation (to which the child almost invariably had responded by crying or screaming, thus indicating their discomfort that their carer was no longer with them). In 2011, Solomon, the original collaborator with Main, with whom she analyzed a large number of SSP tapes, wrote (referring to Bowlby's interest in children being separated from a parent under adverse circumstances):

> Maternal separation and deprivation are, however, usually not the common causes of disorganised attachment. A recent meta-analysis of the conditions under which disorganised attachments are most likely points strongly to families in which there has been maltreatment or where there is high cumulative stress.
>
> (Cyr, Euser, Bakermans-Kranenburg, & Van Ijzendoorn, 2010,
> cited in Solomon & George, 2011, p. 14)

Until relatively recently, many authors have tended to view disorganized attachment in the SSP as likely to be the result of child maltreatment, as this leaves the child frightened of a carer in situations when they need comfort, protection and reassurance. This can be marked if the carer is perceived as more frightening than the external source of the child's fear (for example, a large spider, a barking dog, a loud bang etc.). Indeed, in the meta-analysis referred to, it needed all of five stressful socio-economic factors studied (e.g. unemployment, drug abuse, domestic abuse . . .) to produce the same effect as child maltreatment on its own.

While Solomon and George (2011) go on to consider other explanations, by 2016–17 they, Mary Main and others wanted to clarify their original explication of the concept and history of the concept to take account of other 'pathways to D' (Granqvist et al., 2016). But some of the confusion around the aetiology of 'D behaviour' centres on whether the 'maltreatment' being referred to is understood as being 'intentionally' caused (e.g. sexual abuse) or whether it happened 'unintentionally' (e.g. from 'frightening [FR] caregiving'), perhaps as a result of a parent having experienced unresolved trauma themselves. Either way, it is now acknowledged that there exist several different 'pathways to D', including frequent placement moves, scenarios in which the child is frightened *of* – or *for* – a primary caregiver and even excessive exposure to the SSP (for more detail see Shemmings, 2016b). But whatever the pathway, a child who regularly experiences marked distress from which there is little or no prospect of relief is in a precarious psychological predicament. To change such a pattern, the parents will need help and support to provide more nurturing, and certainly less frightening, responses. The prospect of such help and support being effective is high, often within short timescales. For example, increased sensitivity and reduced FR were noted after only a few sessions in attachment and bio-behavioural catch-up (ABC) (Dozier & Roben, 2014).

Contemporary attachment theory

A modern reading of attachment theory and research now re-emphasizes John Bowlby's (1982) original concept of a 'goal-corrected partnership' as a baby approaches toddlerhood. Infants up to about six to nine months mostly gain the attention of their primary carers by actions such as crying, screaming, cooing or smiling. But by around nine months, they adjust their responses in accordance with the carer's behaviour. The dyad becomes more reciprocal, including more conditional responses by the child: there is now more of a 'dance', but it isn't always synchronized. So, for example, excluding the cluster of D behaviours, when a toddler was reunited with the temporarily absent parent in the SSP, three different, organized patterns were noted, each aimed at ensuring that the parent stays in the room (because it was clearly distressing for the child when they left). That is the 'goal' . . . but the child's behaviour is 'corrected', depending on their experience of what is perceived as 'working'. So some children show their feelings and are comforted (secure attachment), while others defensively exclude their feelings by pretending they are 'OK' (insecure *avoidant* attachment) – but of interest here is that, while they look unphased on the surface, underneath, their cortisol levels are often alarmingly high (Spangler & Grossmann, 1993). The third group escalate their emotional reaction to ensure that the carer's attentional resources are focused on them rather than the parent (the insecure *ambivalent* attachment pattern). But because the insecure patterns account for such a large percentage of any population, we believe that social workers should divert their attention to more rewarding areas of attachment theory and research.

Refinements of Bowlby's original ideas are constantly producing exciting findings, each of which has applications to social work practice. We consider four of these contemporary developments.

1 The concept of 'mentalisation'

When trying to assess what is 'going on' in close, caregiving relationships – whether involving infants, toddlers, teenagers or adults when they are cared for by other adults – a central construct that emerges is individuals' appreciation that others have different experiences, wishes, hopes and expectations than themselves. We have always known this intuitively, often indicated by phrases such as 'He doesn't seem to understand the child's needs', or 'She seems to meet her own needs, often at the expense of the person being cared for'.

As it turns out, this idea of being curious about another person's perspective is at the root of all attachment relationships because they are essentially about 'mind-to-mind' connections. It was first called 'mentalisation' by Fonagy in 1989. Other terms, all relevant to social workers, have similar resonances with 'mentalisation', such as 'mind-mindedness' (Meins, 2013) and 'reflective function' (Fonagy & Target, 1997; see Chapter 9). For example, the ability of a carer to understand the perspective of an older person in the early stages of dementia can help inoculate them from inappropriate attributions such as 'She's doing this deliberately'. It might also help relatives understand why asking older people if they remember who they are is likely to be very distressing for them both.

Individuals who have secure, or at least organized, attachment biographies tend to be more capable of mentalization, whereas individuals who have been neglected or abused are wary or even fearful of 'other's minds'. This is for the obvious reason that the 'mind of another' is not somewhere they feel comfortable or safe. Consider the dynamics of sexual abuse, and it is easy to appreciate why this is the case: the abuser's mind is the last place a survivor wants to visit.

With a contemporary knowledge of 'mentalisation', social workers aim to bring the 'inside out' (a deliberate reference to the Disney/Pixar film of the same name). Practitioners known to us in the field of child protection often use the following film clip from *Inside Out* (see www.youtube.com/watch?v=_MC3XuMvsDI). They show the extract and then ask a couple of questions to establish whether the idea of 'mentalisation' is understood. For example, they will ask an adult or teenager why Riley's mother is annoyed with her father. The answer is that he asked the same question that she did. She doesn't know he is thinking about a football match – some family members will need this explained – and he certainly doesn't know about the 'Brazilian helicopter pilot'. Only the audience knows these things.

Another related concept is that of 'epistemic trust'. 'Episteme' is a Greek word for knowledge and so 'epistemic trust' connotes the 'verifiable' experience of being understood. It is far more than a feeling that 'this social worker seems like someone who understands people'; it's the experience of feeling that they understand *me*. So, if an older person in a residential home said, 'I'm sick of this place. I wish I was back home', it might prompt the following response to develop epistemic trust: 'I've seen pictures of your garden, and I can see why you'd miss it. Is that what you miss most?' Such responses help the person feel that they are being listened to, understood and responded to with 'intelligent kindness and unsentimental compassion' (Shemmings & Shemmings, 2014, p. 15). They also encourage the individual to talk more (if, of course, they wish to). The worker might then invite the resident to show them some more photos and maybe pay a visit. If this is not feasible, they could ask a relative to make a short film of the area and then bring it with them next time. A practitioner would need to consider whether this level of 'occasioned nostalgia' could make things worse for the individual.

Another application of practice based on this concept is 'parental-embodied mentalisation' (PEM: Shai & Belsky, 2016). This idea progresses beyond the simple verbalization of implied intentional states of mind to include considering how they manifest bodily, facially and non-verbally within dyadic interactions. So far, PEM has only been applied with parent-child interactions, but there is no reason why such insights cannot be applied to a range of adult-to-adult caregiving situations.

2 Unresolved trauma

At the time of writing, the UK has experienced two terrorism-related incidents as well as an inferno in a London tower block in which over 70 people perished, with hundreds made homeless and others who suffered serious injuries. Many will remember the images of archetypically 'tough' and resilient fire-fighters breaking down in tears at what they witnessed. The effects of such 'event-based' trauma are well documented, whereas the downstream consequences of chronic sexual, physical and emotional maltreatment are only just being acknowledged. But the 'body keeps the score' (van der Kolk, 2015, title), often for many years in situations when a carer is at the same time a source of terror. 'Attachment-based' trauma is no less debilitating and draining of attentional, cognitive and emotional resources than 'event-based' trauma, but it tends to elicit far less sympathy and understanding. Social workers are now beginning to develop 'trauma-informed' practice with children and families. Enlightened leaders and managers see that, for their staff to undertake this demanding work and act as a secure base and safe haven with those they work with, they, as professionals, have the right to expect the same from the organizations employing them. Consequently, we are seeing the fledgling shoots of 'trauma-informed' organizations and management practice beginning to take root in parts of the country (see also Chapters 33–34).

From an attachment-perspective:

> . . . if . . . trauma (is) 'resolved', the original memory is eventually integrated within its original context in such a way that makes sense in the present. If the original memory remains disjointed and partitioned from the present, intrusive half-remembered images may return unannounced, often as a result of sights, smells and sounds alongside thoughts and emotions accompanied by physiological responses.
>
> *(Fearon & Mansell, 2001)*

This is why a traumatized individual finds it difficult to concentrate and stay emotionally available to a demanding infant, a challenging teenager or a dependent and frightened older relative. An individual traumatized by events becomes over-sensitized and hypervigilant to anxiety and stress, especially memories that remind them of the original event. With attachment-based trauma, on the other hand, it will be subconscious recollections of the *abuser* – for example, their clothing, tone of voice, favourite food – that will plunge the victim or survivor into a frightening abyss. But the main problem for them is that their trust in humans has been fractured and, in some cases, seemingly destroyed altogether.

According to Main and Hesse (1990), a vicious cycle is soon established in which the sensitivity of the parent to the child's needs is compromised, and 'dysregulation manifests if the unresolved loss or trauma in the parent has been triggered by the infant's signals for comfort' (Main & Hesse, 1990). They can't find the inner resources to calm or soothe the child. This leaves the parent feeling very frightened which, in turn, frightens the child, who reacts by being more and more demanding, or, worse still, switching off and dissociating. The final phase in the cycle involves the parent avoiding the child whenever they are even minimally distressed or in need of comfort, reassurance and protection: in other words, the child's most basic attachment needs are overlooked or even punished.

This mostly unconscious process is what we called elsewhere 'repeating what we can't remember' (Shemmings & Shemmings, 2011, p. 109). It has many similarities to post-traumatic stress disorder (PTSD), for example re-experiencing the trauma through flashbacks, nightmares and intrusive waking thoughts or emotional numbness. There are differences, however, in that it tends to be potentially trustworthy people, typically social workers, teachers or sports coaches who can become the trigger. This is because the child's central nervous system is operating from a basic 'I'm unlovable' script, and they unconsciously devote considerable attentional resources in the short term to lassoing the unsuspecting, well-meaning practitioner into maintaining the model ... by rejecting the child.

One of the important findings from research into attachment-based trauma is that it is not the severity of abuse that causes emotional problems later; it is the meaning behind it. This is not a new idea; over 2000 years ago the Greek philosopher Epictetus concluded that: 'In a word, neither death, nor exile, nor pain, nor anything of this kind is the real cause of our doing or not doing any action, but our inward opinions and principles' (Long, 1904, p. 36). We hope that without too much infidelity to his sharp-wittedness, this could be amended slightly to: 'It is not the past that's the problem; it's the sense we make of it'. As if to underline the ubiquity, timelessness and universality of these insights, Lyons-Ruth and Jacobvitz (2008) found they applied over time and across cultures.

Social workers are key people in helping, either directly or indirectly, a child or adult 'make better sense of the past' and become a more resilient individual, as we shall see in the next section. But practitioners need to know precisely how to become a trusted secure base and safe haven to create and sustain such a working alliance, while continually being placed under considerable relational pressure to reject the very individual who needs it most.

3 Secure-base priming and its applications

The third strand of contemporary research findings directly relevant to social work practice is the notion of 'secure base priming' (Carnelley & Rowe, 2007). This is at first sight a remarkably simple and practical idea, and it is surprising that it has only recently entered the social work dictionary.

When any of us struggle emotionally, if we don't have a trusted attachment figure available, we tend to 'call up' thoughts, images or transitional objects that have offered us comfort and reassurance in the past. They might include, for example, photos of loved ones, teddy bears or dolls or a piece of music. Trauma workers in the British army speak frequently of patiently sitting with a traumatized soldier as he clutches his favourite childhood teddy, wrapped in a duvet, weeping uncontrollably: a part of the process of coming to terms with his 'in theatre' demons. He needs to find a 'safe place and a safe person' (the trauma worker) to 'walk through the trauma' so as to create, to quote the clinical psychologist Trickey (2009), 'an insulation to encase the live wire of the trauma'. By finding words to describe the unprocessed 'sights, smells and sounds', the trauma survivor is slowly released from the intrusive memories, flashbacks and unwanted reminders. But there are two preconditions for this to happen without the survivor ending up re-traumatized; this is often an unintended outcome of 'talking cures' when deployed in isolation. Firstly, the worker needs to 'calm the body', which is often achieved by using a 'relaxation' technique such as eye movement desensitization and reprocessing (EMDR), rhythmic tapping, controlled diaphragmatic breathing or mindfulness training. Secondly, the ability of the worker to act as a container of anxiety (Bion, 1962) is crucial to the survivor's ability eventually to reprocess the trauma. These two conditions apply equally to event-based and attachment-based trauma. With this notion of containment, we see resonances with Bowlby's belief that an adult attempting to act as a safe haven and secure base would need to act but, more importantly, be *perceived* as acting in a 'bigger, stronger, wiser and kind' manner. Here we see resonances with 'epistemic trust'.

It was only a matter of time before Carnelley and her colleagues thought of reversing the process. Could we not 'call to mind' a secure base object, on demand and when the need arises?

As a consequence, we are now seeing the use of reassuring and comforting Paro robot seals (see www.pararobots.com/) with older people with early onset dementia and the 'proof-of-concept' development of a responsive, interactive avatar (RITA) (see www.kent.ac.uk/sspssr/ccp/Rita-mrs-jones-video.html) as a 'virtual companion', again with people in the early stages of dementia. There is also an exciting innovation being pioneered at Imperial College London, where an avatar is created with children who have experienced attachment-based trauma (Cittern, Edalat, & Ghaznavi, 2017). The avatar represents their 'inner child', who they are then shown how to nurture and then finally to re-parent. The inner child avatar is, of course, meant to represent a 'synth' of themselves. If this sounds fanciful, we can assure readers it isn't; it merely represents the general trend towards the incorporation of machine learning, artificial intelligence and animated robotic holograms.

But, to return to a more analogue-based present reality, there is a more mundane implication for social workers offering a secure base and safe haven to children and adults. In 2014, we wrote a chapter with Sonya Falck, a psychotherapist based in Harley Street, called 'Fake it till you make it' (Shemmings & Shemmings, 2014 pp. 212–213). It refers to research that argues that the more we act as a secure base, the more we become securely attached ourselves. In the attachment literature this is called 'earned security' (Roisman, Padrón, Scroufe, & Egeland, 2002). That looks and sounds like the ultimate 'win-win' situation for social work. Of course, to become a secure base and safe haven for family members requires practitioners to be aware of their own attachment history and organization. Without this knowledge, they can easily be lassoed into rejecting a traumatized individual with an 'I'm unloveable' script, as we saw in the previous section.

4 Attachment-based social work in later life relationships

In this final section we explore how contemporary attachment theory contains profound insights into work with older people (see also Chapters 7 and 40–41). The first two examples are both focused on people with dementia, whereas the third looks at how practitioners can support adult children caring for their ageing parents through an understanding of later life filial attachments. The teams conducting the first two studies each benefitted from experienced attachment theorists and researchers, respectively Everett Waters and Rudi Dallos.

Attachment and dementia

Chen et al. (2013) asked 87 primary caregivers to construct three stories around three different themes (for example, 'Your parent gets lost'), using 12 to 14 prompt words suggesting a beginning, middle and end. With the 'parent gets lost' example, the prompt words were as follows:

your parent	worried	tears
driving	telephone	dinner
lost	calls your home	talk
getting late	directions	smile

Their efforts were analyzed with the discourse analytic method used in the *Adult Attachment Interview* (AAI: George, Kaplan, & Main, 1996). Clark Baim and Lydia Guthrie (2017) have recently been promoting the use of the AAI with social workers in adult services. This approach produces what are termed 'attachment representations' (i.e. access to an individual's internal working model of relationships). The resulting stories were used to assess whether the content carried an implied concept of a 'secure-base script' (see our Section 3). The quality of interactions between the carer and the older person were also measured using the *Level of Expressed Emotions Scale* (Cole & Kazarian, 1988), alongside self-report measures of caregivers' perception of caregiving as being 'difficult'. Experienced social workers will recognize the implications for working with primary caregivers in this challenging role:

> Caregivers' secure base script knowledge predicted lower levels of negative expressed emotion. This effect was moderated by the extent to which participants experienced caring for elderly parents as difficult. Attachment representations played a greater role in caregiving when caregiving tasks were perceived as more difficult. These results support the hypothesis that attachment representations influence the quality of care that adults provide their elderly parents'.
>
> *(Cole & Kazarian, 1988, p. 392)*

The second study by Kokkonen, Cheston, Dallos, and Smart (2013) looked at the role of staff attachment style, geriatric nursing self-efficacy and approaches to dementia in burnout with 77 members of dementia care staff working in an inpatient ward. This research is primarily concerned with how individuals deal with stress and emotion, as most attachment researchers now conceptualize the theory as one of 'affect regulation'. The article makes an important contribution because of its unexpected findings, each of which offers important insights to social workers in this field.

The authors expected, entirely understandably, that 'less positive attitudes would be related to higher levels of burnout'. But they found that 'insecure attachment, lower levels of self-efficacy, and *more optimistic attitudes in staff* were related to *higher* levels of burnout' (p. 544, emphases added). Their explanation of the 'more hope, more burnout' finding was that 'staff with more optimistic attitudes give more of themselves in their work, and as a consequence are more likely to experience burnout in some settings' (p. 562).

The authors acknowledge that further research is required to explore the relationship between a sense of optimism and burnout of dementia care staff. It may be that a design is needed to separate and isolate the intervening, moderating and mediating effects of different influencing factors. For example, the 'more hope, more burnout' finding may be a function of the attachment organization of each individual.

Adult carers of ageing parents

Attachment theory in general implies that one of the primary reasons for the maintenance of this bond in later life concerns the protection of the attachment figure. But adult sons and daughters and their parents are aware, consciously or unconsciously, that this relationship is moving inexorably towards its end, and hence, relational stress may be experienced by both parties. Such stress may be compounded when middle-generation adults invite their parent to live with them, especially if personal and intimate care involving role reversal are provided.

One of us considered filial attachment relationships from the perspective of the adult 'child' (Shemmings, 2006a). The overarching research question was 'How do adult children mentally represent their past, present and future attachment relationships with a parent'? Participants were selected using the *Attachment Style Questionnaire* to include equal numbers of the three main attachment styles. Firstly, *Q Methodology* (Shemmings, 2006b) was used to factor analyze a Q-sort of 44 attachment-specific statements concerning this relationship. Secondly, an extended version of the *Adult Attachment Interview* acted as a guided conversation from which transcripts were examined to illuminate the results of the factor analysis.

Six robust factors emerged, accounting for 71 percent of the variation. The first two, *Confident Resolution* and *Resolved Yearning* ('Things are not great between us, but we're resigned to it – it works, and that's OK') incorporate the *secure* attachment organization. The division of the secure attachment organization into two factors constitutes a new finding in attachment theory. The third and fourth factors – *Distant Irritation* and *Dutiful Loyalty*, respectively – capture the *avoidant* style, with the remaining two factors – *Unresolved Yearning* and *Entangled Resentment* – comprising *ambivalent* individuals. Here is an example of 'Dutiful Loyalty':

Respondent   *I think 'hot coals' would describe my relationship to her really. I think she is super-sensitive about lots of things and yet very dominant, you know there's that sort of conflict there so you went around a bit on eggshells for a lot of the time. I don't ever want to upset her; there were times when I could scream and yell as one does and swear at her and call her names . . . but I never do. I don't think I have ever answered her back in my life . . . about anything . . . for as long as I can remember, you know you always had to treat Mummy a bit carefully, you were wary of what you said and what you did and how you did it.*

Interviewer   And that's still true?

Respondent   *Oh, yeah . . . it's still true! She's sort of an emotional bombshell, I think. So, you see, when I see her etc., it's out of loyalty, not love.*

It is easy to see how such information can help social workers advise adult sons and daughters contemplating having their parents live with them, a situation likely to increase considerably as we live longer, especially if dependents become concerned that they might lose large amounts of their inheritance if parents have to sell their house to pay for residential care. But the intensity of the relationship may prove to be very stressful if carers are unaware of how their attachment histories may play out in daily caregiving tasks.

Conclusion

If social workers avoid the misconceptions, myths and misuses of attachment theory identified in this chapter, it will continue to provide a prism through which to make sense of relationships which are, after all, the cornerstone of work with family members of all ages. And if practitioners keep up to date with contemporary developments, they will find in attachment research fascinating insights into what a secure base is and why it is so crucial in helping regulate emotion.

References

Baim, C., & Guthrie, L. (2017, May). *Using attachment theory to enhance your interviews: Lessons from the Adult Attachment Interview*. Manchester: Community Care Live.

Bion, W. (1962). *Learning from experience*. London: Heinemann.

Bowlby, J. (1982). Attachment and loss: Retrospect and prospect. *American Journal of Orthopsychiatry, 52*(4), 664–678.

Carnelley, K. B., & Rowe, A. C. (2007). Repeated priming of attachment security influences immediate and later views of self and relationships. *Personal Relationships, 14*(2), 307–320.

Chen, C. K., Waters, H. S., Hartman, M., Zimmerman, S., Miklowitz, D. J., & Waters, E. (2013). The secure base script and the task of caring for elderly parents: Implications for attachment theory and clinical practice. *Attachment and Human Development, 15*(3), 332–348.

Cittern, D., Edalat, A., & Ghaznavi, I. (2017, April). *Applying relationships science to contemporary interventions*. Artificial Intelligence and Simulation of Behaviour Annual Convention, Bath: Bath University.

Cole, J. D., & Kazarian, S. S. (1988). The level of expressed emotion scale: A new measure of expressed emotion. *Journal of Clinical Psychology, 44*(3), 392–397.

Crittenden, P. M. (1995). Attachment and psychopathology. In S. Goldberg, R. Muir, & J. Kerr (Eds.), *John Bowlby's attachment theory: Historical, clinical, and social significance* (pp. 367–406). New York: Analytic Press.

Cyr, C., Euser, E. M., Bakermans-Kranenburg, M. J., & Van Ijzendoorn, M. H. (2010). Attachment security and disorganization in maltreating and high-risk families: A series of meta-analyses. *Development and Psychopathology, 22,* 87–108.

Dozier, M., & Roben, C. (2014). Attachment related preventive interventions. In J. Simpson & W. S. Rholes (Eds.), *Attachment theory and research: New directions and emerging themes* (pp. 374–392). New York: Guilford.

Falck, S., & Shemmings, D. (2014). Fake it till you make it. In D. Shemmings &. Y. Shemmings (Eds.), *Assessing disorganised attachment behaviour in children: An evidence-based model for understanding and supporting families* (pp. 212–223). London: Jessica Kingsley.

Fearon, R. M. P., & Mansell, W. (2001). Cognitive perspectives on unresolved loss: Insights from the study of PTSD. *Bulletin of the Menninger Clinic, 65,* 380–396.

Fonagy, P., & Target, M. (1997). Attachment and reflective function: Their role in self-organization. *Development and Psychopathology, 9,* 679–700.

George, C., Kaplan, N., & Main, M. (1996). *The attachment interview for adults* (3rd ed.). (Unpublished Manuscript). Department of Psychology, University of California, Berkeley.

Granqvist, P., Hesse, E., Fransson, M., Main, M., Hagekull, B., & Bohlin, G. (2016). Prior participation in the strange situation and overstress jointly facilitate disorganized behaviours: Implications for theory, research and practice. *Attachment & Human Development, 18*(3), 235–249.

Howe, D. (1995). *Attachment theory for social work practice.* London: Palgrave Macmillan.

Howe, D. (2011). *Attachment across the lifecourse: A brief introduction.* Basingstoke: Palgrave Macmillan.

Kokkonen, T., Cheston, R., Dallos, R., & Smart, C. (2013). Attachment and coping of dementia care staff: The role of staff attachment style, geriatric nursing self-efficacy, and approaches to dementia in burn out. *Dementia.* doi:10.1177/1471301213479469

Long, G. (Tr.) (1904). *Discourses of epictetus.* New York: Appleton.

Lyons-Ruth, K., & Jacobvitz, D. (2008). Attachment disorganisation: Genetic factors, parenting contexts, and developmental transformation from infancy to adulthood. In J. Cassidy & P. R. Shaver (Eds.), *Handbook of attachment: Theory, research and clinical applications* (2nd ed., pp. 666–697). New York: Guilford.

Main, M., & Hesse, E. (1990). Parents' unresolved traumatic experiences are related to infant disorganized attachment status: Is frightened and/or frightening parental behavior the linking mechanism? In M. T. Greenberg, D. Cicchetti, & E. M. Cummings (Eds.), *Attachment during the preschool years: Theory, research and intervention* (pp. 161–182). Chicago: University of Chicago Press.

Main, M., Hesse, E., & Hesse, S. (2011). Attachment theory and research: Overview, with suggested applications to child custody. *Family Court Review, 49,* 426–463.

Meins, E. (2013). Sensitive attunement to infants' internal states: Operationalising the construct of mind-mindedness. *Attachment & Human Development, 15*(5), 524–544.

Roisman, G. I., Padron, E., Sroufe, L. A., & Egeland, B. (2002). Earned-secure attachment status in retrospect and prospect. *Child Development, 73*(4), 1204–1219.

Shai, D., & Belsky, J. (2016). Parental embodied mentalizing: How the nonverbal dance between parents and infants predicts children's socio-emotional functioning. *Attachment and Human Development, 19*(2), 191–219.

Shemmings, D. (2006a). Using adult attachment theory to differentiate adult children's internal working models of later life filial relationships. *Journal of Aging Studies, 20,* 177–191.

Shemmings, D. (2006b). 'Quantifying' qualitative data: An illustrative example of the use of Q methodology in psychosocial research. *Qualitative Research in Psychology, 3,* 147–216.

Shemmings, D., & Shemmings, Y. (2011). *Understanding disorganized attachment: Theory and practice for working with children and adults.* London: Jessica Kingsley.

Shemmings, D. (2016a, 15 February). A quick guide to attachment theory. *The Guardian,* Online.

Shemmings, D. (2016b). Making sense of disorganised attachment behaviour in pre-school children. *International Journal of Birth and Parent Education, 4* (1), 21–26.

Shemmings, D., & Shemmings, Y. (Eds.). (2014). *Assessing disorganized attachment behaviour in children: An evidence-based model for understanding and supporting families.* London: Jessica Kingsley.

Solomon, J., & George, C. (2011). The disorganized attachment-caregiving system: Dysregulation of adaptive processes at multiple levels. In J. Solomon & C. George (Eds.), *Disorganized attachment and caregiving* (pp. 3–24). New York: Guilford.

Spangler, G., & Grossmann, K. E. (1993). Biobehavioral organization in securely and insecurely attached infants. *Child Development, 64*, 1439–1450.

Trickey, D. (2009, October). *Child abuse: Neuroscience and intervention.* London: Anna Freud Centre.

van der Kolk, B. (2015). *The body keeps the score: Brain, mind, and body in the healing of trauma.* New York: Viking.

Wilkins, D., Shemmings, D., & Shemmings, Y. (2015). *The A-Z of attachment.* London: Palgrave Macmillan.

How green is social work? Towards an ecocentric turn in social work

John Coates and Mel Gray

The environmental crisis is not just having an impact on our lives. It is our way of life. It is the advancement of the industrial enterprise through the consumption of nature and the exploitation of people.

(Coates, 2005, p. 31)

Growing worldwide concern for climate change and environmental decline has spawned much scholarship in social work, where attention to ecological approaches has increased due to global awareness of these issues and their anticipated catastrophic consequences. Advocates suggest that these approaches provide a foundation of values, assumptions and practices for the profession to contribute effectively to the struggle to counter climate change and environmental degradation. Despite some notable exceptions, ecological articulations, however well intended, have proved ineffective in garnering sufficient endorsement and adherence to move the profession away from the dominant individualistic, deterministic and clinical or direct practice focus. Many of these articulations deal with causal connections as they add additional layers of services and skill-sets, while the core foundation remains unexamined and unchanged. Any hope of positive long-term change is minimized as interventions, to be effective, must operate from a value base different from that from which the problem arises (Einstein, n.d.).

The wealth of scholarly thought provides the opportunity for a deep review of social work's traditional theoretical foundations. If social change were, indeed, a central task of social work, then clearly one of the profession's tasks would be to 'expose the values, beliefs and destructive practices' (Coates, 2016, p. 70) that have contributed to the exploitation of people and the planet. To do this effectively, or at least adequately, social work would have to decolonize itself and operate from a theoretical foundation that enables well-rounded, critical assessment, as well as consideration of alternatives.

Most scholarship is consistent with a conventional environmental consciousness (Christopher, 1999), which adheres to mechanistic and rationalist thinking and an over-reliance on technological solutions to the problems of waste and over-harvesting. Coates (2012) argues that such conventional thinking is consistent with what other scholars have labelled human welfare ecology (Eckersley, 1992), resourcist (Howard, 2008), and conventional environmentalist

(Wapner, 2003) understandings of nature. What follows from such approaches are technological efforts to reduce the effects of global warming through *inter alia* more efficient use of resources, resource conservation, waste reduction and technological advances. This is consistent with the resource conservation movement (see Pinchot, 1947) that emerged in the US in the early 20th century as a way to conserve nature for human use. Such measures may reduce the negative impact of climate change and over-harvesting, but, at best, they are mere symptom reduction. Environmental and social problems are not outliers or miscalculations; they are built-in consequences of 'modern capitalism, industrial technology, individualistic morality, and mechanistic science' (Christopher, 1999, p. 361). Long-term, effective solutions will not occur when exploitative, extractive and anthropocentric principles and actions remain dominant. A truly effective response can only come about when we expunge and replace dualistic, anthropocentric thinking, where Earth is viewed as a resource for human use and garbage can for human waste.

To be truly transformative and effective, the profession would first have to explore its foundational theories, decolonize itself from modernist worldviews and, rather than fit in with anthropocentric perspectives, work through a metamorphosis consistent with the 'transitional discourses' (Escobar, 2011). The 'transitional discourses' critique the discontinuities that are the most central feature of the modern world view – the disconnections between people and nature, self and other, social and environmental and spiritual and material (Escobar, 2011). Bridging the divide with principles of interdependence and interconnection, self-organizing and complexity, point to a relational world view that offers a 'different way of imagining life' (Escobar, 2011, p. 139) and the human role on the planet. Such a transitional view informs the work of Berry (1988), Coates (2003, 2005), Gibson-Graham (2006), Hathaway and Boff (2009), Hopkins (2009), and Shiva (2005, 2008), among others. A transitional discourse transforms the dominant, anthropocentric, individualistic and materialist understanding of progress and well-being to one that is ecocentric and deeply communal and sees relationships of interdependence and, for some, a spiritual connection among all life on the planet. Such an 'ecocentric turn' (Escobar, 2011) would enable a transition to new foundational assumptions, values and beliefs in keeping with the universe's creative processes. It would lead to a radical transformation of understanding of society, the planet and the human role therein.

The ecological approach, when based on a non-modern, ecocentric world view, offers a different way of imagining well-being and a society that supports it. This is similar in many ways to traditional indigenous thought and is evident, for example, in Hart's (2002) notion of 'the good life' and Escobar's (2011) idea of 'living well', where economic issues are subservient to ecological justice. Such a view does not accept the inevitability and universality of globalization based on capitalist modernity. It argues for the benefit of a new economy (Korten, 2009), based *inter alia* on economic localization (Mander & Goldsmith, 1996), sustainable consumption (Heap & Kent, 2000; Hoque, 2014; Jackson, 2005), limited growth (Meadows, Meadows, Randers, & Behrens, 1972), food security (Polack, Wood, & Bradley, 2008), reducing the human ecological footprint (Wackernagel & Rees, 1996) and the inseparability of social and environmental justice (Rixecker & Tipene-Matua, 2003).

Tracing social work's ecological turn

Social work emerged in modern society to deal with the families and individuals who suffered the ill effects of industrialization, urbanization and war. In ecological language, these people (victims perhaps) did not 'fit in' with the developments that were taken to be progressive in modern society. In the years that followed, social work strengthened its professional place in modern society by adopting a therapeutic focus that concentrated, in practice though not in theory, on work with individuals and families. In its early years, social work looked to the scholarship of other professions and disciplines. Thus, the work of Freud, Rank, Rogers and Skinner, *inter alia*, found its way into social work theory, education and practice. As distinct social work scholarship evolved, various ways of conceptualizing social work developed, such as the functional and diagnostic schools, and different approaches emerged – psychoanalytic, psychosocial and problem solving. Still other more structured methods came forward, such as task-centred practice (Reid, 1978; Reid & Epstein, 1972a, 1972b) and the cognitive behavioural approach (Berlin, 1982) and, more recently, several other intervention models emerged, such as narrative and strengths-based practice.

Some of these developments came out of the push for research-based practice and were clearly models for direct practice situated within broader theoretical frameworks, such as cognitive behavioural and empirically based practice (Fischer, 1976, 1978; Gambrill, 1977). Still others emerged that were primarily theoretical, such as anti-racist, structural, feminist, systems and ecological perspectives, and practice skills were articulated over time. Many of these developed in response to changes in the academic community and larger society, such as the Frankfurt School, racial unrest and feminist and postmodern critiques.

Systems theory's strong influence on social work began in the 1970s (Hearn, 1969, 1974; Payne, 2002; see Chapter 15). The integrated ecosystems approach arose primarily from attempts to overcome the specialized methods approach to social work and the situation wherein casework, group work and community work were each developing their own theory and practice, giving social work a fragmented appearance (Germain, 1979, 1981, 1985; Greif & Lynch, 1983; Siporin, 1980; Gilgun, 1999). Systems theory and the ecosystems perspective reflected the search for a unitary or integrated approach to social work (Germain, 1991; Goldstein, 1973; Gray & Bernstein, 1994; Pincus & Minahan, 1973). While most influential in the US, however, it had minimal influence on social work in the UK (Payne, 2002).

How green is social work?

Despite using the language of ecology and recognizing the important role of the social environment in people's lives, consideration of the environment in social work scholarship was restricted to the sociocultural environment. Despite recent efforts to rewrite social work history by noting the long-standing inclusion of the natural environment in social work's ecological approach (Germain & Gitterman, 1980; Meyer, 1983; Meyer & Mattaini, 1998), reviews of scholarly social work literature indicated that, with some exceptions (Hoff & McNutt, 1994; Soine, 1987; Tester, 1994), there was only cursory reference to nature and the physical environment, especially in practice (see for example, Besthorn, 1997, 2014; Coates, 2003, 2005; Zapf, 2009). As the environmental movement grew and scientific research on global warming confirmed the devastating long-term impacts of climate change (World Commission on Environment and Development (WCED), 1987), social work scholarship shifted with calls for attention to this area and claims of how well situated social work was to play a major role. However, despite this scholarly literature and media attention to the environmental crisis, professional practice remains reactionary and primarily ameliorative (Coates, 2012). Dewane (2011) points out that, despite the centrality of the person-in-environment perspective in 'courses on human behavior and the social environment, which are strongly recommended by the CSWE . . . little can be found about the natural or physical environment in these courses' (p. 5). While recent publications have sought to address this imbalance (Gray, Coates, & Hetherington, 2013; McKinnon & Alston, 2016), impactful and effective interventions will only come about when the profession shifts to a foundation of values and principles that enable practice to challenge the root causes of exploitation, poverty and inequality. The constraints of modernity domesticate the social work profession to the degree that it is unable to solve wicked problems. These include poverty, exploitation and inequality embedded within, and created by, the dominant collective world view: 'Unmitigated environmental destruction, social injustice and poverty are societal problems that are linked directly to the values and beliefs inherent in the structure of modern society' (Coates, 2012, p. 64). Why does poverty persist and the income gap increase steadily despite a generation of policies and programmes that seek to address them?

The myth that material progress and abundance, technological development and industrial growth and lower taxes and tariff-free trade will solve the problems of marginalization, exploitation and destitution underlies and sustains modernity's dysfunctional values and beliefs.

Rather than sustainability, however, successive post-war policies, including the UN Millennium Development Goals (MDGs), like those of social work, have followed the modernizing path of social and economic development and a pattern of relationships to create conditions that give priority to constant industrial progress and economic growth. As already argued, development policy has focused mainly on economic growth, notwithstanding the various shifts in focus from industrialization and modernization to human development and poverty reduction with the advent of the MDGs. The argument has been that economic growth is the best way of achieving a better quality of life and poverty reduction, but history has proved that instead it has brought gross inequality with many millions of people still mired in poverty worldwide.

Unrestrained modernity, and the economic, social and industrial processes that support it, are exploitation in practice. It remains a challenge to shift our thinking away from the domination of self-interest and individualism, the dualism of nature and markets and the domination by and surrender of creativity to market forces. Modernity has brought many benefits to the world but, to overcome its limitations, it must be transcended and incorporated into a larger and more inclusive world view that offers the potential to create a world where social and ecological justice prevail. An inclusive and holistic framework, a whole-system consciousness, builds on the interdependence and connectedness of all people and all life forms. Such a world view or global consciousness is not in opposition to modernity for it builds upon earlier knowledge and advancements, but it does subject the assets and processes of modernity to a new set of beliefs and values. Self-interest expands to include the interests of all people and all things. Personal well-being is dependent upon the well-being of others.

Green social work is environmentally friendly social work. It goes beyond human rights and social justice and, of necessity, considers issues of poverty and inequality in relation to climate change and environmental decline. It has synergies with the discourse on sustainable social development but goes further in its quest for ecological justice (Haberl, Fischer-Kowalski, Krausmann, Martinez-Alier, & Winiwarter, 2011; see Chapter 25). Hence, green politics and, by extension, green social work argue for 'an epochal transition' (Escobar, 2011, p. 138). This is informed by the transition discourses that have emerged from 'social movements, some civil society NGOs, and from intellectuals with significant connections to environmental and cultural struggles . . . in several fields, including those of culture, ecology, religion and spirituality, and alternative science (e.g. living systems and complexity)' (Escobar, 2011, p. 138; see also Escobar, 1996). Transition discourses posit 'radical cultural and institutional transformations' (p. 138). They promote values and beliefs of interdependence, community, belonging and participation that conjure a very different world. Such a world is characterized by 'decentralized, biodiversity-based organic food and energy systems that operate on the basis of grassroots democracy, place-based knowledge, local economies, and the preservation of soils and ecological integrity' (Escobar, 2011, p. 138). It is an 'ecology of transformation' (Hathaway & Boff, 2009), 'a transition to a worldview grounded in ecological justice, in which humans are part of our ecosystems' (Cox-Shrader, 2011, p. 270).

The transition discourses see no other alternative to the consequences of the contemporary *anthropocene* era than an ecocentric one (Crutzen & Stoermer, 2000), in which humans recognize they have caused climate change and environmental damage on an unprecedented scale. Hence, humans' relationship with the environment and the interdependence between human behaviour and the physical environment have become central to the normative vision of ecological justice. Living in harmony with the environment as a condition of human well-being and that of all living and non-living things has long been a central tenet of indigenous cosmologies. For indigenous peoples, 'sustainability is circular, complex; it is about harmony, relationships and rhythms. It is not an accounting exercise for rationing how we use the planet's resources' (Bullard, 2011, p. 142). Ecosocial work, whereby human well-being is contingent on protecting or replenishing Earth's fragile ecosystems and finite resources, holds potential for progressive, modernizing approaches to be brought into line with age-old ecocentric indigenous perspectives (Coates, Gray, & Hetherington, 2006). As Brundtland (1989) observed:

> The gross mismanagement of our planet has much to do with an inequitable distribution of the benefits of development. Perpetuating this inequity can only mean a continuing drawdown on the world's natural resources and the environment. After a century of unprecedented growth, marked by scientific and technological triumphs that would have been unthinkable a century ago, there have never been so many poor, illiterate and unemployed people in the world, and their number is growing. Close to a billion people live in poverty and squalor, a situation that leaves them little choice but to go on undermining the conditions of life itself, the environment and the natural resource base.
>
> *(cited by Estes, 1993, p. 2)*

The goals of ecological justice align with those of sustainability. These are 'equity within and across generations, places and social groups; ecological integrity; and human well-being and quality of life' (Sneddon, Howarth, & Norgaard, 2006, p. 264). They are similar to the goals of social development, as laid out in the Copenhagen Declaration (United Nations, 1995), to which latterly social work has expressed a great deal of allegiance in its Global Agenda (Gray & Webb, 2014). Here, ecocentric green social work necessarily means grappling with the politics of social development and poverty alleviation and the dismal progress toward environmental sustainability by an intransigent focus on economic development (Sachs, 1999). However, its interests are environmental. Its concern includes the consequences of poverty and inequality *on the environment*.

Though, since the Brundtland Commission (WCED, 1987), scientific research has increased our knowledge of sustainability, a major focus of Brundtland, recent scholarship (Dylan, 2012; Luke, 2005) argues that sustainable development is neither sustainable nor development. Bullard (2011) wonders, 'confronted with collapsing ecosystems, toxic environments, soil depletion, climate chaos, disappearing species and finite fossil fuels, does sustainability even make sense when there is so little left to sustain?' (p. 141). As Bullard (2011, p.141) noted:

> Perhaps the greatest challenge we face is not so much about how we understand sustainability, but rather how we understand development. When we consider the state of the world and the routine failure of 'development' to feed, house, clothe, educate and care for the invisible majority, the word no longer has any moral or even practical content.

Acero's (2011, p. 205) view of development as 'equitable and sustainable growth. . . [based on the] expansion of human capacities. . .' makes its success unattainable, since it requires '. . . the transformation of social gender relations, and transversally, racialism, sexism and all forms of discrimination'. The intractability of patriarchal relations in the Global South, like economic growth, is based on exploitation, and this has made progress on 'women's political participation and visible organized engagement' (Acero, 2011, p. 207) challenging, at best. The priority of development has to take place within a framework that prioritizes a sustainable environment, social and ecological justice and global equity. It blends social and economic policy with environmental health, fostering eco-friendly social policy and incorporating environmental well-being in therapeutic interventions. Working cooperatively with communities and nations on the struggle to find trade and political arrangements that promote both human and ecological well-being. Modelling policy on the principles that fit in with Earth's processes rather than subverting them for exclusive economic benefit.

However, there has been a lack of political will to pursue models of development that would guarantee the invisible majority a decent quality of life and address inequalities or make the kind of decisions that would lessen the uninterrupted downhill slide of environmental degradation (Sneddon et al., 2006). Likewise, the lack of political will extends to social policies that act as investments in long-term well-being but are seen as costs or debits against short-term profit. As long as economic development trumps environmental sustainability, sustainable social development – in policy discourse and development practice – will remain an unworkable ideal. The language of and thinking behind sustainable development must be replaced. Using Brown's (1991) distinction between four types of sustainability, sustainable economic progress would take account of: (i) *ecological sustainability* and ensure that Earth's renewable and non-renewable resources would not be depleted for the sake of short-term improvement; (ii) *economic sustainability* and ensure equity in resource distribution to minimize poverty; (iii) *political sustainability* and strive for the maintenance of power relations supportive of sustainability; and (iv) *cultural sustainability* and ensure local cultural values, expectations, norms and practices support improvement (see Hawkes, 2001). The world view of modernity cannot meet the requirements for sustainability – inclusiveness, connectivity, equity, prudence and security (Gladwin, Newburry, & Reiskin, 1997).

There is a need to be deeply critical of social work's stance and to deconstruct initiatives to open the door for discussion on an ecocentric foundation that places priority on environmental justice when approaching equity, poverty reduction and social development. Rather than study these issues in their broader context, social work tends to take a normative stance and this, too, is how issues of environmental sustainability and ecological justice are being approached (Besthorn, 2012, 2013, 2014). The problem with this normative stance is there is little room for serious debate and critique, for social workers pursue the cause with missionary zeal rather than informed scholarly enquiry and critical debate. Areas of environmental and climate change science are hotly debated. In books, in conferences and on electronic discussion lists, there is an element of preaching to the converted and a great deal of within-group encouragement and promotion such that a climate change denier would be a pariah. There are, within social work, people with left- and right-wing leanings, yet its discourse carries a largely leftist, emancipatory ethos that for green social work does not go far enough. For change to take place, social workers of diverse political persuasions need to be involved in the discussion, and concerns about the environment need to move from the margins to the mainstream.

Much of this hortatory discourse is evident in contemporary social work literature on social development, environmental sustainability and ecological justice. The latter is related to, but is far more ecologically radical than, social work's notions of social and environmental justice, which are based on human rights and needs and reflect social work's humanistic ethos (Besthorn, 2013; Dominelli, 2012; Miller, Hayward, & Shaw, 2011). Ecological or deep justice attributes inalienable rights to non-human entities in the natural world. As Besthorn (2012) explained, this kind of deep justice is 'the proper and necessary framework for social work as it moves into the troubled waters of a world on the edge of environmental and economic collapse' (p. 255). Green social work necessarily is political – its goal is well-being for all and ecological justice. These objectives are achievable only by radical social change informed by a foundation of values and beliefs based on equity, interdependence and ecological justice.

For green social work to emerge as a solid area of theory and practice, we need to move beyond hortatory, apocalyptic, environmental moralism and policy incrementalism to an alternative framework (Yanarella & Bartilow, 2000). Further, a reality test is needed as to what social workers might conceivably achieve. In Gray (2017), contributors writing about social work and social development in Africa wrote repeated accounts of how they were trying to embed developmental social work hampered by legislative environments, where social workers lacked a collective voice and professional legitimacy. Though undoubtedly poverty exists in the Global North, the bulk of the world's poor lives in the Global South, and social development and environmental sustainability have as their main objective the struggle against poverty and inequality, not least because of the consequences for the environment (Agyeman, Bullard, & Evans, 2003; Glasmeier & Farrigan, 2003). It is essential that ecological justice and social justice are considered jointly, and, until they are, it is highly likely that neither poverty nor ecological destruction will be alleviated. Without an ecocentric transition, a narrow and limited understanding of social justice and human interest will prevail in social work. Thus, green social work, like its predecessor the ecological paradigm, is a misnomer, and environmental social work is a more accurate description of the direction in which the profession is currently heading in addressing environmental concerns. Are the modern values underpinning social work and its humanistic interests too deeply rooted and an ecocentric turn too radical for the profession today?

Conclusion

In this chapter, we have reviewed the ecological approach in recent iterations of green, ecosocial and environmental social work, most of which are strongly embedded in anthropocentric, individualistic and deterministic – or modern – foundational beliefs and values. However, the ecological approach, we argue, is situated more appropriately among transitional discourses that, unlike other theoretical approaches, are based on an ecocentric foundation and can be truly transformative for both individuals and societies. We argue that green social work demands attention to sustainability, poverty and inequality and their consequences for the natural environment. We see environmental social work as a more accurate description of social work's current engagement, motivated as it is by human interests and the impact of climate change, environmental decline and natural disasters on human beings. Time will tell whether the profession is prepared to take the radical ecological turn or 'epochal transition' (Escobar, 2011) ecocentric green social work necessarily entails in its concern with the consequences of social development, poverty and inequality *on the environment*.

References

Acero, L. (2011). Pathways towards sustainability, participatory human development and the state. *Development, 54*(2), 205–208.

Agyeman, J., Bullard, R. D., & Evans, B. (Eds.). (2003). *Just sustainabilities: Development in an unequal world.* Cambridge, MA: MIT Press.

Berlin, S. B. (1982). Cognitive behavioral interventions for social work practice. *Social Work, 27*(3), 218–226. doi:https://doi.org/10.1093/sw/27.3.218

Berry, T. (1988). *Dream of the Earth.* San Francisco: Sierra Club.

Besthorn, F. H. (1997). *Reconceptualizing social work's person-in-environment perspective: Explorations in radical environmental thought.* (Unpublished doctoral dissertation). Lawrence: University of Kansas.

Besthorn, F. H. (2012). Deep ecology's contribution to social work: A ten-year retrospective. *International Journal of Social Welfare, 21,* 248–259.

Besthorn, F. H. (2013). Radical equalitarian ecological justice: A social work call to action. In M. Gray, J. Coates, & T. Hetherington (Eds.), *Environmental social work* (pp. 31–45). London: Routledge.

Besthorn, F. H. (2014). Ecopsychology, meet ecosocialwork: What you might not know – A brief overview and reflective comment. *Ecopsychology, 6*(4), 199–206. doi:10.1089/eco.2014.0024

Brown, L. D. (1991). Bridging organizations and sustainable development. *Human Relations, 44*(8), 807–831.

Brundtland, G. H. (1989). Sustainable development: An overview. *Development, 1989,* 2/3.

Bullard, N. (2011). It's too late for sustainability: What we need is system change. *Development, 54*(2), 141–142. doi:10.1057/dev.2011.29

Christopher, M. (1999). An exploration of the 'reflex' in reflexive modernity: The rational and pre rational social causes of the affinity for ecological consciousness. *Organization and Environment, 12*(4), 357–400.

Coates, J. (2003). *Ecology and social work: Toward a new paradigm.* Halifax, NS: Fernwood Press.

Coates, J. (2005). The environmental crisis: Implications for social work. *Journal of Progressive Human Services, 16*(1), 25–49.

Coates, J. (2012). Prisoners of the story: A role for spirituality in thinking and living our way to sustainability. In J. Groen, D. Coholic, & J. R. Graham (Eds.), *Spirituality in social work and education: Theory, practice and pedagogies* (pp. 57–76). Waterloo, ON: Wilfred Laurier University Press.

Coates, J. (2016). Ecospiritual approaches: A path to decolonizing social work. In M. Gray, J. Coates, M. Yellow Bird & T. Hetherington (Eds.), *Decolonizing social work* (pp. 88–112). London: Routledge.

Coates, J., Gray, M., & Hetherington, T. (2006). An 'ecospiritual' perspective: Finally, a place for indigenous approaches. *British Journal of Social Work, 36*(3), 381–399.

Cox-Shrader, K. (2011). Notes on the transition: Globalization, (re)localization, and ecological justice. *Development, 54*(2), 265–267. doi:10.1057/dev.2011.1

Crutzen, P. J., & Stoermer, E. F. (2000). The 'Anthropocene'. *Global Change Newsletter, 41,* 17–18.

Dewane, C. (2011). Environmentalism and social work: The ultimate social justice issue. *Social Work Today, 11*(5).

Dominelli, L. (2012). *Green social work: From environmental crises to environmental justice.* Bristol: Polity.

Dylan, A. (2012). Rethinking sustainability on planet Earth: A time for new framings. *Electronic Green Journal, 1*(34). Retrieved from https://escholarship.org/uc/item/8wm6s8s2

Eckersley, R. (1992). *Environmentalism and political theory: Towards an ecocentral approach.* Albany, NY: SUNY Press.

Einstein, A. (n.d.). *Einstein quotes.* Retrieved 7 March 2017 from www.alberteinsteinsite.com/quotes/einsteinquotes.html

Escobar, A. (1996). Constructing nature. In R. Peet & M. Watts (Eds.), *Liberation ecologies: Environment, development, social movements* (pp. 46–68). New York: Routledge.

Escobar, A. (2011). Sustainability: Design for the pluriverse. *Development, 54*(2), 137–140. doi:10.1057/dev.2011.28

Estes, R. (1993). Towards sustainable development: From theory to praxis. *Social Development Issues, 15*(3), 1–29.

Fischer, J. (1976). *The effectiveness of social casework.* Springfield, IL: Charles C. Thomas.

Fischer, J. (1978). *Effective casework practice: An eclectic approach.* New York: McGraw-Hill.

Gambrill, E. (1977). *Behavior modification: A handbook of assessment, intervention and evaluation.* San Francisco: Jossey-Bass.

Germain, C. B. (Ed.). (1979). *Social work practice: People and environments, an ecological perspective.* New York: Columbia University Press.

Germain, C. B. (1981). The ecological approach to people-environmental transactions. *Social Casework, 62*(6), 323–331.

Germain, C. B. (1985). The place of community work within an ecological approach to social work practice. In S. H. Taylor & R. W. Roberts (Eds.), *Theory and practice of community social work.* New York: Columbia University Press.

Germain, C. B. (1991). *Human behaviour in the social environment: An ecological view.* New York: Cambridge University Press.

Germain, C. B., & Gitterman, A. (1980). *The life model of social work practice.* New York: Columbia University Press.

Gibson-Graham, J.K. (2006). *A postcapitalist politics.* Minneapolis, MN: University of Minnesota Press.

Gilgun, J. F. (1999). An ecosystemic approach to assessment. In B. G. Compton & B. Galaway (Eds.), *Social work processes* (6th ed., pp. 66–82). Chicago: Dorsey Press.

Gladwin, T. N., Newburry, W. E., & Reiskin, E. D. (1997). Why is the northern elite mind biased against community, the environment and a sustainable future? In M. H. Bazerman, D. M. Messick, A. E. Tenbrunsel, & K. A. Wade-Benzni (Eds.), *Environment, ethics and behavior: The psychology of environmental valuation and degradation.* San Francisco: The New Lexington Press.

Glasmeier, A. K., & Farrigan, T. L. (2003). Poverty, sustainability, and the culture of despair: Can sustainable development strategies support poverty alleviation in America's most environmentally challenged communities? *The ANNALS of the American Academy of Political and Social Science, 590*(1), 131–149.

Gray, M. (Ed.). (2017). *The Routledge handbook of social work and social development in Africa.* London: Routledge.

Gray, M., & Bernstein, A. (1994). Integrated practice: A misnomer in social work. *Social Work / Maatskaplike Werk, 30*(1), 199–208.

Gray, M., Coates, J., & Hetherington, T. (Eds.). (2013). *Environmental social work.* London: Routledge.

Gray, M., & Webb, S. A. (2014). The making of a civil society politics in social work: Myth and misrepresentation in the global agenda. *International Social Work, 57*(4), 346–359.

Greif, G. L., & Lynch, A. (1983). The ecosystems perspective. In C. Meyer (Ed.), *Clinical social work in the ecosystems perspective.* New York: Columbia University Press.

Goldstein, H. (1973). *Social work practice: A unitary approach.* Columbia: University of South Carolina Press.

Haberl, H., Fischer-Kowalski, M., Krausmann, F., Martinez-Alier, J., & Winiwarter, V. (2011). A sociometabolic transition towards sustainability? Challenges for another great transformation. *Sustainable Development, 19*, 1–14.

Hart, M. A. (2002). *Seeking mino-pimatisiwin: An aboriginal approach to helping.* Halifax, NS: Fernwood.

Hathaway, M., & Boff, L. (2009). *The tao of liberation: Exploring the ecology of transformation.* Maryknoll, NY: Orbis.

Hawkes, J. (2001). *The fourth pillar of sustainability: Culture's essential role in public planning.* Melbourne: Cultural Development Network Victoria. Retrieved 22 January 2017 from www.culturaldevelopment.net. au/community/Downloads/HawkesJon(2001)TheFourthPillarOfSustainability.pdf

Heap, B., & Kent, J. (Eds.). (2000). *Towards sustainable consumption: A European perspective.* London: The Royal Society.

Hearn, G. (Ed.). (1969). *The general systems approach: Contributions toward an holistic conception of social work.* New York: Council on Social Work Education.

Hearn, G. (1974). General systems theory and social work. In F. J. Turner (Ed.), *Social work treatment: Interlocking theoretical approaches* (pp. 343–372). New York: The Free Press.

Hoff, M., & McNutt, J. (Eds.). (1994). *The global environmental crisis: Implications for social welfare and social work.* Brookfield, VT: Ashgate Publishing.

Hopkins, R. (2009). *The transition handbook: From oil dependency to local resilience.* White River Junction, VT: Chelsea Green Publishing.

Hoque, N. (2014). Analysing sustainable consumption patterns: A literature review. *Development, 56*(3), 370–377. doi:10.1057/dev.2014.13

Howard, P. (2008). Ecology, phenomenology, and culture: Developing a language for sustainability. *Diaspora, Indigenous, and Minority Education, 2*(4), 302–310.

Jackson, T. (2005). Live better by consuming less? Is there a 'double dividend' in sustainable consumption. *Journal of Industrial Ecology, 9*(1/2), 19–36.

Korten, D. C. (2009). *Agenda for a new economy: From phantom wealth to real wealth.* San Francisco: Barrett-Koehler.

Luke, T. W. (2005). Neither sustainable nor development: Reconsidering sustainability in development. *Sustainable Development, 13*(4), 228–238.

Mander, J., & Goldsmith, E. (Eds.). (1996). *The case against the global economy: And for a turn toward the local.* San Francisco: Sierra Club Books.

McKinnon, J., & Alston, M. (Eds.). (2016). *Ecological social work: Towards sustainability.* London: Palgrave Macmillan.

Meadows, D. H., Meadows, D. L., Randers, J., & Behrens, W. W. (1972). *The limits to growth.* New York: Universe Books.

Meyer, C. (Ed.). (1983). *Clinical social work in the ecosystems perspective.* New York: Columbia University Press.

Meyer, C. H., & Mattaini, M. A. (1998). The ecosystems perspective: Implications for practice. In M. A. Mattaini, C. T. Lowery, & C. H. Meyer (Eds.), *The foundations of social work practice* (pp. 3–19). Washington, DC: NASW Press.

Miller, S. E., Hayward, R. A., & Shaw, T. V. (2012). Environmental shifts for social work: A principles approach. *International Journal of Social Welfare, 21,* 270–277.

Payne, M. (2002). The politics of systems theory within social work. *Journal of Social Work, 2*(3), 269–292.

Pinchot, G. (1947). *Breaking new ground.* Washington, DC: Island Press.

Pincus, A., & Minahan, A. (1973). *Social work practice: Model and method.* Ithaca, IL: F. E. Peacock Publishing.

Polack, R., Wood, S., & Bradley, E. (2008). Fossil fuels and food security: Analysis and recommendations for community organizers. *Journal of Community Practice, 16*(3), 359–375. doi:10.1080/10705420802255114

Reid, W. J. (1978). *The task-centered system.* New York: Columbia University Press.

Reid, W. J., & Epstein, L. (1972a). *Task-centered casework.* New York: Columbia University Press.

Reid, W. J., & Epstein, L. (Eds.). (1972b). *Task-centered practice.* New York: Columbia University Press.

Rixecker, S. S., & Tipene-Matua, B. (2003). Maori Kaupapa and the inseparability of social and environmental justice: An analysis of bioprospecting and a people's resistance to (bio)cultural assimilation. In J. Agyeman, R. D. Bullard, & B. Evans (Eds.), *Just sustainabilities: Development in an unequal world* (pp. 252–268). Cambridge, MA: MIT Press.

Sachs, W. (1999). *Planet dialectics: Explorations in environment and development.* Halifax, NS: Fernwood Publishing.

Shiva, V. (2005). *Earth democracy: Justice, sustainability, and peace.* Cambridge, MA: South End Press.

Shiva, V. (2008). *Soil not oil: Environmental justice in an age of climate crisis.* Boston: South End Press.

Siporin, M. (1980). Ecological systems theory in social work. *Journal of Sociology and Social Welfare, 7*(4), 507–532.

Sneddon, C., Howarth, R., & Norgaard, R. (2006). Sustainable development in a post-Brundtland world. *Ecological Economics, 57,* 253–268.

Soine, L. (1987). Expanding the environment in social work: The case for including environmental hazards content. *Journal of Social Work Education, 23*(2), 40–46.

Tester, J. F. (1994). In an age of ecology: Limits to voluntarism and traditional theory in social work practice. In M. Hoff & J. McNutt (Eds.), *The global environmental crisis: Implications for social welfare and social work* (pp. 75–99). Brookfield, VT: Ashgate Publishing.

United Nations. (1995). *Copenhagen declaration on social development.* Retrieved from https://www.un.org/en/development/desa/population/migration/generalassembly/docs/globalcompact/A_CONF.166_9_Declaration.pdf

Wackernagel, M., & Rees, W. (1996). *Our ecological footprint: Reducing human impact on the earth.* Gabriola Island, BC: New Society Publishers.

Wapner, P. (2003). *Tikkun environmentalism: Towards a new realism. Tikkun, 18*(5), 41–44.

World Commission on Environment and Development (WCED). (1987). *Our common future.* Oslo, Norway: United Nations.

Yanarella, E. J., & Bartilow, H. (2000). Beyond environmental moralism and policy incrementalism in the global sustainability debate: Case studies and an alternative framework. *Sustainable Development, 8*(3), 123–134.

Zapf, M. K. (2009). *Social work and the environment: Understanding people and place.* Toronto: Canadian Scholars' Press.

15

Theory on systems, complexity and chaos

Christopher G. Hudson

Introduction

This chapter introduces an emerging theoretical framework for assessing a wide range of personal and social systems that social workers are regularly asked to work with. This framework includes elements of traditional structural-functional general systems, and ecosystems theories that became popular in the latter half of the 20th century. It also incorporates several newer theories, collectively termed complex systems theory. These include chaos, self-organization, and autopoietic theories (Hudson, 2010). Unlike the earlier functional and general systems perspectives that focus on understanding the conditions for the maintenance of stable or equilibrium conditions, complex systems theories focus on systems that function at 'far from equilibrium' conditions, which are also, alternatively, referred to as the 'edge of chaos' (Richards, 1996). In this respect, they focus on how systems change, on the *dynamics* or processes by which systems move from one state to another, how they disintegrate or develop greater levels of adaptability and creativity. These newer theories extended rather than replacing the earlier general systems model. That can now be understood as describing a special but ubiquitous type of system embedded in a broader array of social, biological and physical systems.

First generation systems theory: general systems

Parts of this section have been adapted from Hudson (2010, pp. 9–16).

Many social workers are committed to the notion of understanding the 'total situation' of their clients, a term first used by Sheffield (1937). They have not only been influenced by structural-functionalism in sociology, but also been drawn to notions of emergence, holism and systems. Bertalanffy's definition of a system established the foundation for general systems theory (GST) and its applications in the human services as follows:

> a complex of components in mutual interaction . . . Concepts and principles of systems theory are not limited to material systems, but can be applied to any [whole] consisting of interacting [components].
>
> *(1974, p. 1100)*

General systems theory represents an attempt to integrate the perspectives and findings from such diverse fields as organismic social theories of the 19th century, the social survey movement, human ecology, information theory and cybernetics (Leighninger, 1977; Siporin, 1980). Although the concept of general systems theory was initially introduced in 1937 and first published in 1945 (Hearn, 1979), it was not until the 1950s that it was popularized in psychology by Miller (1955) and introduced to social work by Hearn (1969). In the 1960s, general systems achieved popularity in social work, mostly through family systems therapy and the community mental health movement (Siporin, 1980). The 1970s saw a substantial growth in the applications of GST in the profession, and numerous social work texts began to include it.

General systems theory is premised on the assumption that there are universal rules, laws or processes that govern systems in a wide range of domains and scales. It focuses on single well-defined systems, such as a person, family, organization or community. Systems have been defined as collections of interacting elements that have a meaningful boundary separating them from their various environments (Bertalanffy, 1974). The most essential characteristics of this boundary is that it may be either permeable or impermeable, flexible or rigid, often permitting influences to pass into and out of the focal system. What passes into and out of every system is some combination of information, energy and matter, whether these involve verbal or nonverbal statements; reports, electricity, funds or motivation; waste; food; air and so on. The essential paradigm for understanding what happens within a system is a three-part process: input, process and output. Inputs in social systems may involve people, whether clients or workers; intervening processes may include therapies, support groups and administrative procedures and outputs might involve clients with better parenting skills, successfully adjudicated housing claims or students with marketable competencies.

A particularly important part of systems theory is the way that the intervening processes are conceptualized. These processes are often thought of as being controlled by implicit or explicit rules that control various procedures or algorithms. With many social systems, such as those driven by professional social workers, these processes are usually both iterative and transactional. They are iterative in that many actions are repeated until some goal or desired state is successively approximated. They are transactional in that they involve back and forth communications, often referred to as feedback loops.

Transactional patterns usually consist of some combination of positive and negative feedback loops. The more common involve negative feedback loops that operate like the proverbial thermostat that turns a furnace on or off, depending on the temperature, bringing the temperature within a pre-set acceptable range. Many biological and social processes follow this pattern (e.g. thirst, hunger, bodily temperature control, responses to group clients who talk too little or too pattern or supervisory responses to workers who deviate too far from their expected caseload size). Such processes serve to maintain equilibrium and have traditionally been emphasized in general systems explanations of dynamic processes, often at the expense of understanding how systems change. In contrast, the often-neglected positive feedback loops are interactive patterns in which processes become amplified (Arthur, 1990). One problem inflames another until there is a complete breakdown, or clients learn new problem-solving skills that reinforce one another and permit them to transition to a more effective level of adaptation, breaking out of lower equilibria governed by positive feedback loops. A frequent point of confusion involves the fact that 'positive' or 'negative' feedback loops do not mean good or bad, functional or dysfunctional loops. Either may be desirable or undesirable. Instead, positive loops are those that are deviation-amplifying, and negative loops are those that are deviation-dampening.

Other concepts are used to characterize and understand systems. Also of importance is the differentiation or specialization of functions that may or may not be developed and that may be effective or ineffective. Families may differentiate between the responsibilities of children, parents and grandparents, and organizations may have various departments. Related is the recognition that systems typically have multiple levels of organization: for example, in education, there are systems involving individual students, classrooms, schools and larger school systems, each system nested within a more encompassing system. In social work, microsystems refer to individuals and families; meso- or mezzo-systems, larger groups, organizations and local communities; and macro-systems, larger policy-making and other national and international systems, each with associated practice methods (see Bronfenbrenner, 2005; see also Chapters 25 and 27).

Because of the intellectual origins of general systems theory, which include cybernetics, there are several assumptions that tend to underlie many of the applications of this approach. These often assume local causation and emphasize the maintenance of equilibrium conditions or, alternatively, suggest that the only ways to break out of dysfunctional equilibria may be through confrontation, rather than facilitation, redirection or strengthening of existing growth and change processes. They tend to emphasize systematic and objective approaches to analysis and knowledge building, often at the expense of an intersubjective and phenomenological understanding of clients' experiences and attitudes, important in the social work profession. Nonetheless, general systems theory, in its aim to holistically understand the dynamic processes that govern entire systems, has established an invaluable foundation for the second generation of systems theory which addresses many of its shortcomings.

The second generation: complex systems theory

Parts of this section have been adapted from Hudson (2010, pp. 23–38).

In the final years of the 20th century, several new approaches have been developed that have been collectively termed theories of 'complex systems' (CS), theories of 'complex adaptive systems' (CAS) or non-equilibrium theories. These provide a richer source of models for the understanding of human and larger system behaviour than general systems theory. Most well-known among these are nonlinear dynamics and chaos theory; also of central importance are self-organization and autopoeitic theory, which will be highlighted in this section.

Defining complex adaptive systems is not straightforward and typically uses general systems theory as an essential backdrop. A fairly generic definition is that of Varela and Coutinho (1991), who define them as ones 'formed by a large number of discrete elements that are highly interconnected in non-trivial forms'. In contrast, Ahl and Allen (1996) characterize complex systems as 'those that require fine details to be linked to large outcomes'.

There have been many attempts to categorize the various kinds of complex systems theories. The major approaches draw on notions of the *periodicity* of process, the *connectivity* of the component elements and the *direction* of change. The use of *periodicity* to understand types of complex systems consists of identifying processes that either (i) settle into a steady non-changing state; (ii) are periodic in a simple rhythmic manner (e.g. circadian or sleep rhythms); (iii) are periodic, but in a more complex manner (e.g. the sinus rhythm of heart beats); (iv) are non-repeating, but exhibit a degree of order (e.g. chaotic strange attractors); or (v) are non-repeating and apparently random. This typology focuses on individual processes rather than systems as a whole (see Çambel, 1993).

In contrast, several theorists emphasize the extent of *connectivity* between the components of systems and define it in terms of the ratio of internal interconnections (k) to total units (n). When k is very small in relation to n, a 'sub-critical system' develops that exhibits little adaptability and an excessively steady state. When the ratio of k to n increases beyond a certain threshold, the system enters a pattern referred to as the 'edge of chaos', in which there are elements of periodicity as well as chaos and randomness and maximum adaptability. Finally, if the number of interconnections (k) approaches or exceeds the number of component parts (n), a system will develop which is 'super-critical', highly unstable, and best described by chaos theory (Sole, Manrubia, Benton, Kauffman, & Bak, 1999).

Finally, the various kinds of systems and associated theories have also been classified based on the *direction* of change, on whether they involve the development of order out of disorder or, conversely, disorder from order. Some of the theories, such as chaos theory, concern the conditions and processes involved in the development of disorder, of the various pathways to chaos. In contrast, self-organization theory is concerned with how it is that organization appears to emerge spontaneously from apparent disorder. Traditional equilibrium theories (i.e. structural-functional and general systems theories), in contrast, are primarily concerned with the maintenance of order. Another theory to be presented, that of autopoiesis, focuses on the maintenance of complex systems, particularly on their capacity to adapt and replicate.

Thus, the field of complex systems theory encompasses approaches that cover both non-adaptive and adaptive, equilibrium and far-from-equilibrium, periodic and non-periodic, sparsely connected and highly interdependent systems, as well as those that are moving toward and away from order. While the complexity of these systems involves both the multiplicity of their component parts and their interactive nonlinear relationships, their adaptability involves their capacity to self-organize and replicate.

Nonlinear dynamics

Complex systems theories are built on an understanding of dynamic processes, which refer to the study of the ways that systems change (Devaney, 1992). Given specified conditions and forces, what are the expected sequences of states that will follow? How can dysfunctional sequences be influenced to generate growth or problem resolution? The field of dynamics has a long history in the natural sciences. Early concepts, such as that of Laplace's (1749–1827) vision of the universe as a clock-like machine, which when wound up or initialized runs in an entirely predictable manner. Generations of both physical and social scientists have implicitly subscribed to this classical paradigm, consistently excusing their failure to predict by citing the lack of sufficient data on initial conditions. Poincare (1854–1912), regarded as the father of nonlinear dynamics, demonstrated toward the end of the 19th century that even with planetary orbits, systems with three or more moving objects involve equations that are unsolvable and, thus, inherently unpredictable.

Traditional evaluations of human services typically examine linear changes in some condition of interest after an intervention or service has been provided. In contrast, nonlinear dynamicists are interested in the processes of change before, during and after intervention. These are typically understood as involving various types of feedback loops and other interactions. Clients, with continuing feedback, attempt to approximate desired behaviours. Such multi-step processes are often modelled using the mathematical technique of *iteration*. The term 'iteration' refers not only to the general processes of repetition, feedback or approximation, but also a mathematical technique of feeding back the results of solving an equation, one which describes an ongoing relationship, into a repeated calculation of the same equation for subsequent time periods.

Growth and development: self-organization theory

Self-organizing systems are those that exist at far-from-equilibrium conditions and do not follow the general rules of the classical sciences (Bütz, 1997). There have also been several scientists who have identified what they consider to be the 'spontaneous appearance of organized structure throughout biological evolution and social development' (Hayles, 1990, p. 21). Kauffman, for instance, argues that self-organization is the 'great undiscovered principle of nature' and that it and natural selection are the twin engines of the biosphere (Kauffman, 1995).

A review of commonly used definitions of self-organization suggests that it has three primary components that distinguish it as a particular type of emergent phenomenon: (i) Characteristic *structures* or organizations are created: 'Self-Organization is a process whereby, in effect, components at one level interact and amalgamate to create a structure at a higher level. Components at that higher level interact and combine to again create an even higher level' (Merry, 1995, pp. 172–174). (ii) Such creation occurs with a minimum of external interference: a system is defined as self-organizing 'if it acquires a functional, spatial, or temporal structure without specific interference from the outside' (Haken, 1988). Finally, (iii) The foregoing happens with apparent spontaneity: 'Self-organization – A spontaneously formed higher-level pattern of structure or function that is emergent through the interactions of lower-level objects' (Flake, 1998).

The literature advances several explanations for the dynamics of self-organizing processes that involve (i) dissipative structures, (ii) 'edge of chaos' phenomena, (iii) the operation of local activity rules, and (iv) the structural coupling of lower-order systems (Hudson, 2004). Some theorists have also emphasized the need for minimum levels of redundancy and reliability, the presence of noise or the amplification of random fluctuations through positive feedback loops, semi-permeable system boundaries and systemic correlation or coherence (Goldstein, 1995).

Prigogine established that the input of energy into and its passage through dissipative systems is a prerequisite for self-organization (Çambel, 1993, p. 128). The example most commonly cited of a dissipative structure is the whirlpool, in which energy is sucked in from the environment, becomes organized and is dissipated or dispersed at a higher or lower level. For example, Zohar and Marshall (1994, p. 198) explain: 'Self-organizing systems are like whirlpools. They take material or information from the surrounding environment and form it into a dynamic pattern. In the case of biological systems, they take material and form it into patterns of tissue or organism. In the case of mind, information is formed into patterns of thought, patterns of meaning'.

Another commonly cited dynamic in many self-organizing systems is that involving the *structural coupling* of lower-order systems (Merry, 1995; Maturana & Varela, 1987). While Margulis (1981) is well-known for her identification of such processes in cellular evolution, Laszlo extensively cites examples of the linkage of lower-order systems that he suggests are a function of the lower bonding energies that exist on the more complex system levels (1996).

Most approaches to understanding self-organization emphasize interactions between local component parts or systems as the basis for emergent forms of organization. While there are theories about how and why this happens, such as Kauffman's ideas involving an optimal level of component interrelationships (k) in relation to the number of components (n), the exact principles remain elusive. Much observed self-organization is no doubt a function of local interactions; one of the great discoveries in contemporary physics is the phenomenon of nonlocality that involves relationships in which characteristics of systems change in concert with one another without any external or local interactions (see Goswami, 1993). Even if nonlocality takes place only on the microphysical level (for instance, within the human brain), commonly observed chaotic feedback processes, characterized by 'sensitivity to initial conditions', can be expected to amplify, in parallel fashion, non-local processes that first manifest on the microphysical level to larger scale self-organized patterns. Such *non-local self-organization*, in combination with the more well-known instances of *local self-organization*, is most likely to represent some of the central dynamics governing transitions from disorder to order in psychological and social systems that social workers constantly work with (see Hudson, 2004).

Maintenance and reproduction: autopoiesis

Some theorists have narrowed the concept of self-organization, isolating a particular kind referred to as autopoiesis or social autopoiesis. Humberto Maturana (1928–) and Francisco Varela (1946–2001) have classified complex adaptive systems into those that are allopoietic and autopoietic (Maturana & Varela, 1987). Unlike allopoietic systems, which are pre-programmed, autopoietic systems – most life forms are examples – are self-organizing and self-regulated. They exhibit the capacity not only to alter their internal instructions to adapt to new conditions, but also to self-produce and to self-replicate. Thus, while self-organization and chaos theories are concerned with transitions either out of or into apparently disordered states, autopoiesis theory focuses on the maintenance of order. Maturana and Varela applied autopoiesis theory to both biological organisms and human psychology; however, they were uncertain about its application to society.

In contrast, the sociologist Niklas Luhmann (1927–1998) has extensively researched social autopoiesis, applying the theory to such diverse areas as law and social ecology (Bailey, 1997; Villadsen, 2008). He (1986) specifically applied it to the problem of defining what the constituent elements are that a social system 'self-produces'. Like Maturana he argued that the essential components or units of a society are not individual persons, but instead, communications. For example, he suggested that communications, and particularly legal systems, are self-producing, as well as self-referential.

Luhmann emphasizes the circular, tautological and self-referential aspects of systems of meaning, within which each element defines the other elements, but none have independent meaning outside the particular system under consideration. As self-referential processes, communication systems define, maintain, self-produce and replicate themselves, much as living organisms do. Predating Maturana's work, the work of R. D. Lang (1961) on the communication patterns associated with schizophrenia clearly exemplifies the self-referential character of many complex meaning systems, how communications define each other in a circular fashion.

In recent years, the theory of social autopoiesis has been applied in a variety of domains in addition to the law. Several theorists have used it to understand cognition, organizational dynamics, accounting, narrative therapy and family dynamics. As a relatively recent addition to the array of complex systems theories, social autopoiesis fills an important gap, in that it focuses not only on higher-level systems, but also on their phenomenology as it is experienced internally by its participants through its self-referential systems of meaning.

Concluding comments

Complex systems theory builds on traditional social science and general systems theories and focuses on multiple interacting systems with large numbers of parts and variables, interconnected in non-trivial ways, that are not understandable in terms of linear relationships between their components. Complex systems theory is a collection of theories that have been categorized based on the degree of periodicity of change, the level of interconnectedness and the direction of change.

Applications of systems theories and impact on social work

Types of applications

The applications of systems theory in social work are diverse and still emerging, existing on several levels of development. For some, systems theory represents merely a general perspective that emphasizes the need to consider a broad array of considerations in assessment and intervention planning. For others, it represents a specific conceptual framework that is used as an active guide for integrating professional social work. And, for a few, it also is used to inform the use of a variety of methodological tools to support evidence-based practice. For many years now, traditional systems theories have been actively used in family systems approaches and in several varieties of the biopsychosocial model. Applications of the more recently developed complex systems theories are only emerging, with limited published reports, a few of which will be commented on in this section. Applications of both general systems and complex systems theories can be classified into the following four levels, which are defined by their conceptual, theoretical and methodological sophistication, each of which builds on the foundational level, which commences with:

Level 1: metaphoric

Some attempted applications rely on metaphor to think about the operation of key systems affecting social work clients. For example, Kurt Lewin (1951) suggests that those working with organizational systems need to be concerned with periodic *unfreezing*, *change* and *refreezing* of these systems, with the need to capitalize on the opportunities for change found while systems are unfrozen. The importance of such metaphors as an aid to abstract thought should not be diminished; many argue that they are essential guides to applying formal theories. However, without systematic and formal analysis, over-reliance on metaphor can lead to stereotypical and formalistic approaches.

Level 2: conceptual and theoretical

Upon introduction to any promising theoretical approach, there are many who, impressed with enticing-sounding concepts and theoretical propositions, fail to consider their empirical grounding, need for further testing and practical applications. Such concepts are often used to characterize informal and anecdotal observations, often clinical, and to argue for particular interventions. To the extent that these concepts are not rigorously operationalized, they too often may be used to justify any preferred intervention. While such interpretations can sometimes be justified on exploratory and heuristic grounds, theories ultimately thrive or wither based on their ability to guide practical actions that are successful in achieving commonly valued ends.

There are many examples of the applications of systems theory to families in social work. One of the most popular is Hartman's popularization of ecomaps (1995) in the analysis of family interactions. These unfortunately ignore most of the critical concepts, even from general systems theory, and merely identify domains to be considered involving the environments of client families. The functions of these charting techniques are similar in their intent to many biopsychosocial assessments in their listing of 'factors' within the domains of interest in an assessment (Engel, 1977). There are, however, many more well-developed family systems approaches that are rooted in general systems theory: for instance, the Double ABCX Family Crisis Model (McCubbin & Patterson, 1983), the Circumplex Model of Marital and Family Systems (Olson & Gorall, 2003) and Beaver's Systems Model (Sutphin, McDonough, & Schrenkel, 2013). Others, such as Kantor and Lehr's Distance-Regulation Model (1975), more specifically apply concepts from complex systems theory. Some of these have developed useful instruments for assessing hypothesized dimensions of family functioning that may be relevant for intervention.

There have been a wide range of discussions of the application of complex systems concepts to various areas of social systems and social work. For example, Fish and Hardy (2015) suggest that social work activities need to be plotted on a complexity continuum that differentiates those that need to be proceduralized – ones involving greater predictability – and those for which professional judgement needs to be supported: namely, those involving complex systems and minimal predictability.

Complex systems theory has also been used as an interpretive framework in the analysis of large-systems issues, especially those involving social networks, social service delivery and social policy. Michailakis and Schirmer (2014) draw on Luhmann's theory of social autopoeisis (1982) to argue that priority needs to be given to how those from alternative social systems construct social problems above and beyond their objective indices: for example, suicide. Such examples illustrate a few of the applications of key concepts and propositions from complex systems theory to social work, ones that have some exploratory and heuristic value.

Level 3: single method and perspective

In addition to the metaphoric and theoretical dimensions (Levels 1 and 2), specific research and practice methodologies are sometimes used in isolation to study aspects of complex systems and to plan interventions. Such methods may include nonlinear modelling, system dynamics, agent-based modelling, Delphi, concept mapping and other modelling and mathematical techniques.

For example, Fitch and Jagolino (2012) review a range of studies on the use of system dynamics modelling as an aid to clarifying complex interactions in social service delivery systems. Some of these have focused on formulating models that incorporate diverse stakeholders (Smith, Wolstenholme, McKelvie, & Monk, 2004), while others have focused on the impact of system dynamics modelling as a complement to statistical analyses. System dynamics modelling has a long history of use in business and management literature (Senge, 1980; Sterman, 2000). It has its own journal, *System Dynamics Review*, while the methodology is used in hundreds of management, operations research, healthcare and environmental journals. In social work, Peter Hovmand, director of the Social System Design Laboratory at Washington University, has used system dynamics modelling as an essential part of his studies in the area of domestic violence (Hovmand & Ford, 2009; Hovmand, Ford, Flom, & Kyriakakis, 2009).

Social network analysis, a set of research techniques, is sometimes cited as an application of complexity theory. For instance, Quinn, Woehle, and Tiemann (2012) review this literature and demonstrate one such application with a support group for closeted individuals, arguing that 'the power of complexity theory lies in theory and modelling of practice-like processes'. In contrast, Ihara, Horio, and Tompkins (2012) use agent-based modelling (ABM) to assess the effects of policy changes among caregivers of older adults. Wolfe-Branigan points out: 'Because this study used an existing large data set and varying assumptions of the behaviour of caregivers, it provides a direction for social work researchers to consider as ABM has become common in the physical and social sciences. Because of the use of policy as a boundary, this reveals how complex systems reveal complexity as we move from a solely metaphorical to a mixed-methods approach'.

Level 4: multiple methods and multiple perspectives

Such applications are sometimes employed within a programme of research and practice that links and attempts to reconcile systematically diverse perspectives and mixed methodologies of knowledge building and integrative practice related to complex systems. Especially important is the integration of first, second and third order accounts; accounts of clients and participants; direct observations and indirect sources of data, such as large archival data sets. It is rare that such multiple or mixed methods can be employed within a single project. More typically, they are implemented through a series of linked studies that draw on both quantitative modelling methodologies, often using time series, and qualitative studies that emphasize first-person accounts. For example, Bay (2016) draws on not only complex systems theory, but also deep ecology, as well as a 'biopolitical lens' based on the work of Michel Foucault, as a means of developing change processes involving the transnational Transition Town movement.

Extent of application

There is considerable rhetoric about systems theory and its importance in social work; however, both among academics and practitioners, its penetration into practice as an actual theory is very limited. When it is used, it is predominately on the metaphoric and conceptual/theoretical levels (Levels 1 and 2). Rarely are the concepts sufficiently operationalized or is data collected to permit its use on Levels 3 and 4. As indicated earlier, some of the most common applications involve family systems therapy and, more broadly, the tasks of conducting biopsychosocial assessments and planning interventions based on them. There are various reasons for this that range from inadequate understanding of the theory itself to lack of familiarity with key and the methodologies costs of collecting data over multiple time points. There are excellent examples, even of the application of chaos theory to psychosocial problems, but more typically from the field of psychology (see Fredrickson & Losada, 2005). One of the few Level 4 applications within the field of family systems therapy is the work of John Gottman (Gottman, Murray, Swanson, Tyson, & Swanson, 2002), who has used extensive time series data collection, including videotaping, to predict reliably marital dissolution and identify family interventions.

The extent of application of systems theory in social work has also varied based on the national environment. In an analysis of the differential histories of the first generation of systems theory in the UK and the US, Payne (2002) found that political factors played a substantial role in the diverging trajectories of systems theory in social work within these two nations. Specifically, he examined the reasons for its dominance in the US and decline in the UK, reporting that in the US, systems theory was yoked to the needs of direct practitioners, whereas in the UK, interest in the theory was initially based on the emergence of new organizational contexts, but he explains, 'When further changes arose, systems theory therefore had less of a hold and declined in importance' (pp. 258–266).

Neglected dimensions and further directions

Systems theory, particularly the newest generation of complex systems theory, is among the most holistic theoretical approaches in social work and beyond that promises to guide both social work research and practice on the micro and macro levels. Because of its comprehensiveness, it has been tempting for some to only make rhetorical reference to it or to use it only on a metaphorical or conceptual level. In addition, there are several important dimensions that have historically been neglected in this field, not because of any inherent incompatibility with systems theory.

Social workers have too often interpreted the profession's historic mandate to address problems in the person-environment interface, or their 'goodness-of-fit', as a mandate to simply assist individuals to adjust to non-supportive environments, no matter how dysfunctional. Achieving equilibrium, sometimes a laudable goal, should never be assumed. One of the lessons of complex systems theory and extensive research on its applications in human development, learning and problem solving is that individuals are rarely at equilibrium, and, in fact, much learning thrives at far-from-equilibrium or 'edge of chaos' conditions. Social work macro practitioners often understand this, whereas many clinicians are quick to assume individuals require a return to former states of adjustment, rather than discovering new and better patterns of adaptability and development.

Those who rely only on the first generation of general systems theory tend to emphasize the analysis of negative feedback loops which bring about equilibrium, rather than recognizing the ubiquity of positive feedback loops (deviation-amplifying) which are more useful in explaining change, whether for the better or worse. These are more specifically used in the newest renditions of systems theory but still only occasionally in social work.

Although applications of evolutionary theory have expanded dramatically in recent years in most areas of the social sciences, including psychology, it rarely receives mention in social work. Historically, there have been considerable applications of both general and complex systems theory to evolutionary problems. Yet many in social work do not consider any of the insights of evolutionary theory to be relevant. There are many reasons for this, not the least of which is the focus in social work on self-determination and planned, intentional change. An exclusive focus on natural selection does minimize the importance of human choice and action. However, the importance of selection for human behaviour, including development and problem solving, is better conceptualized as also including the combined impact of social selection, and of especially self-selection, in addition to natural selection (see Hudson, 2004). Increasingly, humans are self-determining in both the immediate and long range through their own self-selections for environmental opportunities. Despite the limitations of evolutionary theory, any theory of individual or collective human behaviour and action must necessarily situate itself within one of the primary processes that have brought us to where we are in our biological and social development.

Just as self-selection and self-determination are neglected by many systems theorists, a more fundamental gap involves the expanding theory and research on human consciousness. To the extent that traditional notions of an atomistic and clockwork, predictable material world predominate, consciousness is regarded as an epiphenomenon, a 'secretion of the brain', a convenient fiction most hold, that is incidental to understanding human behaviour. Just as many in fields such as biological psychiatry and the cognitive sciences are vulnerable to such dysfunctional reductionism, many advocates of systems theory, both old and new, too often neglect the role of consciousness.

Systems theory has also neglected the role of non-local causation, particularly as one of the possible origins of self-organization. Social science assumptions inherited from bygone generations of physics, known as the classical Newtonian perspective, involve the exclusive primacy of local atomistic interactions in an essentially billiard ball–like universe. Of course, many contemporary theorists within the social sciences recognize the importance of long-distance effects (both spatial and temporal), but these are typically viewed as ones that are mediated through traditional mechanisms of local influence. Many biologists and some psychologists, including some researchers in the field of consciousness studies, now have repeatedly confirmed the relevance of quantum non-local effects in the self-organization of higher-order systems, especially those involving human consciousness.

Because of its interdisciplinary nature, such gaps in the development of systems theory do not represent any inherent limitation in the theory, but rather in the particular areas of knowledge of those who seek to understand and apply this theory, including some in social work. Despite these limitations, systems theory, especially as it is currently being developed in the field of complex systems, represents one of the most promising of the holistic theories that can be used not only to guide the integration of lower-level theories, but also to generate a variety of promising interventions in social work and beyond.

Further reading

Hudson, C. G. (2010). *Complex systems and human behaviour.* Chicago: Lyceum.

Warren, K. (2017). Chaos theory and complexity theory. In C. Franklin (Ed.), *The encyclopedia of social work.* Oxford: Oxford University Press.

Wolf-Branigin, M. (2013). *Using complexity theory for research and program evaluation.* Oxford: Oxford University Press.

References

Ahl, V., & Allen, T. F. H. (1996). *Hierarchy theory: A vision, vocabulary and epistemology.* New York: Columbia University Press.

Arthur, W. B. (1990, February). Positive feedbacks in the economy. *Scientific American,* 92–99.

Bailey, K. D. (1997). The autopoiesis of social systems: Assessing Luhmann's theory of self-reference. *Systems Research and Behavioural Science, 14,* 83.

Bay, U. (2016). Biopolitics, complex systems theory and ecological social work: Conceptualising ways of transitioning to low carbon futures. *Aotearoa New Zealand Social Work, 28*(4), 89–99.

Bertalanffy, L. (1974). General systems theory and psychiatry. In S. Arieti (Ed.), *American handbook of psychiatry* (vol. 1. 2nd ed., pp. 1095–1120). New York: Basic Books.

Bronfenbrenner, U. (2005). *Making human beings human: Bioecological perspectives on human development.* Thousand Oaks, CA: Sage.

Bütz, M, R. (1997). *Chaos and complexity: Implications for psychological theory and practice.* Washington, DC: Taylor & Francis.

Çambel, A. B. (1993). *Applied chaos theory: A paradigm for complexity.* San Diego: Academic Press.

Devaney, R. L. (1992). *A first course in chaotical dynamic systems: Theory and experiment.* Reading, MA: Addison-Wesley.

Engel, G. L. (1977). The need for a new medical model: A challenge for biomedicine. *Science,* 196, 29–136.

Fish, S., & Hardy, M. (2015). Complex issues, complex solutions: Applying complexity theory in social work practice. *Nordic Social Work Research, 5*(sup1), 98–114.

Fitch, D., & Jagolino, N. C. (2012). Examining organizational functioning through the lens of complexity theory using system dynamics modeling. *Journal of Social Service Research, 38*(5), 591–604.

Flake, G. W. (1998). *The computational beauty of nature: Computer explorations of fractals, chaos, complex systems, and adaptation.* Cambridge, MA: Bradford Books.

Fredrickson, B. L., & Losada, M. F. (2005). Positive affect and the complex dynamics of human flourishing. *American Psychologist, 60*(7), 678.

Goldstein, J. (1995). Emergence as a construct: History and issues. *Emergence, 1*(1), 49–71.

Goswami, A. (1993). *The self-aware universe.* New York: Penguin-Putnam.

Gottman, J. M., Murray, J. D., Swanson, D. D., Tyson, R., & Swanson, K. R. (2002). *The mathematics of marriage: Dynamic nonlinear models.* Cambridge, MA: MIT Press.

Haken, H. (1988). *Information and self-organization: A macroscopic approach to complex systems.* Berlin: Springer-Verlag.

Hartman, A. (1995). Diagrammatic assessment of family relationships. *Families in Society, 30*(1), 111–122.

Hayles, N. K. (1990). *Chaos bound: Orderly disorder in contemporary literature and science.* Ithaca, NY: Cornell University Press.

Hearn G. (Ed.) (1969). *The general systems approach: Contributions toward an holistic conception of social work.* New York: Council on Social Work Education.

Hearn, G. (1979). General systems theory and social work. In F. J. Turner (Ed.), *Social work treatment: Interlocking theoretical approaches* (2nd ed., pp. 333–59). New York: Free Press.

Hovmand, P. S., & Ford, D. N. (2009). Sequence and timing of three community interventions to domestic violence. *American Journal of Community Psychology, 44*(3), 261–272.

Hovmand, P. S., Ford, D. N., Flom, I., & Kyriakakis, S. (2009). Victims arrested for domestic violence: Unintended consequences of arrest policies. *System Dynamics Review, 25*(3), 161–181.

Hudson, C. G. (2004). The dynamics of self-organization: Neglected dimensions. *Journal of Human Behaviour in the Social Environment, 10*(4), 17–38.

Hudson, C. G. (2010). *Complex systems and human behaviour.* Chicago: Lyceum.

Ihara, E., Horio, B., & Tompkins, C. (2012). Grandchildren caring for grandparents: Modeling the complexity of family caregiving. *Journal of Social Service Research, 38*(5), 619–636.

Christopher G. Hudson

Kantor, D., & Lehr, W. (1975). *Inside the family: Toward a theory of family process.* New York: Harper.

Kauffman, S. (1995). *At home in the universe: The search for the laws of self-organization and complexity.* New York: Oxford University Press.

Laing, R. D. (1961). *Self and others.* New York: Random House.

Laszlo, E. (1996). *Evolution: The general theory.* Cresskill, NJ: Hampton Press.

Leighninger, R. D. (1977). Systems theory and social work: A reexamination. *Journal of Education for Social Work, 13*(3), 44–49.

Lewin, K. (1951). *Field theory in the social sciences: Selected theoretical papers* (D. Cartwright, ed.). New York: Harper & Row.

Luhmann, N. (1982). *The differentiation of society.* New York: Columbia University Press.

Luhmann, N. (1986). The autopoiesis of social systems. In F. Geyer & J. van der Zouwen (Eds.), *Sociocybernetic paradoxes: Observation, control and evolution of self-steering systems* (pp. 172–192). London: Sage.

Margulis, L. (1981). *Symbiosis in cell evolution.* San Francisco: Freeman.

Maturana, H. R., & Varela, F. J. (1987). *The tree of knowledge: The biological roots of human understanding.* Boston: Shambhala.

McCubbin, H. I., & Patterson, J. M. (1983). Family transitions: Adaptations to stress. In H. I. McCubbin & C. R. Figley (Eds.), *Stress and the family: Volume I: Coping with normative transitions* (pp. 5–25). New York: Brunner/Maazel.

Merry, U. 1995. *Coping with uncertainty: Insights from the new sciences of chaos, self-organization, and complexity.* Westport, CT: Praeger.

Michailakis, D., & Schirmer, W. (2014). Social work and social problems: A contribution from systems theory and constructionism. *International Journal of Social Welfare, 23*(4), 431–442.

Miller, J. (1955). Toward a general theory of the behavioral sciences. *American Psychologist, 10,* 513–31.

Olson, D. H., & Gorall, D. M. (2003). Circumplex model of marital and family systems. In F. Walsh (Ed.), *Normal family processes* (3rd ed., pp. 514–547). New York: Guilford.

Payne, M. (2002). The politics of systems theory within social work. *Journal of Social Work, 6*(2), 269–292.

Quinn, A., Woehle, R., & Tiemann, K. (2012). Social network analysis for analyzing groups as complex systems. *Journal of Social Service Research, 38*(5), 605–618.

Richards, R. (1996, Spring). Does the lone genius ride again? Chaos, creativity, and community. *Journal of Humanistic Psychology, 36*(2), 44–60.

Senge, P. M. (1980). A system dynamics approach to investment-function formulation and testing. *Socio-Economic Planning Sciences, 14*(6), 269–280.

Sheffield, A. (1937). *Social insight in case situations.* New York: Appleton Century.

Siporin, M. (1980). Ecological systems theory in social work. *Journal of Sociology and Social Welfare, 7*(7), 507–532.

Smith, G., Wolstenholme, E. F., McKelvie, D., & Monk, D. (2004, July). *Using system dynamics in modeling mental health issues in the UK.* Paper presented at the 22nd international system dynamics society conference, Oxford, England.

Sole, R. V., Manrubia, S. C., Benton, M., Kauffman, S., & Bak, S. (1999). Criticality and scaling in evolutionary ecology. *Trends in Ecology and Evolution, 14,* 156–160.

Sterman, J. D. (2000). *Business dynamics: Systems thinking and modeling for a complex world.* Boston: Irwin McGraw-Hill.

Sutphin, S. T., Mcdonough, S., & Schrenkel, A. (2013). The role of formal theory in social work research: Formalizing family systems theory. *Advances in Social Work, 14*(2), 501–517.

Varela, F. J., & Coutinho, A. (1991). Second generation immune networks. *Immunology Today, 12,* 159–166.

Villadsen, K. (2008). 'Polyphonic' welfare: Luhmann's systems theory applied to modern social work. *International Journal of Social Welfare, 17*(1), 65–73.

Zohar, D., & Marshall, I. (1994). *Quantum society: Mind, physics and new social vision.* New York: Quill.

16

Cognitive-behavioural therapy and social work practice

A. Antonio Gonzalez-Prendes and C. M. Cassady

Cognitive behavioural therapy

Cognitive behavioural therapy (CBT) is a system of psychotherapies that integrate behavioural and cognitive theories and therapies. CBT is not a single approach to psychotherapy. Rather, CBT is an umbrella under which one finds various evidenced-based approaches and strategies to work with individuals, groups, couples and families. Some of these approaches (e.g. contingency management, systematic desensitization) emphasize the behavioural aspects of CBT while others (e.g. cognitive therapy, rational emotive-behaviour therapy, self-instructional training) emphasize the cognitive aspects. CBT approaches rest on the fundamental principle that cognitive processes (e.g. appraisals, meanings, judgements, assumptions) associated with life events are the primary, although not the only, determinants of one's emotional and behavioural responses to those events. Other factors such as illnesses, injuries, exposure to environmental toxins and cultural norms and display rules may influence how one expresses emotions and behaviours. Consequently, even though in CBT cognitions may play a primary role in this process, it is important that we recognize that human problems are often complex and multi-layered. For this reason, Greenberger and Padesky (2017) suggest that to get an accurate understanding of a presenting problem, we must consider the reciprocal interaction that takes place between thoughts, moods, behaviours, physical reactions and environmental factors.

Dobson and Dobson (2009) offer three fundamental hypothetical assumptions that underscore most CBT approaches: the *access* hypothesis, the *mediation* hypothesis and the *change* hypothesis. The *access* hypothesis suggests that the content of our thoughts is accessible and can be known. Even when the content of our thoughts is not in our immediate awareness, with proper effort we can recall such content. The *mediation* hypothesis suggests that our beliefs mediate how we interpret events in our lives and the meaning that we attach to those events. For instance, our core beliefs, those central, absolute and definitive views that we have internalized about ourselves, about people in general and about life or the world can be conceptualized as forming a 'filter' through which we look at life. Life experiences are then processed through that filter and are interpreted according to the existing content of those core beliefs. For example, a person who thinks they are 'useless' and 'incompetent' goes for a job interview and gets the job. As that experience is filtered through their core beliefs (i.e. mental filter), they are likely to reach a conclusion that is consistent with the content of such beliefs. Therefore, they may conclude that they got the job because 'they were desperate' or 'they felt sorry for me', and in the process, they will fail to recognize whatever positive qualities might have persuaded the interviewer to offer them the position. In CBT, this tendency to selectively focus on factors or environmental cues that are consistent with our beliefs and discard those that are not is known as 'cognitive bias' or 'selective abstraction': a form of cognitive distortion or error in thinking. The third assumption, the *change* hypothesis, suggests that cognitions can be intentionally identified, targeted and modified or changed and that changing our thinking in a more realistic, rational and healthy direction leads to a reduction in symptoms and increased adaptation and functionality.

Characteristics of CBT

CBT is a structured, time-limited, collaborative, problem-oriented and solution-focused-in-the-here-and-now psychotherapy that provides deeper insight into and understanding of the presenting problem, as well as cognitive and behavioural skills to manage such problems effectively. J. Beck (2011) outlines ten basic principles of CBT:

1 Involves a fluid conceptualization of the problem in cognitive terms.
2 Requires a sound therapeutic alliance.
3 Emphasizes collaboration and active participation from client and social worker.
4 Goal-oriented and problem-focused.
5 Present-oriented.
6 Educates clients about their problems and how to prevent relapse by teaching the client therapeutic strategies so that they can become their own therapist.
7 Time-limited.
8 Structured sessions.
9 Teaches clients how to recognize, assess and respond to their thoughts.
10 Makes use of a variety of cognitive, behavioural and affective strategies.

The therapeutic relationship is an important aspect of CBT as underlined by Gilbert and Leahy (2007), who provide a comprehensive discussion of the role of the therapeutic relationship in CBT, which forms the backbone of what A. Beck (1976) and Beck, Rush, Shaw, and Emery (1979) described as 'collaborative empiricism'. This concept assumes an active partnership between the client and social worker to help the client identify, evaluate and challenge dysfunctional thinking (i.e. challenge the validity and functionality) and develop more balanced, healthier and more functional views that will contribute to a resolution of the presenting problem. It is also important to understand that although CBT is a present-oriented therapy, it does not ignore the past. An assessment of the client's history (e.g. experiences of abuse, neglect or trauma) helps the social worker understand the impact that such experiences might have had in the formation of the client's core beliefs about self, the world/life and others. Nonetheless, the focus of CBT is on the specific problem that the client is struggling with in the here and now. Past experiences may contribute to the internalization of dysfunctional and self-defeating messages that the client continues to replay mentally in their present life. However, CBT shies away from revisiting those experiences that cannot be changed and rather aims to help the client rewrite the script of those messages and beliefs in the present, in more functional, realistic and self-enhancing ways (see Chapter 3). Another key factor of CBT is that it is a structured, not rigid, approach. This structure provides a framework for the effective and efficient use of the time spent with clients. A typical CBT session should flow seamlessly through a series of steps:

(1) First step: *Setting an agenda.* In a collaborative fashion, the client and social worker identify the problem that the client wants to address in the session. The agenda may also include important issues that the social worker wants to discuss with the client as well as a general overview of what will transpire during the session. Newman (2013) indicates that setting an agenda conveys to the client that therapy involves plan and direction. (2) Second step: *Review of homework assignments and mood check.* The social worker and the client review the mutually agreed-upon homework and check how the client has been doing since the last visit. (3) Third step: *Working on the presenting problem.* This takes the most time as the social worker and the client use various strategies to implement solutions to the presenting problem. (4) Fourth step: *New homework assignment.* The client and social worker collaborate to design homework, including behavioural experiments that help reinforce the gains made in the session. (5) Fifth step: *Eliciting feedback.* Throughout the session, a spirit of collaboration and partnership guides CBT where the client is fully involved in the decision-making, from identifying the targeted problem to the formulation of the homework assignments.

Variations of CBT

Under the umbrella of CBT, the social worker will find a wide range of approaches and strategies to work effectively with various populations and a wide range of presenting problems. Some approaches, such as *cognitive therapy* (CT; Beck, 1976; Beck, Rush, Shaw, & Emery, 1979) and *rational emotive behaviour therapy* (REBT; Ellis, 1962), assume the individual to have a certain level of cognitive ability or development to allow for the process of introspection, abstract/ hypothetical thinking and critical or analytic thinking that forms the basis of cognitive disputation and restructuring. In these approaches, clients are expected to be able to evaluate evidence for or against a given dysfunctional thought and synthesize such evidence into a more balanced, rational and realistic perspective. However, some individuals, due to either maturation, illness, accidents or developmental derailments, may lack such cognitive abilities. In such cases, CBT offers other strategies, such as *stress-inoculation training* (SIT; Meichenbaum, 1985) and *problem-solving therapy* (D'Zurilla & Nezu, 2007), which use a more concrete, self-directed approach emphasizing the use of 'self-talk' to guide the individual in a step-by-step process to the resolution of a problem. Other approaches under the CBT umbrella include *dialectical-behaviour therapy* (DBT), *acceptance and commitment therapy* (ACT; Hayes, Strosahl, & Wilson, 2011) and *mindfulness-based cognitive therapy* (MBCT; Segal, Williams, & Teasdale, 2013), where the focus of mindfulness is not to modify or challenge cognitions, but to adopt a new way of being with one's thoughts through non-judgemental awareness and acceptance (Carlson & González-Prendes, 2016).

The behavioural influence on CBT can be seen in strategies such as behaviour modification and contingency management that are often woven into CBT approaches to work with children (see Kendall, 2012) and adults. The behavioural approach also forms the basis of *exposure therapies*, which have been found to be effective in the treatment of anxiety and trauma-based disorders (Cahill, Rothbaum, Resick, & Follette, 2009; Dobson & Dobson, 2009). Exposure therapies help individuals activate the fear-inducing structures by revisiting the traumatic experience, thus facilitating the therapeutic emotional and cognitive processing of the memory. This process results in relief from the fear and anxiety as the individual learns that the memory of a trauma, albeit unpleasant and uncomfortable, is not dangerous. Variations of exposure therapy include (1) *Prolonged imaginal exposure* for the treatment of PTSD, which uses imagery to help the person revisit and process the traumatic event (Foa, Hembree, & Rothbaum, 2007); (2) *Virtual reality exposure* creates exposure through computer-animated programs and is particularly helpful for those individuals who have difficulties activating the traumatic memory by imagery (Rothbaum,

Ruef, Litz, Han, & Hodges, 2003); (3) *Systematic desensitization* combines gradual exposure to the feared object with relaxation (Wolpe, 1990); (4) *Cognitive processing therapy* involves exposure through detailed writing of a narrative describing the trauma (Resick & Schnicke, 1992). In addition, trauma-focused CBT (TF-CBT) is used to treat PTSD in children and adolescents (Cohen, Mannarino, & Dablinger, 2012).

Empirical support

CBT has generated such a large empirical support base that a detailed discussion of the accumulated evidence is beyond the scope of this chapter. Nonetheless, the evidence behind CBT has been documented by Hofmann, Asnaani, Vonk, Sawyer, and Fang (2012, p. 434), who suggest, 'CBT is arguably the most widely studied form of psychotherapy'. In their study on the efficacy of CBT, the authors reviewed over 269 meta-analytic studies that examined the use of CBT with a wide spectrum of disorders and concluded that, despite weaknesses in some areas and variability in the efficacy of CBT across disorders, CBT has a strong evidence base of support. Other meta-analyses (Butler, Chapman, Forman, & Beck, 2006; Tolin, 2010; Windsor, Jemal, & Alessi, 2015) lend additional support for the efficacy of CBT. However, some gaps in the CBT research literature exist, and as Hofmann et al. (2012, p. 436) indicate in their meta-analysis 'no meta-analytic studies of CBT have been reported on subgroups such as ethnic minorities and low-income samples'. This view is supported by Windsor et al. (2015), who, in their study on the use of CBT to treat substance use disorders, reported that the overwhelming research generated in this area has included predominantly white samples.

CBT and social work

Over the past three decades, there has been a steadily growing relationship between CBT and social work practice (Thyer & Myers, 2011). The influence of cognitive and behavioural theories on social work practice is reflected in the works of social work scholars such as Berlin (2002), Gambrill (2013), Granvold (2011), Lantz (1978), Steketee (1988), Sundel and Sundel (2005), Thomlison and Thomlison (2011), and Thyer (1991, 2011) among others. Although information on the use of CBT among social workers around the world is not readily available, the limited available data suggests that the use of CBT is popular among social workers. For instance, a survey of randomly selected licensed social workers in the United States (Pignotti & Thyer, 2009) revealed that, of 193 respondents, 45 percent listed 'cognitive-behavioural' as their main theoretical orientation, with an additional 6 percent listing either 'cognitive' or 'behavioural' orientations separately. Moreover, CBT was listed by 43 percent of respondents as the most widely used intervention. Other interventions that fall under the CBT umbrella include cognitive restructuring (18.5 percent), behaviour modification (12.6 percent), mindfulness (4.6 percent) and rational-emotive behaviour therapy (3.3 percent).

The practice of CBT has gained global acceptance evident by the presence of cognitive behavioural organizations across all continents encompassing diverse cultures and nationalities. Similarly, social work is a global profession, and issues of diversity are at the core of social work practice. The International Federation of Social Workers (IFSW, 2017) lists 110 social work associations across Africa, Asia, Europe, North America and Latin/South America. In countries around the world, social workers with the proper credentials provide mental health and substance abuse services to persons in need, particularly to disenfranchised populations. In the United States, social workers make up the largest segment of substance use disorder treatment providers (Dilonardo, 2011), as well as 60 percent of mental health professionals (National

Association of Social Workers, NASW, 2017). In Canada, according to the Canadian Association of Social Workers (CASW, 2016), there are approximately 50,000 social workers, with 93 percent of those employed either in the health and social services or government industries, with 74 percent in the former and 19 percent in the latter. Similarly, in the United Kingdom and Australia, social workers with the proper credentials engage in providing therapy and counselling services to clients in need.

CBT, social work and culture

Given the global nature of CBT and its popularity among social work practitioners, it is imperative that social workers consider the fit of CBT with issues of critical importance to social work, such as cultural diversity, empowerment and social work values (see Chapters 28–29). An understanding of cultural diversity is likely to result in more accurate and culturally congruent use of clinical strategies (Beshai, Clark, & Dobson, 2013). The proliferation of CBT organizations across the world suggests that the fundamental principle of CBT – that is, the notion that cognitions affect emotional and behavioural responses – resonates well across nationalities and cultures. However, CBT practitioners must recognize the strong influence that cultural beliefs and traditions exert on the way emotions and behaviours are expressed and interpreted. While discussing multiculturalism in CBT practice, Pantalone, Iwamasa, and Martell (2010) encourage CBT practitioners to be aware of cultural norms that influence behaviour and how they may differ from group to group. Similarly, Hays (2006) suggests that attitudes such as assertiveness, individualism, open self-disclosure and the desire for immediate change, which are common in CBT and other mainstream psychotherapies, reflect Eurocentric perspectives that may not fit well with other cultural views. Consequently, when working with clients whose culture differs from their own, social workers should strive to (1) Evaluate the presenting problem against the framework of the client's cultural background, as this may avoid pathologizing an issue that is not pathological in the client's culture and (2) Develop culturally congruent adaptations of mainstream CBT strategies, as these may increase the effectiveness of such interventions (Griner & Smith, 2006; Hwang et al., 2015).

Culture can be defined as *the heritage of a people characterized by shared beliefs, values meanings and symbolic representations, transmitted from generation to generation and manifested in traditions, behaviours, standard practices and individual and social interactions between people* (Ashford, LeCroy, & Lortie, 2006; Cormier, Nurius, & Osborn, 2017; Geertz, 1973; Maddux & Winstead, 2016). In the context of this definition, we see factors such as beliefs, values, meanings, symbolism and behaviours, which are the subject matter of CBT. Broadly, culture encompasses a wide range of varying identities that include ethnicity, race, heritage, religion, nationality, sexual orientation, gender, age, disability and other ways and practices that mark specificity and differences from the dominant norm (Morton & Meyers, 2016). Where the meaning of culture has broadened generally, it has also become more inclusive in conceptualizing CBT's applicability to specific groups. In recent years, we have seen adaptations of CBT to address the needs of diverse populations including, among others: lesbian, gay and bisexual individuals (Martell, Safren, & Prince, 2004); gay and bisexual men using methamphetamine (Reback & Shoptaw, 2014); sexual minority youth (Craig, Austin, & Alessi, 2013); Hispanic/Latinos (González-Prendes, Hindo, & Pardo, 2011; Interian & Diaz-Martínez, 2007; Kanter, Santiago-Rivera, Rusch, Busch, & West, 2010; Shatell, Quinlan-Colwell, Villalba, Ivers, & Mails, 2010); African Americans (Kelly, 2006; Zigarelli, Jones, Palomino, & Kawamura, 2016); Chinese Americans (Chen & Davenport, 2005; Hwang et al., 2015) and persons with physical, cognitive and developmental disabilities (Kroese, 2014; Radnitz, 2000). As social work researchers and practitioners continue to strive for cultural competence that incorporates the complexities of the individual and intersectional identities (Danso, 2016), CBT is adapting as well, both within social work and without. Nonetheless, a logical question to ask is how well CBT models work with persons of non–European American cultures or members of minority groups.

We know that psychological/emotional disorders are experienced, explained and labelled differently by different cultures (Hinton & LaRoche, 2013), so how does this affect the delivery of CBT? As previously indicated, in their review of meta-analytic studies of CBT, Hofmann et al. (2012) were unable to find one study that reported on ethnic or income minority sub-groups. The more recent meta-analysis by Windsor et al. (2015) begins to answer this gap by looking at several studies using CBT to treat substance abuse in white, black, or Hispanic groups. The authors found that CBT appeared effective for all three populations by measuring overall effect sizes across 16 studies. However, their analysis also revealed that pre-post-test measure effect sizes for CBT were significantly less for studies of Hispanic and black substance use than those of white substance use (Windsor et al., 2015). These mixed results suggest the need for more research involving larger-sample randomized controlled trials (RCT), focusing on specific minority populations to establish firmly the evidence-based effectiveness of CBT adaptations.

At the same time, it is important that social work practitioners and researchers encourage culturally adapted CBT strategies to evolve not solely from empirical data derived from large samples, but also from indicatively derived limitations and disparities between some cultural values and CBT's Eurocentric value roots (Hays, 2009; González-Prendes, Hindo, & Pardo, 2011; Husain & Hodge, 2016). For instance, Hays (2009) notes that CBT, with its focus on the here and now, may influence some practitioners to undervalue or fail to address the cultural context of client behaviours and beliefs. Another challenge to culturally competent CBT is the primary focus on the individual as the locus for change (as in cognitive reframing), to the possible exclusion of external factors that might be modified (Hays, 2009). Quoting Albert Ellis, Husain and Hodge echo Hays's concerns about the individual as the 'change engine' (Husain & Hodge, 2016, p. 396). They note that commonly held Islamic values do not reflect the autonomous individual but the family as the source of authority for what is good or should be (Husain & Hodge, 2016). González-Prendes et al. (2011) voice a similar perspective about the relative importance of family over individual in the study of the use of CBT to treat depression in a Mexican American man.

Several studies have discussed the importance of considering the individualistic-collectivistic orientation of clients' cultures when developing culturally responsive interventions. In one study, Zigarelli et al. (2016, p. 247) argue for a 'culturally responsive' CBT approach in a case of a 15-year-old African American girl with dysthymia and generalized anxiety disorder. In this case, the authors used multicultural strategies in the assessment and treatment of the client, rooted in values such as 'mothering community', collectivism and accountability. The authors argue that the information gleaned from culturally informed assessment and treatment is integral to a competent cognitive behavioural social work approach that avoids pathologizing cultural values, such as the 'mothering community', as a lack of parenting resources. In their case study, González-Prendes et al. (2011) discuss the use of a collectivistic approach, rooted in the traditional concept of *familismo*, to frame the CBT treatment of a Mexican American client with depression. *Familismo* refers to the primary role that the family has for some Latino groups, serving as a source of support, protection and caretaking (Garcia-Preto, 2005). Shifting the focus from individual to collective (i.e. family) perspective resulted in the culturally congruent development of a treatment plan, as well as adaptations of CBT strategies that helped the client recognize how individual gains ultimately had a greater value by benefitting his family.

For many, culture and religion are not separately learned or implemented constructs but overlapping, imbricated ways of being and deciding how to live that are ever present at conscious or pre-conscious levels. While certainly some persons will differ in their commitment to enacting religious principles in their lives, it is important to consider the ways in which religion affects our thoughts, choices and judgements in everyday life, whether or not we have our religious principles in mind at the time. For instance, Husain and Hodge (2016) discuss the interwoven nature of living and Islamic values. The authors point out that for Muslims, Islam is not a part of life but a way of life, offering guidance for their public and private lives, where a duty to worship Allah is central. They also argue that, for Muslims, traditional CBT's self-actualizing statements, often used to enhance autonomy in restructuring cognitive schema may be uncomfortable or counterintuitive to Islamic values of community actualization that support social interdependence and encourage self-restraint in expression. Husain and Hodge offer ways to modify self-statements for restructuring using a three-step process: (1) Identifying key therapeutic precepts within the self-statement (the authors use a representative example from Albert Ellis); (2) Ensuring the values implicit in the self-statement are congruent with Islamic values and (3) 'Repackaging' the therapeutic concept using terminology consistent with Muslim values and narratives. Hodge (2008) offers a similar three-step process for culturally sensitive cognitive reframing with persons from other religious backgrounds. In a critical analysis of the use of CBT with religious and spiritual clients, Carlson and Gonzalez-Prendes (2016) suggest ways for social workers to adapt traditional CBT, as well as the use of mindfulness strategies, when working with such individuals (see Chapter 22).

Dominant culture and intersecting identities also come into play for persons considered sexual minority or non-heterosexual persons who are often coping with feeling outside of, or disconnected from, dominant cultural expectations. Sexual minority persons are more likely to lack support from their own family, in contrast to those whose minority status is solely based on ethnic background or identification (Craig et al., 2013). In their adaptation of CBT designed specifically for sexual minority youth, Craig et al. suggest tailoring CBT interventions for sexual minority youth in a way that 'integrates gay affirmative practices' (2013, p. 258) common in LGBTQ culture such as coming out, seeking support from the LGBTQ community and addressing stigmatization. Further, the authors note that traditional CBT should be adapted specifically for sexual minority youth in identification of dysfunctional thoughts, addressing client reports of discrimination, approaching cognitive restructuring and creating homework assignments that are congruent with LGBTQ culture (Craig et al., 2013). Like the other models suggested here, CBT for sexual minority youth needs much more research.

CBT and social work values

CBT has been described as an empowering and strength-based psychotherapy that aims to help individuals internalize cognitive and behavioural skills to effectively become their own therapists and reduce or eliminate reliance on the social worker (J. Beck, 2011; Lantz, 1996; Ronen, 2007; Van Wormer & Davis, 2018). The empowering and strength-based nature of CBT makes it an appropriate intervention for social workers who often are working with disenfranchised and disempowered populations. Strength-based social work is rooted in the belief that individuals can change, make choices and enhance self-determination. Moreover, González-Prendes and Brisebois (2012) argue that CBT is a good fit with values such as the importance of human relationships, dignity and worth of the person, competence and social justice identified in the NASW Code of Ethics (NASW, 2008).

Importance of human relationships

In CBT, the importance of human relationships is embodied in the concept of collaboration that defines the therapeutic relationship in CBT (Beck 2011; Gilbert & Leahy, 2007). In the spirit of 'collaborative empiricism' (A. Beck, 1976), the client and the social worker establish a partnership that guides the process of treatment from the identification of the problem to be addressed in therapy to the goal to be attained, the evaluation of evidence to test the validity and functionality of dysfunctional thoughts and the formulation of homework assignments. This collaboration actively elicits the participation of the client and empowers the individual to make choices regarding the direction of therapy.

Dignity and worth of the client

CBT recognizes the inherent worth of individuals and thus avoids labelling individuals as 'good' or 'bad' (see Chapter 9). This view is clearly elucidated in the words of Albert Ellis, who stated that in CBT '. . . therapists fully accept their clients no matter how poor their behaviour and they practice tolerance and unconditional positive regard' (1979, p. 3). In CBT, judgemental, pejorative and stereotypical views that devalue self-respect/worth or the worth of others are seen as 'labelling', which is considered a cognitive distortion or 'error in thinking'.

Competence

The value of competence compels social workers to practice within their scope of knowledge and skills and encourages them to enhance their skills set and expand the body of knowledge of the profession (NASW, 1996). CBT, with its focus on evidence-based practices and extensive empirical support base (Butler et al., 2006; Hofmann et al., 2012), offers social workers a broad selection of evidence-based strategies to use with a wide range of presenting problems and clients from diverse backgrounds. In addition, many CBT organizations offer continuing education and certification opportunities for social workers to enhance their CBT skills level.

Social justice

Although social justice (see Chapter 10) is often associated with macro-level social work practice, Rawls (1999) and Wakefield (1988a, 1988b) argue that clinical social work meets the social justice mission of the profession when it strives to help clients restore 'self-respect', a primary social good essential for the pursuit of a rational course of action and one's life goals. Gonzalez-Prendes and Brisebois (2012) suggest that CBT, with its strength-based, non-judgemental, accepting, empowering and collaborative nature, helps individuals eliminate pejorative labels and self-defeating thoughts and behaviours and engender self-acceptance and self-respect, thus helping social workers meet the social justice mission of social work.

Conclusion

In this chapter, we presented an overview of CBT and discussed the fit of CBT with social work to help the reader understand the potential of using CBT in social work practice. We offer that CBT is a good fit for social workers who provide services in the areas of mental health, substance use disorder or other forms of clinical practice. In these realms, CBT provides social workers with treatment options that are cost effective, efficient, relatively brief and supported by extensive empirical research. However, as we also alluded, there are gaps in the CBT research that need attention; specifically research that targets minority populations. This is an issue not only for CBT, but also for most mainstream psychotherapies. However, as González-Prendes and Brisebois (2012) suggest, social work practitioners and researchers, given their work with minority and disenfranchised populations, are uniquely positioned to help fill this specific gap in the knowledge base and thus enhance the future of CBT.

Further reading

Beck, J. (2011). *Cognitive behaviour therapy: Basics and beyond* (2nd ed.). New York: Guilford
This is a must-have book for social workers who want to learn about CBT. The author lays out in a very clear and informative manner the theory and practice of CBT. The book contains an array of examples and case histories to illustrate the process of case conceptualization, as well as the use of various strategies.

Newman, C. (2013). *Core competencies in cognitive-behavioural therapy: Becoming a highly effective and competent cognitive-behavioural therapist.* New York: Routledge.
This book is an excellent resource for beginning as well as experienced CBT practitioners who want to enhance their competency in cognitive behavioural therapy. The author expands on key competencies such as understanding the conceptual basis of CBT, the therapeutic alliance within the CBT framework, conducting integrative assessments, developing accurate case formulations, effective use of CBT strategies, monitoring and evaluation of practice, planning for termination and cultural and ethical issues.

Ronen, T., & Freeman, A. (Eds.). (2007). *Cognitive behaviour therapy in clinical social work practice.* New York: Springer.
In this edited book, the authors discuss various aspects of the application of cognitive behavioural therapy to clinical social work practice. Of particular interest for social work practitioners are chapters that address cultural diversity and cognitive behavioural therapy and chapters addressing the application of cognitive behavioural strategies with children, adults, couples and families.

References

Ashford, J. B., LeCroy, C. W., & Lortie, K. L. (2006). *Human behaviour in the social environment: A multidimensional perspective* (3rd ed.). Belmont, CA: Thomson/Brooks Cole.

Beck, A. T. (1976). *Cognitive therapy and the emotional disorders.* New York: International Universities Press.

Beck, A. T., Rush, A. J., Shaw, B. F., & Emery, G. (1979). *Cognitive therapy of depression.* New York: Gilford.

Beck, J. (2011). *Cognitive behaviour therapy: Basics and beyond* (2nd ed.). New York: Guilford.

Berlin, S. (2002). *Clinical social work practice: A cognitive-integrative perspective.* New York: Oxford.

Beshai, S., Clark, C. M., & Dobson, K. S. (2013). Conceptual and pragmatic considerations in the use of cognitive-behavioural therapy with Muslim clients. *Cognitive Therapy and Research, 37*(1), 197–206. doi:10.1007/s10608-012-9450-y

Butler, A. C., Chapman, J. E., Forman, E. M., & Beck, A. T. (2006). The empirical status of cognitive-behavioural therapy: A review of meta-analyses. *Clinical Psychology Review, 26*(1), 17–31. doi:10.1016/j.cpr.2005.07.003

Cahill, S. P., Rothbaum, B. O., Resick, P. A., & Follette, V. M. (2009). Cognitive-behavioural therapy for adults. In E. B. Foa, T. M. Keane, M. J. Friedman, & J. A. Cohen (Eds.), *The effective treatment of PTSD: Practice guidelines from the international society for traumatic stress studies* (pp. 139–222). New York: Guilford.

Canadian Association of Social Workers. (2016). *What is social work?* Retrieved from www.casw-acts.ca/en/what-social-work

Carlson, K. M., & González-Prendes, A. A. (2016). Cognitive behavioural therapy with religious and spiritual clients: A critical perspective. *Journal of Spirituality in Mental Health, 18* (4), 253–282. doi:10.1080/19349637.2016.1159940

Chen, S., & Davenport, D. (2005). Cognitive-behavioural therapy with Chinese American clients: Cautions and modifications. *Psychotherapy: Theory, Research, Practice, Training, 42*(1), 101–110. doi:10.1037/00333204.42.1.101

Cohen, J. A., Mannarino, A. P., & Dablinger, E. (2012). *Trauma-focused CBT for children and adolescents: Treatment applications.* New York: Guilford.

Cormier, S., Nurius, P. S., & Osborn, C. J. (2017). *Interviewing strategies for helpers* (8th ed.). Boston: Cengage Learning.

Craig, S. L., Austin, A., & Alessi, E. (2013). Gay affirmative cognitive behavioural therapy for sexual minority youth: A clinical adaptation. *Clinical Social Work Journal, 41*, 258–266. doi:10.1007/s10615-012-0427-9

Danso, R. (2016). Cultural competence and cultural humility: A critical reflection on key cultural diversity concepts. *Journal of Social Work, 0*(0), 1–21. doi:10.1177/1468017316654341

Dilonardo, J. (2011). *Workforce issues related to physical and behavioural healthcare integration specifically substance use disorders and primary care: A framework.* Retrieved from www.integration.samhsa.gov/resource/workforce-issues-related-to-physical-and-behavioural-healthcare-integration-specifically-substance-use-disorders-and-primary-care-a-framework

Dobson, D., & Dobson, K. S. (2009). *Evidence-based practice of cognitive behavioural therapy.* New York: Guilford.

D'Zurilla, T. J., & Nezu, A. M. (2007). *Problem-solving therapy: A positive approach to clinical intervention* (3rd ed.). New York: Springer.

Ellis, A. (1962). *Reason and emotion in psychotherapy.* New York: Citadel Press.

Ellis, A. (1979). Rational-emotive therapy. In A. Ellis & J. M. Whitley (Eds.), *Theoretical and empirical foundations of rational-emotive-therapy* (pp. 1–60). Monterey, CA: Brooks/Cole Publishing Company.

Foa, E. B., Hembree, E. A., & Rothbaum, B. O. (2007). *Prolonged exposure therapy for PTSD: Emotional processing of traumatic experiences.* New York: Oxford University Press.

Gambrill, E. (2013). *Social work practice: A critical thinker's guide.* New York: Oxford University Press.

Garcia-Preto, N. (2005). Puerto Rican families. In M. McGoldrick, J. Giordano, & N. Garcia-Preto (Eds.), *Ethnicity and family therapy* (3rd ed., pp. 242–265). New York: Guilford.

Geertz, C. (1973). *The interpretation of cultures.* New York: Basic Books.

Gilbert, P., & Leahy, R. L. (Eds.). (2007). *The therapeutic relationship in the cognitive behavioural psychotherapies.* New York: Routledge.

González-Prendes, A. A., & Brisebois, K. (2012). Cognitive behavioural therapy and social work values: A critical analysis. *Journal of Social Work Values and Ethics, 9*(2), 21–33.

González-Prendes, A. A., Hindo, C., & Pardo, Y. (2011). Cultural values integration in cognitive behavioural therapy for a Latino with depression. *Clinical Case Studies, 10*(5), 376–394.

Granvold, D. K. (2011). Cognitive-behavioural therapy with adults. In J. R. Brandell (Ed.), *Theory and practice in clinical social work* (2nd ed., pp. 179–212). Thousand Oaks, CA: SAGE Publications.

Greenberger, D., & Padesky, C. A. (2017). *Mind over mood: Change how you feel by changing the way you think* (2nd ed.). New York: Guilford.

Griner, D., & Smith, T. B. (2006). Culturally adapted mental health interventions: A meta-analytic review. *Psychotherapy: Theory, Research, Practice, Training, 43*(4), 531–548. doi:10.1037/0033-3204.43.4.531

Hayes, S. C., Strosahl, K. D., & Wilson, K. G. (2011). *Acceptance and commitment therapy: The process and practice of mindful change.* New York: Guilford Press.

Hays, P. A. (2006). Introduction: Developing culturally responsive cognitive-behavioural therapies. In P. A. Hays & G. Y. Iwamasa (Eds.), *Culturally responsive cognitive-behavioural therapy: Assessment, practice, and supervision* (pp. 3–19). Washington, DC: American Psychological Association.

Hays, P. A. (2009). Professional psychology, research and practice: Integrating evidence-based practice, cognitive – Behaviour therapy, and multicultural therapy: Ten steps for culturally competent practice. *Professional Psychology, Research and Practice, 40*(4), 354–360. doi:10.1037/a0016250

Hinton, D. E., & La Roche, M. (2013). Cultural context. In S. G. Hoffman & D. J. A. Dozois (Eds.), *The Wiley handbook of cognitive behavioural therapy Volume I* (pp. 399–433). Chichester, West Sussex, UK: John Wiley & Sons, Ltd.

Hodge, D. R. (2008). Constructing spiritually-modified interventions: Cognitive therapy with diverse populations. *International Social Work, 51*(2), 178–192. doi:10.1177/ 0020872807085857

Hofmann, S. G., Asnaani, A., Vonk, I. J. J., Sawyer, A. T., & Fang, A. (2012). The efficacy of cognitive behavioural therapy: A review of meta-analyses. *Cognitive Therapy and Research, 36*, 427–440. doi:10.1007/s10608-012-9476-1

Husain, A., & Hodge, D. R. (2016). Islamically modified cognitive behavioural therapy: Enhancing outcomes by increasing the cultural congruence of cognitive behavioural therapy self-statements. *International Social Work, 59*(3), 393–405. doi:10.1177/0020872816629193

Hwang, W., Myers, H., Chiu, E., Mak, E., Butner, J., Fukimoto, K., ... Miranda, J. (2015). Culturally adapted cognitive behavioural therapy for depressed Chinese Americans: A randomized controlled trial. *Psychiatric Services*, *66*(10), 1035–1042. doi:10.1176/ appi.ps.201400358

Interian, A., & Díaz-Martínez, A. M. (2007). Considerations for culturally competent cognitive-behavioural therapy for depression with Hispanic patients. *Cognitive and Behavioural Practice*, *14*(1), 84–97. doi:10. 1016/j.cbpra.2006.01.006

International Federation of Social Workers. (2017). *Our members*. Retrieved from http://ifsw.org/member ship/our-members/

Kanter, J. W., Santiago-Rivera, A. L., Rusch, L. C., Busch, A. M., & West, P. (2010). Initial outcomes of a culturally adapted behavioural activation for Latinas with depression at a community clinic. *Behaviour Modification*, *34*(2), 120–144. doi:10.1177/ 0145445509359682

Kelly, S. (2006). Cognitive-behavioural therapy with African Americans. In P. A. Hays & G. Y. Iwamasa (Eds.), *Culturally responsive cognitive-behavioural therapy: Assessment, practice, and supervision* (pp. 97–116). Washington, DC: American Psychological Association.

Kendall, P. C. (Ed.). (2012). *Child and adolescent therapy: Cognitive-behavioural procedures* (4th ed.). New York: Guilford.

Kroese, B. S. (2014). CBT with people with intellectual disabilities. In A. Whittington & N. Grey (Eds.), *How to become a more effective CBT therapist: Mastering metacompetence in clinical practice* (pp. 225–238). Malden, MA: John Wiley & Sons.

Lantz, J. (1978). Cognitive theory and social casework. *Social Work*, *23*(5), 361–366.

Lantz, J. (1996). Cognitive theory and social work treatment. In F. J. Turner (Ed.), *Social work treatment: Interlocking therapeutic approaches* (pp. 94–115). New York: Free Press.

Maddux, J. E., & Winstead, B. A. (Eds.). (2016). *Psychopathology: Foundations for a contemporary understanding* (4th ed.). New York: Routledge.

Martell, C. R., Safren, S. A., & Prince, S. E. (2004). *Cognitive-behavioural therapies with lesbian, gay, and bisexual clients*. New York: Guilford.

Meichenbaum, D. (1985). *Stress inoculation training*. New York: Pergamon Press.

Morton, J., & Meyers, S. (2016). Identity, difference, and the meaning of 'Culture' in health and social care practice. In A. Ahmed & M. Rogers (Eds.), *Working with marginalised groups: From policy to practice* (pp. 21–36). London: Palgrave Macmillan.

National Association of Social Workers. (2008). *Code of ethics*. Retrieved from www.socialworkers.org/ pubs/code/code.asp

National Association of Social Workers. (2017). *Mental health*. Retrieved from www.socialworkers.org/ pressroom/features/issue/mental.asp

Newman, C. F. (2013). *Core competencies in cognitive-behavioural therapy: Becoming a highly effective and competent cognitive-behavioural therapist*. New York, NY: Routledge.

Pantalone, D. W., Iwamasa, G. Y., & Martell, C. R. (2010). Cognitive-behavioural therapy with diverse populations. In K. Dobson (Ed.), *Handbook of cognitive-behavioural therapies* (pp. 445–462). New York: Guilford Press.

Pignotti, M., & Thyer, B. A. (2009). Use of novel unsupported and empirically supported by licensed clinical social workers: An exploratory study. *Social Work Research*, *33*, 5–17. doi:10.1093/swr/33.1.5

Radnitz, C. L. (Ed.). (2000). *Cognitive-behavioural therapy for persons with disabilities*. Northvale, NJ: Jason Aronson.

Rawls, J. (1999). *A theory of justice*. Cambridge, MA: Harvard University Press.

Reback, C. J., & Shoptaw, S. (2014). Development of an evidence-based, gay-specific cognitive behavioural therapy intervention for methamphetamine abusing gay and bisexual men. *Addictive Behaviours*, *39*, 1286–1291. doi:10.1016/j.addbeh.2011.11.029

Resick, P. A., & Schnicke, M. K. (1992). Cognitive processing therapy for sexual assault victims. *Journal of Counseling and Clinical Psychology*, *60*, 748–756.

Ronen, T. (2007). Clinical social work and its commonalities with cognitive behaviour therapy. In T. Ronen & A. Freeman (Eds.), *Cognitive behaviour therapy in clinical social work practice* (pp. 3–24). New York: Springer.

Rothbaum, B. O., Ruef, A. M., Litz, B. T., Han, H., & Hodges, L. (2003). Virtual reality exposure therapy for combat-related PTSD: A case study using psychophysiological indicators of outcome. *Journal of Cognitive Psychotherapy: An International Quarterly*, *62*, 617–622. doi:10.1891/jcop.17.2.163.57438

Segal, Z. V., Williams, J. M. G., & Teasdale, J. D. (2013). *Mindfulness-based cognitive therapy for depression*. New York: Guilford Press.

Shattell, M. M., Quinlan-Colwell, A., Villalba, J., Ivers, N. N., & Mails, M. (2010). A cognitive-behavioral group therapy intervention with depressed Spanish-speaking Mexican women living in an emerging immigrant community in the United States. *Advances in Nursing Science, 33*(2), 158–169.

Steketee, G. (1988). Behavioral social work with obsessive-compulsive disorder. *Journal of Social Service Research, 10*, 53–72. doi:10.1300/J079v10n02_04

Sundel, M., & Sundel, S. (2005). *Behaviour change in the human services: Behavioural and cognitive principles and applications* (5th ed.). Thousand Oaks, CA: Sage.

Thomlison, R. J., & Thomlison, B. (2011). Cognitive behaviour theory and social work treatment. In F. J. Turner (Ed.), *Social work treatment: Interlocking theoretical approaches* (pp. 77–102). New York: Oxford University Press.

Thyer, B. A. (1991). Behavioural social work: It is not what you think. *Aret/Graduate School of Social Work, University of North Carolina, 16*(2), 1–9.

Thyer, B. A. (2011). Social learning theory and social work treatment. In F. J. Turner (Ed.), *Social work treatment: Interlocking theoretical approaches* (pp. 437–446). New York: Oxford University Press.

Thyer, B. A., & Myers, L. L. (2011). Behavioural and cognitive therapies. In J. R. Brandell (Ed.), *Theory & practice in clinical social work* (pp. 21–40). Thousand Oaks, CA: Sage.

Tolin, D. F. (2010). Is cognitive-behavioural therapy more effective than other therapies? A meta-analytic review. *Clinical Psychology Review, 30*, 710–720. doi:10.1016/j. cpr.2010.05.003

Van Wormer, R., & Davis, D. R. (2018). *Addiction treatment: A strengths perspective* (4th ed.). Boston: Cengage Learning.

Wakefield, J. C. (1988a). Psychotherapy, distributive justice and social work, Part 1: Distributive justice as a conceptual framework for social work. *Social Service Review, 62*, 187–210.

Wakefield, J. C. (1988b). Psychotherapy, distributive justice and social work, Part 2: Psychotherapy and the pursuit of justice. *Social Service Review, 62*, 353–382.

Windsor, L. C., Jemal, A., Alessi, E. J. (2015). Cognitive behavioural therapy: A meta-analysis of race and substance use outcomes. *Culture Diversity and Ethnic Minority Psychology, 21*(2), 300–313. doi:10.1037/a0037929

Wolpe, J. (1990). *The practice of behaviour therapy* (4th ed.). New York: Pergamon Press.

Zigarelli, J. C., Jones, J. M, Palomino, C. I., & Kawamura, R. (2016). Culturally responsive cognitive behavioural therapy: Making the case for integrated cultural factors in evidence based treatment. *Clinical Case Studies, 15*(6), 427–442. doi:10.1177/ 1534650116664984

17

Task-centred practice

Simon Cauvain

Introduction

Task-centred practice is a research-informed, problem-focused intervention aimed at helping service users achieve positive personal outcomes. This practice model guides a relationship-based approach between service users and social workers, in which the concept of partnership is central. A well-known and internationally popular approach, it offers social workers a carefully constructed framework that distinguishes task-centred practice from practice involving tasks. This important distinction illustrates the effective combination of evidence-based *and* person-centred practice. It is, however, argued to fall within the individualist-reformist tradition (Payne, 2005, p. 14) due to a lack of focus on social change.

Its social work research underpinning is of equal importance to the centrality of partnership in task-centred work. Doel and Marsh (1992) noted the strength of the approach being so firmly rooted in the early days of social work research and having been developed further from *within* the profession (Reid & Epstein, 1972; Goldberg, Walker, & Robinson, 1977; Gibbons, Butler, Urwin, & Gibbons, 1978; Goldberg, Gibbons, & Sinclair, 1984; Reid, 1978, 1985, 2000; Fortune, 1985; Rooney, 1988). The solid research base and easily measurable achievement of goals support a continually refined model of intervention informed by empirical research (Stepney & Ford, 2000). Doel and Marsh (1992), Marsh and Doel (2005) and Payne (2014) observed the development of the task-centred model reflecting societal and political change that influence service user problems and social work practice.

The time-limited focus of task-centred practice makes the approach more appealing in a present-day context of social work where scarcity of resources (including time and social workers) is widely reported in:

- The US, where the situation is frequently described as being in crisis (Alliance for Children and Families [Alliance], American Public Human Services [APHSA], & Child Welfare League of America [CWLA], 2001; Alwon & Reitz, 2000; Graef & Hill, 2000; United States General Accounting Office, 2003)
- Australia (Wagner, Van Reyk, & Spence, 2001; Lonne, 2003)
- Sweden (Tham, 2007; Tham & Meagher, 2009)

- The Republic of Ireland (Loughran, 2000; McGrath, 2001; Burns & Murray, 2003); Burns (2009)
- The UK (Laming, 2003, 2009); Baginsky et al., 2010; Munro, 2011; Association of Directors of Children's Services [ADCS], 2018)

This popular and effective model is not, however, claimed to be an approach that meets all needs in all situations; the complexity of social work dictates that there is no such thing. This chapter reflects on the compatibility of task-centred practice with a modern climate of enduring austerity in the UK and similar challenges internationally. I explore the question of influence and argue that within the English context, at least, little remains known about the actual work social workers do with their service users.

History

Social work theory literature consistently identifies historical and global development of the task-centred model. That development also provided insights into its practical application and associated technology (Marsh & Doel, 2005).

The task-centred model, created within the social work profession, has a history of over 50 years. It was developed in North America during the 1960s, due to growing dissatisfaction with the lengthy psychodynamic approaches dominant at that time. The drive for effective and economical models resulted in Reid's (1963) extended four-year PhD research, an experimental study of casework treatment methods. Reid and Shyne's (1969) follow-up study of brief and extended casework then laid the foundations of task-centred practice. The subsequent body of associated studies, referred to in the Introduction, further embedded the centrality of research.

Developmental milestones were Reid and Shyne's (1969) study establishing that short-term interventions were just as effective as long-term work, and Reid and Epstein (1972) produced a guide to task-centred practice, which Doel and Marsh (1992) developed further. Epstein and Brown (2002) define task-centred practice as a technology designed to relieve problems that are, crucially, service user–identified, understood and acknowledged as something they wish to address.

Doel and Marsh (1992) and Marsh and Doel (2005) highlight key principles of task-centred work. These include the development of partnership between worker and service user through an empowering approach and rapport building. The worker adopts a participative approach working with the service user, who is recognized as an expert in their own situation. The focus of the work is on small visible successes, not large hidden failures. The intervention is negotiated, measurable and time limited, lasting up to three months. Anti-oppressive practice is upheld through an open, honest and transparent approach by the social worker. The approach is also educative and requires skills of reflection and reflexivity.

The task-centred framework is envisaged as a 'shell' within which other compatible theories can be used (Healy, 2014). Motivational interviewing is identified as one such model that can support task-centred practice (see Chapter 20). Originally created for behavioural psychology, it is used when working with individuals and in interpersonal helping and problem-solving (Healy, 2014) and shares the social work values of partnership and power-sharing with service users (Hohman, 2012).

Payne (2014) convincingly justifies presenting task-centred practice next to crisis intervention within each edition of his ground-breaking *Modern Social Work Theory* textbook through a catalogue of authors and associated connections:

- Golan (1986): task-centred practice research supports crisis intervention.
- Gray (1987): practice structure, action planning, contracts or agreements used.
- Roberts and Dziegielewski (1995): crisis intervention as a brief solution therapy.
- MacNeil and Stewart (2000): task-centred practice can support planning for crisis work.
- Epstein and Brown (2002): each approach adopts brief treatment methods.
- Reid (1992): influence of crisis intervention on task-centred practice.

However, Reid and Epstein (1972), again cited in Payne (2014), identify a clear distinction between task-centred practice and crisis intervention; the scope of problems in task-centred practice are wider, and their definitions, tasks and timescales are more clearly defined. The task-centred focus on goal-setting is shared with solution-focused practice in social work, as noted by Shennan in this edition (see Chapter 19). A fundamental difference between methods is, however, that in task-centred practice, goal-setting is preceded by the retrospective exploration of problems. Solution-focused practice, conversely, is forward looking and future focused (de Shazer, 1985).

Highly structured process

Trevithick identifies social work intervention:

> the purposeful actions we undertake as professionals in a given situation, based on the knowledge and understanding we have acquired, the skills we have learned and the values we adopt. Interventions are, therefore, knowledge, skills, understanding and values in action.
>
> *(2005, p. 66)*

Doel and Marsh's (1992) highly structured practice model is used to illustrate the general approach: an intervention that underpins the distinction between 'task-centred practice' and merely 'practice involving tasks'. I have frequently made this important distinction with social work students on practice placements where they mistakenly described a loosely defined intervention as task-centred practice. A challenge to educators is posed in ensuring theory is not only explored critically but also understood and subsequently applied as theorists intended. Blind faith in applying theory is inappropriate, but deviation should be justified and consciously applied.

This is complex and particularly demanding of the skills of student and social worker alike in its application (Doel & Marsh 1992; Trevithick, 2012). Practical challenges include limitations of time, policy, and that it is service user–led, not worker-led, demands an anti-oppressive approach, needs to be well understood by workers and requires good communication skills, including the ability to listen. Students sometimes note the prescriptive feeling associated with following the process that I summarize in the following section. I argue the art of good practice is to strive to achieve a sense of balance for all involved in its use.

Key stages of task-centred practice

Doel and Marsh (1992) build on the work of their predecessors to include a helpful newspaper metaphor. They also dismiss Reid's (1978) 'verbal contract' between social worker and service user, in favour of a written agreement. Highlighting the power of language, 'contract', they argued, implied it was legally binding and non-negotiable. The intervention is underpinned by the basic principle that a service user's expressed and considered wishes control the work.

Task-centred practice involves four key stages, set out in Table 17.1:

Table 17.1 Key stages of task-centred practice

1 Developing a focus on the problem
2 Reaching agreement: goals and written agreements
3 Developing goals into manageable tasks
4 Ending and reviewing the work

1 Developing a focus on the problem

The first exploring-problems stage is completed across two levels: firstly, the initial expression of problems by the service user and, secondly, the considered expression of the problem by the person. Stage one begins with a scan of the 'newspaper headlines'. Here the range of problem areas are considered in broad terms, not in any specific detail. Any additions to this are used with caution; there may, for example, be a reason for the social worker to explain any important mandatory issues. Having collected the range of problems, the service user and social worker then investigate each problem area in more detail to get the 'inside story' using keywords: what, where, when, who, why and how? The service user summarizes each problem area with a single statement in the form of a 'quote'. They are supported in prioritizing the problems, arriving at a 'lead problem' which will be the first, and possibly only, focus of the work.

2 Reaching agreement: goals and written agreements

The 'problem' on which to work needs to be explicitly acknowledged by the service user as something that they wish and are able to work on, with or without the help of others, including the social worker. The associated 'goal' should be desirable and require service user motivation and ability to actually achieve it. It should be clear, specific and realistic. Also, the achievement of the goal should also be clearly connected to solving, or at least alleviating, the selected problem. The estimated and agreed time limit and frequency of contact will depend on the size of the goal and the resources available. Time therefore provides a framework within which progress is measured.

The written agreement is negotiated and completed in written form to provide formality and a sense that it is to last the duration of the work, whilst implying flexibility through negotiation. A specific problem and its associated 'quote' are selected for central focus. This is followed by an agreed statement beginning with 'I want to . . .', focusing on a goal to work towards.

3 Developing goals into manageable tasks

As the title of the model implies, tasks, identified and agreed on collaboratively between social worker and service user, play a central role. Sessions are used to plan tasks that, mirroring the approach with the goal, are clear, specific and realistic; when completed, they should lead incrementally towards the goal and, eventually, problem solution or alleviation. Within this transparent process, reasons for specific tasks and how they should be achieved are considered. Tasks are varied: session tasks can be completed within the session, homework tasks outside sessions. They may be unique or recurrent or both. They can be completed individually by those involved; reciprocally, as allocated to those involved and shared with participants working together on the same thing.

Session time is spent reviewing and scoring, out of ten, each associated task agreed on in the previous session. This provides a good opportunity for exploratory reflection and learning from reactions, actions and inactions and associated judgements. What obstacles exist, and why were tasks incomplete or unsuccessful? What strengths seemed to support the successful completion of tasks and why? Tasks are then developed further or repeated if necessary, and new tasks created for review at the next session.

4 Endings and evaluations

The agreed on and clearly identifiable final session built into the approach, adhering to the fundamental time-limited principle, offers the opportunity to jointly review and evaluate progress made. The endpoint evaluation helps those involved to manage expectations and appreciate the boundary of time. Achievement against the set of tasks and overarching goal can be measured and judgement made about problem resolution. Social workers can give positive feedback and encouragement for the future with the aim that the service user is better equipped to deal with a recurrence of the same or similar problems.

These four key stages need to be considered within the context of practice. Social workers, and of course students, need to know and understand the mechanics of task-centred practice in order to be able to describe it to those they work with before its implementation. Success in problem-solving seems unlikely without this necessary degree of transparency and ability to communicate effectively and reassuringly. The challenge in adopting this seemingly simple approach might easily be missed by the uninitiated practitioner. Griffith's (2017) argument for the enduring relevance of existentialist philosophy to social work practice acknowledges '. . . that social work processes are messy and . . . while all approaches have some usefulness, none offer a complete answer' (p. 102). Task-centred practice offers a great deal to social workers and service users within a broad range of practice areas. In addition to its versatility, Doel and Marsh (1992) summarize particular strengths:

- It is person-centred and involves close collaboration.
- Problems are defined by person seeking help.
- Tasks and goals are achievable.
- It is time-limited, usually up to three months.
- It is easy to evaluate.

Limitations include:

- It is problematic if service users are reluctant to work collaboratively.
- It often involves a great deal of service user motivation and effort.
- Underlying problems may not be identified.
- It is easy to lose the political and social dimensions of the problem.

Global reach

Doel and Marsh (1992) identify that a particular strength of task-centred practice is that it meets the requirements when tested against three key criteria for practice model evaluation:

- Ethical: a service user–centred approach is adopted.
- Research-based: at the heart of practice development of the model lie research and research-minded practitioners.
- Practical: it can be used in the real world of practice.

The ethical dimension here connects strongly to the co-production concept of the modern social work practice narrative considered in the next section. The research-based dimension highlights the complexity of the method and associated skills required, despite the model's apparent simplicity. On a practical front, whilst the model was developed as an effective brief intervention, social workers require the necessary time for reflection. They need professional motivation and autonomy within an organizational context that can facilitate the model. Social workers *may* also struggle to adopt the method in its intended form, at least Doel and Marsh's (1992) model, where other 'innovations' are prioritized, such as 'signs of safety' in child protection (Turnell & Edwards, 1999; see Chapters 18 and 33–35), the lifespan approach in developmental disabilities (Quinn, 1998) and the strengths-restorative approach in criminal justice (Van Wormer, 2001).

'Signs of safety' is more closely aligned to strengths and solutions-focused theories than problem-solving theories (Healy, 2014; see Chapters 18 and 19), yet similarities with task-centred work exist; it is strengths based and systematic (Featherstone, Gupta, Morris, & White, 2018), humanizing responses to risk and service user engagement (Keddell, 2014). Doel and Marsh (2006) aired their concern at the dearth of literature informing intervention in UK and US literature. Yet they optimistically forecast that by 2020, 14 years from their *Community Care* magazine article, social workers would have returned to more direct practice in which the grey area of uncertainty can be positively engaged. They believed the futile 'search for risk-free practice' and associated procedure and documentation-heavy practice would be more fully understood to be counterproductive, even 'dangerous' (Doel & Marsh, 2006). Rather disappointingly, little remains known about the extent of the use of task-centred practice in social work.

Practice context

The context of current English social work appears increasingly bleak as austerity bites, evidently more stretched than within the somewhat stark 'practice realities' described by Lymbery and Butler (2004); indeed, it is in crisis (ADCS, 2018). Featherstone et al. (2018) note that families in need have been denied the most since 2010. The ADCS sixth annual report on safeguarding pressures (ADCS, 2018). informed by research covering the financial year 2017–18 concludes that over the previous ten years:

- Initial contacts with children and families increased by 78 percent.
- Referrals increased by 22 percent.
- Child protection enquiries increased by 159 percent.
- Children subject to child protections plans increased by 87 percent.
- Children looked after by the local authority increased by 24 percent.

(ADCS, 2018, p. 119)

The report identifies that such demand is well beyond population growth and results from entrenched national actors (poverty, homelessness, job insecurity) outside the control of local authorities, despite all the efforts made. Such effort to meet demand is increasingly presented as creative, innovative, transformative and undoubtedly focused on child well-being. The combination of increasing demand and devastating cuts in budgets culminates in a reported 'tipping point' having been reached (ADCS, 2018, p. 120). Little evidence exists to indicate that this will change in the near future with early intervention preventative services being cut most severely.

The concepts of social worker/service user partnership, advocacy and representation has been a central theme of professional values for nearly 40 years (Foucault, 1981; Ahmed, 1985;

Dominelli, 1990; Hersov, 1992; Social Care Institute for Excellence [SCIE], 2004; Beresford & Hoban, 2005; Doel & Best, 2008). The status of the service user within some areas of social work practice has, however, shifted more significantly, though too slowly for many, over the last two decades, from recipients to participants, then partners and most recently collaborators and co-producers. This is arguably more apparent within learning disabilities and mental health studies (Beresford & Carr, 2012), whereas an uneven picture is reported within child welfare (Featherstone et al., 2018).

So what is being co-produced within this context of increased emphasis on collaboration and co-production? Rather than a tokenistic term, task-centred practice is, and always has been, used as an intervention where co-production in essence *produces* a resolution to a problem or problems identified by the service user in collaboration *with* the social worker.

Featherstone et al. (2018) argue this is bolstered by an increasingly neoliberal, individualistic political context where austerity and cuts in resources negatively impact service user well-being. The relationship between state and citizens is described as '. . . undermined, if not broken, by a variety of economic and social developments' (Davies, 2017, p. 2). Citizens, especially the poor, have become mistrustful, alienated and disconnected as the result of an 'intrusive and neglectful' state, unable or unwilling to live up to expectations in basic living (Davies, 2017; Monbiot, 2017; Peston, 2017). The prevailing UK government Department for Education and Department of Health narrative incentivizing innovation in current practice (see https://whatworks-csc.org.uk/ for example) arguably implies that interventions perceived to be more traditionally enshrined in the social work lexicon are outmoded and less effective.

Ferguson (2013) notes the dearth of literature informed through evaluation of what social workers do in face-to-face practice with service users. He calls for critical best practice, where careful analysis of the minutiae of social work interaction informs practitioners through a critical lens what supports best service user outcomes. This should ultimately present empirical evidence to inform what social workers should do rather than what they should not (Ferguson, 2013) within the messy, highly complex reality of practice (Tobin, 2003).

Conditions in social work organizations, within which practice is always embedded (Ferguson, 2013), are increasingly managerial, procedural, regulated and bureaucratized (Munro, 2011; ADCS, 2018). This represents a far-from-new concern, however, with Doel and Marsh (1992, p. 3) professing that practitioners were constrained by the 'actions and styles . . . policies and procedures' of their associated organizations and institutions. They conclude that practice development, most recently badged as innovation, should be influenced by the strengths and limitations of practicality within the practice context.

The realities of current practice influenced by socio-political and organizational environments challenge social workers to retain their values and ideals (Lymbery & Butler, 2004; Featherstone et al., 2018) and are intertwined with the care and control debate in safeguarding related practice. Power invariably lies with the social worker in the 'professional/client' relationship. Social workers, however, often report feeling powerless within organizational and societal contexts (Tham, 2007). Empathy for the client's sense of powerlessness should arguably therefore be within easy reach.

Not always hitting the mark

> '. . . [I]t is argued that social work in the UK has been systematically reshaped and effectively re-branded within the modernized welfare state, only to become politically compromised and compliant: 'the dog that didn't bark'.
>
> *(Stepney, 2006, p. 1290)*

211

Stepney (2006) observed the erosion of UK social work as a force for positive social change and progressive policy where emancipatory practice, the bastion of preventative social work, is curtailed. Key to this destructive shift were the influence of New Labour, globalization, erosion of public services and marketization (Ife, 1997). This rebranding of the welfare state was observed within Europe and, perhaps more surprisingly, Scandinavia (Lorenz, 2001). Stepney (2006, 2014) reports on the UK, European and US decimation of preventative work and advanced marginality where mainstream services remain 'preoccupied with protection and risk management' (2014, p. 1). This political context seemingly threatens the future, at least in the short term, of task-centred practice. Stepney's (2006) optimistic call to resist dominant discourses, reopen professional boundaries and uphold traditional values of prevention and social justice within a 'critical practice' framework offers hope for enhancing the rights of service users. Despite the current climate of austerity, where welfare demand unfailingly exceeds resource and practitioners respond to one crisis after another, a small-scale English and Finnish study found '. . . quite a lot of preventive work is actually being done in mainstream agencies' (Stepney, 2014, p. 316).

Whilst Doel and Marsh (1992) argue that task-centred practice *can* be used in 'child protection', now most frequently referred to in the UK as 'safeguarding', there is little evidence to suggest this is the case. The Australian import, 'signs of safety' (Turnell & Edwards, 1999), appears to have become a dominant approach (Baginsky, Moriarty, Manthorpe, Beecham, & Hickman, 2017) in some UK local authorities. Task-centred practice, with its underpinning strengths-based and person-centred approach, is arguably more closely aligned to, and effective in, preventative work.

Conclusion: looking to the future

A wealth of core textbooks map development and practical use of task-centred practice, reinforcing its universal appeal and popularity within qualifying social work courses. It cannot be assumed, however, that this is necessarily translated into contemporary global practice. This chapter explored the question of influence, and I argue that within the English context, at least, more needs to be known about the actual work social workers do with their service users. Social work involves a complex interplay of often unique issues and competing demands; the political climate of enduring austerity conflicts with any call for increasing investment in preventative work (Romeo, 2018), time to develop relationships with service users and time to think (Munro, 2011; Ferguson, 2013; Morris, White, Doherty, & Warwick, 2017).

The future of task-centred practice can only be realistically considered when more is known about the present, the ability to see beyond what is familiar, easily forgotten and taken-for-granted (Doel's wallpaper) (Taplin, 2018). Task-centred practice has a solid evidence-informed foundation and adheres to the professional social work values. It seems sensible to ensure it has the opportunity to thrive alongside the range of other approaches available. This individualized practice approach arguably reflects an increasingly individualized global political climate, one that perhaps loses sight of structural challenges. It is, however, an empowering method that can contribute to real and positive personal change and as such can, in turn, influence progressive collective action.

Further reading

Marsh, P., & Doel, M. (2005). *The task-centred book*. London: Routledge.
Shaw, I., & Gould, N. (2001). *Qualitative research in social work*. London: Sage.
Witkin, S. L. (2017). *Transforming social work*. London: Palgrave Macmillan.

References

Ahmed, B. (1985). *Black perspectives in social work*. Birmingham: Venture Press.

Alliance for Children and Families, American Public Human Services Association & Child Welfare League of America. (2001). *The child welfare workforce challenge: Results from a preliminary study*. New York: Alliance, APHSA and CWLA.

Alwon, F. J., & Reitz, A. L. (2000). Empty chairs: As a national workforce shortage strikes child welfare, CWLA responds. *Children's Voice, 9*(6), 35–37.

Association of Directors of Children's Services. (2018). *Research report: Safeguarding pressures phase 6: November 2018*. Manchester: ADCS.

Baginsky, M., Moriarty, J., Manthorpe, J., Beecham, J., & Hickman, B. (2017). *Evaluation of signs of safety in 10 pilots*. London: Department for Education.

Baginsky, M., Moriarty, J., Manthorpe, J., Stevens, M., MacInnes, T., & Nagendran, T. (2010). *Social workers' workload survey: Messages from the frontline: Findings from the 2009 survey and interviews with senior managers*. London: Department for Children, Schools and Families, Department of Health.

Beresford, P., & Carr, S. (Eds.). (2012). *Social care, service users and user involvement*. London: Jessica Kingsley.

Beresford, P., & Hoban, M. (2005). *Participation in anti-poverty and regeneration work and research: Overcoming barriers and creating opportunities*. New York: Joseph Rowntree Foundation.

Burns, K. (2009). *Job retention and turnover: A study of child protection and welfare social workers in Ireland*. (PhD thesis). National University of Ireland.

Burns, K., & Murray, B. (2003). Child protection in crisis: Growing pains from a rapid period of expansion or back pain from the increased burden? *Irish Social Worker, 21*(1–2), 13–16.

Davies, W. (2017). *The limits of neoliberalism: Authority, sovereignty and the logic of competition*. London: Sage.

de Shazer, S. (1985). *Keys to solution in brief therapy*. New York: Norton.

Doel, M., & Best, L. (2008). *Experiencing social work: Learning from service users*. London: Sage.

Doel, M. & Marsh, P. (1992). *Task-centred social work*. Aldershot: Ashgate.

Doel, M., & Marsh, P. (2006). Across the divide. *Community Care*. Retrieved from: https://www.communitycare.co.uk/2006/06/08/across-the-divide/.

Dominelli, L. (1990). *Women and community action*. Birmingham: Venture Press.

Epstein, L., & Brown, L. B. (2002). *Brief treatment and a new look at the task-centered approach* (3rd ed.). Boston: Allyn & Bacon.

Featherstone, B., Gupta, A., Morris, K., & White, S. (2018). *Protecting children: A social model*. Bristol: Policy Press.

Ferguson, H. (2013). Critical best practice. In M. Gray & S. A. Webb (Eds.), *The new politics of social work* (pp. 116–127). Basingstoke: Palgrave Macmillan.

Fortune, A. E. (1985). *Task-centred practice with families and groups*. New York: Springer.

Foucault, M. (1981). *Remarks on Marx*. New York: Semiotext.

Gibbons, J. S., Butler, J., Urwin, P., & Gibbons, J. L. (1978). Evaluation of a social work service for self-poisoning patients. *British Journal of Psychiatry, 133*(2), 111–118.

Golan, N. (1986). Crisis theory. In F. J. Turner (Ed.), *Social work treatment: Interlocking theoretical approaches* (3rd ed., pp. 296–340). New York: Free Press.

Goldberg, E. M., Gibbons, J., & Sinclair, I. (1984). *Problems, tasks and outcomes: The evaluation of task-centred casework in three settings*. London: Allen & Unwin.

Goldberg, E. M., Walker, D., & Robinson, J. (1977). Exploring task-centred casework. *Social Work Today, 9*(2).

Graef, M. I., & Hill, E. L. (2000). Costing child protective services staff turnover. *Child Welfare, 79*(5), 517–533.

Gray, E. (1987). Brief task-centred casework in a crisis intervention team in a psychiatric setting. *Journal of Social Work Practice, 3*(1), 111–128.

Griffith, M. (2017). *The challenge of existential social work practice*. London: Palgrave Macmillan.

Healy, K. (2014). *Social work theories in context: Creating frameworks for practice* (2nd ed.). London: Palgrave Macmillan.

Hersov, J. (1992). Advocacy – Issues for the 1990s. In T. Thompson & P. Mathias (Eds.), *Standards in mental handicap*. London: Bailliere and Tindall.

Hohman, M. (2012). *Motivational interviewing in social work practice*. New York: Guilford.

Ife, J. (1997). *Rethinking social work: Towards critical practice*. Melbourne: Longman.

Keddell, E. (2014). Theorising the signs of safety approach to child protection social work: Positioning, codes and power. *Children and Youth Services Review, 47*, 70–77.

Levin, E. (2004). *SCIE guide 4: Involving service users and carers in social work education*. London: SCIE.

Lonne, R. L. (2003). Social workers and human service professionals. In M. F. Dollard, A. H. Winefield, & H. R. Winefield (Eds.), *Occupational stress in the service professions* (pp. 281–310). London: Taylor and Francis.

Lord Laming. (2003). *The Victoria Climbié inquiry – Report of an inquiry*. Norwich: TSO.

Lord Laming. (2009). *The protection of children in England: A progress report* (HC. 330). Norwich: TSO.

Lorenz, W. (2001). Social work responses to 'New Labour' in continental Europe. *British Journal of Social Work, 31*(3), 595–609.

Loughran, H. (2000). Social work into the future. *Irish Journal of Social Work Research, 2*(2), 5–6.

Lymbery, M., & Butler, S. (Eds.). (2004). *Social work ideals and practice realities*. Basingstoke: Palgrave Macmillan.

MacNeil, G., & Stewart, C. (2000). Crisis intervention with school violence problems and volatile situations. In A. R. Roberts (Ed.), *Crisis intervention handbook* (pp. 229–249). New York: Oxford University Press.

Marsh, P., & Doel, M. (2005). *The task-centred book*. Abingdon: Routledge.

McGrath, J. (2001). Crisis in health board child protection services – Time to tell the truth. *Irish Social Worker, 19*(2–3), 3.

Monbiot, G. (2017). *Out of the wreckage: A new politics for an age of crisis*. London: Verso.

Morris, K., White, S., Doherty, P., & Warwick, L. (2017). Out of time: Theorizing family in social work practice. *Child and Family Social Work, 22*(S3), 51–60.

Munro, E. (2011). *Munro review of child protection: Final report – A child-centred system*. London: Department for Education.

Payne, M. (2005). *Modern social work theory* (3rd ed.). Basingstoke: Palgrave Macmillan.

Payne, M. (2014). *Modern social work theory* (4th ed.). Basingstoke: Palgrave MacMillan.

Peston, R. (2017). *What have we done? Why did it happen? How do we take back control?* London: Hodder and Stoughton.

Quinn, P. (1998). *Understanding disability: A lifespan approach*. Thousand Oaks, CA: Sage.

Reid, W. J. (1963). *An experimental study of methods used in casework treatment*. (PhD dissertation). University of Columbia.

Reid, W. J. (1978). *The task-centred system*. New York: Columbia University Press.

Reid, W. J. (1985). *Family problem-solving*. New York: Columbia University Press.

Reid, W. J. (1992). *Task strategies: An empirical approach to clinical social work*. New York: Columbia University Press.

Reid, W. J. (2000). *The task planner: An intervention resource for human service professionals*. New York: Columbia University Press.

Reid, W. J., & Epstein, L. (1972). *Task-centered casework*. New York: Columbia University Press.

Reid, W. J., & Shyne, A. W. (1969). *Brief and extended casework*. New York: Columbia University Press.

Roberts, A. R., & Dziegielewski, S. P. (1995). Foundation skills and applications of crisis intervention and cognitive therapy. In A. R. Roberts (Ed.), *Crisis intervention and time-limited cognitive treatment* (pp. 3–27). Thousand Oaks, CA: Sage.

Romeo, L. (2018). *Social work safeguards freedom, compassion and respect*, Online. Retrieved from https://lynromeo.blog.gov.uk/2018/12/05/social-work-safeguards-freedom-compassion-and-respect/

Rooney, R. H. (1988). Measuring task-centred training effects on practice: Results of an audiotape study in a public agency. *Journal of Continuing Social Work Education, 4*(4), 2–7.

Stepney, P. (2006). Mission impossible? Critical practice in social work. *British Journal of Social Work, 36*(8), 1289–1307.

Stepney, P., & Ford, D. (Eds.). (2000). *Social work models, methods and theories: A framework for practice*. Lyme Regis: Russell House.

Stepney, P. (2014). Prevention in social work: the final frontier? *Critical and Radical Social Work, 2*(3), 305–320.

Taplin, S. (Ed.). (2018). *Innovations in practice learning*. St. Albans: Critical Publishing.

Tham, P. (2007). Why are they leaving? Factors affecting intention to leave among social workers in child welfare. *British Journal of Social Work, 37*(7), 1225–1246.

Tham, P., & Meagher, G. (2009). Working in human service: How do experiences and working conditions in child welfare social work compare? *British Journal of Social Work, 39*, 800–827.

Tobin, M. (2003). The role of a journal in scientific controversy. *American Journal of Respiratory and Critical Care Medicine, 168*, 511–515.

Trevithick, P. (2005). *Social work skills: A practice handbook* (2nd ed.). Maidenhead: Open University Press.

Trevithick, P. (2012). *Social work skills: A practice handbook* (3rd ed.). Maidenhead: Open University Press.

Turnell, A., & Edwards, S. (1999). *Signs of safety: A solution and safety oriented approach to child protection case-work*. New York: Norton.

United States General Accounting Office. (2003). *Child welfare: HHS could play a greater role in helping child welfare agencies recruit and retain staff*. Washington, DC: Author.

Van Wormer, K. (2001). *Counselling female offenders and victims: A strengths-restorative approach*. New York: Springer.

Wagner, R., Van Reyk, P., & Spence, N. (2001). Improving the working environment in children's welfare agencies. *Child and Family Social Work, 6*, 161–178.

18

Strengths perspective
Critical analysis of the influence on social work

Robert Blundo, Kristin W. Bolton and Peter Lehmann

> Practicing from strengths perspective requires that we shift the way we think about, approach, and relate to our clients. Rather than focusing exclusively or dominantly on problems, your eye turns toward possibilities. In the thicket of trauma and trouble you see blooms of hope and transformation. The formula is simple: Rally clients' interests, capacities, motivations, resources, and emotions in the work of reaching their hopes and dreams, help them find pathways to those goals, and the payoff may be an enhanced quality of daily life for them.
>
> (*Saleebey, 2013a, p. 1*)

The strengths perspective

The strengths perspective has had a profound impact on the lexicon of social work writing since its first tentative acceptance into the literature. The first brief articles were met with some scepticism as they challenged the dominant pathological perspective that 'the individual is the repository of negative baggage' and that the problems in living were somehow the result of the individual's own defects and disease (Weick, 1981, 1983, pp. 140–151). In 1989, the first article to describe an alternative perspective to the medical model was published in the journal *Social Work*, titled 'A strengths perspective for social work practice' (Weick, Rapp, Sullivan, & Kisthardt (1989). Dennis Saleebey (personal communication with co-author Blundo) pointed out that this first article submission to use the term 'strengths perspective' was accepted on the condition it was brief and was published in the 'Briefly Stated' section of the journal. Presently, it is nearly impossible to find any text or article on practice that does not make some mention of client 'strengths', if one includes concepts such as resilience, social support, hope and coping that reflect the possible presence of strengths. At the same time, publications are much less likely to specifically identify the strengths perspective.

Currently, the very idea of considering strengths when working with individuals, families, groups and communities has become axiomatic (Saleebey, 2013a). A present review of the literature on social work practice reveals that in many cases the strengths perspective has been reduced to the social worker finding and listing what they see as the client's strengths. Strengths are often considered as one more section of an intake form. Saleebey (2013a) describes this practice on the part of authors and practitioners as paying lip service to the perspective. Implementing the strengths perspective involves a radical shift away from the problem or pathological perspectives. To start, the very idea of the strengths perspective must assure that 'everything you do as a social worker will be predicated, in some way, on helping to unearth and embellish, explore and exploit client's strengths and resources in the service of assisting them to achieve their goals, realize their dreams, and shed the irons of their own inhibitions and misgivings and society's domination' (Saleebey, 2013a, p. 2).

The strengths perspective is inherently at odds with the typical medical or pathological models of social work practice. The medical model places the worker as the expert and central to defining the problem in terms of a diagnostic category (see Chapters 6, 36 and 38). The worker then defines the method of treatment based on a theory of causation and intervention. To engage in a strengths perspective practice, one must challenge this idea of being the expert who focuses on identifying the deficits and pathologies and labelling or diagnosing the symptom. The strengths perspective sees the social worker as no longer the sole expert who identifies the problem, names it, and then applies a set manner of techniques/theories to dislodge the pathological condition. Weick et al. (1989) noted that 'the strengths perspective is an alternative to a preoccupation with negative aspects of people and society and a more apt expression of the deepest values of social work' (p. 350). It is a fundamental shift in how social work practitioners look at themselves, the client and the world around them. It is not a world without problems but is at the same time a world of possibilities and potentials. It is not a world without pain and suffering but a world where somehow and in some way people keep on going in their own unique ways. Kisthardt (2013) provides six guiding principles of strengths-based helping to give some guidance on how one might compare the focus of a strengths perspective with that of the problem- and disease-focused work with clients:

1   The initial focus of the helping process is on the strengths, interests, desires, hopes, dreams, aspirations, knowledge and capabilities of each person, not on their diagnoses, deficits, symptoms and weaknesses as defined by another (p. 59).
2   The helping relationship becomes one of collaboration, mutuality and partnership – power with another, not power over another (p. 60).
3   All human beings have the inherent capacity to learn, grow and transform. The human spirit is incredibly resilient. People have the right to try, to succeed, and to experience the learning which accompanies falling short of the goal (p. 62).
4   All human beings have the inherent capacity to learn, grow and transform. People have the right to succeed and the right to fail (p. 62).
5   Helping activities in naturally occurring settings in the community are encouraged in a strengths-based, person-centred approach (p. 64).
6   The entire community is viewed as an oasis of potential resources to enlist on behalf of service participants. Naturally occurring resources are considered as a possibility first, before segregated or formally constituted 'mental health' or 'social services' (p. 65).

Saleebey (2013a, p. 11) describes the significance of the language of the strengths perspective as an important element of the working relationship and the impact it has on the client and worker:

> Any approach to practice speaks a language that, in the end, may have a pronounced effect on the way the clients think about themselves and how they act . . ., our professional phraseology has a profound effect on the way we regard clients, their world, and their troubles.

When the language of pathology and diagnostic labels are applied, the focus is on weakness and abnormalities rather than on resilience, health and wellness, hope and meaningful optimism toward achieving goals for a better life. Therefore, how one collaborates with clients and other service providers is an important element that builds trust and a common ground from which to work together.

The strengths perspective does not provide specific techniques to use when working with the person, family, group or community. It offers a way of thinking about oneself as collaborating with another person who can create a better life as they understand what that would look like for themselves. Taking this position means that the worker does not see the problem as constituting all the person's life. Clients are much more than a diagnosis. Looking through the lens of a problem-based diagnostic label magnifies the problem, which soon becomes the name by which the client is known: borderline, schizophrenic, abused. The strengths perspective sees people as much more than their diagnosis and focuses the work on client goals and the many ways that they keep going. The question becomes: how do you use the strengths perspective when working with clients? In general, the types of questions that replace the typical diagnostic and intervention inquiry offer a set of possible questions that would help engage the client in looking at their own potentials and possible outcomes. Uncovering the strengths is accomplished by focusing on the following possible areas of inquiry:

- Given all the challenges you have faced, how have you managed keep going?
- Ask about any type of support that has been helpful to their ability to keep going.
- Ask about those times when the situation was just a little better and what they think was helpful. What did you do that helped to make that happen?

The focus turns toward what this specific client sees as a hoped-for future.

Given these basic ideas, it is easy to see why thinking about problems is a difficult shift to make given problem-focused training, expectations for a DSM diagnosis and worker-designed treatment plans. The *Diagnostic and Statistical Manual of Mental Disorders* (DSM) published by the American Psychiatric Association provides a guide for diagnosing mental disorders and is a tool used by practitioners interested in identifying clinical diagnoses such as depression, anxiety and substance use disorder. The shift to a strengths perspective is not a negation of the existence of a problem, struggle or challenge faced by the client. It does not negate the pain and wounds experienced by the client. The problem and the pain are acknowledged, recognized and clarified by the worker. At the same time, the strengths lens sees that the person has somehow and not without pain managed to keep going. They are doing the best they can at this time. This is the *choice point* where the worker might take the pathological path by identifying or diagnosing the problem according to a predetermined label with corresponding symptoms that need to be addressed by applying a specific set of techniques. Rather, the choice can be made to utilize a strengths perspective. This choice is based on the fundamental idea of respecting what clients reveal about themselves and demonstrating an appreciation for their story and a belief in their ability to create a better life as they understand it to be. Strengths perspective is demonstrated when the client is aware that the worker really believes in their potential for a better life. This position is guided 'first and foremost by a profound awareness of, and respect for, clients' positive attributes and abilities, talents and resources, desires and aspirations. Furthermore, the practitioner must be genuinely interested in, and respectful of, clients' accounts and narratives, the interpretive slant they take on their own lives' (Saleebey, 1992, p. 6). Kisthardt (2002, p. 164) describes the very nature of a strengths perspective that needs to be seen and heard by the client:

Send a clear message that you are not there to make negative judgments, to try to change people, but rather to affirm service participant's own aspirations . . . and to assist individuals, families, and communities within the context of a mutually enriching, collaborative partnership, to identify, secure and sustain the range of resources, both external and internal, needed to live a normally interdependent manner in the community.

Impact on social work interventions

Although misunderstood by many educators and practitioners, the idea of considering a client system's strengths has become a part of the social work language, as noted above. It is most often considered in assessments rather than an actual intervention. The idea of clients having strengths has become just one of many areas of an assessment and evaluation protocol. According to the CSWE list of core competencies, client system strengths are considered a part of the development of 'mutually agreed-on intervention objectives based on the critical assessment of strengths, needs, and challenges within clients and constituencies' (CSWE, 2017). It therefore remains an aspect of assessment but not of a specific practice method.

In a study of 44 out of 180 masters of social work (MSW) programmes in the US, it was found that although there was 'an almost universal awareness of and attention to integrating strengths-based content', few were focused on non-pathological ways of practising (Donaldson, Early, & Wang, 2009, p. 211). The study demonstrated that, although the programmes used the language of a strengths-based practice, there was a strong reliance on pathological and problem-focused practice.

The strengths perspective has had a significant influence on the profession by bringing into prominence the fundamental importance of client strengths and abilities. Other ideas, such as empowerment, resilience, person-centred practice, social justice and human rights, have become more prominent in education, training and practice (see Chapters 10 and 28). The more traditional social work profession was provoked into shining a larger light on the strengths of clients and making client strengths a larger part of assessment and practice. Yet the very idea of not focusing on fixing the problem as defined by the social work theories and practice techniques has led to marginalizing what is fundamental to the strengths perspective. Over the past decades, the idea of client strengths has become an element of theory and practice texts with mixed results. The strengths perspective is acknowledged but is not seen as a viable treatment modality. This situation is demonstrated by the practice work of McMillen, Morris, and Sharraden (2004):

> [The social work practitioner] . . . gets it. She or he understands that strengths are important considerations in intervention planning. She or he likely understands that it is important to inquire about clients' dreams and aspirations as well as their problems. She or he wants and works to empower her or his social work clients. *But she or he also needs to help clients with the problems they confront.*
>
> *(p. 323)*

This example gives acknowledgement to strengths being an important concept to include while, at the same time, the focus turns back to the *problem* as a separate sphere, that of needing to be labelled and applying techniques to 'cure' or fix the client. This is the typical state of most social work practice other than solution-focused and strengths perspective approaches in case management (see Chapter 19). The use of the term 'strengths' has become part of most practice and human development texts over the last decade yet it has not become a specific core *practice* competency requirement for social work education as listed by the Council for Social Work Education (CSWE), the US regulatory organization for social work education. Strengths are now a part of nearly every intake form. Yet asserting the idea of strengths as a part of practice has not necessarily shifted the actual assessments and practice with clients.

What important aspects of these ideas have failed to have an impact in social work?

The lack of a specific set of techniques or skills to implement the fundamental idea has created a vacuum for practitioners. Being without both specific explanations of causalities and the specific interventions required to 'treat' the client or problem leaves practically minded social workers without a way of engaging and working with client strengths. Saleebey (2013b) describes this dilemma by recognizing that:

> . . . [n]ot as elegant nor as opulent as a full-blown theory, the strengths perspective does recognize the fallibilities of people and the grinding problems that they face. It is, however, an attempt to restore, beyond flowery rhetoric, some balance to the understanding of the human condition – as social workers we recognize and respect the strengths and capacities of people as well as their afflictions and agonies.
>
> *(p. 279)*

The simple fact that the strengths perspective is just that, a perspective, and not an *explanatory theory* (see Payne, 2014) of practice has led to misunderstandings in its use for practice. As an *explanatory theory*, it would need to explain or give reasons for a 'problem' to exist. It would need to describe the problem in terms of causes and symptoms and prescribe a treatment or practice to alleviate the problem. Just as cognitive behavioural therapy (see Chapter 16) has a theory of causation and a way to intervene or practice to address those causations that are problems in how the person thinks about themselves and the world, the strengths perspective exists as a *guide* to how the social worker thinks about themselves and those they work with. It does not purport to have a specific set of techniques or interventions that social workers can learn to implement with their client system.

When looked at as a guide or model of practice, such as Rapp's (2006) model working with chronic and persistently mentally ill people and with substance abusers, the viability of its use can be better understood. It is in the interactive work of case management with clients that a way of practising can become clear. Rapp's model of practice makes it easier for practitioners to appreciate the perspective. The idea of a model for practice provides workers with a guide to 'what happens during practice in a general way, in a structured form. This helps to give our practice consistency in a wide range of situations. Models help you to structure and organize how you approach a complicated situation' (Payne, 2014, p. 9). The hard work of creating more models of practice based on the strengths perspective would potentially give better access to using the perspective as a model for working with a wide range of clients.

The key points of the SBCM (strengths based case management) (Rapp, 1998; Arnold, Walsh, Oldham, & Rapp, 2007) provide a guide to practising from a strengths perspective and a guide to outcome research:

- A focus on individual strengths rather than pathology, diagnosis or labels.
- Viewing the community as abundant in resources.
- Interventions based on client self-determination.
- The primary and essential nature of the manager–client relationship.
- Aggressive outreach.

An important contribution to understanding how one might practice from a strengths perspective comes from the work of Turnell (2010) on signs of safety in child protection services (see Chapters 19 and 34). The model moves away from the traditional focus on risk assessment, which Turnell (2010) sees as being overly judgemental, legalistic and intrusive, resulting in depreciating the family members. From a strengths perspective, the family is worked with toward a future with safety in mind. The focus is on what is working well and how the family can define and create a safe environment. Obviously, the collaborative work is focused on safety for the children and what needs to happen to create and maintain a safe environment for the family members.

Significant research and analysis of strengths-based interventions

Several strengths-based interventions have been developed and evaluated. The literature surrounding the evidence of strengths-based practice is surprisingly sparse, given social work's adoption of this perspective. Research on the SBCM approach, already discussed, with adult substance abuse issues revealed a significant positive outcome with respect to drug use, gaining employment and lower involvement with the criminal justice system (Arnold et al., 2007). Arnold et al.'s (2007) research focused on high-risk youth who have run away from home found that these youths made efforts to improve their lives. Tehan and McDonald (2010), utilizing this strengths-based approach with fathers, revealed that when fathers were accepted as the significant player in the work and not the social worker, the father as expert clinician position resulted in greater father participation with young people by improving the father's participation in the programme and improving the effectiveness of the intervention. These findings were supported by the work of Price-Robertson (2010). This study found that using strengths-based practice resulted in a shift from young parents being 'at risk' to being able to achieve positive outcomes. Importantly, they could start to identify their own strengths and work toward positive goals.

Lietz (2007) evaluated the use of the strengths perspective with group work. Its use in a single-parent support group increased attendance and active participation by members. Group work practice in a residential treatment centre with 10- to 13-year-old residents found a decrease in negative behaviour and an increase in prosocial behaviours.

Proyer, Ruch, and Buschor (2012) evaluated what they saw as strengths-based interventions by looking at programmes that focused on curiosity, gratitude, hope, humour and zest as a means of enhancing life satisfaction. These basic ideas are a part of the work being done in positive psychology. Their conclusions were that 'the results point towards a potential in strengths-based interventions for contributing positively to the well-being of people' (published online: 16 March 2012).

Conclusion

The future of the strengths perspective will depend on how this approach or way of thinking and acting with client systems is able to demonstrate its effectiveness as a practice. Given the medical model's requirement for establishing a diagnosis and the utilization of a predetermined technique to treat the client system, it is unlikely that the strengths perspective will be able to meet these artificial requirements. Donaldson et al. (2009) found that the strengths perspective was an '. . . espoused value of [MSW programmes'] culture, but they still lack a fully internalized culture of strengths in which underlying assumptions of strengths become an unconscious "given" that fully accepted by the [faculty] (p. 233). Some faculty – that is, academic staff – saw it as a perspective but were not able to see its implication for changing the work of practice.

Emphasis on the world of evidenced-based practice and requirements that agencies utilize a predetermined intervention model leaves little room for integration of a different approach, much less a strength-based approach. Gergen (2009) describes this dilemma with attempting to embrace a different way of approaching clients:

> Socialized into plausible structures [pathological and problem-solving models] that is, conceptual understandings of the world and rational support of those understandings. As we come to rely on these plausibility structures, so do we develop a natural attitude, that is a sense of a natural, taken-for-granted reality.

(p. 23)

Maintaining the idea that client systems have strengths as one of many ideas about client systems gives a false sense of understanding to those learning and attempting to engage in strengths-based practice. Social work educators have managed to use the language of strengths, empowerment, self-determination and social justice while maintaining the 'prerogative to plan and strategize, direct and control', all the while believing that their practice is built on client strengths (Margolin, 1997, p. 122).

The strengths perspective has introduced an important addition to social work thinking and practice. Challenging the medical model and problem-focused interventions will be difficult given the impact of evidence-based practice and, more importantly, the idea of social work practice taking on the mantle of a medicalized practice model of disease and curing. With the emergence of positive psychology and neuroscience (see Chapters 18–22) as important steps in understanding how people fare in this world might just lead to seeing the strengths perspective as a real alternative to the present attachment to pathologically focused practice.

Further reading

Saleebey, D. (2013). *The strengths perspective in social work practice* (6th ed.). Upper Saddle River, NJ: Pearson.

References

Arnold, E. M., Walsh, A. K., Oldham, M. S., & Rapp, C. A. (2007). Strengths-based case management: Implementation with high-risk youth. *Families in Society*, 88(1), 86–94.

Donaldson, L. P., Early, B. P., & Wang, M-L. (2009). Toward building a culture of strengths in US MSW programs. *Advances in Social Work*, 10(2), 211–229.

Gergen, K. L. (2009). *An invitation to social construction* (2nd ed.). Los Angeles: Sage.

Kisthardt, W. E. (2002). The strengths perspective in interpersonal helping: Purpose, principles, and functions. In D. Saleebey (Ed.), *The strengths perspective in social work practice* (3rd ed., pp. 163–184). Boston: Allyn and Bacon.

Kisthardt, W. E. (2013). Integrating the core competencies in strengths-based, person-centered practice: Clarifying purpose and reflecting principles. In D. Saleebey (Ed.), *The strengths perspective in social work practice* (6th ed., pp. 23–78). Upper Saddle River, NJ: Pearson

Lietz, C. A. (2007). Strengths-based group practice: Three case studies. *Social Work with Groups*, 30(2), 73–87.

Margolin, L. (1997). *Under the cover of kindness: The invention of social work*. Charlottesville: University Press of Virginia.

McMillen, J. C., Morris, L., & Sherradan, M. (2004). Ending social work's grudge match: Problems versus strengths. *Families and Society*, 85(3), 317–325.

Payne, M. (2014). *Modern social work theory* (4th ed.). Chicago: Lyceum.

Proyer, R. T., Ruch, W., & Buschor, C. (2012). Testing strengths-based interventions: A preliminary study on the effectiveness of a program targeting curiosity, gratitude, hope, humor, and zest for enhancing life satisfaction. *Journal of Happiness Studies*, 14, 275–292.

Rapp, C. A. (1998). *The strengths model: Case management with people suffering from severe and persistent mental illness*. Oxford: Oxford University Press.

Rapp, R. C. (2006). The strengths perspective and persons with substance abuse problems. In D. Saleebey (Ed.), *The strengths perspective in social work practice* (4th ed., pp. 77–96). New York: Allyn & Bacon.

Saleebey, D. (1992). *The strengths perspective in social work practice*. White Plains, NY: Longman.

Saleebey, D. (2013a). Introduction: Power to the people. In D. Saleebey (Ed.), *The strengths perspective in social work practice* (6th ed., pp. 1–24). Upper Saddle River, NJ: Pearson.

Saleebey, D. (2013b). The strengths perspective: Possibilities and problems. In D. Saleebey (Ed.), *The strengths perspective in social work practice* (6th ed., pp. 279–303). Upper Saddle River, NJ: Pearson.

Tehan, B., & McDonald, M. (2010). *How to engage fathers in child and family services* (CAFCA Practice Sheet 2). Melbourne: Communities and Families Clearinghouse Australia. Retrieved from www.aifs.gov.au/cafca/pubs/sheets/ps/ps2.html

Turnell, A. (2010). *The signs of safety: A comprehensive briefing paper*. Perth: Resolutions Consultancy.

Weick, A. (1981). Reframing the person-in-the-environment perspective. *Social Work, 26*(2), 140–143.

Weick, A. (1983). Issues in overturning a medical model of social work practice. *Social Work, 28*(6), 467–471.

Weick, A., Rapp, C., Sullivan, W. P., & Kisthardt, W. (1989). A strengths perspective for social work practice. *Social Work, 34*, 350–389.

19

Solution-focused practice in social work

Guy Shennan

Introduction

Solution-focused practice is a forward-looking approach which helps service users move towards futures they want by building on how they are already doing so. First developed at the Brief Family Therapy Center (BFTC) in the US in the 1980s by a group of therapists, many of whom originally trained as social workers (Lee, 2013), its use dates from the late 1980s onwards. A case has been made for a good fit in principle between solution-focused practice and social work (Wheeler, 2003; Walsh, 2010; Greene & Lee, 2011; Corcoran, 2016), which is supported in part by the numerous applications of the approach by social workers, some surveyed in this chapter. There are also, however, aspects of solution-focused practice that present challenges for its use in present-day social work, and it is important we also give these clear-eyed consideration.

Neither solution-focused practice (Miller & de Shazer, 1998) nor social work (Cree, 2009) are monolithic and unchanging activities, which complicates the question of the influence of one on the other. A later streamlined version (Ratner, George, & Iveson, 2012) helps bring some difficulties that social workers face in using solution-focused practice into sharper relief. Having considered these challenges, I will provide examples where social workers have risen to meet them, beginning in the field of children and families. As with other therapeutic practice models, it has been difficult to fit unadorned solution-focused practice into certain functions that dominate modern social work, such as assessment, risk management and care planning. This has led to some creative adaptations, where solution-focused ideas have been drawn upon to create new models, including the signs of safety approach to child protection practice (Turnell & Edwards, 1999). I shall consider the relationship between the solution-focused and signs of safety approaches, as there is scope for confusion between them. A look at some uses of the solution-focused approach with other service user groups will lead us to examine its current positioning within social work in the US as part of the strengths perspective (see Chapter 18).

The challenges in using solution-focused practice also relate to aspects of present-day social work, and I shall end with a note of encouragement to those embarked on the project to 'reimagine social work' (Featherstone, White, & Morris, 2014; RSW Collective, 2015; Walden,

2015) that they might usefully embrace solution-focused practice in all its radical simplicity and genuine transfer of power from professional to service user.

A developing model

Solution-focused brief therapy (SFBT) grew from the discovery that whatever problems people brought to therapy, there were invariably *exceptions* to them, when the problem did not happen or happened less often or with less intensity. The discovery of exceptions led the BFTC team to focus on what their clients were doing that *was* working. The therapists' task shifted from creating change to uncovering change already underway and amplifying it. The goal focus of brief therapy was utilized to ensure that change was heading in the right direction and further developed via the 'miracle question' (de Shazer, 1988), which invited clients to describe a post-miracle problem-free future in more detail. The new SFBT approach was set out by the BFTC team in a landmark paper (de Shazer et al., 1986), later developed in ways that had implications for its use within social work.

As the approach was increasingly disseminated by its founders, it began to be used in professional contexts outside therapy, including social work. Influential in this were the accounts of its various applications by Insoo Kim Berg and collaborators in substance misuse, children's services and coaching (Berg & Miller, 1992; Berg, 1994; Berg & Reuss, 1997; Berg & Kelly, 2000; Berg & Steiner, 2003; Berg & Szabo, 2005). In the UK, the approach was taken up most influentially by a team of social workers who were also family therapy practitioners and teachers (George, Iveson, & Ratner, 1990). At their solution-focused clinic and training centre, BRIEF, they honed an influential version of solution-focused practice (Ratner et al., 2012; Shennan, 2014). The most striking features of this are its streamlining of the approach, the lack of any reference point to the client's problems, a clearer opening focus on what the client wants and the dropping of any intervention by the worker. The approach was distilled to three activities:

- Establishing the outcome the client hopes for from the work.
- Eliciting a detailed description of the realization of this hoped-for outcome.
- Eliciting a description of progress the client is making towards realizing their hopes.

The minimalism of the BRIEF version brings out clearly some of the aspects of solution-focused practice that make it usable by social workers (Shennan, 2014, pp. x–xiii). The daily round of social workers and their contacts with their service users is typically not as structured as for therapists and their clients, and the flexibility of BRIEF's solution-focused practice provides a good fit with this. Its use does not require a pre-programmed number of sessions, with clients being invited to carry out tasks in between, and conversations containing descriptions of hoped-for futures and progress towards them can take place anywhere at any time. Not only is a one-off session seen as potentially useful (Hogg & Wheeler, 2004, p. 306), but also occasional questions used in brief contacts – 'How would you know the situation was improving?' 'What have you done that's helped his behaviour to improve?' – create possibilities for social workers on duty or in crisis situations to use the approach.

Challenges for social work

By the same token, the distilled nature of the BRIEF version also highlights some features that present challenges to social workers using the approach: the lack of active exploration of the client's problems, the absence of an assessment component and the strong focus on what the client wants from the work. Let us examine these in turn.

The need for problem talk

An attachment to exploring problems runs deep in social work, as can be seen in a classic British text on task-centred social work (Doel & Marsh, 1992). Being organized around goals rather than problems, this approach shares similarities with solution-focused practice (Bucknell, 2000). However, before goal-setting in task-centred work, there is a problem exploration stage, with problems being scanned and detailed before one or more are selected to work on. Doel and Marsh see a criticism that task-centred work does not get to the roots of problems as a misconception, stating that 'it is a fallacy to suppose that change is necessarily dependent on a "knowledge of the history"' (1992, p. 94). They cite de Shazer (1985) to support their point, as a brief therapist who 'starts with the goal and leaves the problems untouched'. Notwithstanding this approving reference, there is no suggestion that they had considered dropping problem exploration from their model.

This problem attachment can also be detected in a trenchant critique of the solution-focused approach (Stalker, Levene, & Coady, 1999). These critics mention research showing that brief therapies are less effective than longer-term ones in relation to severe problems but provide no references, and the evidence base for solution-focused practice is now quite solid (Franklin, Trepper, Gingerich, & McCollum, 2012; Gingerich & Peterson, 2013; Macdonald, 2017). Stalker et al. (1999, p. 473) also refer to 'clinical wisdom', which 'challenges SFBT's precepts that one does not need to know anything about how the problem developed', and critique a piece of solution-focused work with a young mother whose two children had been removed from her care and its neglect of 'client history and broader assessment'. This work was said to be naive and to illustrate 'SFBT's disregard of a gender-sensitive perspective and of large-systems factors'. The authors do not report the outcome of this work, which was that the mother had her children returned to her care (Berg & de Jong, 1996), suggesting that their difficulties with the approach are more ideological than empirical. The idea that people need to talk about their problems is a normative one and is challenged by the growing evidence base for solution-focused practice.

However, it is a misconception that solution-focused practice does not allow problem talk. Not asking about problems does not preclude people talking about them, and careful thought has been given to how to respond in these situations. A position of 'acknowledgement and possibility' (O'Hanlon, 1992, p. 138) shows that the worker is hearing the difficulty – 'things are really tough at the moment . . .' – while at the same time is aware that the service user has resources, opening up possibilities for change – '. . . what are you doing that is getting you through?' Such 'coping questions' were first mentioned in the solution-focused literature in Berg's early accounts of using the approach with particular groups: people with alcohol problems (Berg & Miller, 1992) and families at risk of breakdown (Berg, 1994), and I suspect their introduction followed the approach, moving beyond the therapy room into contexts familiar to social workers, whose caseloads do not include many people not dealing with severe difficulties (Shennan, 2014, p. 122).

The need for assessment

Another reason for talk about problems might be that workers need to hear about them to form their assessments, which has taken on more force as the assessment role has grown in social work (Asquith, Clark, & Waterhouse, 2005). Here also solution-focused practice challenges received ideas (Shennan, 2003). There are several reasons for engaging in assessment, perhaps most importantly where there needs to be a risk assessment due to concerns that someone might come to harm. Assessments are also carried out to judge whether someone needs help and the type of help they might need. These judgements will be affected by the helping resources available, with shortages increasing the gatekeeping function of the assessment. Where someone is seeking help for themselves, a solution-focused practitioner will question whether an assessment is required, for 'if a parent was asking for help, then they must need help . . . the parent had carried out their own assessment, the conclusion of which led to their request for a service' (Shennan, 2003, p. 79). An assessment might still be needed for gatekeeping, but as assessment itself is resource intensive, reducing the amount of assessing done would free up more resources to provide help and support.

The focus on what the client wants

The clarity with which solution-focused practice starts with what the client wants might also put it at odds with much modern social work, insofar as it is dominated by statutory functions of investigating, assessing, policing and protecting over help and support. This is associated with a growth of involuntary over voluntary clients, especially in children's services, so that the work cannot be directed by what the client wants. Furthermore, asking someone what they want assumes motivation, and many helping professionals view their service users as not motivated or ready to change, which has contributed to the growing use of motivational interviewing (Miller & Rollnick, 2013; see Chapter 20).

In response, first, it is important not to make exaggerated claims for a therapeutic practice model; solution-focused practice is not designed to be used in all situations faced by social workers. When, for example, concerns about a child's safety have been raised and need to be investigated, the starting point for the social worker will not be to ask the parent what their desired outcome is. While this may be asked at a later stage, if there are concerns about the child's safety, social work will not be directed by the parents' hopes but by the need to secure safety for the child and so will not be solution-focused practice in any strict sense.

Second, to use the approach, social workers need to both look for and actively create contexts where it is legitimate and potentially useful to ask clients what they want and through talking help them move towards this (Shennan, 2014, p. 183). Duty teams have used the approach by first separating self-referrals from third-party referrals reporting concerns and then determining whether practical support, advice or advocacy was required or the issue was such that talking might help (Hogg & Wheeler, 2004; Shennan, 2014, pp. 185–186). A context for solution-focused practice can be created where the client has been externally mandated to see the social worker by drawing on the principles of the 'non-treatment paradigm' for probation practice (Bottoms & McWilliams, 1979). In that instance, the mandate for supervision, ordered by the court, is separate from the mandate for help given by the client; a similar distinction in mandate applies in other situations. A solution-focused opening invitation in probation might be 'Though it was not your idea to see me, and in fact the court has ordered you to, I hope our meetings can still be useful for you. What would need to be happening in your life so that they were useful?' On the question of whether the client is ready to change, solution-focused practitioners assume that if someone is talking to them, then they must want *something* to come from this, even if that is for the work to come to an end and the worker go away. Motivation for something is assumed.

In its transparent focus on what the client wants and ensuring this is what always drives the work forward, solution-focused practice stands out among other therapeutic modalities.

However, the multiplicity of roles and tasks of a social worker make keeping the client's hopes at the forefront a particular challenge, as Sundman (1997, p. 166) found when researching the use of solution-focused practice by social workers in Helsinki: 'The key solution-focused concept 'goal' is, in social work practice, a complicated ongoing negotiation, if done at all'. Sundman was not always clear, listening to tapes of client-worker meetings, when there was agreement on goals or what the goals were. The radical nature of asking a client what they want, and the difficulty levels involved in maintaining a focus on this, should not be underestimated.

Solution-focused social work with children and families

Social work with children and families is often divided into two main functions, child protection and family support, and we have seen that solution-focused practice is not straightforwardly applicable to the former, at least in its 'front end' stages. It has, however, been successfully applied in family support teams in the UK (Vostanis, Anderson, & Window, 2006; Forrester et al., 2008; Shennan, 2008; Stancer, 2008; Thom, Delahunty, Harvey, & Ardill, 2014; Fernandes, 2015; Turney & Merchant, 2017). There is evidence that the approach is proving effective in this context, in improving children's well-being (Fernandes, 2015) and in contributing to a reduction in the numbers of children entering care (Thom et al., 2014; Fernandes, 2015; Turney & Merchant, 2017). It is not always possible to isolate one factor as responsible for such outcomes, and in two of the services listed here, solution-focused practice was used alongside motivational interviewing (Forrester et al., 2008; Thom et al., 2014). We shall return later to the issue of integrating approaches.

Overall, these studies add to the growing evidence for solution-focused practice's effectiveness with children and families (see Chapters 32–34). A systematic review of studies between 1990 and 2010 found the evidence to generally support SFBT (Bond, Woods, Humphrey, Symes, & Green, 2013). The studies were of work with both families and children on an individual basis and showed that solution-focused work could be effective in each case. The approach may be adapted to apply to children (Berg & Steiner, 2003; Hackett & Shennan, 2007; King, 2017), and social workers in a service for children in or on the edge of care (Fernandes, 2015) produced their own variations later made available as a 'toolkit' (NSPCC, 2015). In the evaluation of this service, both children and carers suggested the potential usefulness of parents or carers being involved in the sessions too. Users also welcomed a family-centred approach in a service across Wales (Thom et al., 2014). Both studies therefore support calls for a return to family-based social work practice with children (Featherstone et al., 2014).

Solution-focused practice and child protection

The Bond review studies, while instructive for social work with families, were not in the main of work done by social workers, but the review's origins nevertheless make it of interest in studying connections between solution-focused practice and social work (see also Chapter 32). It was commissioned by the government in England to review the effectiveness of SFBT with children and families and to consider its use in safeguarding children from harm, after comments made in the second Serious Case Review into the death of Peter Connelly: 'SFBT is not compatible with the authoritative approach to parents in the protective phase of enquiries, assessment and the child protection conference if children are to be protected' (Haringey LSCB, 2009, para. 3.16.7). That the authors of the review then found it difficult to find studies where the focus was directly on child protection issues is unsurprising, given that solution-focused practice is not used to do child protection work, certainly in its 'protective phase', the comment of the Serious Case Review above being no more than a truism The first of the two studies that were found relating to child protection was a single case study which suggested that solution-focused therapy was used, to good effect, to help a mother find alternatives to physical punishment in managing her son's behaviour (Corcoran & Franklin, 1998). The second concerned an approach called solution-based casework (Antle, Barbee, Christensen, & Sullivan, 2009), which, while including the use of solution-focused methods, 'does not exclude formal risk assessment and incorporates other more "instructional" and directive intervention strategies' and 'provides a case planning framework which includes the use of safety plans' (Woods, Bond, Humphrey, Symes, & Green, 2011, p. 38).

This approach seems to share features with those of the signs of safety model, another approach to child protection that draws upon solution-focused practice and which necessarily added other features to apply it to child protection contexts. Initially, the model consisted of 'practice elements' and an assessment and planning framework (Turnell & Edwards, 1999). The solution-focused influence was explicit in the practice elements, which included finding exceptions to the maltreatment, discovering family strengths, focusing on goals and scaling safety and progress. It was also implicit in aspects of the assessment and planning framework, in its attention to signs of existing safety as well as to danger and harm and in its future orientation and use of scaling, though here there are crucial differences with solution-focused practice. First, in child protection work, the agency with its statutory responsibilities to protect children will need to judge that a child is safe; hence the future-focused question that signs of safety is organized around is 'What do we need to see before we are able to close the case?' Second, the different use of scaling relates to whose agenda and judgements are central, with the client's rating of progress being of sole importance in solution-focused work, whereas the child protection worker necessarily rates the child's safety in the signs of safety assessment.

The signs of safety model has continued to develop, and while the influences of the solution-focused and brief therapy traditions remain, they are perhaps more implicit than showing up as specific techniques. For example, while the assessment and planning framework is similar to its original form, the 'practice elements' are not referred to in the latest account of the approach, with more attention paid to safety planning (Turnell & Murphy, 2017). There are still strong ties between the approaches, as evidenced by the inclusion of a chapter on signs of safety in a major text on the evidence base of SFBT (Wheeler & Hogg, 2012), while some agencies preparing their staff to use signs of safety provide solution-focused training (Baginsky, Moriarty, Manthorpe, Beecham, & Hickman, 2017). It is important, though, to be clear that they are quite distinctive in aim and scope and to beware of talking loosely about 'using solution-focused practice in child protection'. The signs of safety approach has also spread beyond child protection to other contexts where attention to risk is central, sometimes modified as Signs of Wellbeing (Wheeler, Hogg, & Fegan, 2006; Bunn, 2013, p. 9; Stanley, Keenan, Roberts, & Moore, 2017). It is possible to use this approach in other contexts, such as early intervention, at the same time believing that a fully solution-focused alternative could be used. This would have the advantages, from a solution-focused perspective, of dispensing with problem exploration and worker assessment and keeping clients in charge of the work's direction.

Solution-focused social work with adults

The flexibility of solution-focused practice, together with its lack of concern with identifying problems, means that it is used widely across many service user groups. The following examples demonstrate this and also show how social workers manage more roles than that of 'therapist'.

Gaiswinkler and Roessler (2009) show, for example, how a solution-focused approach was used in Austria in a social work service to prevent homelessness. A simple framework accommodated the social work tasks of decision-making (for example, about whether to provide financial support), information giving and liaison and advocacy with other agencies alongside psychosocial counselling. This framework was built around two kinds of social work knowledge. First, an 'expertise of knowing' allowed social workers to draw upon knowledge about agency policies, community facilities, law and legal procedures. This assisted clients towards goals established through the use of the social workers' other kind of knowledge, an 'expertise of not knowing'. This expertise, based on the use of solution-focused skills, ensured that the work was taking place within the client's frame of reference. It also helped build and maintain the client-worker alliance.

Effective use has been made of solution-focused practice with court-mandated domestic violence offenders in the US (Lee, Sebold, & Uken, 2012). Offenders are held accountable for solutions rather than focusing on responsibility for problems. This contrasts with other work in this field, typically psychoeducational programmes using a cognitive behavioural approach or drawing on a feminist perspective (see, for example, Pence & Paymar, 1993). In Bottoms and McWilliams's (1979) tradition, already discussed, social control and treatment functions are separated, with self-determined goals being a central component. Insisting on specific goals being developed by a certain point in the programme and regular checking on progress towards them make this a more instrumental solution-focused practice than the BRIEF version and fits with the judicial context. Programme completion rates and levels of recidivism compare favourably to other approaches (Lee et al., 2012). Solution-focused approaches have also been used in youth justice (Clark, 1996; Corcoran, 1997), though these early developments have since been widened to include motivational interviewing and a broader strengths-based model (Clark, 2005, 2009). Common ground has been found between solution-focused practice and restorative justice (Lehmann, Jordan, Bolton, Huynh, & Chigbu, 2012; Walker, 2008).

The solution-focused approach has been little used in social work services for disabled people, at least in the UK, though the Care Act 2014 has increased attention to strengths-based approaches (Gollins et al., 2016). Smith's (2011) reflections on the limited impact of solution-focused training for social workers with adults with learning disabilities echo the role constraints facing children's social workers. The introduction of care management (Department of Health, 1990) separated assessment and service provision, encouraging a directive, task-focused stance and reducing the focus on emotional support to service users. The social workers on this course thus questioned the relevance of training in a therapeutic practice model to their role and found solution-focused practice hard to use. They reported, however, some shifts in practice, including increased listening and a less directive and more reflective approach.

There has been greater use of the approach in the mental health field, though most published accounts of this have not been within social work (Vaughn, Young, Webster, & Thomas, 1996; Hawkes, 2003; Hosany, Wellman, & Lowe, 2007; Simon & Nelson, 2007). Greene et al. (2006, p. 347) writing in the US, report that 'case managers can use the interviewing and intervention tools of solution-focused therapy to further operationalize strengths-based case management'.

The strengths perspective

Greene et al.'s comment illustrates the positioning of solution-focused practice within social work in the US, where it is seen as part of the strengths perspective (Cynthia Franklin, personal communication; see Chapter 18). This support calls for an integrative approach, the possibility of which had been rejected by de Shazer (O'Connell, 2000), as it would involve importing problem-focused concepts. Beyebach (2009), however, suggests supplementing solution-focused techniques with others from conceptually linked fields, which could include other approaches that share the strengths perspective as a metatheory (Simmons et al., 2016). Specific connections include with motivational interviewing (Lewis & Osborn, 2004) and narrative and other models (Parton & O'Byrne, 2000; Greene & Lee, 2011). The latest edition of a standard UK text on social work assessment groups solution-focused and narrative approaches with the 'resilience model' in a chapter on strengths-based approaches to assessment (Milner, Myers, & O'Byrne, 2015).

Narrative practices (see Chapter 21) can enrich the constructive descriptions of service users' lives elicited by solution-focused practice. The idea of preferred states of identity, incorporating a person's values, principles and commitments can link together episodic accounts of exceptions into stories that can reverberate through a whole life. While White (2007) named his approach according to the story metaphor, at one point he considered naming it 'linking lives therapy' (Hugh Fox, personal communication). Its non-individualized focus has recommended it to radical social workers (Turbett, 2014, pp. 132–134), and the efforts of narrative practitioners to connect their clients with other people are reflected in the creation of a 'lifelong network' around a child that has become an important part of safety planning in the signs of safety approach (Turnell & Murphy, 2017). Saleebey (2012, p. 302) criticized solution-focused practice for not as yet paying sufficient attention to resources in the environment; bringing narrative practice alongside it is a means of addressing this.

A couple of caveats may be noted concerning the idea of strengths and some practical applications of the strengths perspective. Strengths assessments (Rapp, 1998) help clients notice and amplify their strengths in developing personal plans and so can be congruent with a wholly client-led approach, but introducing a notion of assessment may run the risk of workers adopting an expert position even if unintentionally. Moreover, where worker-led assessments are required, Brandon et al. (2009, p. 47) warn that strengths-based approaches that emphasize focusing on positive aspects of families – for example, the Common Assessment Framework – might endanger children if they discourage workers from making judgements about parental deficits. Brandon et al. (2009) comment positively on signs of safety as an approach that focuses on danger and harm as well as strengths and safety. Writing in Australia, Durrant (2016) summarizes other concerns about 'strengths', noting their static nature and suggesting the solution-focused emphasis on outcome injects movement into the perspective. He, like Greene and Lee (2011), also points out that the strengths perspective does not have a model of practice to guide work with clients.

Conclusion

While social workers are undoubtedly making use of solution-focused practice, many face challenges in doing so, in part due to certain aspects of modern social work. The calls for a 'reimagined social work' are coming from those concerned that it has become increasingly authoritarian, especially in children's services and in those 'Western' countries where neo-liberalism has held sway (Featherstone et al., 2014; Parton, 2014). This authoritarian tendency is seen in over-intrusive responses to families in need of help, due to an excessive use of assessments designed for situations where children are at risk of suffering significant harm but which have spread to other cases where families require support (Devine, 2015).

Recognizing this in her review of child protection in England, Munro (2011, p. 80) stated that 'the right approach (for most) is to offer services to children and families where they are able to make a voluntary choice to receive them', and Devine (2015) is concerned that it should be clear where support is intended to be consensual. A solution-focused approach, with its focus on what the service user wants, can help provide this clarity. It can go further, seeing service users as more than passive recipients and consenters, but as active requesters of help. In this way, it can help create social work services which are actively wanted and used by those who might benefit from them.

Further reading

Greene, G., & Lee, M. Y. (2011). *Solution-oriented social work practice: An integrative approach to working with client strengths*. New York: Oxford University Press.
   This book, which integrates elements from the strengths perspective, solution-focused therapy, narrative therapy, and the strategic therapy of the Mental Research Institute into an eclectic framework, is aimed primarily at clinical social workers in the US, but it is packed with useful ideas and a huge number of references that can be drawn on by social workers anywhere.

Hogg, V., & Wheeler, J. (2004). Miracles R them: Solution-focused practice in a social services duty team. *Practice, 16*, 299–314.
   This is a valuable account of research into what helped a Social Services children's duty team incorporate the solution-focused approach into its everyday practice.

Macdonald, A. (2017). *Solution-focused brief therapy evaluation list*. Retrieved from http://solutionsdoc.co.uk/sfbt-evaluation-list/

Shennan, G. (2019). *Solution-focused practice: Effective communication to facilitate change* (2nd ed.). London: Palgrave Macmillan.
   In my book I provide a systematic account of how to use the solution-focused approach, using numerous illustrative real-life case examples, including some drawn directly from social work.

References

Antle, B., Barbee, A., Christensen, D., & Sullivan, D. (2009). The prevention of child maltreatment recidivism through the solution-based casework model of child welfare practice. *Children and Youth Services Review, 31*(12), 1346–1351.

Asquith, S., Clark, C., & Waterhouse, L. (2005). *The role of the social worker in the 21st century: A literature review*. Edinburgh: Scottish Executive. Retrieved from www.gov.scot/Publications/2005/12/1994633/46334

Baginsky, M., Moriarty, J., Manthorpe, J., Beecham, J., & Hickman, B. (2017). *Evaluation of signs of safety in 10 pilots: Research report*. London: Department for Education.

Berg, I. K. (1994). *Family-based services: A solution-focused approach*. New York: Norton.

Berg, I. K., & de Jong, P. (1996). Solution-building conversations: Co-constructing a sense of competence with clients. *Families in Society, 77*(6), 376–391.

Berg, I. K., & Kelly, S. (2000). *Building solutions in child protective services*. New York: Norton.

Berg, I. K., & Miller, S. (1992). *Working with the problem drinker*. New York. Norton.

Berg, I. K., & Reuss, N. (1997). *Solutions step by step: A substance abuse treatment manual*. New York: Norton.

Berg, I. K., & Steiner, T. (2003). *Children's solution work*. New York: Norton.

Berg, I. K., & Szabo, P. (2005). *Brief coaching for lasting solutions*. New York: Norton.

Beyebach, M. (2009). Integrative brief solution-focused family therapy: A provisional roadmap. *Journal of Systemic Therapies, 28*(3), 18–35.

Bond, C., Woods, K., Humphrey, N., Symes, W., & Green, L. (2013). Practitioner review: The effectiveness of solution focused brief therapy with children and families: A systematic and critical evaluation of the literature from 1990–2010. *Journal of Child Psychology and Psychiatry, 54*(7), 707–723.

Bottoms, A., & McWilliams, W. (1979). A non-treatment paradigm for probation practice. *British Journal of Social Work, 9*(2), 160–201.

Brandon, M., Bailey, S., Belderson, P., Gardner, R., Sidebotham, P., Dodsworth, J., Warren, C., & Black, J. (2009). *Understanding serious case reviews and their impact – A biennial analysis of serious case reviews 2005–2007*. London: Department for Schools, Children and Families.

Bucknell, D. (2000). Practice teaching: Problem to solution. *Social Work Education, 19*(2), 125–144.

Bunn, A. (2013). *Signs of safety in England: An NSPCC commissioned report on the signs of safety model in child protection*. London: NSPCC.

Clark, M. (1996). Brief solution-focused work: A strengths-based method for juvenile justice practice. *Juvenile and Family Court Journal, 47*, 57–65.

Clark, M. (2005). Entering the business of behavior change: Motivational interviewing for probation staff perspectives. *Journal of the American Probation & Parole Association, 30,* 38–45.

Clark, M. (2009). The strengths perspective in criminal justice. In D. Saleebey (Ed.), *The strengths perspective in social work practice* (5th ed., pp. 122–145). New York: Longman.

Corcoran, J. (1997). A solution-oriented approach to working with juvenile justice offenders. *Child and Adolescent Social Work Journal, 14*(4), 277–288.

Corcoran, J. (2016). Solution-focused therapy. In N. Coady & P. Lehmann (Eds.), *Theoretical perspectives for direct social work practice: A generalist-eclectic approach* (3rd ed., pp. 435–450). New York: Springer.

Corcoran, J., & Franklin, C. (1998). A solution-focused approach to physical abuse. *Journal of Family Psychotherapy, 9*(1), 69–73.

Cree, V. E. (2009). The changing nature of social work. In R. Adams, L. Dominelli, & M. Payne (Eds.), *Social work: Themes, issues and critical debates* (3rd ed., pp. 26–36). Basingstoke: Palgrave Macmillan.

de Shazer, S. (1985). *Keys to solution in brief therapy.* New York: Norton.

de Shazer, S. (1988). *Clues: Investigating solutions in brief therapy.* New York: Norton.

de Shazer, S., Berg, I. K., Lipchik, E., Nunnally, E., Molnar, A., Gingerich, W., & Weiner-Davis, M. (1986). Brief therapy: Focused solution development. *Family Process, 25*(2), 207–221.

Department of Health. (1990). *Caring for people in the next decade and beyond: Policy guidelines.* London: HMSO.

Devine, L. (2015). Considering social work assessment of families. *Journal of Social Welfare and Family Law, 37*(1), 70–83.

Doel, M., & Marsh, P. (1992). *Task-centred social work.* Farnham: Ashgate.

Durrant, M. (2016). Confessions of an unashamed solution-focused purist: What is (and isn't) solution-focused. *Journal of Solution-Focused Brief Therapy, 2*(1), 40–49.

Featherstone, B., White, S., & Morris, K. (2014). *Re-imagining child protection: Towards humane social work with families.* Bristol: Policy Press.

Fernandes, P. (2015). *Evaluation of the face to face service: Using a solution-focused approach with children and young people in care or on the edge of care.* London: NSPCC.

Forrester, D., Pokhrel, S., McDonald, L., Giannou, D., Waissbein, C., Binnie, C., Jensch, G., & Copello, A. (2008). *Final report on the evaluation of 'Option 2'.* Cardiff: Welsh Assembly Government.

Franklin, C., Trepper, T., Gingerich, W., & McCollum, E. (Eds.). (2012). *Solution-focused brief therapy: A handbook of evidence-based practice.* New York: Oxford University Press.

Gaiswinkler, W., & Roessler, M. (2009). Using the expertise of knowing and the expertise of not-knowing to support processes of empowerment in social work practice. *Journal of Social Work Practice, 23*(2), 215–227.

George, E., Iveson, C., & Ratner, H. (1990). *Problem to solution: Brief therapy with individuals and families.* London: BT Press.

Gingerich, W., & Peterson, L. (2013). Effectiveness of solution-focused brief therapy: A systematic qualitative review of controlled outcome studies. *Research on Social Work Practice, 23*(3), 266–283.

Gollins, T., Fox, A., Walker, B., Romeo, L., Thomas, J., & Woodham, G. (2016). *Developing a wellbeing and strengths-based approach to social work practice: Changing culture.* London: Think Local Act Personal.

Greene, G., Kondrat, D., Lee, M. Y., Clement, J., Siebert, H., Mentzer, R., & Pinnell, S. (2006). A solution-focused approach to case management and recovery with consumers who have a severe mental disability. *Families in Society, 87*(3), 339–350.

Greene, G., & Lee, M. Y. (2011). *Solution-oriented social work practice: An integrative approach to working with client strengths.* New York: Oxford University Press.

Hackett, P., & Shennan, G. (2007). Solution-focused work with children and young people. In T. Nelson & F. Thomas (Eds.), *Handbook of solution-focused brief therapy: Clinical applications* (pp. 191–212). New York: Haworth.

Haringey Local Safeguarding Children Board (LSCB). (2009). *Serious case review 'CHILD A'.* London: Department for Education.

Hawkes, D. (2003). A solution-focused approach to 'psychosis'. In B. O'Connell & S. Palmer (Eds.), *Handbook of solution-focused therapy* (pp. 146–155). London: Sage.

Hogg, V., & Wheeler, J. (2004). Miracles R them: Solution-focused practice in a social services duty team. *Practice, 16,* 299–314.

Hosany, Z., Wellman, N., & Lowe, T. (2007). Fostering a culture of engagement: A pilot study of the outcomes of training mental health nurses working in two UK acute admission units in brief solution-focused therapy techniques. *Journal of Psychiatric and Mental Health Nursing, 14*(7), 688–695.

King, P. (2017). *Tools for effective therapy with children and families: A solution-focused approach.* New York: Routledge.

Lee, M. Y. (2013). Solution-focused brief therapy. In C. Franklin (Ed.), *Encyclopedia of social work.* Washington, DC and New York: National Association of Social Workers and Oxford University Press. doi:10.1093/acrefore/9780199975839.013.1039

Lee, M. Y., Sebold, J., & Uken, A. (2012). Solution-focused model with court-mandated domestic violence offenders. In C. Franklin, T. Trepper, W. Gingerich, & E. McCollum (Eds.), *Solution-focused brief therapy: A handbook of evidence-based practice* (pp. 165–182). New York: Oxford University Press.

Lehmann, P., Jordan, C., Bolton, K. W., Huynh, L., & Chigbu, K. (2012). Solution-focused brief therapy and criminal offending: A family conference tool for work in restorative justice. *Journal of Systemic Therapies, 31*(1), 49–62.

Lewis, T., & Osborn, C. (2004). Solution-focused counseling and motivational interviewing: A consideration of confluence. *Journal of Counseling and Development, 82*(1), 38–48.

Macdonald, A. (2017). *Solution-focused brief therapy evaluation list.* Retrieved from www.solutionsdoc.co.uk/sft.html

Miller, G., & de Shazer, S. (1998). Have you heard the latest rumor about . . .? Solution-focused therapy as a rumor. *Family Process, 37*(3), 363–377.

Miller, W., & Rollnick, S. (2013). *Motivational interviewing: Helping people change* (3rd ed.). New York: Guilford.

Milner, J., Myers, S., & O'Byrne, P. (2015). *Assessment in social work* (4th ed.). Basingstoke: Palgrave Macmillan.

Munro, E. (2011). *Munro review of child protection final report: A child-centred system.* Norwich: The Stationery Office (TSO).

NSPCC. (2015). *Solution-focused practice: An NSPCC toolkit for working with children and young people.* London: NSPCC. Retrieved from www.nspcc.org.uk/services-and-resources/research-and-resources/2015/solution-focused-practice-toolkit/

O'Connell, B. (2000). Solution focused brief therapy: Bill O'Connell talks to Steve de Shazer. *Counselling, 11*(6), 343–344.

O'Hanlon, B. (1992). History becomes her story: Collaborative solution-oriented therapy of the after-effects of sexual abuse. In S. McNamee & K. Gergen (Eds.), *Therapy as social construction* (pp. 136–148). London: Sage.

Parton, N. (2014). *The politics of child protection: Contemporary developments and future direction.* Basingstoke: Palgrave Macmillan.

Parton, N., & O'Byrne, P. (2000). *Constructive social work: Towards a new practice.* Basingstoke: Palgrave Macmillan.

Pence, E., & Paymar, M. (1993). *Education groups for men who batter: The Duluth model.* New York: Springer.

Rapp, C. (1998). *The strengths model: Case management with people suffering from severe and persistent mental illness.* New York: Oxford University Press.

Ratner, H., George, E., & Iveson, C. (2012). *Solution focused brief therapy: 100 key points and techniques.* Hove: Routledge.

RSW Collective. (2015). *Re-imagining social work in Aotearoa New Zealand* (Blog post). Retrieved from www.reimaginingsocialwork.nz/2015/04/an-open-letter-to-all-progressive-organisations-in-aotearoa-new-zealand

Saleebey, D. (2012). *The strengths perspective in social work practice* (6th ed.). Boston: Pearson.

Shennan, G. (2003). Solution-focused practice and assessment. *Journal of Primary Care Mental Health, 7,* 78–81.

Shennan, G. (2008). Solution focused practice in a family support team. *Solution Focused Research Review, 1*(1), 11–15.

Shennan, G. (2014). *Solution-focused practice: Effective communication to facilitate change.* London: Palgrave Macmillan.

Simon, J., & Nelson, T. (2007). *Solution-focused brief practice with long-term clients in mental health services: 'I am more than my label'.* New York: Haworth.

Simmons, C., Shapiro, V., Accomazzo, S., & Manthey, T. (2016). Strengths-based social work: A meta-theory to guide social work research and practice. In N. Coady & P. Lehmann (Eds.), *Theoretical perspectives for direct social work practice: A generalist-eclectic approach* (3rd ed., pp. 131–154). New York: Springer.

Smith, I. (2011). A qualitative investigation into the effects of brief training in solution-focused therapy in a social work team. *Psychology and Psychotherapy, 84*(3), 335–348.

Stalker, C., Levene, J., & Coady, N. (1999). Solution-focused brief therapy: One model fits all? *Families in Society, 80*(5), 468–477.

Stancer, M. (2008). Family solutions: From 'problem families to families finding solutions'. In P. De Jong & I. K. Berg (Eds.), *Interviewing for solutions* (3rd ed., pp. 279–286). Belmont, CA: Thomson/Brooks Cole.

Stanley, T., Keenan, K., Roberts, D., & Moore, R. (2017). Helping Birmingham families early: The 'signs of safety and well-being' practice framework. *Child Care in Practice.* doi:10.1080/13575279.2016.1264369

Sundman, P. (1997). Solution-focused ideas in social work. *Journal of Family Therapy, 19*, 159–172.

Thom, G., Delahunty, L., Harvey, P., & Ardill, J. (2014). *Evaluation of the integrated family support service: Final year 3 report.* Cardiff: Welsh Government Social Research.

Turbett, C. (2014). *Doing radical social work.* Basingstoke: Palgrave Macmillan.

Turnell, A., & Edwards, S. (1999). *Signs of safety: A solution and safety oriented approach to child protection case-work.* New York: Norton.

Turnell, A., & Murphy, T. (2017). *Signs of safety: Comprehensive briefing paper* (4th ed.). Perth: Resolutions Consultancy.

Turney, D., & Merchant, W. (2017). *A review of the divisional-based intervention team (D-BIT) service.* Chelmsford: Essex County Council.

Vaughn, K., Young, B., Webster, D., & Thomas, M. (1996). Solution-focused work in the hospital: A continuum-of-care model for inpatient psychiatric treatment. In S. Miller, M. Hubble, & B. Duncan (Eds.), *Handbook of solution-focused brief therapy* (pp. 99–127). San Francisco: Jossey-Bass.

Vostanis, P., Anderson, L., & Window, S. (2006). Evaluation of a family support service: Short-term outcome. *Clinical Child Psychology and Psychiatry, 11*(4), 513–528.

Walden, D. (Ed.). (2015). *Reimagining social care: Evidence review executive summary.* Dartington: Research in Practice for Adults. Retrieved from www.ripfa.org.uk/resources/publications/evidence-reviews/reimagining-social-care-evidence-review-2015-executive-summary-download/

Walker, L. (2008). Implementation of solution-focused skills in a Hawaii prison. In P. De Jong & I. K. Berg, *Interviewing for solutions* (3rd ed., pp. 302–308). Belmont, CA: Thomson/Brooks Cole.

Walsh, T. (2010). *The solution-focused helper: Ethics and practice in health and social care.* Maidenhead: Open University Press.

Wheeler, J. (2003). Solution-focused practice in social work. In B. O'Connell & S. Palmer (Eds.), *Handbook of solution-focused therapy* (pp. 106–117). London: Sage.

Wheeler, J., & Hogg, V. (2012). Signs of safety and the child protection movement. In C. Franklin, T. Trepper, W. Gingerich, & E. McCollum (Eds.), *Solution-focused brief therapy: A handbook of evidence-based practice* (pp. 203–215). New York: Oxford University Press.

Wheeler, J., Hogg, V., & Fegan, G. (2006). Signs of wellbeing: A tool for early intervention. *Context, 86*, 5–8.

White, M. (2007). *Maps of narrative practice.* New York: Norton.

Woods, K., Bond, C., Humphrey, N., Symes, W., & Green, L. (2011). *Systematic review of Solution Focused Brief Therapy (SFBT) with children and families.* London: Department for Education.

20

Motivational interviewing's theory of practice for social work

Promises and pitfalls

Lori L. Egizio, Douglas C. Smith,
Stéphanie Wahab and Kyle Bennett

Introduction

Motivational interviewing (MI) continues to evolve and be disseminated for use with different social work target populations. It places high importance on the relationship between the practitioner and the client, utilizing very specific communication skills to enhance relationships and promote clients' advocating for their own change. The resulting outcomes are often positive. This chapter will reflect on the practice theory of MI. First, we describe the clinical components of MI to further illuminate its theoretical underpinnings. Then, we turn our attention to how widely MI has been adopted within the social work profession. Finally, we highlight potential limitations associated with MI's practice theory.

Definition and theoretical foundations

Motivational interviewing is currently defined as 'a collaborative, goal-oriented style of communication with particular attention to the language of change. It is designed to strengthen personal motivation for and commitment to a specific goal by eliciting and exploring the person's own reasons for change within an atmosphere of acceptance and compassion' (Miller & Rollnick, 2013, p. 29). Initially developed in the substance use treatment field, MI has since been applied to many contexts where individuals are ambivalent about making health behaviour changes. For example, it has been used by clinicians to help individuals resolve ambivalence about exercise behaviours (Smith et al., 2012), engagement in treatment programs (Smith, Ureche, Davis, & Walters, 2015) and obtaining colorectal cancer screens (Menon et al., 2011). There are hundreds of clinical trials on MI's efficacy (Miller & Rose, 2009).

Quite to the contrary of recent critiques that MI is an atheoretical practice (Atkinson & Woods, 2017), MI represents a fundamental theoretical shift in thinking about client behaviour change. With roots in humanistic and cognitive behavioural therapy, the seminal article on MI opposed the then-contemporary views that individuals with alcohol problems were inherently resistant to change at best and personality disordered at worst (Miller, 1983). Miller (1983) proposed the radical idea that lacking motivation was not a personal attribute, but rather a product of clinical interactions where clients reacted to harsh confrontation.

MI's clinical method is based on a communication theory assuming that some patterns of clinician-client communication are counterproductive to making decisions about change. Rather than conceptualizing individuals as being in denial or lacking motivation, MI conceptualizes individuals as naturally ambivalent about change, typically weighing the costs and potential benefits of change when making decisions about it. Thus, the clinical method, described further below, emphasizes clinician use of empathy, a deep respect for client autonomy, and specialized strategies to influence and reinforce clients' in-session pro-change statements, referred to as *change talk*. *Discord* refers to conflict which may occur within the practitioner-client relationship (Miller & Rollnick, 2013; Arkowitz, Miller, & Rollnick, 2015). Discord can occur when the relationship is not aligned with the client's needs and may lack harmony. This is an important time for the practitioner to join with the client in an effort to build the relationship even if it results in more *sustain talk*, which refers to language used by the client expressing the client's desires not to change the target behaviour.

MI was never based on nor intended to comprise a grand theory of behaviour change (Miller & Rollnick, 2009). Yet the core premises of the practice model, that clinicians should both be empathic and attend to shaping client language in favour of change, have been subject to extensive empirical studies (Miller, Benefield, & Tonigan, 1993; Amrhein, Miller, Yahne, Palmer, & Fulcher, 2003; Apodaca et al., 2016). So the MI's practice theory assumptions are in fact testable and falsifiable, long considered to be features of sustainable theories (Popper, 1959). In that regard, the MI's practice theory has remained largely coherent since 1983, and adherents appear open to refining the model when new empirical data emerges, as has recently been the case with revisions associated with refraining from using a decisional balance activity (i.e. making a pros and cons list about behaviour change) to explore ambivalence (Miller & Rose, 2015).

In the remainder of this chapter, we continue to reflect on the practice theory of MI. First, we describe the clinical components of MI to further illuminate its theoretical underpinnings. we Then turn our attention to how widely MI has been adopted within the social work profession. Finally, we highlight potential limitations associated with MI's practice theory.

Clinical components

To fully understand MI's underlying practice theory, one should understand the skills used in MI. We will briefly explain some of the most important components, but to truly use MI, a practitioner would be advised to be fully trained. Let's begin with some of the more significant, yet basic, aspects of MI.

The spirit of MI

The *spirit of MI* can be described as its heart and soul. This concept reveals the overall mood that is present when MI is being successfully utilized. Miller and Rollnick (2013) wanted to make certain that the spirit of MI is clearly not the act of manipulating people to do as the practitioner would like them to do.

Forged from training experiences and concerns that clinicians would use MI techniques robotically and devoid of the overall purpose of creating an accepting and empathic environment, Miller and Rollnick describe what the overall feel of the intervention should be, referring to it as the 'spirit' of motivational interviewing. This MI spirit is often difficult to conceptualize, yet Miller and Rollnick (2013) speak of it as one of the most important facets of MI.

The MI spirit consists of four aspects: *partnership, acceptance, compassion,* and *evocation.* First, partnership is the coming together of the client and practitioner to form a team. The practitioner's task is to assist clients with expressing themselves by establishing a comfortable and accepting environment. In addition, it is to guide the client, never becoming forceful or falling into the role of an expert. An example of an expert role would be a practitioner giving unsolicited advice by saying, 'When managing your diabetes, it is best to check levels three times a day'. In MI, the practitioner strives to move away from this expert language and instead state, 'If it's okay, I can share a couple of things that have worked with some of my previous clients when managing their diabetes'.

The second dimension of the MI spirit is acceptance. This acceptance is not the same as agreeing with or approving of the client's actions, but simply finding the value and worth in the client. This is very similar to social work's concept of strengths-based perspectives (Manthey, Knowles, Asher, & Wahab, 2011; see Chapter 18). Included in this concept of acceptance are absolute worth, affirmation, empathy and support of autonomy. Much as Rogers (1959) explained, Miller and Rollnick's (2013) practice theory assumes that a 'critical condition for change is accurate empathy, an active interest in and effort to understand the other's internal perspective' (p. 18). Empathy is often demonstrated through using reflections. This microskill is simply the action of repeating back what the client has already stated (Miller & Rollnick, 2013; Hohman, 2011; Moyers, Manuel, & Ernst, 2014), perhaps in a more complex manner reflecting underlying emotion and/or meaning. Unfortunately, further discussion of all MI microskills is beyond the scope of this chapter.

The third aspect of the MI spirit is compassion. It refers not only to focusing on the client's feelings and needs, but also to placing them as a priority over one's own needs. This element was added to ensure that the trust that is created between practitioner and client is authentic.

The final concept is evocation. This concept shares similarities with social work's strengths-based approach by relying on the assumption that individuals have all they need inside them to make change happen. Unlike other approaches, which assume that clients are missing tools or skills and requires a practitioner to give them these skills, MI recognizes that the client is their own expert.

The four processes of MI

The four processes help us break down the different foci of MI practice; they include *engaging, focusing, evoking* and *planning* (Miller & Rollnick, 2013). Elwyn et al. (2014) summarized these processes. Engaging includes the time spent between the practitioner and client when the trusting relationship is developed. It is the initial relationship-building portion of the conversation. Focusing attends to practitioner and client working together to identify a target of change. Evoking refers to periods in which practitioners intentionally mine for desire, ability, reasons, need, commitment, activation and taking steps from client statements. Planning is the final process, in which practitioners assist clients with moving toward changes that have been reported to be desirable. Practitioners then assist clients with developing a concrete plan and committing themselves to the plan of change.

Change talk

In addition to demonstrating the MI spirit in clinical interactions, MI practitioners also attend to change talk. This is the language spoken by the client during the session that demonstrates a desire for change (Miller & Rollnick, 2013). On the other hand, sustain talk occurs when clients express a desire to remain in the status quo. The simultaneous presence of change talk and sustain talk is conceptualized not as client resistance, but rather as client ambivalence, feeling two ways about change (Miller & Rollnick, 2013). MI is only indicated in situations where client ambivalence is present and because clinicians differentially elicit and reinforce change talk. That is, they make direct and strategic attempts to encourage change talk through very nuanced types of open questions and reflections (e.g. elicit change talk). Further, when they hear change talk, they also make attempts to reinforce it and grow it. That is, they use strategies to pinpoint parts of client's speech that indicate any desire, ability, reasons, needs and commitments to change. For example, clients often make statements that contain both sustain and change talk such as 'I know I should change, but it is really hard'. Clinicians trained in MI are taught to selectively reinforce the change talk component. Here, an example of a reflection to do this may be 'You know it will be tough, yet it is getting a little more urgent for you to change'. This is called a *double-sided reflection* because it acknowledges both the sustain and change talk components of the statement. However, by ending on the change talk part of the statement, it is thought that the client will usually offer more change talk, which is the goal of a good MI session, to progressively and selectively reinforce change language. Although it may convey empathy, selectively reinforcing sustain talk is contraindicated in MI. So practitioners are discouraged from reflecting back: 'You aren't looking forward to jumping through these hoops again', referring to this same client statement. Thus, currently, a key theoretical tenet of the MI model is that we selectively reinforce change talk and attempt to steer gently away from sustain talk when it arises. Thus, making pros and cons lists about change, called a decisional balance activity, is not currently considered contemporary MI practice. Additionally, for ethical reasons, selective reinforcement of change talk is contraindicated for some client decisions (e.g. whether to get divorced). In such situations, the practitioners utilize equipoise, or neutral, client-centred communication (Miller & Rollnick, 2013). The practice of selectively reinforcing change talk is grounded in research showing that change talk predicts positive outcomes longitudinally (Amrhein et al., 2003), and sustain talk predicts more negative outcomes (Magill et al., 2014). Theoretically, there is disagreement about how this process works to produce change. Some authors suggest it may work due to Bem's self-perception theory (Bem, 1972) as people may believe more firmly what they say out loud. Alternatively, there may be a biological process that explains this as people subsequently exposed to their own sustain talk from an MI session experience brain activation in response to substance use triggers, whereas those exposed to change talk do not (Feldstein-Ewing, Filbey, Sabbineni, Chandler, & Hutchison, 2011). Explaining why and how change and sustain language influence outcomes represents one major theoretical frontier for MI practice.

Adoption of motivational interviewing

Adoption within social work

To determine the scope of MI's influence in social work, we undertook a search of top social work journals based on their overall impact factors (see Figure 22.1). Using each journal's internal search feature, we used the following keywords: 'motivational interviewing', 'motivational enhancement', and 'motivational enhancement therapy'. Articles were excluded from the results if these keywords were not mentioned explicitly in the title or the abstract or if the article was a book review.

The earliest article referencing MI was from 2000, appearing in the *British Journal of Social Work* (Harper & Hardy, 2000). For the total number of articles in each journal, see Figure 22.1.

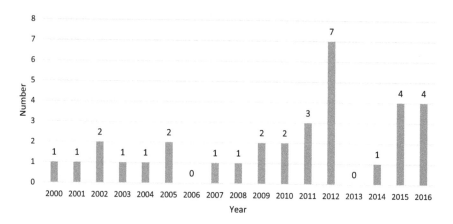

Figure 20.1 Motivational interviewing focused articles in top-ranked social work journals.

Note: N= 33. Journals included *British Journal of Social Work* (3), *Research on Social Work Practice* (11), *Journal of Social Work Practice* (8), *Social Work* (2), *Journal of Social Work* (1), *Children and Schools* (1), *Health and Social Work* (3), *Children & Youth Service Review* (2) and *Child and Family Social Work* (2).

The majority (58 percent) of MI-focused articles from the past 17 years were from *Research on Social Work Practice* and the *Journal of Social Work Practice in the Addictions*. The 33 articles have been cited an average of 44 times (median number of citations = 14), and most of them (55 percent) were outcome or trial studies. Notably, Lundahl, Kunz, Tollefson, and Burke's (2010) meta-analysis published in *Research on Social Work Practice* is the top-cited article, accruing over 600 citations. Of the remaining articles, 36 percent were identified as theoretical or descriptive studies, 12 percent were identified as meta-analyses, and 3 percent were identified as 'other empirical' studies, that is articles that did not fit neatly into the previous three categories. In our search, 27 percent of all articles we located were produced via internationally based research (i.e. outside the United States). Figure 22.1 illustrates the number of journals presenting MI over the past 17 years.

MI and social work ethics and values

The United States' National Association of Social Workers (NASW) Code of Ethics describes six values, including service, social justice, value of dignity, importance of individuals, relationships and the social worker's integrity (NASW, 2017). 'Service' refers to social workers placing the needs of others before themselves, thus working to assist those in need using the skills afforded to the social worker. One basic requirement for successful MI is the use of empathy. Within an MI session, empathy is used to demonstrate to clients that the practitioner is listening and understanding what they are saying (Hohman, 2011). However, the use of empathy goes beyond this by also indicating to the client that the practitioner is relating to what the client is saying and is able to understand the client's emotions on this topic. Miller (2000) explained the impact of empathy on a client when discussing the findings that even one empathic encounter with a client who reports alcohol drinking habits can substantially impact the treatment progress. This powerful skill is aligned with this code of service in that conveying empathy sometimes requires putting clients' needs and feelings above those of practitioners. The degree to which practitioners can set aside personal biases and communicate an understanding of the other's experience is critical. The practice of MI also requires that the provider acknowledge that they are not an expert on the client, but rather have the capacity to bring skills to the interaction (Miller & Rollnick, 2013). The service code of ethics mandates that social workers use their skills to help their clients (NASW, 2017). Both MI and the social work Code of Ethics expect humility and prioritizing the other over the practitioner (Wahab, 2005).

The second social work Code of Ethics principle relates to social justice (NASW, 2017; see Chapter 10). The primary purpose of this code is to guide social workers to focus efforts toward social injustices, including discrimination, oppression and other injustices. While the focus of practice in MI typically rests at the micro level with a focus on individual change, MI is a useful tool for working across social group differences in a way that attends to various forms of power. The client-centred elements of MI, coupled with the need to resist our own 'righting reflex', require practitioners to strive to understand and work with the world view, needs, language, beliefs and values of the individual, rather than imposing the practitioners' own on clients. This approach to communication and practice consequently requires a type of practitioner reflexivity around power, positionality and privilege consistent with anti-oppressive practices.

The third social work Code of Ethics principle of dignity pertains to social workers valuing the dignity of all individuals (NASW, 2017; see Chapter 9). This principle also involves respecting individuals' right to self-determination and striving to 'enhance clients' capacity and opportunity to change and to address their own needs' (NASW, 2017, para. 15). MI-consistent practice shares this ideal (Wahab, 2005), as it has been grounded in the idea of self-efficacy (Miller, 1983) and aligned with self-determination theory (SDT) (Markland, Ryan, Tobin, & Rollnick, 2005). SDT is the idea that people desire to move toward growth and better life choices yet may need guidance or support to begin the process. MI was found to offer this support with the move toward self-determination through the practitioner's use of evocation of change talk (Miller & Rollnick, 2013). It is the position of the practitioner to activate the clients' knowledge of themselves that desires change.

The NASW Code of Ethics also recognizes the need for social workers to develop relationships (NASW, 2017). This ethical principle guides social workers to 'understand that relationships between and among people are an important vehicle for change' (NASW, 2015, para. 16). Miller and Rollnick (2013) describe MI as something that is done *with* a client: 'it is an active collaboration between experts' (p. 15). They use this description to explain what they call the dance between practitioner and client (Arkowitz, Miller, & Rollnick, 2015). Both participants are necessary to create the plan for change, but most importantly, the ideas of how and why must come from the clients, who know their options and situations. In MI, it is critical to establish collaborative relationships which are highly consistent with the NASW Code of Ethics.

The ethical principle recognizes the importance of the social worker's integrity (NASW, 2017). This identifies the need to practice in an ethical and truthful manner. Miller and Rollnick (2013) demonstrate this through their value of research and integrity. They openly acknowledge that MI is not a panacea for all clinical problems and recommend continued research to refine the intervention. In fact, one could argue that the lack of a coherent theory of why MI works is, in fact, driven by humility about what we don't know about how MI works.

The final code of ethics principle states the expectation of social workers to practice within their areas of expertise and continuing advancement of this knowledge (NASW, 2017). Within this code lies the understanding that social workers will continue to develop their skills and knowledge within the field. It expresses the need of social workers to continue to strive to improve their knowledge and skills. Healthy practice of MI requires a similar expectation. Miller and Rollnick (2013) recommend continued coaching and feedback to maintain integrity within MI. In addition, they recognize that individuals may require different amounts of coaching to reach a proficient level. The initial training assists with basic skills, but true MI skill is established from further work in the field (Motivationalinterviweing.org, 2016). Proficient MI skills require ongoing support and feedback (Miller & Rollnick, 2013), much like this code, which expects social workers to continue developing and gaining knowledge. One way or another, this code and MI have expressed the same philosophy of continued skill development.

Where are the theoretical boundaries of MI?

Thinking critically about any widely adapted practice such as MI is of paramount importance. In this final section of this chapter, we address some potential perils of the theoretical assumptions of MI, as well as areas where theory in MI merits additional development. We have already described our theoretical understanding of how the processes through which change and sustain talk affect client outcomes is poorly understood. So we will turn our attention elsewhere. Specifically, we first take a macro-economic focus and view MI from a broad, societal perspective. Next, we critique biological explanations of MI as an authority-based approach and highlight the limitations of these often-exploratory basic research designs. Finally, we note the lack of attention to the role of clients' emotional response to MI interventions and what that may mean for intervention refinement.

Neo-liberalism and individual responsibility

MI may further a neoliberal agenda that privileges individual responsibility as the cause of and resolution for social problems. Carton (2014) argues that MI's strengths-based roots and focus constitute individuals or clients as fully autonomous, capable, 'responsible hyper-economic individual(s)' who can act on their own self-care (p. 203). While certainly strengths-focused, the concerted focus on individual responsibility (to make change happen) in MI obscures the role and influence of institutional and macro forces on individuals' lives, behaviours and choices. Reisch (2009) offers a detailed discussion of the problematics of re-individualized and de-politicized social work practice in its shift away from structural transformation via a focus on resiliency and compliance instead of resistance.

Similarly, Jani and Reisch (2011) have suggested that strengths-based, empowerment and person-in-environment approaches (which include MI) represent some of the most influential theories in social work practice. They also, however, 'include' a linearity of bio-psychosocial and spiritual needs; the notion of fixed boundaries of various environmental systems; the presence of a universal, static hierarchy of human needs' (Jani & Reisch, 2011, cited in Reisch, 2013, p. 723).

> Strength based autonomous subjects freely acting on themselves as rational, balanced and prudential responsible individuals eschew the patrimony of state intervention. Entities such as disease, hurt, lack of education can be deleted from the vocabulary. There is a new freedom, facilitated by the newly embourgoised practitioner, increasingly subsisting in new discourses that reside in networks of professionalization, evidence-base and fiscal concerns.
>
> *(Carton, 2014, p. 203)*

Since MI is designed to effect individual rather than systemic or institutional change, macro oriented social work(ers) may take issue with yet another practice that both holds individuals responsible and accountable for their own well-being and directs the labour and energy of the provider on individual rather than systemic change.

Biology as an authority-based rationale for MI

Large funding agencies have prioritized learning more about biological processes, and some argue that the social sciences could become myopically focused on biological processes operating in psychosocial treatments (Schwartz, Lilienfeld, Meca, & Sauvigné, 2016). Schwartz and colleagues (2016) summarize research on the phenomenon of *neuroseduction*, the process whereby people will accept flawed scientific findings prematurely if they are based on neuroscientific research. We previously discussed a study wherein individuals seeing their own pro-change statements (i.e. change talk) from an MI session paired with substance use triggers did not have as much brain activation in reward centres as those seeing their pro–status quo statements (Feldstein-Ewing et al., 2011). Admit it; did your eyes get big when you read this? Well, let's now note that that study was of a sample of ten people.

Neuroseduction is relevant to MI; there is a growing emphasis on explaining the effects of MI through a neuroscientific lens. Notwithstanding the enormous potential value of this research, the grand irony of going too far in this direction may be that authority-based arguments are made for the adoption of MI. Just as they are contraindicated in the clinical practice of MI, authority-based arguments for adopting MI violate the MI spirit and may hinder its dissemination. Further, social workers appreciate the complex interplay between people and their environments and should advocate that social and environmental research on MI continue despite the current emphasis on biological processes.

Motivational interviewing and emotions

We know practically nothing about individuals' emotional responses to MI. Wagner and Ingersoll (2008) note the limited attention to emotions in MI sessions and describe a theoretical model where increasing positive emotions through the warm accepting behaviours of MI could set the stage for a strong, positive emotional reaction from clients and result in deepened exploration of change. Prior research on mechanisms of change has only coded client language and found that pro-change statements made in sessions (i.e. change talk) mediate substance use treatment outcomes. No study, however, has ever coded emotional response to MI. Increased positive emotion in MI sessions may improve MI treatment efficacy for several reasons. For example, positive emotional responses initially may increase the volume of change talk or pro-change statements. As previously noted, change talk is linked to future client outcomes. Alternatively, in-session positive emotion may make change talk uttered by clients more memorable later, which may buffer against post-intervention substance use. Strong negative emotions that are evoked during discussions of negative consequences of substance use, a form of change talk, may also play a role in determining client outcomes. Thus, one wide-open frontier for MI would be expanding the theoretical base to include emotional processes associated with receipt of MI.

Conclusion: the future of MI in social work

As the practice of MI continues to permeate other areas besides substance use disorder prevention and treatment, it is likely that more social workers will be exposed to MI. Arguably, MI is founded on more extensive research than many clinical methods, especially on its underlying mechanisms of change. That is, extensive research on how empathy and change language influence outcomes provides much support for MI's underlying theoretical assumptions, as well as widely disseminated MI training models. Yet it remains important to be candid about any practice's theoretical assumptions. Social workers should think critically about the limitations of MI practice, being especially mindful of the lack of emphasis on environmental determinants of problems, recently proliferating biological explanations of MI and the lack of emphasis on alternative mechanisms of change, such as emotional response to MI.

Acknowledgement

The development of this article was supported, in part, by the Substance Abuse and Mental Health Service Administration (#1U79TI026046–01, Smith). The opinions expressed, however, are those of the authors and not the federal government of the US.

Further reading

For continued development of knowledge in motivational interviewing, we have listed some great sources.

Miller, W. R., & Rollnick, S. (2013). *Motivational interviewing: Helping people change* (3rd ed.). New York: Guilford.

Miller and Rose's (2009) article outlines the theory behind MI and breaks the concepts down into simplistic ideas. Miller and Rollnick (2013) is the most current edition of the primary source of MI. My advice would include having this text on hand whenever attempting to understand or use the concepts of MI.

Rosengren, D. (2009). *Building motivational interviewing skills: A practitioner workbook*. New York: Guilford.

The final source listed, Rosengren (2009) is a wonderful workbook with many practice examples to develop a solid understanding of the skills utilized within MI.

References

Amrhein, P. C., Miller, W. R., Yahne, C. E., Palmer, M., & Fulcher, L. (2003). Client commitment language during motivational interviewing predicts drug use outcomes. *Journal of Consulting and Clinical Psychology, 71*(5), 862.

Apodaca, T. R., Jackson, K. M., Borsari, B., Magill, M., Longabaugh, R., Mastroleo, N. R., & Barnett, N. P. (2016). Which individual therapist behaviours elicit client change talk and sustain talk in motivational interviewing? *Journal of Substance Abuse Treatment, 61*, 60–65.

Arkowitz, H., Miller, W. R., & Rollnick, S. (Eds.). (2015). *Motivational interviewing in the treatment of psychological problems*. New York: Guilford.

Atkinson, C., & Woods, K. (2017). Establishing theoretical stability and treatment integrity for motivational interviewing. *Behavioural and Cognitive Psychotherapy, 45*(4), 337–350.

Bem, D. J. (1972). Self-perception theory. *Advances in Experimental Social Psychology, 6*, 1–62.

Carton, T. (2014). The spirit of motivational interviewing as an apparatus of governmentality. An analysis of reading materials used in the training of substance abuse clinicians. *Sociology Mind, 4*(2), 192–205.

Elwyn, G., Dehlendorf, C. R., Epstein, R. M., Marrin, M. K., White, J., & Frosch, D. L. (2014). Shared decision making and motivational interviewing: Achieving patient-centered care across the spectrum of health care problems. *Annals of Family Medicine, 12*(3), 270–275. doi:10.1370/afm

Feldstein Ewing, S. W., Filbey, F. M., Sabbineni, A., Chandler, L. D., & Hutchison, K. E. (2011). How psychosocial alcohol interventions work: A preliminary look at what FMRI can tell us. *Alcoholism: Clinical and Experimental Research, 35*(4), 643–651.

Harper, R., & Hardy, S. (2000). Research note. An evaluation of motivational interviewing as a method of intervention with clients in a probation setting. *British Journal of Social Work, 30*(3), 393–400.

Hohman, M. (2011). *Motivational interviewing in social work practice*. New York: Guilford.

Jani, J. S., & Reisch, M. (2011). Common human needs, uncommon solutions: Applying a critical framework to perspectives on human behavior. *Families in Society, 92*(1), 13–20.

Lundahl, B. W., Kunz, C., Brownell, C., Tollefson, D., & Burke, B. L. (2010). A meta-analysis of motivational interviewing: Twenty-five years of empirical studies. *Research on Social Work Practice, 20*(2), 137–160.

Magill, M., Gaume, J., Apodaca, T. R., Walthers, J., Mastroleo, N. R., Borsari, B., & Longabaugh, R. (2014). The technical hypothesis of motivational interviewing: A meta-analysis of MI's key causal model. *Journal of Consulting and Clinical Psychology, 82*(6), 973–983.

Manthey, T., Knowles, B., Asher, D., & Wahab, S. (2011). Strength based practice and motivational interviewing. *Advances in Social Work, 2*(2), 126–151.

Markland, D., Ryan, R. M., Tobin, V. J., & Rollnick, S. (2005). Motivational interviewing and self-determination theory. *Journal of Social & Clinical Psychology, 24*(6), 811–831.

Menon, U., Belue, R., Wahab, S., Rugen, K., Kinney, A. Y., Maramaldi, P., & Szalacha, L. A. (2011). A randomized trial comparing the effect of two phone-based interventions on colorectal cancer screening adherence. *Annals of Behavioural Medicine, 42*(3), 294–303.

Miller, W. R. (1983). Motivational interviewing with problem drinkers. *Behavioural psychotherapy, 11*(02), 147–172.

Miller, W. R. (2000). Rediscovering fire: Small interventions, large effects. *Psychology of Addictive Behaviours, 14*(1), 6–18. Retrieved from http://dx.doi.org/10.1037/0893-164X.14.1.6

Miller, W. R., Benefield, R. G., & Tonigan, J. S. (1993). Enhancing motivation for change in problem drinking: A controlled comparison of two therapist styles. *Journal of Consulting and Clinical Psychology, 61*(3), 455.

Miller, W. R., & Rollnick, S. (2009). Ten things that motivational interviewing is not. *Behavioural and Cognitive Psychotherapy, 37*(2), 129–140.

Miller, W. R., & Rollnick, S. (2013). *Motivational interviewing: Helping people change* (3rd ed.). New York: Guilford.

Miller, W. R., & Rose, G. S. (2009). Toward a theory of motivational interviewing. *American Psychologist, 64*(6), 527.

Miller, W. R., & Rose, G. S. (2015). Motivational interviewing and decisional balance: Contrasting responses to client ambivalence. *Behavioural and Cognitive Psychotherapy, 43*(02), 129–141.

Moyers, T. B., Manuel, J. K., & Ernst, D. (2014). *Motivational interviewing treatment integrity coding manual 4.2.1.* (Unpublished manual). Retrieved from http://casaa.unm.edu/download/MITI4_2.pdf

National Association of Social Workers. (2017). *Code of ethics of the national association of social workers.* Retrieved from www.socialworkers.org/About/Ethics/Code-of-Ethics

Popper, K. (1959). *The logic of scientific discovery.* New York: Basic Books.

Reisch, M. (2009). *Die politik der soziale arbeit in zeiten der globalizierung [The politics of social work in the age of globalization].* In F. Kessl & H-U. Otto (Eds.), *Soziale arbeit ohne wohlfahrtsstaat? Zeitdiagnosen, problematisierungen und perspektiven* (pp. 223–244). Weinheim: Juventa.

Reisch, M. (2013). Social work education and the neo-liberal challenge: The US response to increasing global inequality. *Social Work Education, 32*(6), 715–733.

Rogers, C. R. (1959). A theory of therapy, personality, and interpersonal relationships as developed in the client-centered framework. In S. Koch (Ed.), *Psychology: The study of a science. Vol. 3. Formulations of the person and the social contexts* (pp. 184–256). New York: McGraw-Hill.

Rosengren, D. (2009). *Building motivational interviewing skills: A practitioner workbook.* New York: Guilford.

Schwartz, S. J., Lilienfeld, S. O., Meca, A., & Sauvigné, K. C. (2016). The role of neuroscience within psychology: A call for inclusiveness over exclusiveness. *American Psychologist, 71*(1), 52.

Smith, D. C., Lanesskog, D., Cleeland, L., Motl, R., Weikart, M., & Dlugonski, D. (2012). Motivational interviewing may improve exercise experience for persons with multiple sclerosis: A small randomized trial. *Health and Social Work, 37*(2), 99–109.

Smith, D. C., Ureche, D. J., & Davis, J. P., & Walters, S. T. (2015). Motivational interviewing with and without normative feedback for adolescents with substance use problems: A preliminary study. *Substance Abuse, 36*(3), 350–358.

Wagner, C. C. & Ingersoll, K. S. (2008). Beyond cognition: broadening the emotional base of motivational interviewing. *Journal of Psychotherapy Integration. 18*(2), 1919–206.

Wahab, S. (2005). Motivational interviewing and social work practice. *Journal of Social Work, 5*(1), 45–60. doi:10.1177/1468017305051365

21

Narrative social work

Key concepts

Karen Roscoe

This chapter provides a theoretical map of narrative approaches by drawing on critical theories. Critical social work practice is influenced by a wide range of critical perspectives including feminism, racism, anti-oppressive practice and post-structuralism (Ferguson, 2003; see Chapter 29). According to Ferguson (2003), this influenced a form of practice that seeks to reconstruct the idealized theoretical notions that are available in social work. In other words, it is a branch of theories that seeks to challenge oppressive practices that consist of a variety of fixed ideas of individuals' problems. This chapter frames narrative theories as a form of 'language critique' for practice by drawing on a range of critical social theories in the endeavour to understand how identity is constructed in and through language.

These methods of practice have a very practical application and involve a dialogue between individuals that is based on a way of logic. This type of logic provides a platform for identifying contradictions in ideas concerning the self and our surrounding knowledge. In order to develop a 'language critique', it is vital to understand what a narrative *is*, as we are reminded as practitioners of our own professional knowledge and how the profession encourages us to view 'problems'. Garrett (2017) highlights how the verbal categories that we use as practitioners operate as sources of power that serve to frame identities in particular ways.

Narratives go beyond social constructionism, and narrative analysis can be extended to the wider historical, socio-political, ideological and institutional contexts in which people live their lives (Roscoe & Pithouse, 2016). Developing a 'language critique' in social work is important because language carries considerable power in the constitution and reproduction of our everyday lives (Fairclough & Graham, 2002).

Narratives and social work

Narrative theory is underpinned by the philosophy of language, and so what we say and how we say it matters. This tradition starts from the theoretical assumption that people make meaning because it is constructed socially. Any narrative, therefore, is crafted around events that have been linked into sequence, across time and according to a dominant plot or theme (Morgan, 2000). Narratives are an essential means of human sense-making and are accounts of what happened, to whom it happened and where it happened (Garfinkel, 1967; Squire, 2013). Narratives are also a powerful and early-acquired way of individuals interpreting their identities and those of other people (Bruner, 1990).

These approaches involve re-storying conversations in collaboration with individuals or groups (Ricoeur, 1984). On the surface, this may seem simple, but this perspective puts people in the driving seat of their lives, as any of us co-construct meaning with others and act upon that basis. 'Since individuals are conscious agents, they are able to re-interpret their situation and consider new forms of actions' (King, 2004, p. 71). People have the power to resist their oppression in a variety of ways (Dominelli, 1997). This is because our lives can be multi-storied, and we can draw on a variety of different ways in which to make sense of our world and our identity (Morgan, 2000). Thus, any narrative assumes that commonly accepted conventions or meanings can also vary across cultures and traditions, and people's constructions are partly handed down by cultural heritage.

Critical practitioners also identify how words and language do not exist in themselves but are influenced by ideological forces embedded in powerful social structures (Lemke, 1995). Ideology here derives from Gramsci (1971), who sees it as serving the interests of certain groups with power. Ideologies come to be regarded as legitimate and common sense and inform the way people interpret themselves and the world around them. Social workers who wish to adopt narrative methods will need to consider how they can avoid being seen as lacking political and social awareness if they ignore the politics of narratives and the extent to which they support or contest social structures and practices (Fraser, 2004).

Language and power

We all have stories about ourselves, and these tell us something about our abilities, strengths, actions and desires. Yet the way we have developed these stories is determined by how we have linked specific events together and the meaning we have attributed to each of them. Narrative analysis exposes the power and effects of language by utilizing the concept of *discourse*. As Lemke (1995) points out, the social effects of power are multiplied by our hopes and fears, our beliefs, our expectations and our sensitivities and values. Some take the view that all discourses are ideological and thus viewed as a social practice (Kress & Hodge, 1993).

Discourses are inherent within narratives and present themselves as a set of more or less coherent stories or statements the person tells themselves about the way the world ought to be (Roscoe & Pithouse, 2016). Sexism is an example of a wider social discourse arising as a result of a set of statements and taken-for-granted assumptions about women. Any discourse consists of a 'group of statements which provide a language for talking about – a way of representing the knowledge about – a particular topic at a particular historical moment' (Wetherell, Taylor, & Yates, 2001, p. 72). People draw on these to make sense of themselves and the world around them. Discourse organizes and regulates all aspects of interpersonal relationships because they are considered here as social practices; they are organized ways of behaving and talking and structure our relations with one another (Fairclough, 1995). Some discourses dominate others, whilst others are heard less or marginalized altogether (Fairclough, 1995).

In social work, the narrative practitioner works with the narrative through artful conversations and analyzes what the narrative is and represents (Carson, 2009). We can then engage in a conversation that helps develop an alternative narrative that coexists alongside the dominant story, but this one is based on strengths and other qualities. This understanding and tradition of theories can be aligned with feminist theorizing, radical pedagogy and community activism (Monk, Winslade, Crocket, & Epston, 1997). Here, narratives are concerned with identifying ideologies that enable stories to hold together or to make sense and link to wider social structures and practices. Ideologies will characterize the way that certain discourses become accepted over others in social work such as 'stress' and 'at risk' (Roscoe & Pithouse, 2016).

The role of ideology becomes critical in narrative social work because it has the potential to reveal taken-for-granted 'truths' by critically deconstructing (unpacking) historically conditioned social practices. What enables discourses to remain dominant lies in the extent to which they go unquestioned by the listener and the teller, whilst the potential to disturb the power inherent in these discourses is in our readiness to critically unpack them (Pease & Fook, 1999; Fook, 2016).

Identity positioning: shaping ourselves through language and discourse

Identities are not freely created products of introspection or the unproblematic reflections of the private sanctum of the 'inner self', but are conceived within certain ideological frameworks constructed by the dominant social order to maintain its own interests. Identities in this analysis are profoundly political (Kitzinger, 1994, p. 82).

No one has complete power over their social environment, and we are reminded as social workers that a narrative is only one possible interpretation among many. It may, therefore, always be other than what it is (Carson, 2009). Yet we do shape ourselves and are shaped by discourse. Identity here is therefore partly understood to be an effect of discourse as well as constructed in discourse and is based on the enactment (or avoidance) of specific roles (Fairclough, 2003). The effects of dominant discourses upon identity are profound, bound up with conflicting or contradictory discourses. In narrative analysis, this offers us a type of analysis that is called 'positioning theory' in narrative approaches. Positioning theory is used to explain how people develop and recreate patterns of relationships by drawing on dominant discourses. This is because discourses have a prescriptive function as there are dominant ideas, such as the role of a wife. This shows us where women are positioned in the narrative and what background assumptions there are and locates how people make sense of their lives in the context of their social history. This history shapes our stories about the groups we belong to and about how we have become who we are today (Monk et al., 1997).

Stories give a sense of coherence to our lives, and we (inter)act according to these ideas through our daily practices and routines. If a person does not want to take up the position within the dominant discourses contained within the narrative, and the associated taken-for-granted assumptions, they may have to expect to engage in some difficult conversations with others. Thus, our positioning within the overall narrative is important in our ability to contribute socially. When we speak to or about ourselves to others, we are giving them something about the ideas we draw on about ourselves. We also position ourselves in relation to others in the narrative often recognized using pronouns such as 'we', 'they' 'she' and so on (Roscoe & Pithouse, 2016). Whether we do this implicitly or explicitly in our stories, we often infer characteristics or taken-for-granted assumptions about aspects of identity; these inferences provide ready-made meanings and are brought to all interactions.

Drawing on critical and post-structuralist theories, we do not assume that identities are fixed and stable. White (2005) uses the idea of the thin/thick contrast of identity formation to explain the ideas of post-structuralist theory. Post-structuralist thought in social theory is associated with ideas that identity is a public and social achievement and is based on negotiations with people, communities and institutions (Derrida, 1978, Foucault, 1972). Whereas structuralists view meaning as fixed, poststructuralists argue that meaning is produced in language and discourse, which is unstable and open to interpretation (Lemke, 1995). What this means is that the

Table 21.1 Structuralist and post-structuralist thinking about identity

Structuralist	Post-structuralist
• Elements of people's personality can be classified and categorized. • Constructs systems to treat categorizations/ classifications. • These elements and categorizations are seen as the building blocks to identity. • Identity is the product of the self.	• Encourages the deconstruction of people's negative truths about identity. • Assists people to break free from thin conclusions about their lives and identities. • Supports people in conversations that contribute to a thick description of their lives and identities. • Identity is a public and social achievement.

structuralist strand of linguistics sees these ideas as fixed and tends to give a surface description (thin) of identity. In other words, ideas become all-encompassing labels and a set of discourses that encourage negative truths about the person such as 'depressive'. In contrast, poststructuralists encourage people to break free from 'thin' conclusions about their lives and identities. The narrative practitioner supports conversations and dialogue that are based on a 'rich' description of identity.

The characteristics of structuralist and post-structuralist thought surrounding identity are summarized in Table 21.1.

For White (2007), the extensive use of Foucault's notion of discourse is emphasized in the context of removing relatively fixed qualities which are ascribed to the person's identity (Foucault, 1971; Jessup & Rogerson, 1999). Thus, it is vital that common sense or taken-for-granted assumptions be subject to critical interrogation in social work practice (Gramsci, 1971) so that the individual is able to move away from the 'subjected being' to a subject who authors their own narrative. Althusser (1971[1989]) captures this point succinctly, referring to subjects being the authors of their own actions. The social worker addresses questions about the relationship between our physical and social environments, what we do and say about them and how we live within them (Sims-Schouten, Riley, & Willig, 2007). This is because any 'reality' here is 'understood to be a reflection of external structures . . . as well as internal constructed ways of thinking' (Morley, 2004, p. 299).

Changing positions

Whilst discourse offers prescribed patterns of behaviour, positions or 'thin' descriptions of identity, it is possible for us to hold several positions within the same narrative. For example, a wife can also be a feminist, author, poet or painter. This enables us to draw on alternative discourses that challenge taken-for-granted assumptions about our identities and others'. Narrative theory seeks to harness such ideas about the power of language and how the self is formed and re-formed through language. Thus, our identities comprise an ongoing process and a project which is never finished or complete. Archer (2000) concludes that our social and personal identities are neither guaranteed nor ever confirmed and completed.

Narrative strategies: stories and alternative stories

Narrative approaches assume that we can only speak ourselves into existence with the terms or words or stories that are available to us (Monk et al., 1997). Yet if we were to go through life adopting and accepting the discourses of others about the way of the world or about how we should behave, then we would conclude that this is the natural state of the world. These ways of thinking can mask alternative, new or emergent discourses. The term 'emergence' is what Fairclough (2005) uses to depict the articulation of new, marginalized or alternative discourses that can coexist alongside dominant discourses. The narrative practitioner listens for alternative descriptions that coexist against the dominant plot or discourse (White, 2007). The social worker accepts people's struggle and recognizes that no account or story is so consistent that we cannot find elements that contradict the problematic story. Life is embedded in contradictions and this can be used to the advantage of the narrative and critical practitioner. The opposite is always present in any meaning, and meaning making depends on the possibility of perceiving a different perspective. This perspective embraces a way of logic inspired by Marx, Hegel, Kant, Foucault and Derrida (Harrison-Barbet, 2001). Thus, we can listen for what is not being said in narratives.

Human agency

There is often space for human agency to promote alternative perspectives and strategies in which collective change and progress can be made (Mumby & Stohl, 1991). Agency refers to the extent to which people can act for themselves and speak on their own behalf. The person's capacity for acting freely is more of an achievement than a right as people often feel as if they have lost agency. What is central to these sociological arguments is whether agency is considered to be constrained by larger social structures, such as the church or government (Archer, 2000). The problem of agency is the extent to which individuals are considered capable of pursuing their own objectives and responding to constraints established within the institutional, structural and historical contexts with which they interact (Giddens, 1984).

We can be critical of theorists who reduce social life solely to the effects of powerful social structure and who ignore the possibility of a construing agent (Houston, 2001, 2010). The capacity of narratives and critical theories here to explain sources of oppression in society and take action to transform them is considered a useful tool in the raising of consciousness in social work methods. 'People, in their conscious activity, for the most part unconsciously reproduce (and occasionally transform) the structures governing their substantive activities' (Bhaskar, 1979, p. 44). The process of raising consciousness sees the practitioner and individual co-construct another story with a focus on bringing about change. This is in the context of helping individuals free themselves from oppressive discourses (Creswell, 2007). These theoretical traditions argue that critical awareness can contribute to developing radical change. Giroux (1994), Hall (1985), Freire (1970) and Gramsci (1971) all point out the power of emancipatory pedagogical strategies as ways to engender change and human agency (Sewpaul, 2013). These traditions of theories assume that any reality is derived through language, meaning making and the social context (Oliver, 2011), and this provides a dual focus on agency and structure in a cause and effect way, identified as a key feature of critical social work (Dominelli, 1997; Houston, 2010). While these traditions emphasize the role of human agency in constituting the social world, they do not underestimate the power and role of discourses originating from social structures in shaping experience and the individual (Fairclough, 1995; Archer, 2000).

The narrative practitioner, then, listens and helps uncover an alternative narrative that is enabling, fostering independent thought and practice by thinking about the world in a historical and philosophical way (praxis). This develops an alternative 'scaffold' for the repositioning in the narrative or the individual reclaiming their voice amongst many competing discourses.

Deconstruction: 'problems' revisited

The post-structuralist strand is utilized in narrative theory using *deconstruction*, which is associated with Derrida's method. It involves unpacking, exploring and understanding the unspoken and implicit assumptions that underpin thoughts and language (Harrison-Barbet, 2001). For example, Derrida viewed dualistic ways of thinking as ignoring the diversity within categories (such as masculine or feminine), as well as failing to identify many interpretations lying between those categories. As Fook (2016) points out, binary opposites (dualistic ways) create forced categories of choice in which some discourses are often privileged over others. Derrida pointed to looking at the opposite meaning of the word that is inferred for the word to make sense. For example, if someone says they are 'weak', they are implying that to be 'strong' is the preferred way of being. The opposite is always considered to be present in any meaning, and meaning making depends on our ability to perceive difference in the words that lie between these categories, as well as where these ideas might come from.

Narrative theory also draws on the term 'deconstruction' from the way in which Foucault was concerned with uncovering hidden meanings of the workings of power and questioning claims to knowledge and 'truth' (Monk et al., 1997). As noted by Foucault, power relations characterize all our social interactions. In this way of using deconstruction, the narrative practitioner 'unearths' the ways in which the individual has had access to their own power to speak, often reduced by their acceptance of dominant discourses. These dominant discourses can often reflect the language of authorities (Monk et al., 1997). That said, this shows how people within a culture share a dominant set of discourses or ways of making sense. If we take this together with the notion that the world is constantly changing, we can assume that there is no single 'right' way in which to interpret ideas. Individuals can experience this idea as enormously liberating (Monk et al., 1997).

Externalizing

Through linguistic analysis, it is possible to explore and expose dominant discourses such as gender, depression or anxiety. What this means is that consciousness and agency are experienced and are partly the products of ideology 'speaking through' the subject (Althusser, 1971[1989]). For example, dominant discourses of 20th-century problems such as the notion of 'troubled families' have promoted the view that it is families that need to develop 'resilience'. Such a linguistic analysis here discloses ideas, beliefs, norms and behaviours, which produce normalizations – in effect, expression of and [re]production of prevailing power structures around race, class, gender, poverty, sexuality and so on. As social workers, 'we can collude with this or attempt to shift discourses and their outcomes for individuals' (Pease & Fook, 1999, p. 171). In careful discussion, the narrative practitioner can open possibilities for individuals to rethink whole social categories (Jessup & Rogerson, 1999). The use of externalizing conversations through deconstruction of the narrative creates an alternative space for a different type of understanding in which discourses are accorded more influence in the shaping of experience (Monk et al., 1997).

The deconstruction process involves the use of externalizing conversations in narrative approaches. This is called 'mapping the effects of the problem in the narrative' (Morgan, 2000, p. 20). The aim of externalizing conversations is to encourage individuals to consider themselves and their problems as separate and *not* the same thing. This is achieved through asking questions in which the adjectives that people use to describe themselves are changed into nouns. Hence,

Table 21.2 Internalizing and externalizing

Internalizing	Externalizing
• Don't you think your behaviour does not help? • Do you think that you are depressed? • Are you unhappy and unmotivated? • You're a bit of a worrier, aren't you? • Are you an alcoholic?	• How has *the* behaviour affected your relationships? • What control does *the* depression have over you? • How does motivation affect confidence on the course? • In what way does *the* worry stop you from doing the things you want to do? • How has *the alcohol* influenced your decisions in your life?

instead of 'how long have you been stressed', we ask: 'How long has the *stress* influenced you?' There are four general questions that we use:

- How has {**the problem**} affected your life?
- How long has {**the problem**} affected your relationships?
- How has {**the problem**} affected your view of yourself?
- Are these {**effects/influences**} helpful or unhelpful?

(Roscoe et al., 2011, p. 15)

The device of externalizing helps reverse the trend in individualist thought toward seeking more and more deficits in individual character. This contemporary emphasis on individualism creates the view that structural inequalities can be reduced to individual deficits (Scharff, 2011). We encourage individuals to see themselves as defiant and victors against the problem. The following table illuminates how individualist and internalizing ways of thinking can reinforce social problems through processes of categorization.

Discourses that have been located in our culture and taken-for-granted notions, such as notions of 'stress', 'at risk' or 'depression' can often restrict other ways in which to think about alternative interpretations. The process of externalizing conversations serves the purposes of deconstruction. Internalizing conversations sees the person as the problem, with it becoming a central core of the self. Externalizing conversations explore the person's *relationship* to the problem. This is then located in a context that is external and outside of their identity (Morgan, 2000).

Positioning ourselves differently – re-authoring processes

Re-authoring conversations is an invitation to individuals to do what they usually do: that is, to link events of their lives in sequences through time according to an alternative plot or theme. Alternative narratives can be found in what is called 'unique outcomes' in White's (1995, 2007) work. Here we see these as emergent discourses and we can call these *contradictions*. White (1995) argues that no single story of life can be free of ambiguity or contradiction; contradictions are aspects of a person's lived experience that lie outside the dominant story and its associated discourses. White (2007) suggests practitioners listen with a view to identifying these contradictions which encourage a 'thick' description of people's lives, identity, values and aspirations. These begin separating the thin description of identity with a thick description, hence beginning to co-author an alternative story. In any narrative, there will be instances where the problem was less influential, and these instances may stand out in contrast to the dominant story. Contradictions, however, can go unnoticed without careful listening from the practitioner as people can place less significance on events that do not support the dominant story. Themes or patterns of contradictions such as 'bravery', 'compassion' and, 'determination' can emerge. These in turn can provide a type of scaffolding to re-author an alternative story. The contradictions provide a conduit for exploring identity.

A practical application

Learning a set of skills and language critique techniques is vital in relation to the 'use of self' in social work, and so we must view ourselves as a key resource when drawing on narrative ideas for practice. Viewed as a strengths-based approach (Payne, 2014), narrative methods and theories can be applied to a variety of practice contexts and conversations. For example, narratives are often used for conflict resolution, enabling both parties to reconstruct both sides of the argument, and then the social worker helps facilitate and co-author an alternative position in the narrative (White, 2005). Narrative ideas are particularly useful for social work assessments as well as methods of intervention. In assessment, whether with children or adults, narrative theory enables us to understand identity politics and how an individual has internalized their wider social and cultural context. We may engage in educational processes with parents about the power and impact of language on a child's sense of self by using visual cards with positive images such as 'courage' and 'bravery' to help re-author an alternative story. This shows how developing parenting solutions can help in child in need or child protection contexts. Similarly, we might work with women around notions of 'domestic violence', co-authoring alternative stories surrounding 'self-blame', 'guilt' or duty.

In educational terms, the use of narratives with women with 'eating disorders' in the form of group work is a powerful strategy for raising consciousness of the power of media and capitalism in defining what women 'should' look like. Similarly, group work can be used with men around notions of masculinity and how this affects the family's roles, responsibilities and expectations.

With older adults, or adults with disabilities or mental health problems, we can encourage the externalization of totalizing descriptions of identities to reveal and uncover hidden competencies and values. In community care, narrative approaches can help us determine what the individual's goals and aspirations are, and in co-authoring notions of 'disability' with notion of 'ability', both the worker and individual can unite against the problem and question the power of psychiatric or disability discourses in determining and restricting what we 'think' we can or cannot do.

We can conclude this chapter by encouraging the practitioner to move beyond the notion of 'therapy' and focus on the use of acquiring narrative skills and techniques in their use of self and for everyday critical practice, as well as considering narrative theories and methods as specialist forms of intervention targeting a particular 'problem' in individuals' or families' lives.

Further reading

Morgan, A. (2000). *What is narrative therapy?* Adelaide: Dulwich Centre Publications.
Roscoe, K. D., Carson, A. M., & Madoc-Jones, I. (2011). Narrative social work: Conversations between theory and practice. *Journal of Social Work Practice*, 25(1), 47–56.
White, M. (2007). *Maps of narrative practice.* New York: Norton.

References

Althusser, L. (1971[1989]). Ideology and ideological state apparatuses (pp. 123–175). In L. Althusser (Ed.), *Lenin and philosophy and other essays.* New York: Monthly Review Press.

Archer, M. (2000). *Being human: The problem of agency*. Cambridge: University Press.

Bhaskar, R. A. (1979). *The possibility of naturalism*. Brighton: Harvester.

Bruner, J. (1990). *Acts of meaning*. Cambridge, MA: Harvard University Press.

Carson, A. M. (2009). Narrative practice. *International Journal of Narrative Practice, 1*(1), 1–9.

Creswell, J. W. (2007). *Qualitative inquiry and research design: Choosing among five traditions* (2nd ed.). Thousand Oaks: Sage.

Derrida, J. (1978). *Writings and difference*. Chicago: University of Chicago Press.

Dominelli, L. (1997). *Sociology for social work*. Basingstoke: Macmillan.

Fairclough, N. (1995). *Critical discourse analysis: The critical study of language*. London: Longman.

Fairclough, N. (2003). *Analysing discourse: Textual analysis for social research*. London: Routledge.

Fairclough, N. (2005). Peripheral vision: Discourse analysis in organization studies: The case for critical realism. *Organization Studies, 26*(6), 915–939.

Fairclough, N., & Graham, P. (2002). Marx as critical discourse analyst. *Estudios de Sociolinguistica, 3*(1), 185–229.

Ferguson, H. (2003). Outline of a critical best practice perspective on social work and social care. *British Journal of Social Work, 33*(8), 1005–1024.

Fook, J. (2016). *Social work: A critical approach to practice* (3rd ed.). London: Sage.

Foucault, M. (1971). Orders of discourse. *Social Science Information, 10*(2), 7–30.

Foucault, M. (1972). *The archaeology of knowledge*. New York: Pantheon.

Fraser, H. (2004). Doing narrative research: Analysing personal stories line by line. *Qualitative Social Work, 3*(2), 179–201.

Freire, P. (1970). *Pedagogy of the oppressed*. New York: Herder and Herder.

Garfinkel, H. (1967). *Studies in ethnomethodology*. Englewood Cliffs, NJ: Prentice-Hall.

Garrett, P. M. (2017). *Welfare words: Critical social work and social policy*. London: Sage.

Giddens, A. (1984). *The constitution of society: Outline of the theory of structuration*. Cambridge, UK: Polity Press.

Giroux, H. A. (1994). *Disturbing pleasures: Learning popular culture*. New York: Routledge.

Gramsci, A. (1971). *Selections from the prison notebooks*. London: Lawrence and Wishart.

Hall, S. (1985). Signification, representation, ideology: Althusser and the post structuralist debates. *Critical Studies in Mass Communication, 2*(2), 91–114.

Harrison-Barbet, A. (2001). *Mastering philosophy*. Basingstoke: Palgrave Macmillan.

Houston, S. (2001) Beyond social constructionism: Critical realism and social work. *The British Journal of Social Work, 31*(6), 845–861.

Houston, S. (2010). Prising open the black box: Critical realism, action research and social work. *Qualitative Social Work, 9*(1), 73–91.

Jessup, H., & Rogerson, S. (1999). Postmodernism and the teaching and practice of interpersonal skills. In B. Pease & J. Fook (Eds.), *Transforming social work practice: Postmodern critical perspectives* (pp. 161–178). St. Leonards: Allen & Unwin.

King, A. (2004). *The structure of social theory*. Routledge: London.

Kitzinger, C. (1994). The discursive construction of identities. In J. Shotter & K. Gergen (Eds.), *Texts of identity* (pp. 82–98). London: Sage.

Kress, G., & Hodge, B. (1993). *Language as ideology* (2nd ed.). London: Routledge.

Lemke, J. (1995). *Textual politics: Discourse and social dynamics*. London: Taylor and Francis.

Monk, G., Winslade, J., Crocket, K., & Epston, D. (1997). *Narrative therapy in practice: The archaeology of hope*. San Francisco: Jossey-Bass.

Morgan, A. (2000). *What is narrative therapy?* Adelaide: Dulwich Centre.

Morley, C. (2004). Critical reflection in social work: A response to globalization? *International Journal of Social Welfare, 13*, 297–303.

Mumby, D. K., & Stohl, C. (1991). Power and discourse in organization studies: Absence and the dialectic of control. *Discourse and Society, 2*, 313–332.

Oliver, C. (2011). Critical realist grounded theory: A new approach for social work research. *British Journal of Social Work, 42*(2), 371–387.

Payne, M. (2014). *Modern social work theory* (4th ed.). Basingstoke: Palgrave Macmillan.

Pease, B., & Fook, J. (1999). *Transforming social work practice: Postmodern critical perspectives*. London: Routledge.

Ricoeur, P. (1984). *Time and narrative*. Chicago: Chicago University Press.

Roscoe, K. D. (2014). *Social work discourses: An exploratory study*. (PhD thesis). University of Chester, Chester.

Roscoe, K. D., Carson, A. M., & Madoc-Jones, I. (2011). Narrative social work: Conversations between theory and practice. *Journal of Social Work Practice, 25*(1), 47–61.

Roscoe, K. D., & Pithouse, A. (2016). Discourse, identity and socialization: A textual analysis of the 'accounts' of student social workers. *Critical and Radical Social Work*. Retrieved from https://doi.org/10.1332/204986016X14761129779307

Sewpaul, V. (2013). Inscribed in our blood: Challenging the ideology of sexism and racism. *Affilia, 28*, 116–125.

Scharff, C. (2011). Disarticulating feminism: Individualization, neoliberalism and the othering of Muslim women. *European Journal of Women's Studies, 18*(2), 119–134.

Sims-Schouten, W., Riley, S. C. E., & Willig, C. (2007). Critical realism in discourse analysis: A presentation of a systematic method of analysis using women's talk of motherhood, childcare and female employment as an example. *Theory and Psychology, 17*(1), 101–124.

Squire, C. (2013). From experience-centred to socioculturally-oriented approaches to narrative. In M. Andrews, C. Squire, & M. Tamboukou (Eds.), *Doing narrative research* (pp. 47–71). London: Sage.

Wetherell, M., Taylor, S., & Yates, S. J. (Eds.). (2001). *Discourse theory and practice: A reader*. London: Sage.

White, M. (1995). *Re-authoring lives: Interviews and essays*. Adelaide: Dulwich Centre Publications.

White, M. (2005). *Narrative practice and exotic lives: Resurrecting diversity in everyday life*. Adelaide: Dulwich Centre Publications.

White, M. (2007). *Maps of narrative practice*. New York: Norton.

22

Mindfulness and social work

Yuk-Lin Renita Wong

Originating in the teachings of Siddhārtha Gautama (or Gautama Buddha; c. 563 BCE/480 BCE–c. 483 BCE/400 BCE), over the past two decades mindfulness practice has been secularized and has grown in popularity in the fields of social work, psychology, health and mental health. To date, most of the research and writings have been in psychology and medicine. This chapter focuses primarily on research and publications by social work scholars, researchers, educators and practitioners. It highlights the unique contributions of social work in integrating mindfulness into practice on multiple levels to bring about individual and social change.

This chapter will anchor the understanding of mindfulness in its Buddhist roots, hoping to address some of the confusion surrounding the secular use of mindfulness and issues of cultural appropriation. It will call for a paradigm shift in our knowledge construction and application of mindfulness in the field and identify where social work uniquely stands in relation to mindfulness practice in our commitment to social justice.

What is mindfulness?

What is mindfulness? Thich Nhat Hanh (1996) tells a story to illustrate its meaning. Once Gautama Buddha was asked, 'What do you and your students practice?' He replied, 'We sit, we walk and we eat'. The questioner continued: 'But everyone sits, walks and eats'. The Buddha then said, 'When we sit, we know we are sitting. When we walk, we know we are walking. When we eat, we know we are eating'.

Mindfulness is an experiential and embodied state of being. It must be experienced to be understood. Defining mindfulness using just words fails to grasp its essence. Nonetheless, the foregoing story emphasizes three important qualities of mindfulness. First, it is an everyday practice to be carried out during our mundane activities. Everyone has the capacity to do it. It is about how we stay aware of each moment of our lives. Second, the mind is connected to the body in 'knowing' what is happening. Quite often these days, when we eat, we eat with our cell phone, while the mind travels miles away in cyberspace or virtual networking. We do not really 'know', nor are we aware, that we are eating or what we are eating. When we walk, we often walk with our head filled with many projects or running into the future. We are not aware that we are walking or how we are walking. The characteristic of mindful 'knowing' as embodied challenges the Western Cartesian epistemology in which the function of knowing is in the mind that is separate from and elevated above the body. Third, mindful 'knowing' is an equanimous, or non-reactive, awareness of what is going on in the present moment. When we pay attention to our mental activities, it is common to notice that the mind constantly labels, categorizes or comments on what we are experiencing: good or bad, pleasant or unpleasant, liking or disliking. We cling to what feels pleasant or what we like and reject what feels unpleasant or what we dislike. Mindfulness brings our awareness to our conditioned reactivity that colours our perceptions and keeps us from seeing clearly what is happening.

Mindfulness in Pali is *sati* (Sanskrit: *smṛti*), which means 'remembering', 'recollecting', 'bearing in mind'. It involves remembering to come back to the present moment (Nhat Hanh, 1999). Bhikkhu Bodhi (2011) asserts that in the Buddha's teaching, *sati* has acquired a new application based on the older meanings. He argues that mindfulness is best characterized as 'lucid awareness', which includes recognition of objects pertaining to the past as well as awareness of present happenings. The English translation, 'mindfulness', can be misleading, as it seems to focus exclusively on the mind. On the contrary, we can be present only when we are grounded in the body. The body anchors us in the here and now while the mind often takes us into the past or the future. When the mind is not present, we are more likely to go on autopilot without being fully aware of what we are doing or experiencing. In the *Satipaṭṭhāna Sutta* (*Discourse on the Foundations of Mindfulness*), a classic Buddhist text on mindfulness, 'observation of the body in the body' is the first foundation of mindfulness, followed by observation of 'the feelings in the feelings', 'the mind in the mind' and 'the objects of mind in the objects of mind' (Nhat Hanh, 2002). Mindfulness supports a non-reactive observation of and inquiry into our habitual thinking, feeling and action. When the mind is connected to the body in the present, we are less carried away by our mental chatter, especially our conditioned reactivity of attachment and aversion that causes much suffering (Teasdale & Chaskalson, 2011a, 2011b). Instead, we gain a steadier awareness of the arising, unfolding and passing of phenomena as they happen and greater understanding of the causes and conditions of things and how they exist in relation to each other. With this clear seeing, we are more able to discern skilful from unskilful action in response to what is happening.

In their introductions to mindfulness and social work, Hick (2009) and Dylan and Coates (2016) find core similarities among a variety of definitions of mindfulness. Many researchers refer to the definition of Kabat-Zinn (1994, p. 4), a forerunner to the movement to secularize mindfulness practice in Western society: 'mindfulness means paying attention in a particular way, on purpose, in the present moment, and nonjudgmentally'. Using the work of Shapiro, Carlson, Astin, and Freedman (2006) and Baer (2006), Hick (2009) identifies the three components of mindfulness as attention, intention and attitude.

Garland (2013), on the other hand, finds mindfulness research within and outside social work lacking in conceptual clarity and precise operationalization. Other researchers have made similar observations (Chiesa, 2013; Dylan & Coates, 2016). When mindfulness is divorced from its Buddhist roots, it is not surprising to find authors formulating their own definition to fit their purpose. Within social work, for example, Potter (2009) identifies mindfulness as a 'specific and effective method of focusing the mind on the essence of experience' and points out that 'versions of this practice are common among the spiritual traditions of the world' (p. 45). Dylan and Smallboy (2016) share the idea that aspects of mindfulness are similar to practices in other spiritual traditions and liberally construct a 'broader definition' of mindfulness as 'more generally . . . a state of keen awareness' (p. 108). Many use mindfulness primarily as 'a tool' or a 'skills training' method (Trowbridge & Lawson, 2016; Turner, 2009), ignoring that what is integral to mindfulness is the orientation of the mind and ethical stance (Bodhi, 2011; Sharf, 2015; Nhat Hanh, 1999).

Garland (2013) is concerned that such a wide range of definitions and imprecise operation-alization of the construct of mindfulness seriously threaten its validity and that empirical studies of supposedly identical phenomena may result in inconsistent outcomes. He argues that advancing mindfulness research within social work requires establishment of a uniform and coherent set of definitions. Many researchers in other fields are similarly keen to measure mindfulness (Baer, 2007, 2011; Cardaciotto, Herbert, Forman, Moitra, & Farrow, 2008; Feldman, Hayes, Kumar, Greeson, & Laurenceau, 2007; Lau et al., 2006). Despite urging a uniform definition, Garland nonetheless acknowledges that for vulnerable people facing poverty, homelessness, violence and trauma, mindfulness may indeed have a different meaning. He notes that most studies on mindfulness have been conducted with samples of white, middle- to upper- class individuals and cautions social work researchers to 'remain mindful of the cultural and contextual forces' that influence the state of mindfulness (p. 446).

Hick (2009) contends that the abstract conceptualization, objectification and standardized measurement of mindfulness based on positivist research methodologies is antithetical to its embodied and experiential nature. They constitute a form of epistemic violence (Rosch, 2007, cited in Gause & Coholic, 2010). Hick invites mindfulness researchers to consider other paradigms of inquiry into mindfulness that 'proceed from an embodied, open-ended, reflective mode. *Embodied mode* refers to reflection that brings mind and body together. *Open-ended reflection* itself is a form of experience that can be done mindfully'. Rather than seeing 'reflection as just *on* experience', as in positivistic research, mindfulness-based research examines 'reflection as *in* the experience itself' (italics original, p. 16). Hick argues that this can disrupt our habitual way of thinking in research. As Rosch (2007) writes, 'there may be levels (or modes of functioning) of the mind below the surface level of reason, emotion, and ego which are not approachable through the assumptions and logic of our present research . . . What we need at this point is not conceptual closure about mindfulness but openness, wisdom, and creative ferment' (p. 263).

In a methodical explication of the nuanced meanings of *sati* in the Buddhist canonical texts, Bhikkhu Bodhi (2011) reminds us that what must not be overlooked in determining the meaning of *sati*, and what remains consistent across the diverse renderings of mindfulness, is that it is embedded in, and constitutive of, the Noble Eightfold Path central to Buddhist teaching. It is oriented towards developing an ethical stance of non-harm to self and others, animate or inanimate (Nhat Hanh, 1999).

The eight practices in the Noble Eightfold Path are right view, right intention, right speech, right action, right livelihood, right effort, right mindfulness, and right concentration. The concept of 'right' (Pali: *sammā*; Sanskrit: *samyak*) in Buddhist thought is not based on prescriptive or moralistic rules but emerges from ethical considerations of what is wholesome and unwholesome. Thoughts or actions that cause harm are considered unwholesome, whereas those that are benevolent to or supportive of life are considered wholesome. In some translations, the word 'wise' is used instead of 'right'. The *Majjhima Nikāya* (Middle Length Discourse) contains a clear stipulation as to how these eight path factors occur in association with each other. As part of the Four Noble Truths (suffering, roots of suffering, cessation of suffering, and the path to the cessation of suffering), the Noble Eightfold Path is the path leading to the elimination or reduction of suffering on the individual and collective levels. Thus, Bhikkhu Bodhi rejects the popular description of mindfulness as 'bare attention' that is pre-conceptual and devoid of evaluation or judgement. Such a depiction of mindfulness does not correspond to the canonical texts and may even lead to a misguided view of how mindfulness is to be practised.

Divorced from its roots, especially its ethical stance, the secularization of mindfulness in Western society has been appropriated to perpetuate the harm militarization and capitalist-driven productivity has caused in people's lives. Mindfulness has been commoditized as a 'cheap' tool for the healthcare system to treat modern and urban ailments such as stress and mental distress (Bunting, 2013) without examining the socio-economic-political conditions that produce the stress and mental health issues so common in the global capitalist era. Corporate employees are offered mindfulness trainings to enhance productivity (Purser & Forbes, 2017; Purser, Ng, & Walsh, Forthcoming). A version of mindfulness has also been adopted to train soldiers to cope better with stress in the US military (Watson, 2013). As a discipline and profession with core values of service and social justice, it is very important for social work that we critically reflect on how we engage with mindfulness practice.

Mindfulness applications in social work

Mindfulness has been used within social work in four major ways: (1) an intervention in micro-, mezzo- and macro-practice; (2) practitioners' self-care; (3) cultivation of presence and therapeutic relationship and (4) cultivation of self-awareness and critical reflection.

Practitioners in various helping professions have shown extraordinary interest in mindfulness-based therapy because it affects their practice, both for themselves and for their clients. A number of benefits of mindfulness have been identified in the literature, such as clear awareness of thoughts and emotions, new ways of relating to pain and difficulties, regulation of affect, development of self-awareness, more effective response to stress, greater clarity and awareness in making choices and an improved sense of well-being (Hick, 2009). A growing number of neuroscience studies seem to support these findings (Davidson et al., 2003; Siegel, 2007). The question remains, however, whether the experience of mindfulness and its effects can be fully captured and understood by observing the brain function.

Mindfulness has been used as a clinical intervention with a variety of populations. Developed by Kabat-Zinn (1990), mindfulness-based stress reduction (MBSR) is probably the most widely adopted mindfulness intervention in the UK and North America. It is a non–religious structured group programme comprising eight weekly two- to three-hour classes and one day-long retreat. It includes formal guided mindfulness meditation and body scan and movement practices. It also introduces daily mindfulness exercises to enhance moment-to-moment awareness of bodily sensations, emotions and thoughts and, ultimately, of communication and life in general. A conceptual and empirical review by Baer (2003, 2006), as well as a meta-analysis by Grossman, Niemann, Schmidt, and Walach (2004), suggests the health benefits of MBSR in terms of relieving anxiety and depression, as well as enhanced coping with stress, pain, and physical impairment and improved quality of life.

The MBSR approach has been adapted to various forms of mindfulness-based therapy (MBT). Among the best known are mindfulness-based cognitive therapy (MBCT) (Segal, Williams, & Teasdale, 2013), acceptance and commitment therapy (ACT) (Hayes & Lillis, 2012), and dialectical behaviour therapy (DBT) (Linehan, 1993). Khoury et al. (2013) conducted a meta-analysis of 209 MBT intervention studies enrolling 12,145 participants with various health and mental health issues. Similarly, MBT is found to be an effective intervention in various psychological issues, especially for reducing anxiety, depression and stress. Social workers use MBT in groups with older adults (Foulk, Ingersoll-Dayton, Kavanagh, Robinson, & Kales, 2014), immigrants (George, 2009), homeless youth (Bender et al., 2015), survivors of interpersonal violence (Kelly, 2015), vulnerable children (Coholic & Eys, 2016), people with addictions

Garland, Schwarz, Kelly, Whitt, & Howard, 2012; Larkin, Hardiman, Weldon, & Kim, 2012) and caregivers (Minor, Carlson, MacKenzie, Zernicke, & Jones, 2006). Hick (2009) calls the impact of mindfulness on psychology the 'third wave in western psychology', and sees a similar effect on clinical social work. The first wave was behaviour therapy in the 1960s, followed by cognitive therapy in the 1970s; more recently, mindfulness practice is directed toward the cultivation of qualities such as awareness, acceptance, compassion and openness to new experience (p. 9).

A distinct feature of social work lies in its commitment to social justice and its position on how personal troubles are embedded in and constructed by dominant discourses and the larger historical and structural contexts (International Federation of Social Workers [IFSW], 2017; see various codes of ethics, IFSW, 2018; see Chapters 10 and 26–28). Social workers are more likely than other helping professions to provide services to disadvantaged populations and to engage in mezzo and macro levels of intervention to bring about institutional, policy and social change (Boone, 2014; Dylan & Coates, 2016; Hick, 2009). The resonance between this social work orientation and the ethical foundation of mindfulness goes beyond the individualist view of human suffering. This is where social work can make its unique contribution among other helping professions in extending mindfulness-based interventions beyond micro clinical practice.

Hick and Furlotte (2009) integrate mindfulness into social justice approaches to social work, such as structural, critical and anti-oppressive social work (see Chapters 26–31), as a method to link the personal and political in direct practice. Involving people who experience severe socio-economic disadvantage and social isolation as well as significant medical, psychological, physical and learning challenges, they have developed a 'radical mindfulness training' (RMT) that explores mindfulness practice on the personal, interpersonal and structural levels (Hick & Furlotte, 2010). The quantitative and qualitative findings of their study demonstrate that the participants showed a reduction in self-judgement and an increase in self-kindness. Participants also felt more connected to others, less isolated and better able to effect change in the institutions that were challenging their lives.

Todd (2009) brings mindfulness practice to community work (see Chapter 25). She argues that it is important to attend to the interior lives of community members and activists. Todd explores how mindfulness can support community members in negotiating passionate and difficult emotions during community mobilization under the burden of oppressive relations and in reconnecting with our sense of curiosity and compassion for self and others. She believes this enhances people's ability to listen to each other, to find common ground and to broaden opportunities for 'a more centered, self-reflective and creative approach to community change' (p. 173). Similarly, London (2009) sees mindfulness as foundational to work for social justice. An activist's work has the potential to be 'poetic and courageous or destructive and blind in its intent and consequences' (p. 188). They thus need to direct purposively their intent and actions congruently with social justice goals. London's approach to mindfulness in social activism echoes the ethical grounding of non-harm integral to mindfulness practice.

Mindfulness practice has also been identified as beneficial in ecosocial work (see Chapter 14). As we witness the increasing impact of environmental crises on the clients we serve, eco or green social work has emerged as a vital new area of practice. Indigenous peoples have always honoured the centrality of the natural world to all existence and have been at the forefront of environmental struggles (Kino-nda-niimi Collective, 2014; Associated Press, 2017; see Chapter 23). Within ecosocial work, Lysack (2009) calls for the 'ecological self' as the object of mindfulness in environmental activism. Crews and Besthorn (2016) argue that the priority of ecosocial work is the transformation of consciousness toward more earth-friendly actions and attitudes. They see mindful engagement with the silence of the natural world as an important strategy in assisting this transformational process. Here we see the potential of mindfulness practice to address the Eurocentric bias in social work that heretofore has excluded the natural world from our practice.

Uebel and Shorkey (2014) go further, shifting the social work perspective from 'person-in-environment' to 'person-as-environment', as they incorporate the Buddhist notion of 'no-self' (Pali: *anattā*; Sanskrit: *anatman*) or no independent existence, an ontological foundation of mindfulness. They contend that at the heart of macro social work is the recognition not only of localized selves embedded in larger systems and environments, but also of the fluidity between and interrelatedness of selves and systems as processes and functions affecting each other. Mindfulness practice supports this awareness of the interdependent nature of reality and existence. Uebel and Shorkey assert, 'This is the point where *ego* becomes *eco*' (p. 218). They argue that the most profound insight from Buddhism for macro social work practice is the realization of 'our non-duality with all "others" such that our own wellbeing is inseparable from their wellbeing' (p. 219).

Social workers also take up mindfulness practice for self-care in an increasingly demanding environment in social service. Research studies show the benefits of mindfulness practice for social work practitioners and students in reducing stress, empathic distress and compassion fatigue and burnout and, consequently, for increasing resilience (Birnbaum, 2009; Botta, Cadet, & Maramaldi, 2015; Crowder & Sears, 2017; McGarrigle & Walsh, 2011; Napoli & Bonifas, 2011; Stickle, 2016; Thieleman & Cacciatore, 2014). Shier and Graham (2011) interviewed 13 respondents with the highest subjective well-being scores from a survey of 700 social workers. These respondents affirmed that being mindful supported their overall subjective well-being and mitigated the stress and negative experiences within the present political and economic environment in social service provision. Shier and Graham do not wish to use mindfulness practice as a tool 'to placate workers into subservient acceptance' of the institutional and systemic problems within the field (p. 31). They do, however, see mindfulness as an important resource that can help social workers practise more effectively and critically.

Trowbridge and Lawson (2016) conducted a systematic review of quantitative and qualitative studies that examined mindfulness-based interventions with social work practitioners or students. They discovered the potential of mindfulness not only to enhance social workers' coping skills, but also to improve and sustain their engagement with clients and families. Researchers and practitioners note how mindfulness practice enhances the practitioner's qualities of attention, deep listening, affect regulation, attunement, empathy (Hick & Bien, 2008; Turner, 2009) and compassion (Stickle, 2016). The benefits of mindfulness practice for practitioners' self-care, self-awareness, and building positive therapeutic relationships have led many social work educators to include mindfulness practice in clinical practice education and practitioner training (Gockel, 2010; Gockel, Cain, Malove, & James, 2013; Lynn, 2010; Mishna & Bogo, 2007; Paré, Richardson, & Tarragona, 2009).

Research studies have consistently shown the importance of relationships for effective therapy and group work (Hick & Bien, 2008). This is where we find the unique contribution of mindfulness practice. Within the client-practitioner relationship, mindfulness practice shifts the practitioner from 'doing' mode to 'being' mode (Hick, 2009). It is a non-striving and accepting presence with the client and with ourselves as practitioner, without pushing away what is difficult or clinging to what we want. It challenges technique-driven and outcome-focused modes in social work. This seems paradoxical for social work as a profession working for change. Meisinger (2009), however, notes that our full presence in 'witnessing the pain' of a traumatized client, rather than being preoccupied with fixing the client or the 'problem', is one of the most important services social workers can provide. Boone's edited collection (2014) explores how 'mindfulness and acceptance offer a flexible and compassionate context' (p. 4) for the interactions among individuals, groups, families and communities with their social and physical environments.

Lord (2010) finds meditation and mindfulness practice help her and her clients cultivate 'sacred space' where they 'listen attentively in deeply silent open and compassionate ways' (p. 273), where 'pains and joys can be rendered' and 'through which transformation and an awareness of infinite possibilities can emerge' (p. 270). Bein (2008) shares Lord's orientation of honouring the sacred in the therapeutic relationship. Bein finds the demand for spiritual approaches to helping intensifies as the social service environment increasingly objectifies both clients and practitioners. Moving 'beyond familiar and formulaic responses' in social work, he seeks to 'grapple with the real moment-to-moment issues for practitioners', such as how to care while letting go, how to maintain presence, how to cultivate radical acceptance, how to bear witness to client pain and trauma, how to hold contradictions and paradoxes and so on. All are qualities of mindfulness practice.

Mindfulness practice has also been found to enrich critical reflection and reflexivity as an ethic of care. Berés (2009) explores ways in which mindfulness and its ontological foundation of no-self can deepen our critical reflection on power and knowledge in the practitioner-client relationship. In her practice, she notices how our desire to be helpful can keep us from being fully present to the other's experiences. As we are caught up in thinking about what to do, we miss the important information the other is trying to convey. She argues that 'the more we experience mindfulness and the impermanence of our thoughts and feelings, the more apt we are to experience a sense of no-self' (p. 74). Thus, mindfulness practice supports practitioners in deconstructing and disengaging from the desire to help and the associated ideas of the self. Berés believes that this would 'provide a more ethical exchange with the "others"' (p. 59), because we would be more open to different ways of being with the people with whom we work.

In her work with immigrants, George (2009) identifies the role of mindfulness in helping practitioners become aware of stereotypes and biases and how we follow socially constructed standards of behaviour. Paré et al. (2009) further explicate how mindfulness practice promotes 'an exquisitely fine-grained awareness of experience as it unfolds', and 'renders more visible to practitioners . . . the ongoing train of thought that accompanies the outer dialogue of therapeutic conversations' (pp. 76–77). Paré et al. consider this awareness to be crucial to ethical practice. It involves an awareness of not only the verbal communication and the nonverbal cues within the room, but also the broader societal discourses that show up as internal dialogue influencing 'how we go forward at every utterance' (p. 78) in our exchange with the client.

Wong (In Press, 2004, 2013, 2014) advocates an integrated body-heart-mind-spirit engage-ment (see Chapter 41) in critical reflection and critical social work education. She challenges the dominant pedagogy of critical reflection that privileges conceptual-analytical thinking and knowing over other, marginalized ways of knowing through the body-heart-spirit. Wong takes up mindfulness as a contemplative and decolonizing pedagogy that shifts the epistemo-logical ground of knowing and knowledge construction in social work and in Western society. Through various mindfulness practices, her students explored knowing through silence and wholeness. Students were encouraged to embody critical awareness through their five senses, to sit with curiosity with the feeling of discomfort as they reflect on their implication in systemic oppression, to hold space for contradictions and paradox and the fluidity of each moment and each person. Responses from her students show that they came to embody critical reflective practice in a way that is not achieved to the same depth through conventional teaching and learning of critical practice with only cognitive-analytical thinking. Some racialized students, in particular, experienced a decolonizing process through mindfulness: a decolonization from the Eurocentric consciousness that separates the mind from the body, heart and spirit, as well as a decolonization from the essentialist, dualistic and individualist construction of self, separate from others, all things and all relations. As these students restored a sense of wholeness and interconnectedness with their community and history, they experienced a burgeoning inner life force beyond the categories of identities, and discovered new possibilities for action in the world.

Conclusion

Birnbaum and Birnbaum (2008) project that the emergence of mindfulness in social work illustrates an ontological and epistemological shift in the field as social work researchers and practitioners open up to 'holistic and transpersonal theories assuming the existence of a metaphysical reality' (p. 87). This vision might seem optimistic while we see the increasingly dominant approach to mindfulness as mostly a technique or skill to be added to the social work toolbox or as a cognitive behavioural intervention demanding precise measurement for empirical assessment of its effectiveness. Observing this trend, Gause and Coholic (2010) urge researchers and practitioners to grapple with the marginalization of holistic and spiritually sensitive methods within mainstream practices and professions and to return mindfulness to its holistic roots. They believe that mindfulness, when practised holistically, 'might be more creative, attuned to people's specific needs or goals, and open to discourse that is spiritual/holistic and existential' (p. 17). Dylan and Coates (2012) also assert that 'functioning from a spiritual core transforms life, politics, and potentially the social work profession itself, into radical practices of wholeness' (p. 142).

Rooted in Buddhist onto-epistemology, mindfulness is not simply a set of techniques for one to pick up, but rather an experiential and spiritual process of being. It is a radical practice that begins with the self and yet illuminates the illusion of self: that is, the illusion of self as an unchanging, separate and independent entity or existence. As an embodied practice, mindfulness brings forth an embodied awareness of self as process, as relations, as 'interbeing'. 'To be is to inter-be' (Nhat Hanh, 1992, p. 96). As such, mindfulness practice calls for one's ethical engagement with the world, since we both make the world and are made by it.

Social work is distinct among other helping professions in its multilevel interventions and its core values of service, equity and social justice. This chapter is intended to focus primarily on what social work can uniquely offer in applying mindfulness to addressing human suffering. It is up to us to engage respectfully and holistically with the full potential of mindfulness on all levels for the well-being of all. More critically, are we open to the challenge of mindfulness practice to unsettle our metaphysical and onto-epistemological grounding in social work practice and knowledge construction? Or, simply put, in how we know and what we are?

Perhaps the best way to respond to this challenge is to start experiencing mindfulness now for yourself.

Further reading

Bein, A. (2008). *The Zen of helping: Spiritual principles for mindful and open-hearted practice.* Hoboken, NJ: Wiley.
> This book is a pragmatic and self-caring guide that deals with the realities of social work practice and takes us beyond the familiar and formulaic responses to client dilemmas and moment-to-moment issues for helping professionals.

Bodhi, B. (2011). What does mindfulness really mean? A canonical perspective. *Contemporary Buddhism, 12*(1), 19–39.
> This paper provides a methodical exposition of the nuanced meanings of mindfulness (*sati*) in the Buddhist canonical texts that helps address much of the confusion around the secular use of mindfulness.

Hick, S. F. (2009). *Mindfulness and social work*. Chicago: Lyceum.
This is the first book linking mindfulness to social work. It provides a systematic introduction to mindfulness and social work, covering multiple levels of intervention and mindfulness for practitioners' self-care, therapeutic relationship building, and critical reflection.

References

Associated Press. (2017, 23 February). *Standing Rock protestors defy order to leave*. Retrieved from www.cbc.ca/news/world/standing-rock-evacuation-1.3995407

Baer, R. A. (2003). Mindfulness training as a clinical intervention: A conceptual and empirical review. *Clinical Psychology, 10*(2), 125–143.

Baer, R. A. (2006). *Mindfulness-based treatment approaches: Clinician's guide to evidence base and applications*. Burlington, MA: Academic Press.

Baer, R. A. (2007). Mindfulness, assessment, and transdiagnostic processes. *Psychological Inquiry, 18*(4), 238–242.

Baer, R. A. (2011). Measuring mindfulness. *Contemporary Buddhism, 12*(1), 241–261.

Bein, A. (2008). *The Zen of helping: Spiritual principles for mindful and open-hearted practice*. Hoboken, NJ: Wiley.

Bender, K., Begun, S., DePrince, A., Haffejee, B., Brown, S., Hathaway, J., & Schau, N. (2015). Mindfulness intervention with homeless youth. *Journal of the Society for Social Work and Research, 6*(4), 491–513.

Beres, L. G. (2009). Mindfulness and reflexivity: The no-self as reflexive practitioner. In S. F. Hick (Ed.), *Mindfulness and social work* (pp. 67–75). Chicago: Lyceum.

Birnbaum, L. (2008). The use of mindfulness training to create an 'accompanying place' for social work students. *Social Work Education, 27*(8), 837–852.

Birnbaum, L. (2009). The contribution of mindfulness practice to the development of professional self-concept in students of social work. In S. F. Hick (Ed.), *Mindfulness and social work* (pp. 92–102). Chicago: Lyceum Books.

Birnbaum, L., & Birnbaum, A. (2008). Mindful social work: From theory to practice. *Journal of Religion & Spirituality in Social Work, 27*(1–2), 87–104.

Bodhi, B. (2011). What does mindfulness really mean? A canonical perspective. *Contemporary Buddhism, 12*(1), 19–39.

Boone, M. S. (2014). *Mindfulness & acceptance in social work: Evidence-based interventions & emerging applications*. Oakland, CA: Context.

Botta, A. A., Cadet, T. J., & Maramaldi, P. (2015). Reflections on a quantitative, group-based mindfulness study with social work students. *Social Work with Groups, 38*(2), 93–105.

Bunting, M. (2013, 7 April). Zen and the art of keeping the NHS bill under control. *Guardian*. Retrieved from www.theguardian.com/lifeandstyle/2013/apr/07/zen-buddhism-nhs

Cardaciotto, L., Herbert, J. D., Forman, E. M., Moitra, E., & Farrow, V. (2008). The assessment of present-moment awareness and acceptance: The Philadelphia mindfulness scale. *Assessment, 15*(2), 204–223.

Chiesa, A. (2013). The difficulty of defining mindfulness: Current thought and critical issues. *Mindfulness, 4*(3), 255–268.

Coholic, D. A., & Eys, M. (2016). Benefits of an arts-based mindfulness group intervention for vulnerable children. *Child and Adolescent Social Work Journal, 33*(1), 1–13.

Crews, D., & Besthorn, F. H. (2016). Eco social work and transformed consciousness: Reflections on eco-mindfulness engagement with the silence of the natural world. *Journal of Religion & Spirituality in Social Work, 35*(1–2), 91–107.

Crowder, R., & Sears, A. (2017). Building resilience in social workers: An exploratory study on the impacts of a mindfulness-based intervention. *Australian Social Work, 70*(1), 17–29.

Davidson, R. J., Kabat-Zinn, J., Schumacher, J., Rosenkranz, M., Muller, D., Santorelli, S. F., et al. (2003). Alterations in brain and immune function produced by mindfulness meditation. *Psychosomatic Medicine, 65*(4), 564–570.

Dylan, A., & Coates, J. (2012). The spirituality of justice: Bringing together the eco and the social. *Journal of Religion & Spirituality in Social Work, 31*(1–2), 128–149.

Dylan, A., & Coates, J. (2016). Introduction to special issue: Mindfulness and social work. *Journal of Religion & Spirituality in Social Work, 35*(1–2), 1–6.

Dylan, A., & Smallboy, B. (2016). Land-based spirituality among the Cree of the Mushkegowuk territory. *Journal of Religion & Spirituality in Social Work: Social Thought, 35*(1–2), 108–119.

Feldman, G., Hayes, A., Kumar, S., Greeson, J., & Laurenceau, J-P. (2007). Mindfulness and emotion regulation: The development and initial validation of the Cognitive and Affective Mindfulness Scale-Revised (CAMS-R). *Journal of Psychopathology and Behavioral Assessment, 29*(3), 177–190.

Foulk, M. A., Ingersoll-Dayton, B., Kavanagh, J., Robinson, E., & Kales, H. C. (2014). Mindfulness-based cognitive therapy with older adults: An exploratory study. *Journal of Gerontological Social Work, 57*(5), 498–520.

Garland, E. L. (2013). Mindfulness research in social work: Conceptual and methodological recommendations. *Social Work Research, 37*(4), 439–448.

Garland, E. L., Schwarz, N. R., Kelly, A., Whitt, A., & Howard, M. O. (2012). Mindfulness-oriented recovery enhancement for alcohol dependence: Therapeutic mechanisms and intervention acceptability. *Journal of Social Work Practice in the Addictions, 12*(3), 242–263.

Gause, R., & Coholic, D. (2010). Mindfulness-based practices as a holistic philosophy and method. *Currents, 9*(2). Retrieved from https://journalhosting.ucalgary.ca/index.php/currents/article/view/15903

George, M. (2009). Mindfulness-influenced social work practice with immigrants. In S. F. Hick (Ed.), *Mindfulness and social work* (pp. 149–170). Chicago: Lyceum Books.

Gockel, A. (2010). The promise of mindfulness for clinical practice education. *Smith College Studies in Social Work, 80*(2–3), 248–268.

Gockel, A., Cain, T., Malove, S., & James, S. (2013). Mindfulness as clinical training: Student perspectives on the utility of mindfulness training in fostering clinical intervention skills. *Journal of Religion & Spirituality in Social Work, 32*(1), 36–59.

Grossman, P., Niemann, L., Schmidt, S., & Walach, H. (2004). Mindfulness-based stress reduction and health benefits: A meta-analysis. *Journal of Psychosomatic Research, 57*(1), 35–43.

Hayes, S. C., & Lillis, J. (2012). *Acceptance and commitment therapy* (1st ed.). Washington, DC: American Psychological Association.

Hick, S. F. (2009). *Mindfulness and social work.* Chicago: Lyceum.

Hick, S. F., & Bien, T. (2008). *Mindfulness and the therapeutic relationship.* New York: Guilford.

Hick, S. F., & Furlotte, C. (2009). Mindfulness and social justice approaches: Bridging the mind and society in social work practice. *Canadian Social Work Review, 26*(1), 5–24.

Hick, S. F., & Furlotte, C. (2010). An exploratory study of radical mindfulness training with severely economically disadvantaged people: Findings of a Canadian study. *Australian Social Work, 63*(3), 281–298.

International Federation of Social Workers. (2017). *First report of the global agenda: Promoting social and economic equalities.* Retrieved from http://ifsw.org/get-involved/agenda-for-social-work-2/

International Federation of Social Workers. (2018). *National codes of ethics.* Retrieved from http://ifsw.org/publications/national-codes-of-ethics/

Kabat-Zinn, J. (1990). *Full catastrophe living: Using the wisdom of your body and mind to face stress, pain, and illness.* New York: Dell.

Kabat-Zinn, J. (1994). *Wherever you go, there you are: Mindfulness meditation in everyday life* (1st paperback ed.). New York: Hyperion.

Kelly, A. (2015). Trauma-informed mindfulness-based stress reduction: A promising new model for working with survivors of interpersonal violence. *Smith College Studies in Social Work, 85*(2), 194–219.

Khoury, B., Lecomte, T., Fortin, G., Masse, M., Therien, P., Bouchard, V., et al. (2013). Mindfulness-based therapy: A comprehensive meta-analysis. *Clinical Psychology Review, 33*(6), 763–771.

Kino-nda-niimi Collective. (2014). *The winter we danced: Voices from the past, the future, and the Idle No More movement.* Winnipeg: ARP Books.

Larkin, H., Hardiman, E. R., Weldon, T., & Kim, H. C. (2012). Program characteristics as factors influencing the implementation of mindfulness meditation in substance abuse treatment agencies. *Journal of Religion & Spirituality in Social Work, 31*(4), 311–327.

Lau, M. A., Bishop, S. R., Segal, Z. V., Buis, T., Anderson, N. D., Carlson, L., et al. (2006). The Toronto mindfulness scale: Development and validation. *Journal of Clinical Psychology, 62*(12), 1445–1467.

Linehan, M. (1993). *Cognitive behavioral treatment of borderline personality disorder.* New York: Guilford.

London, T. (2009). Mindfulness in activism: Fighting for justice as a self-reflective emancipatory practice. In S. F. Hick (Ed.), *Mindfulness and social work* (pp. 188–201). Chicago: Lyceum.

Lord, S. A. (2010). Meditative dialogue: Cultivating sacred space in psychotherapy – An intersubjective fourth? *Smith College Studies in Social Work, 80*(2–3), 269–285.

Lynn, R. (2010). Mindfulness in social work education. *Social Work Education, 29*(3), 289–304.

Lysack, M. (2009). From environmental despair to the ecological self: Mindfulness and community action. In S. F. Hick (Ed.), *Mindfulness and social work* (pp. 202–218). Chicago: Lyceum.

McGarrigle, T., & Walsh, C. A. (2011). Mindfulness, self-care, and wellness in social work: Effects of contemplative training. *Journal of Religion & Spirituality in Social Work, 30*(3), 212–233.

Meisinger, S. E. (2009). *Stories of pain, trauma, and survival: A social worker's experiences and insights from the field.* Washington, DC: NASW Press.

Minor, H. G., Carlson, L. E., MacKenzie, M. J., Zernicke, K., & Jones, L. (2006). Evaluation of a mindfulness-based stress reduction (MBSR) program for caregivers of children with chronic conditions. *Social Work in Health Care, 43*(1), 91–109.

Mishna, F., & Bogo, M. (2007). Reflective practice in contemporary social work classrooms. *Journal of Social Work Education, 43*(3), 529–541.

Napoli, M., & Bonifas, R. (2011). From theory toward empathic self-care: Creating a mindful classroom for social work students. *Social Work Education, 30*(6), 635–649.

Nhat Hanh, T. (1992). *Peace is every step: The path of mindfulness in everyday life.* New York: Bantam.

Nhat Hanh, T. (1996). *The long road turns to joy: A guide to walking meditation.* Berkeley, CA: Parallax.

Nhat Hanh, T. (1999). *The heart of the Buddha's teaching: Transforming suffering into peace, joy, and liberation* (New ed.). New York: Harmony.

Nhat Hanh, T. (2002). *Transformation and healing: Sutra on the four establishments of mindfulness.* Berkeley, CA: Parallax.

Pare, D. A., Richardson, B., & Tarragona, M. (2009). Watching the train: Mindfulness and inner dialogue in therapist skills training. In S. F. Hick (Ed.), *Mindfulness and social work* (pp. 76–91). Chicago: Lyceum.

Potter, R. (2009). Mindfulness in social work practice: A theoretical and spiritual exploration. In S. F. Hick (Ed.), *Mindfulness and social work* (pp. 45–56). Chicago: Lyceum.

Purser, R., & Forbes, D. (2017, May 30). *How to be mindful of McMindfulness.* Retrieved from www.ora.tv/homepage/2016/8/29/1

Purser, R., Ng, E., & Walsh, Z. (Forthcoming). The promise and peril of corporate mindfulness. In C. Mabley & D. Knights (Eds.), *Leadership matters: Finding voice, connection and meaning in the 21st century.* London: Routledge.

Rosch, E. (2007). More than mindfulness: When you have a tiger by the tail, let it eat you. *Psychological Inquiry, 18*(4), 258–264.

Segal, Z. V., Williams, J. M. G., & Teasdale, J. D. (2013). *Mindfulness-based cognitive therapy for depression* (2nd ed.). New York: Guilford.

Shapiro, S. L., Carlson, L. E., Astin, J. A., & Freedman, B. (2006). Mechanisms of mindfulness. *Journal of Clinical Psychology, 62*(3), 373–386.

Sharf, R. H. (2015). Is mindfulness Buddhist? (and why it matters). *Transcultural Psychiatry, 52*(4), 470–484.

Shier, M. L., & Graham, J. R. (2011). Mindfulness, subjective wellbeing, and social work: Insight into their interconnection from social work practitioners. *Social Work Education, 30*(1), 29–44.

Siegel, D. J. (2007). *The mindful brain: Reflection and attunement in the cultivation of wellbeing* (1st ed.). New York: Norton. Retrieved from www.loc.gov/catdir/toc/ecip0620/2006030093.html

Stickle, M. (2016). The expression of compassion in social work practice. *Journal of Religion & Spirituality in Social Work, 35*(1–2), 120–131.

Teasdale, J. D., & Chaskalson, M. (Kulananda). (2011a). How does mindfulness transform suffering? 1: The nature and origins of dukkha. *Contemporary Buddhism, 12*(1), 89–102.

Teasdale, J. D., & Chaskalson, M. (Kulananda). (2011b). How does mindfulness transform suffering? 2: The transformation of dukkha. *Contemporary Buddhism, 12*(1), 103–124.

Thieleman, K., & Cacciatore, J. (2014). Witness to suffering: Mindfulness and compassion fatigue among traumatic bereavement volunteers and professionals. *Social Work, 59*(1), 34–41.

Todd, S. (2009). Mobilizing communities for social change. In S. F. Hick (Ed.), *Mindfulness and social work* (pp. 171–187). Chicago: Lyceum.

Trowbridge, K., & Lawson, L. M. (2016). Mindfulness-based interventions with social workers and the potential for enhanced patient-centered care: A systematic review of the literature. *Social Work in Health Care, 55*(2), 101–124.

Turner, K. (2009). Mindfulness: The present moment in clinical social work. *Clinical Social Work Journal, 37*(2), 95–103.

Uebel, M., & Shorkey, C. (2014). Mindfulness and engaged Buddhism: Implications for a generalist macro social work practice. In M. S. Boone (Ed.), *Mindfulness & acceptance in social work: Evidence-based interventions & emerging applications* (pp. 215–234). Oakland, CA: Context.

Watson, J. (2013, 20 January). *US Marines studying mindfulness-based training.* Retrieved from https://medical xpress.com/news/2013-01-marines-mindfulness-based.html

Wong, Y. L. R. (2004). Knowing through discomfort: A mindfulness-based critical social work pedagogy. *Critical Social Work*, *5*(1). Retrieved from https://doi.org/http://www1.uwindsor.ca/criticalsocialwork/knowing-through-discomfort-a-mindfulness-based-critical-social-work-pedagogy

Wong, Y. L. R. (2013). Returning to silence, connecting to wholeness: Contemplative pedagogy for critical social work education. *Journal of Religion & Spirituality in Social Work*, *32*(3), 269–285.

Wong, Y. L. R. (2014). Radical acceptance: Mindfulness and reflection in critical social work education. In M. S. Boone (Ed.), *Mindfulness & acceptance in social work: Evidence-based interventions & emerging applications*. Oakland, CA: Context.

Wong, Y. L. R. (In Press, 2018). 'Please call me by my true names': The decolonizing pedagogy of mindfulness and interbeing in critical social work education. In S. Batacharya & Y. L. R. Wong (Eds.), *Sharing breath: Embodied learning and decolonization*. Edmonton: Athabasca University Press.

23

Indigenist social work practice

Michael Anthony Hart

Indigenous understandings of helping that inform social work are based in philosophies that concentrate on spirit, life in natural environments, fluxes, patterns and cycles, holism, diversity, relationships, interdependence, community, egalitarianism and respectful individualism. These philosophies result in a practice orientation referred to as indigenist social work. It focuses on individuals coming together as groups or communities to engage with one another; learn from lands, waters and other life; share historical and cultural understandings of the cycles and patterns around them; participate in practices meant to strengthen and harmonize relationships and acknowledge fluxes and cycles. Indigenous peoples recognize that these philosophical understandings and practices have been and are gravely impacted by the ongoing colonial oppression perpetrated against Indigenous peoples. Therefore, the scope of indigenist social work includes a political focus that directly confronts and challenges this colonial oppression and upholds Indigenous self-determination. It is guided by such values as sharing, reciprocity, kindness and honesty and relies on such processes such as storytelling, rituals and ceremonies.

In this chapter, the spelling 'knowledges' with an 's' is purposeful. It emphasizes the position that knowledge is subjectively impacted by time, place and interactions. Thus, there can be differing sets of knowledge held by people who are of differing time, place or interaction. This point reflects Indigenous philosophical perspectives but is a greater topic than can be addressed here. Also, the adjective 'Indigenous' is capitalized, following the practice of many Indigenous authors, reflecting its equivalence with regional descriptors such as European.

This chapter briefly highlights this philosophical base and the theoretical aspects of indigenist social work and identifies values and processes important to this means of social work practice. It provides an overview of some critical reflections on indigenist social work and closes with a brief discussion regarding its impact on the profession overall.

Context for indigenist social work practice

It is difficult to provide a concise overview of Indigenous theories related to social work for several reasons. First, there is no globally accepted definition of 'Indigenous'. Instead of a definition, the United Nations has offered the following points to support an understanding of the term:

- Self-identification as Indigenous peoples at the individual level and accepted by the community as its member.
- Historical continuity with pre-colonial and pre-settler societies.
- Strong link to territories and surrounding natural resources.
- Distinct social, economic or political systems.
- Distinct language, culture and beliefs.
- Form non-dominant groups of society.
- Resolve to maintain and reproduce their ancestral environments and systems as distinctive peoples and communities.

(www.un.org/esa/socdev/unpfii/documents/5session_factsheet1.pdf, no date)

The primary focus has been on identifying who is Indigenous, with the most prevailing criteria being the act of self-definition. This focus on who self-identifies as Indigenous results in a significant diversity of peoples, contexts and philosophical understandings. Second, this philosophical and contextual diversity in the estimated 370 million people thought to be Indigenous reverberates down to how Indigenous people understand and practice social work at the community level. Third, Indigenous people continue to live under colonial oppression. People outside their societies continue to exercise significant control over their lives and impact what they can say and do. How these other people exercise this control varies, imposing further diversity within and between Indigenous societies. Fourth, Indigenous people have been significantly marginalized in, if not excluded from, the development, administration, practice, teaching and oversight of social work. The majority of Indigenous theories that could relate to social work remain in place at community levels but are not well incorporated in the field or professional literature. Fifth, while some Indigenous peoples of certain global areas have been able to enter academic institutions to study, research and write about their practices, academic institutions in other global areas do not include Indigenous philosophies and voices in social work. Because of this dynamic, the global perspective that is available is skewed towards certain Indigenous perspectives while excluding others.

It is also important to highlight that colonizing efforts in several parts of the world such as Taiwan, Canada and Norway have focused on assimilating Indigenous peoples into the dominating cultures. As a result, there are segments of Indigenous populations in particular nations who are fully absorbed into dominating cultures and do not attempt to maintain connection to their Indigenous cultures. On the other hand, there are also segments of the Indigenous populations who are consistently striving to maintain their traditions, cultures, knowledge systems and values. Individuals from this position seek Indigenous understandings and practice, even from social work practices. In between there are large numbers of people with varying cultural ties who utilize or avoid both Indigenous and settler-based practices. While Indigenous people do not fit neatly into these three identified culturally expressive boxes, since all people culturally express themselves in varying ways for various reasons, this diversity can be understood as a continuum from settler-based ways of being to indigenist-based ones where individuals strive to maintain their sense of indigeneity, and traditional values, beliefs and practices (McKenzie & Morrissette, 2003).

Until recent decades, social work can be seen primarily, if not solely, as an extension of non-Indigenous settler traditions, philosophies, cultures and practices, thus heavily reflecting the assimilationist side of the continuum. Indigenous peoples have been voicing their concerns about this marginalization of their theories, practices and experiences and stressing how colonial oppression has resulted in significant social issues that are too often framed as individual problems (Hart & Lavallee, 2015). While recognition of these concerns resulted in the adoption of such approaches as culturally sensitive, culturally aware and cross-cultural practices in the profession, Indigenous people have been working to expand how social work is practised with Indigenous populations, developing such theories as culturally safe practice and indigenist social work (Hart & Bracken, 2016).

Indigenous philosophies, knowledges and ways of being as the base of indigenist social work

While keeping in mind that there is significant diversity between Indigenous nations and how they understand their worlds resulting from these points, some philosophical understandings have been shared by many Indigenous peoples. Among these understandings is the focus on spirit, the natural environments, patterns, fluxes, and holism. Spirit is that essence which permeates all entities. It is also that aspect of life that is seen as the source of meaning and transcendence (Mark & Lyons, 2010; see Chapter 11). It plays a central role in many Indigenous philosophies, such as those of the Néhiyawak (Cree people), who identify processes to tap into life forces around us as a means to move beyond the ordinary and rethink the world around us (Ermine, 1995; McLeod, 2007). It is through spirit that we are connected to all other aspects of life, including that beyond human life (Hart, 2015). Through the interconnections with other life, Indigenous understandings incorporate and reflect life in natural environments, particularly in their own territories. Lands, waters and other-than-human beings are seen as not only providing sustenance, but offering knowledge, guidance, identity, a sense of belonging and healing (Green & Baldry, 2008; Gross, 2003; Hart, 2015; Mark & Lyons, 2010; McGregor, 2013).

Indigenous philosophical understandings and knowledges reflect a particular dynamic within natural environments, specifically the cycles, fluxes and patterns that take place. Indigenous understandings incorporate these movements and pay attention to the actions and interactions between entities as well as within the various entities themselves, whether they be animals, plants, climate or other aspects of life (Cajete, 2000; Cunningham & Stanley, 2003; Kasirisir, 2016; Little Bear, 2012). As all entities are interconnected through these interactions, people are not considered separate beings; we are part of, and dependent on, these patterns, cycles and changes (Baskin, 2016; Hart, 2015). This recognition of interconnection reflects the philosophical and practical emphasis on holism (Burnette & Figley, 2017; Hart, 2002; Mark & Lyons, 2010). Little Bear (2012) expressed it this way: 'If everything is forever moving and changing, one has to look at the whole of being to discern developing patterns' (p. 523). Thus, Indigenous philosophical orientations tend to be holistic (Absolon, 2010; Mark & Lyons, 2010; Hart, 2015).

These philosophical understandings have led to other foundational points held in many Indigenous societies. These points are diversity, relationship and interdependence. There is recognition that lands, waters and other beings are greatly diverse, including diversity of their actions. There is understanding that parts of the lands, waters and beings are constantly adjusting to the movements of other parts (Cajete, 2000). This diversity is reflected in people and their actions as well, where individuals and groups of people are constantly interacting and adjusting to the actions of others. These actions are what form, shape and end relationships. From this perspective, there are no relationships without action. These interactions support the understanding that all life is interdependent. As people, we demonstrate this interdependence, including mutual responsibility and working together, through such means (Te Momo, 2015).

It is through the understanding of relationships and interdependence that many Indigenous societies have developed ways of being that emphasize community, egalitarianism and respectful individualism. Indigenous societies tend to be communal where there is a desire by community members to be part of their community and contribute to the well-being of the group as a whole. At times, community is a formalized entity with a territory and a politically represented population. At other times, most often due to external colonial forces, community is loosely defined and with a greater focus on social interactions as the key dynamic holding the community together. In either case, many Indigenous communities have a strong sense of working together and providing support to one another to achieve communal goals (Baird, 2013; Hart, 2008, 2009; Novogrodsky, 2012; Zander, Dunnett, Brown, Campion, & Garnett, 2013). Gross (2003) has noted that in addition to the communal focus there is also a focus on individuals that needs to be considered. Some Indigenous nations give individuals great leeway in determining their own actions. It is understood that this leeway is granted since individuals are orientated to contributing to the well-being of the community (Gross, 2003; Brant, 1990; Prowse, 2012). Gross (2003) referred to this symbiotic relationship between individuals and communities as 'respectful individualism' where 'the individual takes into consideration and acts on the needs of the community, and does not act on the basis of selfish interest alone, so the community is willing to grant a given individual great leeway in personal expression' (p. 129). This balance of respectful individualism and communalism emphasizes the egalitarian orientation of many Indigenous societies.

Indigenist social work

Indigenist social work is based on Indigenous philosophies, knowledges and ways of being, as well as the political and social contexts that Indigenous peoples face (Hart, 2007, 2009). It can be symbolically seen as an inner circle with the foundational centre grounded and nurtured by traditional Indigenous values, beliefs, knowledges and practices and an outer circle that confronts and pushes back against the colonial oppression Indigenous societies are facing. This pushback creates more space for Indigenous philosophies, knowledges and ways to exist and operate with less colonial control and imposition.

The inner circle focuses on relationships and the interactions at the individual, familial, group and community levels. Following the holistic understanding of Indigenous philosophies, these relationships are seen contextually in both the traditions and cultures of Indigenous peoples, as well as the lands, waters and other life in the local territory (Green & Baldry, 2008; Mark &

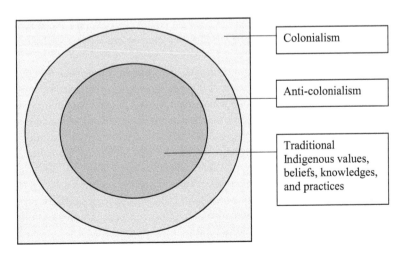

Figure 23.1 Indigenist social work

271

Lyons, 2010). Further, this holistic understanding includes the historic, social, economic and political dynamics, as well as the mental, spiritual, emotional and physical aspects of individuals (Hart, 2002, 2015; Hart & Rowe, 2014; Mark & Lyons, 2010; Mafile'o & Vakalahi, 2016). These entities, relationships and dynamics are considered in terms of how they are impacting or supporting the relationships of the people social workers are serving. As such, individuals are seen as members of families, groups and communities who are interacting in contextualized ways where relational patterns and cycles emerge (Hart, 2015; Weaver, 2008). Ideally, people interact in ways meant to strengthen, balance and harmonize their relationships. However, these interactions also include periods of flux where individuals, families, groups and communities experience significant change, even upheaval, in their cycles and patterns (see Chapter 18). At these times of significant change, people seek to rely on their relationships to re-establish balance and harmony. Alternatively, there are times when people are caught in patterns that are consistent but may not be supporting them to move forward with emerging relationships, changes in their context or growth from within. These patterns are often seen as harmful to individuals, families, communities or peoples.

One of the consistent yet harmful patterns that Indigenous people face is colonialism, represented by the box surrounding the two circles. There are many definitions of colonialism. However, most definitions do not well reflect Indigenous perspectives. An Indigenous definition is more encompassing where colonialism is understood as the processes through which the colonizing group's beliefs, values and practices are imposed on Indigenous peoples at the cost of Indigenous lives, beliefs, values, practices, resources and lands. These oppressive processes seek to hinder, if not stop, Indigenous peoples on individual, family, community and nation levels from making decisions about their own lives including how, if at all, they choose to incorporate the ideas, beliefs, values and practices of other peoples. The implementation of this oppression varies from being outright violent to unconsciously inflicted. Overall, the intent remains where Indigenous people are to be dominated and their exercise of self-determination over their own lives, territories and resources is to be obstructed (Hart, Straka, & Rowe, 2016; Hart & Rowe, 2014). The theme of colonialism from this perspective is separation. Through colonial oppression, Indigenous people face separation from their traditional lands and waters, cultures and histories, families and communities and identities. In addition, colonizing forces separate Indigenous people from their bodies through dismemberment or death (Razack, 2015); their minds by decreeing what to think and predetermining what knowledge is valuable; their hearts by dictating what they can and cannot feel; and their spirits through demonizing their essence, outlawing their spiritual ways of living or killing their spiritual leaders (Hart, 2002).

Anti-colonialism confronts this oppression and the separation processes. Symbolically, it is the outer circle that works to (a) create space for the inner circle that encompasses the traditional practices, beliefs and values of Indigenous peoples and (b) protect the inner circle from colonial oppression. Indigenist social work practice incorporates an anti-colonial stance, where anti-colonialism is defined as colonized peoples' proactive, holistic struggle against the political, economic, social and cultural oppression they experience, including the beliefs, values and practices associated with this oppression (Ashcroft, Griffiths, & Tiffin, 2013; Hart et al., 2016; Smith, 2012). An anti-colonial stance recognizes that colonialism continues today. It resists and challenges the imposition of power and control over Indigenous people and their territories and supports the self-determination of Indigenous individuals and communities and the revitalization of Indigenous cultural, social, economic and political institutions.

Indigenist anti-colonialism recognizes that these power differentials occur on the structural level as well as the individual level. As such, anti-colonialism requires a significant degree of self-reflection to address how structures and individuals access, incorporate, hold and utilize power to confront or support colonialism. The use of power is tied to racism, privilege, whiteness, settler fragility, internalized dominance, micro-oppressions and internalized oppression. Indeed, racism is a vital construct used to maintain colonial oppression on various levels, including the individual and structural levels (Dominelli, 1997; Hart & Lavallee, 2015; Memmi, 1991/1965; Mullaly, 2007). Individuals have to spend time coming to understand these dynamics to change their own actual and potential participation in the colonial oppression of Indigenous peoples. To develop a deeper understanding of colonial oppression, racism and privilege, indigenist social work relies on Indigenous knowledges as well as critical theories and literature on social justice. Literature addressing colonialism, neo-colonialism, anti-colonialism, post-colonialism, and decolonization support the conceptual foundation of anti-colonialism (Green & Baldry, 2008; Hart, 2007, 2009). Further, individuals and institutional structures have to be action orientated; knowledge alone is not enough. There is a focus on moving beyond 'awareness' and 'sensitivity' to working toward a shift of power to increase Indigenous peoples' implementation of self-determining actions. In addressing power distributions on various levels, the matter of rights, including Indigenous rights, human rights and ecological justice plays a central role in working for and supporting Indigenous self-determination.

Guiding values and processes

Indigenist social work relies on several values that stem from Indigenous peoples' ways of being. As previously noted, philosophically, Indigenous peoples have often emphasized interconnection and interdependence, community and respectful individualism. There are values that reflect these central philosophical points and come into indigenist social work practice. These values include sharing and reciprocity (Hart, 2014; Hertel, 2017; Kirkness & Barnhardt, 1991; La & Wasilewski, 2004; Mafile'o, 2008) and respect (Hart, 2009; McAuliffe et al., 2016; Muller, 2014; see also Chapters 7–9). Reflecting a commitment to others, individuals are encouraged to share with others in their families and communities, especially with those who have less and may be struggling. Some Indigenous cultures will have formalized ways to support the redistribution and reciprocity, such as the potlatches of nations in northwest North America (Trosper, 2002), the give-away ceremony of central plains nations (Hallowell, 2010) and the growing and sharing of food in Aotearoa (Ritchie, 2015). The idea of sharing is tied to the idea of reciprocity, where individuals see themselves as giving to and receiving from their communities as well as the land and waters (Kornelsen, Boyer, Lavoie, & Dwyer, 2015/2016; Trosper, 2002). In indigenist social work, practitioners' knowledge and skills are seen as gifts to others, where the idea of gifting reflects an important concept and process for Indigenous peoples in various parts of the world (Kuokkanen, 2007; Whitt, 2004). Respect is also tied to the idea of reciprocity, in that respect of others is important to the collective well-being (Hart, 2008; Mafile'o, 2008). However, respect for others on its own merit is also required as all life deserves respect (Weaver, 2008).

Indigenist social work recognizes that there are values that particular peoples emphasize that should be foundational to practice with them. For example, Tongan values of *fetokoni* (mutual help), *faka'apa'apa* (respect), *'ofa* (love) and *tauhi vā* (nurturing relationships) are incorporated in Tongan social work (Mafile'o, 2008). Another example is the significant importance of the Seven Sacred Grandfather Teachings of *nibwaakaawin* (wisdom), *Zaagi-idiwin* (love), *Manaazodiwin* (respect), *zoongide'ewin* (bravery), *gwekwaadiziwin* (honesty), *dibasendizowin* (humility) and *dibasendisowin* (truth) (Absolon, 2009; Day, 2014) for the Anishinaabek. Munford and Sanders (2011) outline several specific values important to Maori social work, namely *mana* (respect, valuing others' views) *wairuatanga* (the spiritual dimension of life) *whanau* (wider family) and *whakapapa* (geneology). All nations will have values that are central to their cultures. Indigenist social work reflects the specific values of Indigenous nations and peoples being served.

Several Indigenous cultural processes common to many Indigenous cultures are incorporated in indigenist social work. Indigenist practitioners have incorporated storytelling (Adelowo, 2016; Hart, 2014), rituals and ceremonies (Desjarlais, 2012; Moghaddam, Momper, & Fong, 2015; Richardson, 2012), being on the land and waters (Absolon, 2008; Baikie, 2009; Green & Baldry, 2008) and spending time with elders and traditional healers (Absolon, 2010; Day, 2014). While these processes more commonly held across nations are incorporated into indigenism, there is a strong recognition that indigenist social work has to reflect the practices of local people. Consequently, processes of particular Indigenous peoples, areas and cultures are also reflected in indigenist social work. These include *Ho'oponopono*, a family conflict resolution that evolved and is used by native Hawaiians (Hurdle, 2002); the use of medicine wheels and circles by Anishinaabek people (Absolon, 2010), the Murri way found in Australia and Torres Strait islands (Lyn, 2001) and the incorporation of sweat lodges facilitated by highly trained traditional practitioners of particular Indigenous first nations in North America (Schiff & Pelech, 2007).

Critical analysis and the impact on social work

Indigenist social work gives voice to Indigenous peoples on issues on various levels of concern and attempts to link individual experiences with structural issues created by an oppressive framework. As with other broad and multifaceted approaches to social work, indigenist social work theories have several areas that have been or could be critiqued. As an area within social work, indigenism is quite new, and thus has few direct critiques. However, parallel critiques may also relate to indigenist social work. These include key matters around identity, culture and how to support individuals to create change under macro issues of oppression (see Chapter 29). In addition, as indigenist theories are heavily based in perspectives, experiences and practices unfamiliar to settler societies and their dominating epistemological perspectives, there are critiques around its development. These include who can practice from this approach and when they may do so, the research available to support the approach, Indigenous forms of knowledge development and the amount of preparation needed to practise indigenist social work. A significant critique relates to the concept of spirit and its subjective nature that is most often framed within a religious context. This critical analysis begins with a direct critique related to the value base of social work and Indigenous values.

While there is recognition of the hegemonic spread of Western social work (Brydon, 2011), the need for developing Indigenous social work practice is still questioned (Cheng Yuk-Tin, 2011). It has been suggested that social work values are 'normative': in other words, values that are reflected universally by people. The critique goes on to suggest that social work values are based on rationally justified moral principles and that these normative values serve the profession from a moral point of view by providing rational, logical justifications regardless of the social and cultural background of the people involved. Cheng Yuk-Tin goes on to explain that Indigenous values, and in turn Indigenous social work practices, are 'positive' in that they are only upheld by a particular group from particular regions, thus tied to particular social and political realities. They are more about social explanations than they are about normative evaluations. As such, those arguing for Indigenous-based social work are erroneously conflating local positive values with generalized normative values.

On the other hand, there is concern that indigenist social work may not recognize well the differences between Indigenous peoples from various parts of the world, including differences between peoples whose traditional territories are side by side. For example, Chong (2016) has noted the significant diversity in Indigenous peoples in Taiwan recognized by the Taiwanese government. These groups have unique histories, cultures, languages and family structures, and, therefore, the various Indigenous peoples should not be stereotyped together under the conceptual construct of 'Indigenous group' (Chong, 2016). The concern about stereotyping Indigenous people as one group extends to, and within, other regions of the globe. This critique relates to another area of critical analysis: namely, the focus of indigenist social work on concepts around identity and culture.

Indigenous identities have been under scrutiny since early interactions between Indigenous and European peoples, and the concept of identity is itself contested. While the United Nations has provided a non-defining discussion of the concept, many people continue to look at a checkbox means of identifying who is and who is not Indigenous. Part of the rationale for requiring a definition of 'Indigenous' reflects empirical-positivistic efforts to define concepts so the concepts can be 'objectively' measured and re-measured. This need for a clear definition is heavily influenced by political factors, particularly territorial dispossession, how natural resources are to be used and who is to benefit from use or extraction of the natural resources. For many Indigenous peoples, a checkbox approach is seen as continued symbolic and violent search for 'authentic' Indigenous peoples (Maddison, 2013) that is tied to control, if not elimination, of Indigenous people as peoples. As an alternative to the checkbox method, efforts have been made for people to self-identify as Indigenous, such as the discussion provided by the United Nations (n.d.). Overall, debates on stricter definition standards or leaving the matter as a self-determining exercise remain (Lawson, 2014).

These critical debates run parallel to those addressing the concept of culture. Lawson (2014) notes that culture is a contested yet influential term that carries significant normative weight. Practices that are considered part of a 'culture' are often given superior moral consideration and legitimacy. However, the means to determine what are recognized as cultural practices are greatly influenced by individuals external to the cultures being described. Those with greater power are able to shape, create and drop the identification of cultural practices. This power dynamic has led to the appropriation and reconstruction of Indigenous cultural practices by powerful individuals and groups who are not from the culture as a means to uphold a settler society's power (Aldred, 2000; Smits, 2014; Waldron & Newton, 2012). It has also led other powerful individuals within the cultural group to identify narrowly what are 'legitimate' practices, thus limiting who can reflect or access the cultural practices (Lawson, 2014). These critiques around identity and culture lead to questions of who may utilize indigenist social work and which cultural practices may be used in social work. The questioning extends to when indigenist social work could be utilized and with whom. Within this context, the practice of indigenist social work is itself a political act.

This point of indigenist social work being a political act relates to another critique: namely supporting individuals to create change under macro issues of oppression. While many authors have outlined how colonialism has impacted individuals greatly (Hart, 2002; Linklater, 2014; Duran & Duran, 1995), more often the focus remains on the macro level, addressing issues such as economic and political factors, and usually from a position that neglects indigenist perspectives. While indigenism presents explanations of the interconnections between individual experiences and colonial structures of oppression, these explanations are more often seen as anecdotal, if understood at all by people of the dominant society. As a result, indigenist social work may be seen as a macro approach that is not well connected or necessarily relevant to direct practice.

There is also questioning that centres around the development of indigenist theories. Indigenist social work relies on indigenist epistemologies and methodologies (Absolon, 2011; Hart,

2010; Kovach, 2009). These philosophical research orientations may be critiqued for their lack of objectivity and a lack of generalizability. One aspect of this critique exemplifies it over-all. Indigenous epistemologies significantly incorporate the researcher in the research process. Researchers' social locations, such as their positions in their communities and their life experiences, are seen as relevant to and influential on the research. Instead of trying to be 'objective' by disregarding or controlling these influences, Indigenous epistemologies recognize that research-ers are part of how people come to know and expect them to self-examine and identify their social location and to acknowledge the point that they influence the entire research process (Absolon, 2011; Hart, 2010; Kovach, 2009) This incorporation of the researcher's self may be seen by others as a limiting factor that raises questions about the significance of the research for other situations and people.

Another critique relates to the expectation that indigenist practitioners should be deeply versed in indigenist perspectives, experiences and practices. Most social workers, particularly those not from Indigenous societies, are not well-versed in the perspectives, experiences and practices of traditionally based Indigenous people. The expectations placed on indigenist prac-titioners go beyond their social work practice to a scope that encompasses all aspects of their lives (Hart, 2009). It can be argued that such expectations are beyond what a profession should expect. Individuals should be able to determine their own life choices without having to be judged on whether these choices affect their practice. This matter is compounded for individu-als of settler societies and their lack of experience with and understanding of colonial oppres-sion, Indigenous perspectives of social issues and Indigenous-based practices. These expectations placed on potential practitioners mean that indigenist social work requires a degree of education and preparation that is beyond almost all current offerings of social work education and outside the life experiences of many people.

Perhaps one of the elements of indigenist social work that raises the strongest critiques is the incorporation of the concept of 'spirit'. Western ontologies have tended to emphasize the isola-tion of spirit to matters of religion (see Chapter 11). When spirit is incorporated into knowl-edge development and practice, it is seen as religion directing knowledge development, thus emphasizing faith-based actions without empirical support. From this stance, spirit is generally understood as too subjective as it cannot be addressed without a religious context.

A final area of analysis relates to the need for continued critique of indigenist social work. As has been noted (Ugiagbe, 2015), indigenist social work practitioners cannot blindly adhere to Indigenous traditional social and cultural structures. All societies have elements that can be questioned for how they treat their own citizens. Any society has to be able to question, openly and critically, the maintenance of oppressive inequities and injustices within their society. Any society, including Indigenous societies, has to assess critically its values, beliefs and practices about how it upholds such things as the hegemony of patriarchal systems, heterosexuality and physical ability.

Importance of indigenist social work to the profession

Indigenist social work has been important to social work as it provides approaches to work with Indigenous peoples that are consistent with their ways of being in the world, including their values, beliefs and practices. It provides support to people across Indigenous nations while upholding local ideas and the practices of particular peoples. This dynamic has provided a foun-dation for Indigenous social workers from various parts of the world to come together, share their experiences and approaches and support individual Indigenous social workers to work in ways that directly reflect their nations and peoples. Indigenist social work has also provided a framework for settler social workers to understand how to proceed in ways that support the self-determination of Indigenous nations and persons. It has encouraged settler social workers to recognize the need for continuous critical self-reflection and to see how the profession is not free from participating in the oppression of Indigenous peoples. It has also re-emphasized the need for advocacy, supportive practices and making room for other ways of practice beyond those of the dominant theories and practices of settler societies.

While these developments in social work have been important, there remains much work to be done. There is still a tendency to lump Indigenous people together and only have the ideas of particular Indigenous people act as the representative ways for all Indigenous peoples. There is still the tendency to see the issues Indigenous peoples face as individual issues, as opposed to structural concerns impacting the relationship between Indigenous and settler societies. Colonialism is too often seen as over and the remaining concern as being how to help individuals adjust to the past impacts. This concern is also related to many settler social workers who are overwhelmed with the much-needed self-reflection and seeing how they may be participating in the oppression. Such social workers try to find solace by erroneously seeing colonialism as a past issue or by ignoring how they are implicated as social workers. The recent stances of professional bodies such as the International Association of Schools of Social Work, the International Federation of Social Workers and the Canadian Association of Social Workers on Indigenous peoples has not well reached individual social workers, service organizations or education institutions.

The primary strength of these ideas in the future will lie with Indigenous social workers who will undertake the critical self-reflection processes and make the commitment to stand with Indigenous individuals, communities and nations as they push forward for self-determination. The strength will lie in these social workers' ability to consistently reflect the values, beliefs and practices of Indigenous peoples. Thus, as long as Indigenous people continue to enter the social work profession on their own grounds, the strength of these ideas will remain, if not grow. This growth will be supported by settler social workers who learn about the historic and current colonial processes and will ensure that local Indigenous peoples determine how social work knowledge and skills will be utilized by the people. These social workers will be the ones to join Indigenous people in maintaining anti-colonial social work practices in support of indigenist social work. Overall, the future of indigenist social work will depend on the willingness of any social worker to go beyond what is presently taught in social work education to learn how to establish and maintain a culturally based, positive, respectful and safe relationship with Indigenous people, communities, and nations.

Further reading

As an emerging focus in the field of social work, the resources addressing indigenist social work are limited and recent. Some readings to considered by those seeking to learn more about this focus include the following:

Hart, M. A., Burton, A. D., Hart, K., Halonen, D., & Pompana, Y. (Eds.). (2016). *International indigenous voices in social work*. Newcastle-upon-Tyne: Cambridge Scholars Publishing.
    This book, written by Indigenous and non-Indigenous scholars, presents three areas relevant to indigenist social work: resurgence, implementation and collaboration. It gives examples of how Indigenous people have turned to Indigenous values, beliefs and practices and implemented them in practices. It also outlines the anti-colonial perspectives of several settler social workers on how they collaborate with Indigenous peoples as allies.

Mafile'o, T., & Vakalahi, H. F. O. (2016). Indigenous social work across borders: Expanding social work in the South Pacific. *International Social Work, 61*(4), 537–552.
This article exemplifies many points identified here through a particular context, specifically the South Pacific. It demonstrates the importance of understanding local matters while relating across Indigenous nations.

References

Absolon, K. (2008). *Kaandosswin, this is how we come to know: Indigenous graduate research in the academy: Worldviews and methodologies.* (Unpublished doctoral dissertation). University of Toronto.

Absolon, K. (2009). Navigating the landscape of practice: Dbaagmowin of a helper. In R. Sinclair, M. A. Hart, & G. Bruyere (Eds.), *Wicihitowin: Aboriginal social work in Canada* (pp. 172–199). Winnipeg: Fernwood.

Absolon, K. (2010). Indigenous wholistic theory: A knowledge set for practice. *First Peoples Child and Family Review, 5*(2), 74–87.

Absolon, K. E. (2011). *Kaandossiwin: How we come to know.* Halifax, NS: Fernwood.

Adelowo, A. (2016). African oral tradition/narrative as an African paradigm. In M. A. Hart, A. D. Burton, K. Hart, G. Rowe, D. Halonen, & Y. Pompana (Eds.), *International indigenous voices in social work* (pp. 41–60). Newcastle-upon-Tyne: Cambridge Scholars Publishing.

Aldred, L. (2000). Plastic shamans and Astroturf sundances. *American Indian Quarterly, 24*(3), 329–352.

Ashcroft, B., Griffiths, G., & Tiffin, H. (2013). *Postcolonial studies: The key concepts* (3rd ed.). New York: Routledge.

Baikie, G. (2009). Indigenous-centred social work. In R. Sinclair, M. A. Hart, & G. Bruyere (Eds.), *Wicihitowin: Aboriginal social work in Canada* (pp. 42–64). Halifax, NS: Fernwood.

Baird Ian, G. (2013). Indigenous peoples and land: Comparing communal land titling and its implications in Cambodia and Laos. *Asia Pacific Viewpoint, 54*(3), 269–281.

Baskin, C. (2016). Spirituality: The core of healing and social justice from an Indigenous perspective. *New Directions for Adult and Continuing Education, 152,* 51–61. doi:10.1002/ace.20212

Brant, C. C. (1990). Native ethics and rules of behaviour. *Canadian Journal of Psychiatry/Revue Canadienne De Psychiatrie, 35*(6), 534–559. Retrieved from http://uml.idm.oclc.org/login?url=https://search-proquest-com.uml.idm.oclc.org/docview/61260477?accountid=14569

Brydon, K. (2011). Promoting diversity or confirming hegemony? In search of new insights for social work. *International Social Work, 55*(2), 155–167. doi:10.1177/0020872811425807

Burnette, C. E., & Figley, C. R. (2017). Transcendence: Can a holistic framework explain violence experienced by Indigenous people? *Social Work, 62*(1), 37–44. Retrieved from https://doi-org.uml.idm.oclc.org/10.1093/sw/sww065

Cajete, G. (2000). *Native science: Natural laws of interdependence.* Santa Fe, NM: Clear Light.

Cheng Yuk Tin, C. (2011). Is the development of an Indigenous perspective on social work values justified? A preliminary conceptual exploration. *China Journal of Social Work, 4*(1), 83–94. doi:10.1080/17525098.2011.563948

Chong, H. H. (2016). The understanding of Indigenous peoples towards professional relationships: The case of Taiwan. *International Social Work, 59*(2), 235–245.

Cunningham, C., & Stanley, F. (2003). Indigenous by definition, experience, or world view: Links between people, their land and culture need to be acknowledged. *British Medical Journal, 327*(7412), 403–404. Retrieved from www.bmj.com/content/327/7412/403

Day, P. A. (2014). Tradition keepers: American Indian/Alaska Native Elders. In H. N. Weaver (Ed.), *Social issues in contemporary Native America* (pp. 143–156). Burlington, VT: Ashgate.

Desjarlais, S. A. (2012). Emptying the cup: Healing fragmented identity: An Anishinawbekwe perspective on historical trauma and culturally appropriate consultation. *Fourth World Journal, 11*(1), 43–71.

Dominelli, L. (1997). *Anti-racist social work: A challenge for white practitioners and educators.* Basingstoke: Palgrave Macmillan.

Duran, E., & Duran, B. (1995). *Native American postcolonial psychology.* Albany: State University of New York.

Ermine, W. (1995). Aboriginal epistemology. In M. Battiste & J. Barman (Eds.), *First Nations education in Canada* (pp. 101–112). Vancouver: UBC Press.

Green, S., & Baldry, E. (2008). Building Indigenous Australian social work. *Australian Social Work, 61*(4), 389–402. doi:10.1080/03124070802430718

Gross, L. W. (2003). Cultural sovereignty and Native American hermeneutics in the interpretation of the sacred stories of the Anishinaabe. *Wicazo Sa Review, 18*(3), 127–134.

Hallowell, R. (2010). Time-binding in the Lakota sun dance: Oral tradition and generational wisdom, ETC. *A Review of General Semantics, 67*(1), 85–93.

Hart, M. A. (2002). *Seeking Mino-Pimatisiwin: An Aboriginal approach to helping.* Halifax, NS: Fernwood.

Hart, M. A. (2007). *Cree ways of helping: An indigenist research project.* (Unpublished doctoral thesis). University of Manitoba.

Hart, M. A. (2008). Critical reflection on an Aboriginal approach to helping. In J. Coates, M. Grey, & M. Yellowbird (Eds.), *Indigenous social work around the world: Towards culturally relevant education and practice* (pp. 129–140). Aldershot: Ashgate.

Hart, M. A. (2009). Anti-colonial indigenist social work: Reflections on an Aboriginal approach. In R. Sinclair, M. A. Hart, & G. Bruyere (Eds.), *Wicihitowin: Aboriginal social work in Canada.* Winnipeg: Fernwood.

Hart, M. A. (2010). Indigenous worldviews, knowledge, and research: The development of an Indigenous research paradigm. *Journal of Indigenous Voices in Social Work, 1*(1), 1–16.

Hart, M. A. (2014). A brief overview of Indigenous ways of helping. In P. Menzies & L. Lavallee (Eds.), *Journey to healing: Working with Canada's Indigenous peoples with addiction and mental health issues* (pp. 73–85). Toronto: Centre for Addictions and Mental Health.

Hart, M. A. (2015). Indigenous social work. In J. D. Wright (Ed.), *The international encyclopedia of social and behavioral sciences* (2nd ed.). Amsterdam, NL: Elsevier. Retrieved from http://dx.doi.org/10.1016/B978-0-08-097086-8.28041-0

Hart, M. A., & Bracken, D. (2016). Canadian social work and first nations peoples. In G. Palattiyil, D. Sidhva, & M. Chakrabarti (Eds.), *Social work in a global context: Issues and challenges* (pp. 59–73). Oxford: Routledge.

Hart, M. A., & Lavallee, B. (2015). Colonization, racism, social exclusion and Indigenous health. In L. Fernandez, S. MacKinnon, & J. Silver (Eds.), *The social determinants of health in Manitoba* (2nd ed., pp. 145–160). Winnipeg: Canadian Centre for Policy Alternatives.

Hart, M. A., & Rowe, G. (2014). Legally entrenched oppressions: The undercurrent of first nations peoples' experiences with Canada's social welfare policies. In H. N. Weaver (Ed.), *Social issues in contemporary Native America* (pp. 23–41). Burlington, VT: Ashgate.

Hart, M. A., Straka, S., & Rowe, G. (2016). Working across contexts: Considerations of doing indigenist/anti-colonial research. *Qualitative Inquiry, 23*(5), 332–342. doi:10.1177/1077800416659084

Hertel, A. L. (2017). Applying Indigenous knowledge to innovations in social work education. *Research on Social Work Practice, 27*(2), 175–177. Retrieved from https://doi-org.uml.idm.oclc.org/10.1177/1049731516662529

Hurdle, D. E. (2002). Native Hawaiian traditional healing: Culturally based interventions for social work practice. *Social Work, 47*(2), 183–192. Retrieved from http://dx.doi.org.uml.idm.oclc.org/sw/47.2.183

Kasirisir, K. (2016). Indigenous peoples and development of Taiwanese social work: Where are we? In M. A. Hart, A. D. Burton, K. Hart, G. Rowe, D. Halonen & Y. Pompana (Eds.), *International Indigenous voices in social work* (pp. 61–82). Newcastle-upon-Tyne: Cambridge Scholars Publishing.

Kirkness, V. J., & Barnhardt, R. (1991). First nations and higher education: The four R's: Respect, relevance, reciprocity, responsibility. *Journal of American Indian Education, 30*(3), 1–15.

Kornelsen, D., Boyer, Y., Lavoie, J., & Dwyer, J. (2015/2016). Reciprocal accountability and fiduciary duty: Implications for Indigenous health in Canada, New Zealand and Australia. *Australian Indigenous Law Review, 19*(2), 17–33.

Kovach, M. (2009). *Indigenous methodologies: Characteristics, conversations, and contexts.* Toronto: University of Toronto Press.

Kuokkanen, R. (2007). *Reshaping the university: Responsibility, Indigenous epistemes, and the logic of the gift.* Vancouver: UBC Press.

La, D. H., & Wasilewski, J. (2004). Indigeneity, an alternative worldview: Four R's (relationship, responsibility, reciprocity, redistribution) vs. two P's (power and profit). sharing the journey towards conscious evolution. *Systems Research and Behavioral Science, 21*(5), 489–503. doi:10.1002/sres.631

Lawson, S. (2014). The politics of Indigenous identity: An introductory commentary. *Nationalism and Ethnic Politics, 20*(1), 1–9. doi:10.1080/13537113.2014.878609

Linklater, R. (2014). *Decolonizing trauma work: Indigenous stories and strategies.* Winnipeg: Fernwood.

Little Bear, L. (2012). Traditional knowledge and the humanities: A perspective by a Blackfoot. *Journal of Chinese Philosophy, 39*(4), 518–527.

Lyn, R. (2001). Learning the 'Murri way'. *British Journal of Social Work, 31*(6), 903–916.

Maddison, S. (2013). Indigenous identity, 'authenticity' and the structural violence of settler colonialism. *Identities: Global Studies in Culture and Power, 20*(3), 288–303. Retrieved from http://dx.doi.org/10.1080/1070289X.2013.806267

Mafile'o, T. (2008). Tongan social work practice. In J. Coates, M. Grey, & M. Yellowbird (Eds.), *Indigenous social work around the world: Towards culturally relevant education and practice* (pp. 119–127). Aldershot: Ashgate.

Mafile'o, T., & Vakalahi, H. F. O. (2016). Indigenous social work across borders: Expanding social work in the South Pacific. *International Social Work. 61*(4), 537–552.

Mark, G. T., & Lyons, A. C. (2010). Maori healers' views on wellbeing: The importance of mind, body, spirit, family and land. *Social Science and Medicine, 70*, 1756–1764. doi:10.1016/j.socscimed.2010.02.001

McAuliffe, D., Tilbury, C., Chenoweth, L., Stehlik, D., Struthers, K., & Aitchison, R. (2016). (Re)valuing relationships in child protection practice. *Journal of Social Work Practice, 30*(4), 365–377. doi:10.1080/02650533.2015.1116437

McGregor, D. (2013). Indigenous women, water justice, and zaagidowin (love). *Canadian Woman Studies, 30*(2–3), 71–78.

McKenzie, B., & Morrissette, V. (2003). Social work practice with Canadians of Aboriginal background: Guidelines for respectful social work. In A. Al-Krenawi & J. R. Graham (Eds.), *Multicultural social work in Canada: Working with diverse ethno-racial communities* (pp. 251–282). Don Mills, ON: Oxford University Press.

McLeod, N. (2007). *Cree narrative memory: From treaties to contemporary times.* Saskatoon: Purich.

Memmi, A. (1991/1965). *The colonizer and the colonized.* Boston: Beacon.

Moghaddam, J. F., Momper, S. L., & Fong, W. T. (2015). Crystalizing the role of traditional healing in an urban Native American health center. *Community Mental Health Journal, 51*(3), 305–314. Retrieved from http://dx.doi.org.uml.idm.oclc.org/10.1007/s10597-014-9813-9

Mullaly, R. P. (2007). *The new structural social work* (3rd ed.). Don Mills, ON: Oxford University Press.

Muller, L. (2014). *Indigenous Australian health and human services work: Connecting Indigenous knowledge and practice.* Crows Nest, NSW: Allen & Unwin.

Munford, R., & Sanders, J. (2011). Embracing diversity of practice: Indigenous knowledge and mainstream social work practice. *Journal of Social Work Practice, 25*(1), 63–77. doi:10.1080/02650533.2010.532867

Novogrodsky, N. (2012). All necessary means: The struggle to protect communal property in Belize. *Wyoming Law Review, 12*(1), 197–214.

Prowse, C. E. (2012). Applying Brant's 'Native ethics and rules of behavior' in the criminal justice domain. *Canadian Journal of Native Studies, 32*(2), 209–220. Retrieved from http://uml.idm.oclc.org/login?url=https://search-proquest-com.uml.idm.oclc.org/docview/1498365657?accountid=14569

Razack, S. (2015). *Dying from improvements.* Toronto: University of Toronto Press.

Richardson, C. (2012). Witnessing life transitions with ritual and ceremony in family therapy: Three examples from a Metis therapist. *Journal of Systemic Therapies, 31*(3), 68–78.

Ritchie, J. (2015). Food reciprocity and sustainability in early childhood care and education in Aotearoa New Zealand. *Australian Journal of Environmental Education, 31*(1), 74–85. doi:10.1077/aee.2014.456

Schiff, J. W., & Pelech, W. (2007). The sweat lodge ceremony for spiritual healing. *Journal of Religion & Spirituality in Social Work: Social Thought, 26*(4), 71–93.

Smith, L. (2012). *Decolonizing methodologies: Research and Indigenous peoples.* London: Zed Books.

Smits, K. (2014). The neoliberal state and the uses of Indigenous culture. *Nationalism and Ethnic Politics, 20*(1), 43–62. doi:10.1080/13537113.2014.879764

Te Momo, O. H. F. (2015). Maori social work. In J. D. Wright (Ed.), *International encyclopedia of the social & behavioral sciences* (vol. 11. 2nd ed., pp. 505–511). Oxford: Elsevier.

Trosper, R. L. (2002). Northwest coast Indigenous institutions that supported resilience and sustainability. *Ecological Economics, 41*(2), 329–344. Retrieved from https://doi.org/10.1016/S0921-8009(02)00041-1

Ugiagbe, E. O. (2015). Social work is context bound: The need for Indigenization of social work a practice in Nigeria. *International Social Work, 58*(6), 790–780.

United Nations. (no date). *Who are Indigenous people? Fact sheet.* Retrieved from www.un.org/esa/socdev/unpfii/documents/5session_factsheet1.pdf

Waldron, D., & Newton, J. (2012). Rethinking the appropriate of the Indigenous: Critique of the romanticist approach. *Nova Religio: The Journal of Alternative and Emergent Religions, 16*(2), 64–85.

Weaver, H. N. (2008). Indigenous social work in the United States: Reflecting on Indian tacos, Trojan horses, and canoes filled with Indigenous revolutionaries. In J. Coates, M. Grey, & M. Yellowbird (Eds.),

Indigenous social work around the world: Towards culturally relevant education and practice (pp. 71–81). Aldershot: Ashgate.

Whitt, L. A. (2004). Biocolonialism and the commodification of knowledge. In A. Waters (Ed.), *American Indian thought: Philosophical essays* (pp. 188–214). Oxford: Blackwell.

Zander, K. K., Dunnett, D. R., Brown, C., Campion, O., & Garnett, S. T. (2013). Rewards for providing environmental services: Where Indigenous Australians' and Western perspectives collide. *Ecological Economics, 87*, 145–154. doi:10.1016/j.ecolecon.2012.12.029

24

The social pedagogy dimension of social work activity

Ewa Marynowicz-Hetka

Translated by: Magdalena Machcińska-Szczepaniak

Starting point

The social pedagogy interpretation within social work's multiplicity of meanings

To get to know the field of social work and to act in it, we adopt various perspectives, theories and methods (cf. Adams, Dominelli, &Payne, 1998; Labonté-Roset, Marynowicz-Hetka, & Szmagalski, 2003). Each of these modifies how we define social work and creates a specialized discourse relevant to that perspective. Examples are feminist, inclusion, radical, participatory, organization and management, institutional and critical currents in thinking. Social work has a multiplicity of meanings, and adopting a theoretical perspective selects from them and differentiates the scope of our practice. It particularly affects our approach to action, which, depending on the perspective we adopt, shifts:

- from protection, duration, stabilization, normalization (Foucault, 2004, 2012) and standardization, distribution of goods and services, management of problems and excesses of power that we can see in relationships
- through mediation and creating a space of shared experience (Dewey, [1947] 1968, cf. Marynowicz-Hetka, 2014), participation and cooperation
- to change, pursuing a reform perspective, seeking transformation or amelioration of social issues or a radical perspective, involving debate and systemic change

Thus, perceptions of social work and the meanings attributed to it lead to an interaction between practitioners and discourses within the academic discipline. Consequently, we can ask whether social work is, is becoming or should be a practice activity or a disciplinary discourse in which practice is debated as a metatheory of its activities.

Social pedagogy situates social work as a field of activity or practice and conceptualizes itself through description, interpretation and orientation as one metatheory of social work. In the social pedagogy perspective, the basic concept is 'activity'. Consequently, analyzing activity determines how professional practitioners conduct themselves and builds an integrated paradigm or model of the activity entailed by social pedagogical analysis.

Social pedagogy: a theoretical construct situating activity in social work practice

Social pedagogy is a theoretical construct: that is, an idea combining knowledge, understanding and values. It forms an orientation, a direction, for the social activity that practitioners undertake as they practice social work. An activity's orientation is expressed in the practitioner's mental processes, searching for knowledge, ideas and values relevant to the activity. Orientation helps us find possibilities for action by raising questions about why we are acting in this case and points to a strategy for our action: that is, why the activity makes sense and creates significance for the participants in it.

The social pedagogy perspective on practice incorporates:

- Analysis of how the particular practice of social pedagogy is formed, transformed or saturated with the characteristics that make it 'social work' and
- Conceptual ideas that orientate our activity as we practice. These ideas are incorporated as features of social work into practice.

My aim in this chapter is to present the social pedagogy perspective on practice, analyzing its characteristics and mechanisms and how it creates processes and transformation in people's lives. Since the chapter appears in Part 3 of this handbook, I do not consider other aspects of social pedagogy that establish it as an academic discipline or sub-discipline. Instead, I focus on outlining the conceptual framework of social and pedagogical paradigms of activity in the field of social practice. Its use goes far beyond the field of social work and can shape reflection in a range of disciplines on activity with the other.

Social pedagogy is a stream of thinking (Marynowicz-Hetka, 2007) situated 'at the intersection of human sciences, cultural sciences, social sciences and educational sciences' (Radlińska, 1961, p. 361). It refers in its analyses to American philosophical ideas of progressivism (e.g. Dewey ([1947] 1968) and pragmatism (e.g. James, [1910] 1957). The problem of cooperation is one of the most important in its discourse. It is perceived as a 'complete' concept, an intellectually complete system of pedagogy (Witkowski, 2014).

Social pedagogy points to pedagogical and social issues within social work, seeing it as a social activity, but crucially explains mechanisms that help us design change in and transform environments. Because of this, its educational dimension is highlighted, together with an educational approach to social work. Consequently, social pedagogy can be one of the disciplines forming the theoretical foundations of this area of social activity that we define as social work. At the same time, it establishes links among the ensemble of educational, cultural and social sciences.

The social pedagogy paradigm's emphasis on orienting or directing activity in practice develops that ensemble to form a coherent whole to provide the basis for interpreting reality as we observe it. Together, the paradigm and the ensemble constitute ontological, epistemological and axiological sources for our analysis of reality, producing a characteristic belief system and complex of mental imagery. Thus, social pedagogy questions the point of view that practitioners may take on the following issues:

- The meaning or place of individuals, seen as acting subjects in their milieu, and the complexity or duality of the links between subject and milieu;
- The possibilities, limitations or conditions that form or transform that environment: namely, human energy and potential which enable us to take action as well as wider resources; and
- The characteristics of social pedagogy in both its dimensions: as a discipline and as a paradigm for orienting activity.

Conceptual framework of social pedagogy's position on practice

The contemporary 'map' of social pedagogy, its research, practice, language, subjects, modes of operation and theoretical and methodological approaches, is extremely heterogeneous. This reflects its development as both a way of orienting activity and as a discipline or sub-discipline. Here, we focus on that aspect of social pedagogy concerned with constructing principles for orienting the actions of social pedagogues as acting subjects in practice. Other works (for example, Marynowicz-Hetka, 2006, 2007) consider social pedagogy in its disciplinary dimension, where concepts of complexity and transversality are two important features that argue for social pedagogy's claim as an academic discipline, forming an intellectually complete system of pedagogy. Transversality refers to the way in which concepts of social pedagogy are 'cross-cutting': that is, they cut across conventional discipline boundaries in social and other sciences. It also refers to the interlocking of the various dimensions discussed later in this section.

The conceptual framework of social pedagogy's perspective on practice is structured by two principles. The first recognizes that its conceptual whole fits in the mesostructural space: that is, social relations beyond the individual but not extending to the whole society (see also Chapter 15) and is organized around the social pedagogue's activity. The ontological sources of this activity are twofold:

Humanism, in which the concept of man as the subject of activity and as a participant in activity is expressed in a dualistic way, identifying human beings on the one hand as capable of acting (Ricoeur, 2004; Revault d'Allonnes, 2006), and on the other as at risk and sometimes expecting support and help. This meaning of duality identifies the complexity of the human situation viewed in a comprehensive way, rather than expressing a simple bipolarity (Witkowski, 2013).

A relational paradigm of non-strategic activity (Tillmann, [1989]1996), which, unlike strategic activity, focuses on agreement, cooperation, intersubjective sharing of experiences – that is, the people involved working in common with each other – and creating a new quality of relationship accepted by participants. Theoretical sources of these ideas include John Dewey's concept of activity ([1947] 1968) and the concept of intersubjectivity, whose features involve a kind of 'going beyond the subject's horizon' (Czyżewski, 2005, pp. 50–58).

The second principle structuring the social pedagogy perspective on practice is that it is defined by several dimensions: ontological, epistemological, axiological and methodological.

The ontological dimension of the social pedagogy approach is characterized by the capacity to envision the reality dealt with. The most prominent feature of this vision is its complexity and comprehensiveness. This results from:

- The interactive perspective that constructs this approach. This characteristic is present in Radlińska's early work (1935, pp. 15–16); she places the social pedagogy point of view 'at the intersection of other disciplines'.
- The practical dimension, focusing on critical analysis or contestation of reality, justifying the need to transform both it and the activity of the subject acting on practice.
- The degree of complexity of this practice and the extent to which we can expect to develop an overall understanding of individuals' sphere of life in the context of their whole lives.

The axiological dimension of the social pedagogy approach to practice recognizes that symbolic institutions have a special place (Castoriadis, 1975; Marynowicz-Hetka, 2006). The activity of a social pedagogue in practice creates a symbolic institution in the individual's milieu. This new institution is a set of norms and values at the interface of real and imaginary institutions.

The norms and values of symbolic institutions arise in relationships among individuals in the milieu. What Dewey ([1947] 1968, pp. 68–73, 90–92) calls 'shared experience' emerges from the intersubjective sharing of events. Experience, 'a set of sense constructs' (Barbier, [2011] 2017, p. 109), covers three mental and social spaces: experiencing activity, representing oneself and communicating about experiences. All three aspects of the experience are important subjects acting in practice. The space of communication is indispensable because, in the process of shared or intersubjectively common relations, symbolic space is constructed. This is a necessary consequence of creating a symbolic institution in each milieu. It is the essence of transformation that milieux are altered by this process.

While creation of a symbolic institution is the basis of activity in milieux, the second conceptual framework of social pedagogy in the axiological dimension comprises normativity and valuation. At least two aspects of these concepts are relevant:

- They form a reference point, the ultimate goal, of processing milieux – 'with human energy and potential – in the name of the ideal' (Radlińska, 1935, p. 19). Radlińska's concept of the 'ideal' here is of an image of our aims that provides a reference point as we intervene in social situations.
- They justify constructing a variety of evaluation tools that derive from the model and pattern of our work. As with the 'ideal', the model of our work is an idea of all the possibilities that for our intervention, reference points for our imagination in deciding on our actions. The pattern is the process of creating from the model the ideas that we select to work with as we intervene.

Normativity and valuation are important because they are characteristic of the social pedagogy view since they express the intention of interactions. They help us reconstruct and reorganize individual experiences into a whole shared with others. It is at the same time most exposed to controversy.

The axiological dimension social pedagogy in practice requires reflection on epistemological issues, taking into account the construction of:

- Tools for analyzing and defining a situation that requires us to take up an activity and explain and evaluate it.
- Value concepts that characterize the social pedagogy perspective and constitute grounds and reasons for orienting the activity involved. "Concept' is defined as the 'mental expression of one's relationship to the world and its transformation' (Barbier, [2011] 2017, p. 112; cf. Marynowicz-Hetka, 2006, pp. 83–86).
- Anticipatory and optimizing ideas necessary for co-creating projects and optimizing proposals with participants in practice. They direct the interaction by strengthening the human energy and potential present in the environment, anticipating events and setting up a community of activity, thus creating a symbolic institution.

The epistemological dimension of social pedagogy perspective locates activity in practice within its social context. Its characteristic feature is to acquire processuality and complexity, understanding reality and activity as holistic and increasingly complex (Morin, 2007). Social work practice involves a duality: it is concerned both with the empowerment of individuals and collectivities and with increasing individuals' capabilities to operate in their society. Wagner's (1998) 'diseconomic model' focuses on empowering individuals and communities whose environments create diseconomies that increase their difficulties. It is nevertheless important to provide support and assistance, working alongside individuals as they become capable of acting independently. There is a complex relationship between the human object of our interest and concern and the social objectives of the activity; these are equally valued and important.

Activity in practice becomes valued social activity by constructing an intersubjectively shared experience underlying the building of a symbolic institution. The orientation of such activity in social pedagogy aims to use reasoning to support the solutions adopted in the interaction and our interpretation and definition of the situation. The relational model of resolving problems or difficult situations, both individual and collective, is characteristic of this perspective. It underlines the importance of intentional influence, drawing on the conventional expectations of educational activity. Such views also favour exploring mediation among the participants, rather than focusing on problem management and distributing practical assistance. The radical view supporting contestation and struggle also accepts this approach but focuses on the transformational variation of change.

In response to these difficult questions – 'How should I act?' 'How do I act effectively?' – social pedagogy proposes interacting, creating and using the intersubjective space of experience and generating, in a shared way, a new quality of relationship expressed in a community's convictions and concepts concerning the direction of its final goals.

The methodological dimension of the social pedagogy perspective includes questions about the way to get to know and comprehend practice and how, in particular, to study such a complex construct as activity. How is it possible to develop our questioning into critical inquiry in situations as change takes place within them? Processuality brings together the prospects contained in the 'here and now' with a vision of the future. It is difficult in this process of critical inquiry to 'stop the film' and also to incorporate the temporality of activity and experience. The social pedagogy perspective on research requires complex thinking involving a synergy of research and activity, locating research 'within' practice. The concept of experience, not so much that of the individual as that shared by participants in practice, becomes an important element of social pedagogy research. It points to relationships between research and practice and synergy between research and professional activity, such as applied participatory, interactive and action research approaches (Paturel, 2014).

Transversality in social pedagogy: orienting activity in social practice: analytical tools

The starting point of this chapter identified the usefulness within social pedagogy of constructing the orientation of activity in practice, which may also be applied in social work. The most important focus of discussion is activity. Analysis of both activity and its orientation require us to develop an integrated or transversal (cross-cutting) approach because of the complexity of any social practice. Formation and transformation processes are characterized by two important premises:

- Change occurs processually, within a rhythm of ruptures and discontinuity (Bachelard, [1938] 2002).
- Processes of formation and transformation take place in the long term (Braudel, [1958] 1997, 1999) and acquire the qualities relevant for its long-term nature.

Analysis of activity in practice

Interest in the transversal analysis of activity emerges from approaches stressing the importance of activity and its analysis, referred to as 'discovery of activity' (Saussez, 2014, p. 188). It expresses a paradigmatic shift towards 'the inclusion of customary/routine terms into statements with scientific intention' (Barbier, [2011] 2017, p. 12). It is an example of a paradigm shift that has 'broken' the scientific orientation and abolished any demarcation between theory and practice. One of the important effects of this change is that research is positioned as 'accompanying activity' in which the subject, the person who acts, the practitioner modifies how the research is used.

The 'discovery of activity' reveals epistemological difficulties: 'How can one analyze activity within *networks* of connections and *multiplicities* of meanings?' This requires transversal research, breaking disciplinary and paradigmatic boundaries. Penetrating such ideas is not easy: it requires prior preparation but seems an exciting possibility for researchers interested in activity in practice, including social work practice.

My proposed transversal activity analysis includes the following elements:

- Its comprehensiveness, combining various aspects of activity, and its analysis, in which individual 'acts of activity, perception, cognition, displaying emotions and constructing oneself are inseparable' (Barbier, [2011] 2017, pp. 22–23). This achieves an overview activity not only from the point of view of what is seen, but also from that which is not directly seen, even though it is important for the whole process of the activity.

- Dynamics and processuality: how the activity transforms or evolves and how we may recognize this in practice. Activity analysis seeks to construct a configuration; the aim is not simply the limited one of dividing activity into particular fields. Continuing to problematize activity analysis allows us to recognize and accept the transversal perspective, searching for activity analysis tools that may be used in a range of fields and spaces.

- Locating activity in a changing context, subject to further change, means accepting its variability, evolution and transformation. Situating activity in context also requires taking into account many external circumstances. How may we combine the transversal and holistic dimensions of this concept with its singular and unitary dimensions? One way is to see activity as 'unitary activity organization', a category that can be successfully applied in analytical research work. It allows us to shift the meanings of actors' activities.

- Parallel construction of activities and of the subject, the person who acts. This is important for creating knowledge about activity and for constructing reflective practice by the actors.

- Discovery of activity emphasizes convergence, interdependence, reciprocity and articulation. We may describe the richness and complexity of activity occurring in different fields of practice and space. Because 'activity is life', discovery of activity values the intellectual effort involved in giving new meanings to the obvious, customary and routine meanings of concepts present in our lives. This shift is extremely important, friendly to practitioners, and indicates openness. It sensitizes us to how we construct knowledge of activity in practice, capturing how the activity itself works as part of practice.

This approach can be very useful both for research and reflection on practice. Barbier ([2011] 2017) developed transcendental ideas about activity analysis. Our lexicon for processes uses metaphorical wording such as 'spiral', 'loop', 'chain' and 'pair of interdependencies'. Otherwise, it would be difficult to express the complex duality of activity analysis.

In the transversal approach to activity analysis, the heuristic perspective is clearly present, an exploratory problem-solving approach. Consequently, discourse permeates the way we think of transformations of activity as processes that are multi-complex and interrelated. We intentionally attribute a discursive dimension to meanings: 'everything is a statement'. This results from refusing to see expressions as inseparable categories; for example, a concept may be expressed in mental, imaginative and discursive terms. Following this position, 'profession' is defined as a 'discourse on the profession, run by the group that performs it', and a 'professional' is a person 'able to report on the activity that is performed'.

If we say that 'the function of social sciences is to give new meanings', we distinguish two dimensions of analysis and analytic categories around them:

- *Mobilizing* concepts enable us to describe what subjects do in each space. They include the language of the act, defined as the lexicon of activity. These are the concepts that trigger the activity. We must recognize the complexity of such lexicons, which can be expressed in three registers of meanings: mental, affective and cognitive.
- Concepts of *intelligibility* allow us to create knowledge about activity. They are defined as the lexicon of activity intelligibility. These concepts allow us to establish connections between many elements within the activity, or rather their representations.

The transformation category is an important aspect of the heuristic nature of understanding activity in a holistic, transversal and processual way. Reflection on transformation processes – 'thinking of transformations' – occurs in various spaces. These are twofold. First, we generate mental space when we think about the process and course of activity, our own or others'. Second, we create discursive space when we communicate about taking up activity and following its course. Activity analysis uses numerous connections between these spaces. As a result, statements are constructed that, by expressing 'observable regularity', become the knowledge about activity.

The social pedagogy approach to activity in social work practice

The bases of the social pedagogy approach to practice were formulated in the 1930s by Helena Radlińska (1935). They express how we understand activity in an educational practice of social work and social action. In addition, they provide the main ontological and epistemological sources for formulating social pedagogy approaches to activity focused on work 'for' individuals, social groups and communities, 'together' with them and 'through' them. These ideas include social work practice in mediation or conflict roles (Castel, 1998). They are, however, less useful in justifying approaches that involve stabilizing the social order.

Understood in this way, activity in social practice requires reference to humanistic rather than technological paradigms. The social pedagogy perspective enables us to fulfil a principle of social work methods: 'do not give fish, but teach how to catch it'. Note here the educational emphasis. Compared with relational models of social work, educational issues express the specific characteristics of social pedagogical social work as it becomes social work. At the same time, those characteristics also link social work with social pedagogy.

The social dimension of activity in social work practice – elements of the analysis tool

Here, I try to answer the question: 'What is, specifically, the social dimension of social work?' Since the activity 'social work' is located in a social context, the characteristic feature of social pedagogy within social work is building the attributes of processuality and complexity, bearing in mind that the reality of social work activity is of increasing comprehensiveness and complexity (Marynowicz-Hetka, 2016b). The analysis tool helps us analyze the social dimension of social work activity.

Subject: shared experience. The first set of questions concerns the following issues. What is characteristic of practice actions? What are the expectations of and reasons for taking them, both external and in the subject's mind? And what is the best way to do it? These are questions about the subject of activity analysis. Fully answering them would require an extensive response; here I seek to explore the context of the activity.

Social work, from the social pedagogy perspective, is an activity that emphasizes the social dimension. Because it is geared towards a dynamic process of change and transformation, its emphasis on the social means helping individuals and groups engage in relationships with one another, with others and through others. Different models of it are formulated according to whichever theoretical and methodological references are dominant in the perspective that a practitioner is using.

Experiences are constructed and reconstructed in interactions; they move toward commonality with other participants in the practice activity. The process of acting in social practice occurs in a similarly relational or interactive way. Social work practice is recognized as a space within which the actors share experience, and the activity performed in the space is therefore also shared. This sharing is an important benefit of social work practice to social relations.

The focus of the social dimension of practice is relationship activity taken on without strategic aims. It is that aspect of subjects' activity that seeks to create symbolic institutions, the shared values that characterize the activity and its milieu. If we understand social work in this way, it often focuses on individual and collective empowerment in the four dimensions of the *disoeconomicus* model (Wagner, 1998), discussed above. These dimensions are: 'weight (load), support (base), protection and objectification (use)' (Witkowski, 2017). These dimensions fully define the range and complexity of situations which we may encounter in social work practice and identify the elements that interact within the activity.

Ways of analysis. The second element of the tool is the characteristic approach adopted to analyze phenomena within social situations. The social dimension of practice cannot be isolated from the social contexts in which it is situated and the processes used to analyze it. They form its senses and meanings. Locations of the social dimension, social context and processes of analysis in relation to external and internal social spaces are also important in developing credible practice measures. Attributes of the social dimension such as relativity, processuality, temporality, contextuality and location are crucial. These characteristics determine its scope, including limits to possible activity and opportunities and ways of going beyond them. This is also important for defining a situation's specific nature and designing procedures incorporating processuality and interactivity.

When discussing the way social work practice analyses, situations and processes through which milieux are formed and transformed, our method of analysis relates to paradigm shifts away from positivist scientific perspectives towards interpretative, participative approaches. This paradigm shift also permits us to use methods of analysis to disclose important elements of transformation in social work that are silent or noiseless (Jullien, 2009). Formation and transformation in practice are invisible to the participants for a long time. We notice modifications which are only partial outcomes of the processes taking place, those that are visible and easily seen. Other effects of formation and transformation of milieux are only observable in the long term (Braudel, [1958] 1997) and at moments of rupture (Lavelle, [1951] 1991; Bachelard, [1938] 2002). Discontinuity in processes is expressed by new elements interpenetrating old ones. Thus, processes of formation and transformation of milieux are complex, metaphorically depicted in the structure of a braid (Nawroczyński, 1947) or spiral. Transformations in practice are always conjoint (Barbier, [2011] 2017, pp. 69, 195), occurring alongside but affecting each other, and take different forms: construction, destruction and reconstruction.

Conceptual apparatus. Evaluating our own self-awareness of investigatory approaches and their epistemology is key to using the analysis tool to help us understand the social dimension of acting in social work. Participatory, interactive and transversal approaches are important within the conceptual apparatus, building on activity analysis. How we design the apparatus affects the vocabulary used when we take on and analyze activity. This enables us to make the discursive dimension of activity consistent and thus to explain meanings and their significance.

Barbier ([2011] 2017) distinguishes two types of vocabulary: the language of communication and the language that makes our acting intelligible. Subjects acting in practice use a specific language as they communicate with other actors. Characteristically, this type of vocabulary is strongly axiological, expressing values, and its meanings are simultaneously imaginative, affective and cognitive. Most statements in this type of communication in practice aim to assess the effects of activity or to inspire participants to undertake activity. Concepts are thus located in a kind of network with others. Barbier ([2011] 2017, p. 137) describes these as 'inter-semantic relationships of this type of vocabulary'.

Senses of and meanings given to significant concepts are important in social pedagogy approaches to social work practice: for example: 'social work', 'activity', 'formation', 'transformation', 'invisible environment', 'symbolic institution', 'experience'. By locating their meaning and the revealed sense in the humanistic paradigm and the relational model of activity, it becomes possible to move on to defining the social dimension of social work practice. Recognizing experience as subjected to continual reconstruction and reorganization enriches its content and extends our ability to direct further processes of experiencing (Dewey, [1947] 1968).

Understanding the social pedagogy perspective on activity as a process located in time and space allows us to express its elements: defining the situation, orienting the activity and its design and taking the course of activity. They are not stages or phases of activity, but rather ingredients of a spiral process in which they can interpenetrate and transform each other. Focusing on theoretical understanding of activity favours diversification of the perspectives that we use. For example, we can see this in extracting the dichotomous division 'strategic' and 'non-strategic' activity. In the former, we are 'the perpetrators of activity' (Kotarbiński, 1955, p. 22–25), and as we move forward, we are accompanied by the awareness that we have an impact on the natural course of things. We follow rational solutions, which in consequence are relatively easy to assess, by referring to our previously formulated objectives. In non-strategic activity, acting only changes the configuration of the process, its structure, course or the sequence of events. This is important when we experience difficulties in assessing practice activity because clear definition of the factors to evaluate and constant changes in our assessments result from the unpredictability of the course of activity. Here, evaluation changes its role and may be expressed probabilistically or as exploratory and shaped intersubjectively.

The concept of formation and transformation is important in social work because it emphasizes intentionality in practice activity and its location in the environment. It is also a key concept for social pedagogy. The milieu is captured comprehensively, including elements not visible to observers, such as wishes, expectations, feelings and hopes. It refers to the intimate world, named 'spiritual melioration' (Radlińska, 1937, p. 334). This 'melioration' process is facilitated by shared cultural heritage and incorporation of values meaningful for the chosen orientation of activity. Melioration refers primarily to educational processes in which elements invisible to outsiders are important. Both the practice of social work and the practice of education are activities. In both, social pedagogy sensitizes us to discover what is hidden.

The specificity of the social pedagogy point of view. Understanding the social dimension of activity in social work that has been assumed here is expressed in underlining the importance of the relational model of social work. Acting in the field of social work with such awareness allows this process to gradually acquire a social dimension and become social work, oriented on the other and finding the humanistic dimension of the relationship based on searching, revealing the individual and collective forces in the milieu and activity for it, through it, aiming to create a community, understood as a community sharing values. It is a systematic, continuous activity that includes the essential features of the process, such as anticipation of the consequences and rationalization, prior thought and designing transformation-oriented and optimization/melioration activities. The most important features of this activity are three dimensions: acting for the community, with it and through it. Reflection on these processes includes a system of concepts and meanings, which could be a reference for getting to know the activity – education, assistance in development, its orientation and justifying the choice of methods of activity. Appropriate detailed analysis can be ensured by providing for the relationship of social pedagogy as orientation of activity to other proposals of orienting activity present in sociology, psychology, philosophy, anthropology, ethnology and so on. If we accept (Barbier, [2011] 2017) that the paradigm is a set of rules of scientific activity that make up academic culture, then it will encompass both qualities relevant to the activity perceived as the creation of a symbolic institution and to the notion of culture of practice. The transversal approach to social pedagogy is drawn in two dimensions: a meta-concept that explains the real world from a social and pedagogical point of view and a multi-grounds analysis of the field of social practice and interpretation of its relationships directing the activity being undertaken. Such analysis of the field of practice makes the basis for constructing the conceptual framework of reflection on reflection.

Conclusion

In this chapter, we have tried to present, briefly, the original concept of social pedagogy expressed in its transversal paradigm of analysis and orientation of activity. This can provide the theoretical basis for formulating the social dimension of social work practice. It also allows us to analyze the mechanisms of formation, change and transformation of milieux with the aim of saturating social work practice with activity typical of social action. These attributes of the social pedagogy approach are very valuable and worth considering as we consider and seek to optimize social work practice.

In the social pedagogy paradigm focused on analyzing and orientating activity, social work practice is change oriented. This is, however, not a radical change, but rather a gradual shift, optimizing the social. In our conclusion, we would like humbly to sensitize researchers and social work practitioners to the barriers to and limitations of an acting subject making an impact on processes of change in practice. Practitioners should be encouraged to formulate limited expectations of modifying the configuration of the components of change processes and transformation in practice and consent to locating themselves merely in the role of accompanying persons. The focus of activity in the social pedagogy orientation is combining the 'unitary organization of activities' into chains of transformations imperceptible and invisible in practice. The usefulness of the social pedagogy perspective for social work practice perceived in this way enriches it by sensitizing it to the perception of holistic complexity of practice.

The analysis offered here is very much a summary and going further requires exploring the references and deliberation. Social pedagogy as a practical science, oriented towards optimizing reality and designing possible changes, is itself in the process of creating (constructing) and developing. Its heuristic dimension is very clear: it raises questions and builds analysis tools that help to formulate answers. They are not always easy and unequivocal because of the dual factors of the complexity of practice and its social context.

The culture of the social pedagogue's practice is saturated with the idea of cooperation, 'with', 'for', 'together' and 'through and with thanks to others'. A particular advantage of this cooperation is the others: that is, such individuals or communities that we are looking for in the milieu going beyond/growing above the average, thanks to their potential, capabilities and engagement. These are individuals capable of transforming space into a community in which the basic value is sharing of values, emotions, affect, views. The concept of shared experience enriches an important category of social pedagogy, the concept of the invisible environment and the symbolic institution; this underlines the multidimensional nature of space. Thus, social pedagogy understood in such a holistic way can provide a rich proposition, taking a metaphorical view of practice and its transformation for social work.

Further reading

Kornbeck, J., & Jensen, N. R. (Eds.). (2009). *The diversity of social pedagogy in Europe*. Bremen: Europaischer Hochschulverlag.
Hämäläinen, J. (2018). Social pedagogy. In N. Thompson & P. Stepney (Eds.), *Social work theory and methods: The essentials* (pp. 166–179). New York: Routledge.
Storø, J. (2013). *Practical social pedagogy: Theory, values and tools for working with children and young people*. Bristol: Policy Press.

References

Adams, R., Dominelli, L., & Payne, M. (Eds.). (1998). *Social work: Themes, issues and critical debates*. Basingstoke: Palgrave Macmillan.
Bachelard, G. ([1938] 2002). *Kształtowanie się umysłu naukowego Przyczynek do psychoanalizy wiedzy obiektywnej* [*Forming the scientific mind: A contribution to the psychoanalysis of objective knowledge*]. (D. Leszczyński, Trans.). Gdańsk: Wydawnictwo Słowo/Obraz/Terytoria.
Barbier, J-M. ([2011] 2017). *Vocabulaire d'analyse des activités: Penser les conceptualisations ordinaires* (2nd ed.). Paris: Presses Universitaires France.
Braudel, F. ([1958] 1997). *Les écrits de Fernand Braudel, Vol. 2: Les ambitions de l'histoire*. Paris: De Fallois.
Braudel, F. (1999). *Historia i trwanie* [*History and 'longue durée'*]. (B. Geremek, & W. Kula, Trans.). Warszawa: Czytelnik.
Castel, R. (1998). Du travail social à la gestion social du non travail. *Esprit*, 241(3/4), 28–47.
Castoriadis, C. (1975). *L'institution imaginaire de la société*. Paris: Editions du Seuil.
Czyżewski, M. (2005). Intersubiektywność [Intersubjectivity]. In *Encyklopedia Socjologiczna* [*Sociological Encyclopedia, Supplement*] (pp. 50–58). Warszawa: Oficyna Naukowa.
Dewey, J. ([1947] 1968). *Expérience et éducation* (M. A. Carroi, Trans.). Paris: Librairie Armand Colin.
Foucault, M. (2004). *Sécurité, territoire, population: Cours au Collège de France 1977–1978*. Paris: EHESS, coll. Hautes Études.
Foucault, M. (2012). *Du gouvernement des vivants: Cours au Collège de France 1979–1980*. Paris: Gallimard, Seuil.
James, W. ([1910] 1957). *Pragmatyzm: Popularne wykłady z filozofii* [*Pragmatism: Popular lectures on philosophy*] (W. M. Kozłowski, Trans.). Warszawa: Książka i Wiedza.
Jullien, F. (2009). *Les transformations silencieuses*. Paris: Grasset & Fasquelle.
Kotarbiński, T. (1955). *Traktat o dobrej robocie*. [*A treatise on good work*]. Łódź: Ossolineum.
Labonté-Roset, C., Marynowicz-Hetka, E., & Szmagalski, J. (Eds.). (2003). *Social work education and practice in today's Europe: Challenges and the diversity of responses*. Katowice: Wydawnictwo Naukowe Śląsk.
Lavelle, L. ([1951] 1991). *Traité des valeurs, Vol. 1*. Paris: Presses Universitaires de France.
Marynowicz-Hetka, E. (2006). *Pedagogika społeczna: Podręcznik akademicki, t. I*. [*Social pedagogy: An academic text*, Vol. 1]. Warszawa: Wydawnictwo Naukowe PWN.
Marynowicz-Hetka, E. (2007). Towards the transversalism of social pedagogy (B. Przybylska, Trans.). In F. W. Seibel, H-U. Otto, & G. F. Friesenhahn (Eds.), *Reframing the social: Social work and social policy in Europe* (pp. 85–102). Boskovice: Ed. Albert.
Marynowicz-Hetka, E. (2014). *Orientowanie działania: Rama konceptualna pojmowania kultury praktyki* [Orienting activity: A conceptual framework of comprehending a culture of practice]. In E. Marynowicz-Hetka, L. Filion, & D. Wolska-Prylińska (Eds.), *Kultura praktyki przedstawicieli profesji społecznych: Podejścia mediacyjne w działaniu społecznym* [*Culture of the practice of social professions representatives: Mediation approaches in social activity*] (pp. 17–31). Łódź: Wydawnictwo Uniwersytetu Łódzkiego.

Marynowicz-Hetka, E. (2016). Social pedagogy and social work: An analysis of their relationship from a socio-pedagogical perspective. (M. Machcińska-Szczepaniak, Trans.). *Sociální pedagogika* [*Social Education*], *4*(1), 13–24.

Morin, E. (2007). *Vers l'abime*. Paris: L'herne.

Nawroczyński, B. (1947). *Życie duchowe: Zarys filozofii kultury*. [*Spiritual life: Outline of the philosophy of culture*]. Kraków-Warszawa: Księgarnia Wydawnicza F. Pieczątkowski i S-ka.

Paturel, D. (Ed.). (2014). *Recherche en travail social: Les approches participatives*. Nîmes: Champ.

Radlińska, H. (1935). *Stosunek wychowawcy do środowiska społecznego* [*The attitude of the educator to the social environment*]. Warszawa: Nasza Księgarnia.

Radlińska, H. (1937). *Społeczne przyczyny powodzeń i niepowodzeń szkolnych* [*Social causes of school successes and failures*]. Warszawa: Naukowe Towarzystwo Pedagogiczne.

Radlińska, H. (1961). *Pedagogika społeczna* [*Social pedagogy*] Wrocław-Warszawa Kraków: Ossolineum.

Revault d'Allonnes, M. (2006). *Cet Èros par quoi nous sommes dans l'être'*. *Esprit, mars-avril, La pensée Ricoeur*, 276–289.

Ricoeur, P. (2004). *Parcours de la reconnaissance: Trois etudes*. Paris: Gallimard.

Saussez, F. (2014). *Une entrée activité dans la conception d'environnements de formation pour sortir d'une vision fonctionnaliste de la formation: Un essai de conclusion*. *Activités, 2*(11), 188–200. Retrieved from www.activites.org/v11n2/v11n2.pdf189

Tillmann, K-J. ([1989]1996). *Teorie socjalizacji: Społeczność, instytucja, upodmiotowienie* [*Theories of socialization: Community, institution, empowerment*]. Warszawa: PWN.

Wagner, A. (1998). *Debata o pracy socjalnej/pedagogice społecznej- reprezentujemy homogeniczny czy heterogeniczny paradygmat naukowy* [*Debate about social work/social pedagogy – do we represent homogeneous or heterogeneous scientific paradigms*] (D. Urbaniak-Zając, Trans.). In E. Marynowicz-Hetka, J. Piekarski, & E. Cyrańska (Eds.), *Pedagogika społeczna jako dyscyplina akademicka. Stan I perspektywy* [*Social pedagogy as an academic discipline: Status and perspectives*] (pp. 455–468). Łódź-Warszawa: Wydawnictwo UŁ, ŁTN, WSP ZNP.

Witkowski, L. (2013). *Przełom dwoistości w pedagogice polskiej: Historia: Teoria, krytyka* [*Breakthrough of duality in Polish pedagogy: History: Theory, criticism*]. Kraków: Impuls.

Witkowski, L. (2014). *Niewidzialne środowisko. Pedagogika kompletna Heleny Radlińskiej jako krytyczna ekologia umysłu i idei i wychowania. O miejscu pedagogiki w przełomie dwoistości w humanistyce* [*Invisible environment. Complete pedagogy of Helena Radlińska as a critical ecology of mind and ideas and upbringing. About the place of pedagogy in the turn of dualism in the humanities*]. Kraków: Oficyna Wydawnicza Impuls.

Witkowski, L. (2017). *Humanistyka stosowana. Wirtuozeria, pasje, inicjacje: Profesje społeczne* vs. *ekologia kultury*. [*Applied humanities. Virtuosity, passions, initiations: Social professions vs. ecology of culture*]. Kraków: Oficyna Wydawnicza Impuls.

25

Locality-based social development
A theoretical perspective for social work

Abiot Simeon, Alice K. Butterfield and David P. Moxley

Social development offers a singular framework to address the multiple and interrelated needs of not only individuals and groups, but also whole populations within geographies in which poverty is prevalent. Social development intertwines social institutions, policies and programmes to improve human well-being in nations undergoing development. Hobhouse recognized the relevance of social development in the early 1920s, in which mass literacy campaigns were seen as ways of bringing about development. By the 1940s, British colonialists used the term to describe Western efforts to address social unrest and economic issues in West Africa and other European colonies around the world (Midgley, 1995). Since the 1960s, the United Nations has played a key role in popularizing the social development approach. In 2000, the UN developed the Millennium Development Goals (www.un.org/millenniumgoals/) to underline the importance of social development. South Africa has built its national welfare policy on the foundation of social development (Patel, 2015), and work in Asia has emphasized the role of social development in social policy (Desai, 2013). Social development theory has been used in engaged research on human rights in Ghana (Sossou & Yogtiba, 2016) and the development of a professional association for social work in Namibia (Ananias & Lightfoot, 2012). The theory has been used to address the needs of unemployed middle-aged women in China (Sung-Chan & Yuen-Tsang, 2008), to facilitate the well-being of children in child welfare (Schmid, Wilson, & Taback, 2010), to create social entrepreneurship (Van Wyk & Mandla, 2010) in South Africa and to act in response to tsunami recovery in India (Hawkins & Nalini, 2008). Estes (1994) provides an early summary of four models of social development and curricular issues for social work.

Although social development emerged to address socio-economic issues in the Global South, this should not obscure its importance for countries across the globe that are seeking economic development (Midgley & Conley, 2010). Social development within social work is an important theoretical approach, relevant at practice, policy, organizational and community levels of action. What social development introduces to social work is its distinctive aim to improve the well-being of people at whatever level social workers practice.

Poverty alleviation as the cornerstone of social development

Midgley (1995), one of social development's earliest champions, defines social development as a process of planned social change to promote the well-being of populations, in conjunction with a dynamic process of economic development. As such, the cornerstone of social development is poverty alleviation. Social development is progressive and interventionist. It reflects progressive aims by prioritizing the reduction of social distance and disparities in the quality of life between those who enjoy the most and those who possess very little. The interventionist quality of social development means that practitioners, especially social workers, stand ready to act to promote the quality of life of those who possess limited resources, build infrastructure and create what Gil (1976) calls life-sustaining and life-enhancing resources.

Social development serves as a multidimensional, multilevel and value-based approach useful in addressing and resolving complex social issues (Pawar & Cox, 2010). It incorporates a comprehensive and integrated approach to address the economic, political, social, cultural and ecological aspects of society. Some definitions emphasize systematic planning and links between social and economic development. Some focus on structural change as the central element, and others focus on realizing human potential, meeting community needs and helping people increase their quality of life. Some concepts focus on the development process, others on outcomes of development and some on both process and outcomes (Pawar, 2014). Pandey (1981) proposes four types of strategies. The *distributive strategy* emphasizes the equitable distribution of resources and wealth for achieving social equality in the process of national development. The *participative strategy* promotes the involvement of all sections of the population in the development process. The *human development strategy* enhances the productivity and the income-generating capacity of the labour force. Lastly, the *social integration strategy* involves neglected communities and areas in development.

With the overall goal of promoting social welfare, social development has an inter- and transdisciplinary focus. It is strategic, inclusive and universalistic in scope and specifically emphasizes the well-being of all groups, while it prioritizes the advancement of the well-being of those suffering deep poverty. Social development activities frequently occur in societal and community contexts in which poverty and its serious, often debilitating consequences such as unemployment, little income, poor or diminished infrastructure, disease and limited social mobility are too well-rooted. Within such contexts, social institutions may face considerable challenge in advancing the quality of life (Selznick, 2002). Alternatively, local communities engaging in social development may produce considerable innovation, and social development policies at the institutional and government levels may open up opportunities for local communities. For social work, locality-based development is a means for improving the well-being of populations whose members are the most marginalized. Local communities can tap into leadership that can preserve their core values while advancing institutional responsiveness where needs are considerable (Selznick, 1957, 1992).

Another way of viewing social development is through its multiple societal levels (Figure 25.1). At the individual level, welfare as a whole is enhanced when individuals strive to promote their own welfare, typically through sustainable approaches to income generation. Policies and programmes promoting individual welfare include large-scale interventions that create an enterprise culture in the marketplace, as well as small-scale interventions that assist low-income families, small business proprietors and those in the informal sector. In the community strategy, social development is promoted by people working together harmoniously within their local communities. Still another mechanism is an organizational one. The development of local anchor institutions can mediate between individuals and larger social institutions. Anchor institutions may serve to distribute life-sustaining resources, promote life-enhancing opportunities and build strong local capacities for educating people, facilitating health, creating economic opportunities and producing jobs devoted to advancing the collective well-being. At all governmental levels, social development requires responsive institutions that are just and foster the

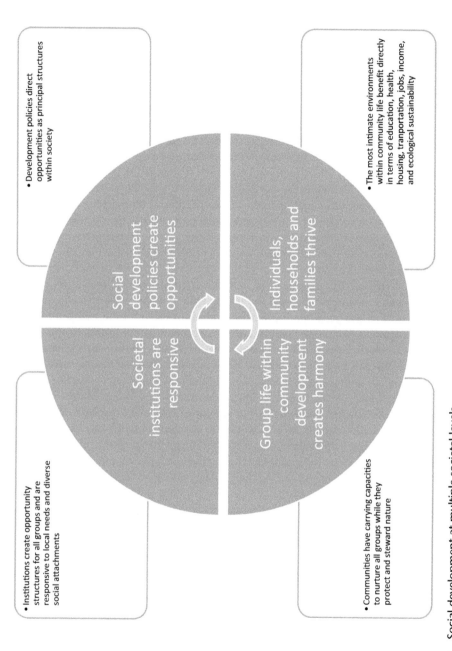

• Development policies direct opportunities as principal structures within society

• The most intimate environments within community life benefit directly in terms of education, health, housing, tranportation, jobs, income, and ecological sustainability

Social development policies create opportunities

Individuals, households and families thrive

Societal institutions are responsive

Group life within community development creates harmony

• Institutions create opportunity structures for all groups and are responsive to local needs and diverse social attachments

• Communities have carrying capacities to nurture all groups while they protect and steward nature

Figure 25.1 Social development at multiple societal levels

quality of life of all groups. Government has a vital role in organizing and promoting social development and ensuring that social development policies are implemented with harmonizing social and economic policies. Since responsive institutions build the fabric of society and its communities (Selznick, 2008), societal institutions and social policies can catalyze locality-based development.

We conceive of social development as the creation of what Huston (2007) and Kegan and Lahey (2009) call holding environments (see also Chapter 13). Such environments nurture human development across the life course, promoting quality of life at each phase of the life course while protecting nature and its own life-sustaining qualities. Thus, social development is complex and multidimensional and forms a space in which human policy interacts with ecological policy as a recognition that humans must live in correspondence with nature.

Locality-based social development

Although local level development can address years of neglect reflected in a community's extreme deprivation and can compensate for failures in development at the national level, little attention has been paid to local-level social development (Pawar & Cox, 2010). Locality-based social development is a neighbourhood-based community improvement strategy used to engage a broad range of key stakeholders in planning change, taking action and evaluating outcomes. Development occurs at the grassroots level and is initiated by leaders, residents and organizations that set out to understand local conditions. These actors establish goals by engaging people and employing specific strategies that align with the overall values, principles and processes of social development. Recognizing that development begins by utilizing local community structures, local communities exercise responsibility for their own development. Locality-based social development draws on theory in five areas of methods. These involve participation, bottom-up development, self-reliance, community capacity building and leadership in framing and enacting local action.

Participation, bottom-up development and self-reliance

Participatory development focuses on people's active involvement and the enhancement of their capacities for engaging in intentional social change. It is a people-driven, pro-poor, pro-vulnerable and pro–marginalized group strategy of development (Osei-Hwedie & Osei-Hwedie, 2010). Participatory development considers that communities have knowledge and awareness of their own conditions, assets and resources, member strengths and capabilities and barriers to development. Participatory development begins with approaching each situation with humility and respect, understanding the power and potential of local knowledge, adhering to democratic practices and acknowledging diverse ways of knowing. For the development practitioner, it requires maintaining a vision of sustainability, putting reality before theory, embracing uncertainty, recognizing the relativity of time and efficiency, taking holistic approaches to the complexity of human interactions and exercising options for the community (Keough, 1998). Weyers' (2011) analysis of published research identifies the habits of highly effective community development practitioners.

Bottom-up development incorporates different strategies that reflect the multidimensional nature of poverty. A bottom-up approach is key to the sustainability of local development since after a project is completed, it has to continue on its own (Akindola, 2010). A bottom-up approach emphasizes the active participation of residents, especially people who are poor, in defining local conditions and in conceiving of and selecting poverty alleviation strategies. For example, bottom-up development can improve income, open credit opportunities, gain health services and improve hygienic conditions and provide access to education. Democratic and participatory governance structures play critical roles in the participation and empowerment of local communities. Social development can enable poor people to participate politically, lead grassroots decision-making processes, and build and use people's capabilities to influence entities that affect their lives, thereby enhancing social productivity, individual autonomy and inclusive action.

Self-reliance is related to the principles of self-help and mutual support (Fonchingong & Fonjong, 2003). Self-reliance is independence and encourages people to improve their living conditions using home-based initiatives and the resources at their disposal (Kim & Isma'il, 2013). Four strategies for achieving self-reliance include rights-based, promotion of resilience, resource mobilization and participatory strategies, which value collective action and build partnerships between people and community institutions (Thomas & Pawar, 2010).

Community capacity building and leadership

Local capacity building is important in addressing poverty, inequalities, social exclusion and poor governance, thereby improving development outcomes in marginal communities. Variations of local capacity building include pathways to economic growth, pro-poor approaches and community-driven approaches (Yadama & Dauti, 2010). Capacity building focuses on participation, local leadership, critical assessment, organizational structure, resource mobilization, external linkages, agency and project management. Partnerships in local social development value the formation of relationships to maximize benefits for the poorest people. Partnerships cover relationships between organizations and their constituents. For productive local social development, an organization must invest in the formation of key relationships, promote participation, create partnerships and engage external power structures linking internal and external stakeholders (Burkett & Ruhunda, 2010).

Locality development brings forth natural leaders from within the community. It identifies, trains and mentors natural leaders so that they can take responsibility and ultimately direct local efforts in concert with other leaders from the locale (Kulkarni & Vaishnav, 2013). Diverse personnel are pivotal in local action: frontline or grassroots workers who are engaged in direct service delivery and mediation, supervisors and administrators, centralized planners, programme designers and policy personnel. Multiple pathways can produce numerous projects, making the field of action the organization supports complex. The complexity of action can require locality-based social development organizations to build numerous competencies and translate them into organizational structures that foster responsiveness and flexibility and in which human need is considerable and deprivation is severe. The social development literature under-appreciates the diversity of organizational forms that locality-based organizations can take in action and how they organize based on the needs, issues and aspirations existing among groups in their geographic place. Due to the lack of trained personnel, leaders often come from a wide range of vocational backgrounds without practice experience or theoretical training in locality-based social development (Cox & Pawar, 2010).

The aims of social development

Quality of environment and standard of living

Holism refers to the multiple processes social development organizations undertake to produce tangible benefits for humans and natural ecologies. The authors conceive of social development as grounded in the aim of promoting the *quality of environment* (or ecology) from which human existence emerges. The quality of environment may concern the quality of soil to stimulate local agriculture or agronomy, weather and climate conditions influencing seasonal shifts in agriculture and the quality of air and water influencing human and animal health. The interactions of human settlements with animal life and biotic species may also be instrumental in health. Social responsibility requires an organization or group or other entity to adopt a local duty to act to bring about conditions in which human beings, groups of human beings and the ecology thrive without the human imprint degrading local flora, fauna, water and soil, aspects of ecology necessary for sustaining human existence. The interactions among the environment and *standard of living* within and between human settlements become an important focus of social development. Standard of living concerns how people earn their livings and provide for their households, families and groups. Improving standards of living deriving from the quality of environment is an increasingly important aim of social development. The realization of a sustainable standard of living that human beings require to thrive is a principal aim of locality-based social development (see also Chapter 14).

Quality of life and quality of day

It is difficult within social development to divorce quality of environment from quality of life. Social development promotes quality of life by recognizing that human populations interact with local ecologies and are a major factor in influencing those ecologies for better or worse. *Quality of life* involves quality of environment, standard of living and quality of day. This subjective assessment focuses on the extent to which people feel a sense of fulfilment in experiencing life-enhancing aspirations. This subjective assessment of quality of life within and across certain domains (e.g. work or housing) is linked to ultimate ends such as personal fulfilment, well-being and a state of health. The *quality of day* is also within the scope of social development aims. Human beings may experience considerable negative consequences from social ecologies that prevent the expression of self, limit work or employment opportunities, degrade nutrition and adequate local food supplies or prevent the acquisition of the knowledge and related competencies to achieve a productive lifestyle. Social isolation, marginalization and displacement can reduce dramatically the quality of day. Proactive social development, with its emphasis on human engagement, can produce quality of day in which people, groups and whole communities engage in activities that can increase productive and self-fulfilling lifestyles. Table 25.1 reveals how the authors order these levels of social development.

Locality-based social development organizations

Temporal frames are pivotal within social development and raise two development questions. What are social development organizations? And what do they do to advance the quality of environment and of life itself?

Social development organizations as alternative organizations

Social development organizations do not have to be large. They can be small organizations, taking action independently of or in concert with other organizations. They are likely to be entrepreneurial in searching for solutions and in building capacities that respond to needs or challenges experienced by the population of a local area. That such organizations are often broader then tall suggests that organizational hierarchy is relatively unimportant to action. Leadership is

Table 25.1 Levels of social development

Level of social development	Social development outcome	Objective of social development
Quality of environment	Positive aesthetic that supports human functioning with minimum disruption of natural ecologies	Integrate infrastructure so that it supports inclusive functioning without degrading natural environments
Standard of living	Achievement of requirements of daily living that meet the needs of individuals, households, groups and communities	Provide conditions of minimal prosperity in which people can sustain a good living, typically involving income and consumption
Quality of day	Rich and engaging settings, infrastructure and opportunities supportive of human development and fulfilment of developmental tasks in daily life	Build settings in which people can fulfil their personal development and experience fulfilling routines
Quality of life	A subjective sense of well-being and satisfaction within individual, group and community life	Assist people to gain the necessary resources, opportunities, roles and identities that support their lives and help them strive towards aspirations they value

a necessity for animating local participation and conceiving of and taking informed collective local action. When social development organizations spread their programmes throughout a region, it heightens ease of access by people. Ease of access is yet another quality that can promote organizational effectiveness as measured by usage of the initiatives the social development organization offers.

When an organization or set of organizations and groups of people accept such responsibility for proactivity, the formation of local alternative institutions is highly likely. For Selznick, the scholar who articulated the institutional school within administration and organizational development (King, 2015), an institution becomes vital when it embodies values that animate the quality of life of a given locale or community. An institution may be an alternative when it replaces public or private ones whose leaders are unwilling or unable to address local needs and bring about the conditions under which ecology and human existence thrive. The local alternative institution becomes a constant in the life of the locality, and it focuses human action on social development.

Social development organizations draw from the wealth of indigenous assets existing within their region (see Chapter 23). People from diverse backgrounds who offer assets that are essential to advancing quality of life may stand out as a distinctive feature of the organization. Knowledge of and skills in crafts, trades, science, technology, economic development, business or enterprise incubation, food propagation, water management, housing construction, disease prevention, literacy, social marketing and group work may be some of the personnel assets of social development organizations. What is significant about personnel is their social capital. They know people within the region and likely have maintained long-term relationships with them, some going back to their childhood or youth (Simeon, 2016). The durability of social networks cutting across the region can strengthen the trust the social development organization commands.

Developmental networks can function 'as holding environments for developing leaders confronted with challenging experiences' (Ghosh, Haynes, & Kram, 2013, p 232). It is this trust that can add to the perceived accessibility of the organization and the willingness among community members to make use of its resources, opportunities and programmes.

Place matters

Place matters in social development. Each local area has its distinctive topology, animal life, vegetation and human geography, which not only influence the formation of social issues such as the spread of disease, but also stimulate creative intergroup interactions that promote social problem solving and quality of life. Attachment to place may further strengthen the attachment of social development organizations to their bioregions and result in the formation of trust between the people and a social development organization. How do such connections evolve? First, the social development organization as an alternative local institution comes to understand the needs, aspirations and strivings of people. Second, as an alternative local institution, the social development organization is rooted in place. Given its distinctiveness, formed principally by its interconnections with immediate place, it is difficult for such an organization to franchise itself, create wholesale solutions for other regions or standardize what it does. Alternative local institutions form in distinctive places, and their actions within those places perpetuate them. They enfold themselves with local cultures, embracing the identities of groups composing the locale, using culture to support local development and stimulating further development or evolution of culture. Given its cultural focus, the alternative institution can stand for the culture that has formed or is forming. This means fostering an identity that can combine with how people live and what they aspire to achieve for themselves, now and into the future. A social development organization of and for a given place will possess continuity in presence and operations and will continue to invest heavily in advancing both the quality of environment and the quality of life of its place or places. Thus, place matters in locality-based social development, and attachment to place among the people living within a given bioregion may be one of the greatest assets of such an organization.

Local leadership, animation and action

Leadership is pivotal in forming and sustaining the social development organization. Two types are salient: transactional leadership and transformational leadership. Transactional leadership ensures that personnel can engage with groups that facilitate action. Such leaders can rally participants' involvement and sustain their productivity and engagement. Sustaining such involvement means that social development personnel are in contact with participants and potential participants, obtaining information about how they wish to proceed in addressing issues and advancing development. Such leaders can negotiate across groups, help those groups form some sense of solidarity, and assist them to overcome cultural or political barriers to cooperation. Transformational leadership is essential to advancing a social development agenda. Transformational leaders can facilitate the formation of vision and organize efforts to translate that vision into action, consequently achieving practical fulfilment of the qualities or values of the vision. For example, moving from a concept or vision of healthy, affordable and adequate housing to realizing an actual housing development is a process through which transformational leaders can make the vision a reality.

Animation and action are two means to advance the participation and involvement of members of the geographic place. *Animation* involves the intentional effort locality-based organizations invest in creating inclusive environments of participation and involvement. The organization seeks to counteract the propensity for groups to pull apart from one another, resulting in the lack of interaction, the creation of negative stereotypes of the other and the potential emergence of intergroup conflict or hostilities. Social development organizations seek collaboration in the pursuit of mutually beneficial ends and conciliation when conditions of intergroup conflict prevail. Although animation may sound somewhat coercive, it is a form of institutional leadership that social development organizations can take when groups will not move towards mutual interaction on their own. And it is an expression of institutional social responsibility when the organization takes on the responsibility for advancing group life, arriving at mutually determined ends that groups find beneficial, catalysing action and augmenting a locality's capacity for self-governance. Linking animation with a strengths perspective (see Chapter 18) can foster inclusion, the investment of energy and the promotion of idealism in which groups and their members co-produce local democracy and the institutions that flow from such democratic involvement.

Action is the practical goal-related institutional behaviour through which social development organizations support the implementation of projects designed to fulfil development aims. Action is purposive, designed to fulfil practical aims and inclusive of individuals and groups. Projects themselves may be complex, spanning broad swathes of geography within the bioregion and various ecologies composing that region. Numerous groups must integrate their actions to bring about aims, as well as dealing with the complicatedness of technologies and methods that a project can incorporate. The aspirations of communities may result in multiple paths of action that locality-based social development organizations and their members adopt. Those pathways can address intersectional issues in which quality of environment interacts with quality of life. When local communities are successful in facing development challenges, a sense of optimism and hope is created. Optimism is immediate, inherent in a positive emotional sense that better circumstances can occur. Hope as a value is anticipatory: it builds awareness of human groups about what needs to be done to anticipate future circumstances that improve upon those operating now, especially for future generations (on action, see also Chapter 24).

Group work, community organizing and pluralism

Given its focus on action animated within localities, social development can set the supportive conditions of group work as an important component of social change. Perhaps one of the most significant qualities of group work is that through participation people form cohesion. Cohesion can reinforce mutual support among members of the community, facilitate the formation of interpersonal bonds and expand familiarity, which itself may mitigate intergroup hostilities. Group work facilitates inclusion that can become a local resource in governing how the geographic area of place will evolve. Successful group work can result in optimism among participants and hope for a future in which subsequent generations experience a better quality of life.

Social development organizations undertaking intrinsic action appreciate group work as a means of involving participants in local problem-solving. Groups may include members who are from the same community, or the members may be quite diverse. This introduces into group projects important values varying by gender, sexual orientation, ethnicity, race and geographic location. Reinventing group life within social development can result in a reinvigoration of group work within social work, moving it from a specialty of clinical social work or interpersonal practice to a discipline of social participation and involvement through democratic engagement. Thus, group life may be a significant contributor to social development in the assessment, design, enactment and evaluation of action.

Another core competency involves organizing at community or neighbourhood levels. The organization functions within a bioregion as the principal institution for getting things done to improve life situations and life circumstances. It anchors social action and serves as the principal convener of local participation. Reminding ourselves that alternative institutions often form when other institutions fail to act or ignore their social responsibility, locality-based social development organizations can activate and animate participation and decision-making across the life course. This would mean that participation and decision-making would not be segregated within any one group whether elite or movement focused or age graded. A participatory ethos incorporates efforts to spread horizontally across the bioregion involving various groups and people. Within local communities, the social development organization can engage groups and people normally isolated from decision-making by class, caste, race, religion and socio-economic status.

Pluralism suggests diversity of group interests and ultimately implicates multiple group identities. If established institutions cannot or are unwilling to address such diversity, alternative institutions can close the potential chasm between groups. The politics of crafting, investing in and enacting intrinsic action indicate that an entity external to a local community can intrude and dictate the terms of development. Ultimately, for social development and social work, such intrusion limits if not undermines self-determination and empowerment.

A good and effective local alternative institution in social development can instil optimism in the now as it fosters hope as a positive cognitive-emotional set for the future. This is the promise of locality-based social development. What is good in this context? The authors suggest five imperatives of the good. The social development organization:

1 Addresses human suffering and does not ignore it in the name of other priorities, such as economic development favouring a certain group.
2 Acts within and on behalf of the bioregion when other institutions fail to take requisite action.
3 Acts mindful of the importance of what is occurring now, mindful that the organization is seeking to bring about a better more sustainable bioregion in the future.
4 Moves beyond a representational approach to organizational action to embrace widespread and meaningful participation within the communities composing the bioregion.
5 Works across sectors to bring about systematic change.

Social work in social development

How can social work embody a framework of social development? Some may argue that social work is developmental in its orientation, a perspective going back to the roots of social work as a profession within Europe and the United States, and now globally. Social workers in social development seek to assess relationships among multiple factors with considerable investment in helping mitigate the severity of issues people experience. At the same time, they invest in helping eliminate or weaken agent factors and eliminate the factors operating in the environment that foster individuals' or groups' susceptibility to social issues and problems (Green & Nieman, 2003). A strong environmental focus will come to characterize social work practice as social workers seek to improve quality of life through the amelioration of environments (see Chapter 14). Alternative institutions, especially those based in localities, seek to integrate efforts within one organization that develops horizontally across a bioregion. Efforts will be focused at sub-regional levels, with teams integrating outreach, engagement, community participation, programme planning, programme implementation and evaluation in various neighbourhoods, particularly those experiencing elevated incidence and prevalence rates for social issues.

Reframing social work practice as social development can also take a proactive stance in which action is a result of the membership's efforts to construe the future direction the community should take to address human needs. Inevitably, this process of discernment occurring within participatory structures imbues social development with values pertaining to involvement or participation of groups whose members normally would be left out of discourse essential to governance. Furthermore, locality-based social development organizations as alternative institutions are characterized by the broad-based inclusion of groups in deliberation, in priority setting, in establishing ultimate direction and aspirations for development outcomes. Such participation elevates the importance of community practice in social work, fusing it with direct practice and group work to make social development a viable alternative to generalist and advanced generalist practice.

A social development organization that embodies an ethos of participation and involvement will make intrinsic action a salient means of the development process. The alternative institution is concerned about the bioregion and the quality of its environment and quality of life. A distinctive approach to social problem-solving emerges when participants prioritize issues that immediate communities face within their daily lives and then identify which creative involvement enables them to address those issues. Creative involvement will make the alternative institution stand out as a generator of positive change. When it can assist the region in generating its own knowledge base, other regions may seek to emulate or at least examine it for potential adoption.

Local social development organizations may stand as alternatives to large-scale public bureaucracies whose leaders may fail to understand fully local desires, aims and cultures. Those local organizations may be very close to the aspirations that local residents hold since their own organizational membership is more likely to comprise individuals who can represent those desires. Such local sensitivity and embodiment of local culture can advance problem-solving, participation and leadership within local communities. Thus, alternative social development organizations may stand as anchor institutions within communities. People can tap them for assistance in addressing the quality of life challenges they face. And they can become involved in decision structures that advance the local community. Thus, not only is social development substantive in that it assists people to get resources they need at individual, group and community levels, but it is also process focused in that people can participate for the sake of their own involvement as change agents.

Theoretical assertions on social work and social development

As we contemplate social development theory in social work, what impresses us most is the distinctive features of locality-based organizations that are devoted to advancing quality of life. Although social development can occur at the institutional and policy levels of a society, what impresses us is the utility of social development organizations as alternative institutions that can offer considerable leadership at local levels. Thus, we make several prescriptive assertions to address this potential utility of locality-based social development organizations and the embrace of social development by social work:

1   It is best to position locality-based social development organizations in communities coping with the numerous and interacting negative consequences of severe poverty. In this sense, locality-based social development organizations embrace survival ethics in which there is an intimate and strong linkage between mobilization of people, the identification

and involvement of natural leaders and investment in human energy in addressing life-sustaining infrastructure.

2   Local control will extend from the scope for participation among people. Participation can occur organically as the locality-based social development organization reaches out and engages individuals and groups that want local solutions to challenging social issues and that want to address proactively the realization of quality of life for all.

3   Collaborative production is a distinctive feature of locality-based social development organizations as alternative social institutions. Thus, residents can look to such organizations as sources of creative solutions that invest in local action, transforming resources that come from outside into energy for addressing locality-based priorities. Assisting residents to direct their energy through collaboration means that a critical mass of human energy can be brought to bear in finding, testing and institutionalizing solutions for a particular community. The strongest, most able locality-based social development organization is one that can overcome group differences, appreciate diversity and form common efforts for social action.

4   Locality-based social development organizations work in real circumstances through direct action with participants, professionals and experts combining their energies to produce a common base of life-sustaining and -enhancing resources.

5   The essential competence of locality-based social development extends from the investments grassroots leaders make in community life through opening opportunity structures, providing life-sustaining and life-enhancing resources and the realization of sustainable ecological capacities.

6   Ultimately, the locality-based social development organization serves as a leading part of social change within a community. Although it can invest in preserving heritage and promoting traditions, its members are also mindful of the potential of the locality and the realization of a future state embedded in current action. Such organizational mindfulness means that locality-based social development organizations honour tradition, solve current challenges and anticipate future conditions. Temporally, the organization anchors itself in these multiple time frames.

In closing, the authors are mindful of the close correspondence between social work and social development. Social work incorporates a strong tradition of development within society at community levels, whether those occur in frontier, rural or urban ecologies; at neighbourhood levels and with groups interacting within conditions of pluralism. Social development as a movement within the developing world presents social work with some important challenges. First, it reminds social work of its historic mission of addressing and resolving the causes and consequences of poverty. From a theoretical stance, social development is about poverty and its alleviation and eradication. It imagines that people mired in poverty are coping with systemic issues that require immediate action. Second, it reminds social work that localities matter, and the development of localities to meet human needs may be one of the most strategic actions social work can take to advance quality of life at individual and group levels. And third, given a focus on the assets and strengths of a locality, an organic evolutionary approach to development holds considerable relevance for social work. Working with indigenous strengths can empower social work itself as a profession in which social solutions require considerable co-production in which the involvement of residents is itself a form of development. Co-production reminds us that, in democratic culture, collaboration in contexts of diversity is the essence of social development. Finding solutions together, despite differences and diversity, requires meaningful action on the part of all. Thus, for social work, unifying action across groups at local levels is an essential aim of social development.

Further reading

Gray, M. (Ed.). (2017). *The handbook of social work and social development in Africa.* New York: Routledge.
  This edited volume draws on educators and practitioners throughout Africa to fill a major gap in the literature on social work and social development in Africa.

Midgley, J., & Pawar, M. (Eds.). (2017). *Future directions in social development.* New York: Palgrave Macmillan.
  This book provides an overview of the history and progress of social development in view of the Millennium Development Goals.

Pawar, M. (2014). *Social and community development practice.* New Delhi: Sage.
  This book covers policy, practice and curriculum development for local-level social development in Asia.

References

Akindola, R. (2010). Importance to poverty alleviation of bottom-up approaches to social development. In M. S. Pawar & D. R. Cox (Eds.), *Social development: Critical themes and perspectives* (pp. 165–182). New York: Routledge.

Ananias, J., & Lightfoot, E. (2012). Promoting social development: Building a professional social work association in Namibia. *Journal of Community Practice, 20*(1–2), 196–210.

Burkett, I., & Ruhunda, A. (2010). Building partnerships for social development. In M. S. Pawar & D. R. Cox (Eds.), *Social development: Critical themes and perspectives* (pp. 118–144). New York: Routledge.

Cox, D. R., & Pawar, M. S. (2010). Personnel for local level social development. In M. S. Pawar & D. R. Cox (Eds.), *Social development: Critical themes and perspectives* (pp. 145–164). New York: Routledge.

Desai, M. (2013). Social policy approaches, human rights, and social development in Asia. *Social Development Issues, 35*(2), 1–17.

Estes, R. J. (1994). Education for social development: Curricular issues and models. *Social Development Issues, 16*(3), 68–90. Retrieved from http://citeseerx.ist.psu.edu/viewdoc/download?doi=10.1.1.544.3937&rep=rep1&type=pdf

Fonchingong, C. C., & Fonjong, L. N. (2003). The concept of self-reliance in community development initiatives in the Cameroon grass fields. *Nordic Journal of African Studies, 12*(2), 196–219.

Ghosh, R., Haynes, R. K., & Kram, K. E. (2013). Developmental networks at work: Holding environments for leader development. *Career Development International, 18*(3), 232–256.

Gil, D. (1976). Social policies and social development: A humanistic–egalitarian perspective. *Journal of Sociology & Social Welfare, III*(3), 242–263.

Green, S., & Nieman, A. (2003). Social development: Good practice guidelines. *Social Work/Maatskaplike werk, 39*(2), 161–181.

Hawkins, C., & Nalini, R. P. (2008). CEDER3: A social development response to the tsunami recovery in Tamil Nadu, India. *Social Development Issues, 30*(1), 29–46.

Huston, T. (2007). *Inside-Out: Stories and methods for generating collective will to create the future we want.* Cambridge, MA: Society for Organizational Learning.

Kegan, R., & Lahey, L. L. (2009). *Immunity to change: How to overcome it and unlock the potential in yourself and your organization (Leadership for the Common Good).* Boston: Harvard Business Press.

Keough, N. (1998). Participatory development principles and practice: Reflections of a western development worker. *Community Development Journal, 33*(3), 187–196.

Kim, I., & Isma'il, M. (2013). Self-reliance: Key to sustainable rural development in Nigeria. *ARPN Journal of Science and Technology, 3*(6), 585–592.

King, B. G. (2015). Organizational actors, character, and Selznick's theory of organizations. In M. S. Kraatz (Ed.), *Institutions and ideals: Philip Selznick's legacy for organizational studies* (pp. 149–174). Bingley: Emerald.

Kulkarni, V. V., & Vaishnav, N. (2013). Locality development through community organization. *Indian Streams Research Journal, 3*(10), 1–8.

Midgley, J. (1995). *Social development: The developmental perspective in social welfare.* Thousand Oaks, CA: Sage.

Midgley, J., & Conley, A. (Eds.). (2010). *Social work and social development: Theories and skills for developmental social work.* New York: Oxford University Press.

Osei-Hwedie, K., & Osei-Hwedie, B. Z. (2010). Participatory development. In M. S. Pawar & D. R. Cox (Eds.), *Social development: Critical themes and perspectives* (pp. 57–75). New York: Routledge.

Pandey, R. S. (1981). Strategies for social development: An analytical approach. In J. F. Jones & R. S. Pandey (Eds.), *Social development: Conceptual, methodological and policy issues* (pp. 33–34–49). Delhi: Macmillan India.

Patel, L. (2015). *Social welfare and social development* (2nd ed.). Cape Town, SA: Oxford University Press Southern Africa.

Pawar, M. S. (2014). *Social and community development practice*. New Delhi: Sage.

Pawar, M. S., & Cox, D. R. (Eds.). (2010). *Social development: Critical themes and perspectives*. New York: Routledge.

Schmid, J., Wilson, T., & Taback, R. (2010). Soul Buddyz Clubs: A social development innovation. *International Social Work, 54*(2), 272–286.

Selznick, P. (1957). *Leadership in administration: A sociological interpretation*. Los Angeles: Harper & Row.

Selznick, P. (1992). *The moral commonwealth: Social theory and the promise of community*. Los Angeles: University of California Press.

Selznick, P. (2002). *The communitarian persuasion*. Washington, DC: Woodrow Wilson Center.

Selznick, P. (2008). *A humanist science: Values and ideals in social inquiry*. Stanford, CA: Stanford University Press.

Simeon, A. (2016). *A case study of mission for community development program as a multifaceted urban social development organization in Addis Ababa Ethiopia*. (Unpublished doctoral dissertation). Addis Ababa University, Addis Ababa, Ethiopia.

Sossou, M., & Yogtiba, J. A. (2016). Promoting social justice and human rights among vulnerable populations: Implications for a social development approach in Ghana. *Social Development Issues, 38*(1), 25–37.

Sung-Chan, P., & Yuen-Tsang, A. (2008). Action research and social development in China. *Action Research, 6*(2), 193–212.

Thomas, M., & Pawar, M. S. (2010). Self-reliant development. In M. S. Pawar & D. R. Cox (Eds.), *Social development: Critical themes and perspectives* (pp. 76–97). New York: Routledge.

Van Wyk, R., & Mandla, A. (2010). Vukani-Ubuntu: A social entrepreneurial answer to social development issues in South Africa. *Social Development Issues, 32*(2), 67–83.

Weyers, M. L. (2011). The habits of highly effective community development practitioners. *Development Southern Africa, 28*(1), 87–98.

Yadama, G. N., & Dauti, M. (2010). Capacity building for local development. In M. S. Pawar & D. R. Cox (Eds.), *Social development: Critical themes and perspectives* (pp. 98–117). New York: Routledge.

26

Critical theory and social work

Historical context and contemporary manifestations

Kenneth McLaughlin

Introduction

Throughout its history social work has been influenced by the wider socio-political environment within which it is located: from the Charity Organisation Society (COS) and the moral reformers of the 19th and 20th centuries, the eugenics policies of the early 20th century and the welfarism of the mid to late 20th century to the neoliberal managerialism of the present day. A cursory glance at these developments shows the influence of various political ideologies, from the left, right and middle ground of British politics.

In this chapter I want to look at one particular political influence on social welfare: 'critical theory', a set of ideas and practices that developed from those on the left of the political spectrum and has subsequently influenced, and been influenced by, other political and theoretical perspectives such as postmodernism and post-structuralism. While there are profound differences between these traditions, engaging with earlier writers, even in critique, has helped clarify the thinking of later theorists, even if the conclusions they reached were different. As these theoretical perspectives interacted with the political struggles of the day (see Chapter 27), they influenced the politics of both identity and difference, perspectives which paved the way for the current popularity within left-wing political thought of intersectional politics. This thinking seeks to understand how various identities intersect and influence the personal and political lives of subjects. We now have, among other things, critical race theory, critical disability studies, critical psychiatry, critical psychology and even, for our purposes, critical social work. Indeed, it would be rare to hear a contemporary social or psychological academic state that they considered themselves to be an *uncritical* theorist.

To illustrate the influence of some of these developments, I first give a summary of key considerations and terms within critical theory. In doing so, I pay particular attention to the thought of a group of theorists who became known as the Frankfurt School and provide further references for readers to gain more detailed engagement with their ideas. This is because critical theory is often associated with Marx's ideas, and indeed he did influence the Frankfurt School. The ideas of these 20th-century social theorists, however, are often summarized as 'critical theory', though they are not necessarily the most influential on critical thought, because such influences are diverse and wide ranging. For example, the thought of those associated with Hall's

Centre for Cultural Studies at the University of Birmingham, UK, may have had more influence on the radical thought of the late 20th century (Hall, Critcher, Jefferson, Clarke, & Roberts, 1978; Hall, 2016).

I then look at the way such thought challenged some key ideas of liberal thought, particularly reason and rationality and how these have been developed by later theorists concerned with challenging social injustice. To demonstrate this, I look at debates within disability and mental health in general and attempts at challenging stigma in particular. In conclusion, I discuss some of the implications for social work and social workers.

What is critical theory?

The Institute for Social Research at Frankfurt University is more commonly known as the Frankfurt School, and from the 1930s, it attracted left-wing intellectuals, such as Horkheimer and Adorno, whose work became known as 'critical theory'. This is an umbrella term that covers the wide-ranging but related theoretical work of the members of the school, although writers such as Ramsey (2000) claim that critical theory was a code name for Marxism.

Critical theory has as its goal human liberation and works 'to create a world which satisfies the needs and powers' of human beings (Horkheimer, 1972, p. 246). The aim is not only to explain but also to transform all the circumstances that limit human freedom. For Horkheimer (1993), a critical theory of society '. . . has as its object human beings as producers of their own historical form of life' (p. 21).

An important concept within critical theory is that of *immanent critique*. If a society has the potential to create a fairer, more just social system and yet fails to do so, then it should be subject to critique from within its own walls. The influence on social work can be seen in the radical social work movement's slogan of 'in and against the state' (London Edinburgh Weekend Return Group, 1980). This emphasized the contradictory aspect of state social work in that it acknowledged that it was a profession embedded within the machinery of the state but that it also had the potential to challenge and change the values and practices of the profession in the pursuit of social justice. Similar criticisms emerged within other disciplines such as psychology and psychiatry. In this respect it is worth noting that despite the varied external critiques of the psy-professions, many of the most perceptive have been from those trained or working in these fields (e.g. Szasz, 1961; Thomas, 1997; Johnstone, 2000; Parker, 2007).

Another important concept is that of *praxis*, which refers to the 'theory-practice' relationship and how social science may serve the goal of social justice. Its emphasis is on theory not being some metaphysical abstraction with guidelines for how we should live and intervene in society, but that people's experiences and subjectivities should influence theoretical insights. To put it in common parlance, there are some things you cannot learn from just reading books; you also need to interact with others. Oliver and Sapey (2006) give the example of the social worker allocated the 'case' of a tetraplegic woman. With limited knowledge of the woman's condition or how it affected her life, the social worker agreed to spend a full day with the woman, from before she got out of bed in the morning to when she got back into it at night. This gave her far more insight into the needs of her client than she would have gained from reading medical books about the causes of and 'cures' for her condition.

This move to acknowledging that many users of services are 'experts by experience' has helped challenge the dominance of professional knowledge. It does not necessarily dismiss the value of medical expertise but rather questions its ability to provide certain insights. So, in the above example, knowing the medical or genetic causes of tetraplegia, whilst important, is of little help in understanding what it is like to confront daily life with it; for that we need experience, not science.

Praxis, in ancient Greece, was a way for practical reasoning to lead to wise action, with the moral disposition to act truly and rightly. In modern times, this moral or ethical component is usually translated as a commitment towards a particular end. With roots in the philosophical work of Aristotle, the notion of praxis has influenced a range of thinkers from all sides of the political spectrum As Karl Marx proclaimed, 'The philosophers have only interpreted the world in various ways; the point is to change it' (Marx, 1845). For the highly influential educationalist and political activist Paulo Freire praxis is reflection and action upon the world in order to transform it (Friere, 1970).

Rather than, as is often the case, practice being seen as separate from theory, praxis aims to bring together practice, reflection, education and research in an integrated whole. One important contribution was by Hannah Arendt, whose book *The Human Condition* criticized much of Western philosophy for being too preoccupied with the contemplative life (*vita contemplativa*) and neglectful of the active life (*vita activa*). For Arendt (1958), the implication of this was missing the relevance of philosophical ideas to daily real life. For her, the mark of human uniqueness was our capacity to grapple with and analyze ideas and engage in active praxis.

Horkheimer's main concern, however, was not a preoccupation with philosophical thought, but rather the lack of reflection within the masses. For him, the instrumentalism of contemporary society brought about by the commodification and classification processes of modernity had turned people into unthinking automatons, looking at the world in quantitative rather than qualitative terms. The creative, freethinking individual is subsumed by the needs of the modern technological age. 'The substance of individuality itself, to which the idea of autonomy was bound, did not survive the process of industrialization' (Horkheimer, 1941, p. 36). Consequently, 'Today, man needs factual knowledge, the automaton ability to react correctly, but he does not need the quiet consideration of diverse possibilities which presupposes the freedom and leisure of choice' (p. 39).

Horkheimer's writing, over 75 years ago, has resonance today in the way that an anti-intellectual attitude prevails within contemporary society and social work. For example, then–Health Minister Jacqui Smith, speaking at the 2002 Community Care Live conference, said that social work '. . . is a very practical job. It is about protecting people and changing their lives, not about being able to give a fluent and theoretical explanation of why they got into difficulties in the first place' (Community Care, 2002). Indeed, the increasing managerialism within social work and the way in which the 'worker-client' relationship is characterized by control and supervision rather than care, on 'doing the job' within the remit of legislation, policy and organizational dictate without active intellectual reflection, on practice, rather than *praxis* has become a concern for some within the profession. Concerned that social work should not be defined by its function for the state but by its value base, Jones, Ferguson, Lavalette, and Penketh (2004; see Chapter 27) exhort the profession to 'coalesce and organise around a shared vision of what a genuinely anti-oppressive social work might be like' (online). Social workers are urged to engage with the 'resources of hope available in the new collective movements for an alternative, and better, world', one based around core 'anti-capitalist' values, such as solidarity and liberty (ibid.). This is, in effect, a contemporary version of the early radical social work movement's call to work both 'in and against the state'.

The popularity of 'evidence-based practice' is an example of instrumental reason, symptomatic of social work being reduced to 'managing' rather than eliminating social injustice. The focus is on what works as opposed to what is being done, why it is being done and whether it should be done or not. Evidence-based practice eliminates the need for moral judgement and reflection; it does not require intellectual thought, just research.

Social workers, then, need to adopt immanent critique and praxis if they are to be more than technicians heeding the calls of their employers.

Critical theory in the contemporary period

The Frankfurt School's thought had a pessimistic slant, influenced by the experience of fascism and the loss of belief in the possibility of working-class emancipation. This saw a turn to culture as a focus for research and potential progressive social change. For the 1960s and 1970s generation of activists, also contending with the defeat of the revolutionary fervour of their own time, critical theory proved influential as they, in turn, began to focus on culture and identity more than on economics and working-class revolution.

A range of at times overlapping and/or competing perspectives has developed from various perspectives on the causes and solutions to humanity's problems. Often these have emerged in conjunction with social movements of the day, such as feminist, anti-racist, disability and queer critiques of normative assumptions and related social oppression. These ideas share a belief that social inquiry should be aimed at decreasing domination and increasing freedom. For many, there was a need to challenge unequal social relations through other means, often within the workplace or the mechanisms of the state: for example, by legislative and social policy means.

In what follows I look at two contemporary tactics by which some attempt to challenge social inequality: anti-stigma campaigns about mental 'disorder' (see Chapter 36) and the embracement of vulnerability with a particular focus on disability (see Chapter 38).

Horkheimer and Adorno were disillusioned with Enlightenment theories of reason and universalism. Reason, for them, leads to the destruction of the subject, with socially constructed inhibitions becoming part of individual consciousness. Horkheimer's critique of reason lay in part on the correct observation that the abstract notion of universality and equality did not fit with a pluralistic and inegalitarian world.

Such sentiments have become increasingly popular within contemporary 'critical' schools of thought. For example, many of the concerns of the earlier critical theorists are incorporated into critical disability studies with society's privileging of rationality, autonomy and competence said to 'other' those subjects who, for whatever reason, fail to live up to this ideal. Influenced by post-structuralism, such critics seek to destabilize binaries and fixed notions of what it means to be human. The idea of the human subject, a key component of liberal thought since the Enlightenment, is not only contested but also stands accused of propagating oppressive social relations both at home and across the globe. The Subject (with a capital S) is a burden of which we would be better relieved as, in actuality, such a Subject is invariably 'man-white-western-male-adult-reasonable-heterosexual-living in towns-speaking a standard language' (quoted in Goodley, 2007, p. 154). For Goodley, this is inevitable as the humanist Subject defines himself by what he excludes.

Those who fail to meet this vision of the human are then classed as 'other', as less human or non-human. Within the field of critical disability studies, biopedagogies are said to 'serve to produce the archetypal (masculine, cisgender, white, non-disabled, middle class, straight) citizen and autonomous human subject under neoliberal capitalism. Those considered other to this limited conceptualization of humanity are positioned to fail' (Rice, Chandler, Liddiard, Rinaldi, & Harrison, 2016, p. 6). In other words, some of us are more human than others, and there are some who are excluded from the category altogether.

Similarly, within the field of critical psychiatry, the distinction between madness and reason, normal and abnormal, illness and health is called into question. For Derrida (1978), even supposedly more progressive attempts to write about madness ended up reinforcing the divide, as such endeavours tended to be written from the perspective of reason. The classification and diagnosis of aspects of human experience as mental disorders is far from an exact science, and the medicalization of distress is a relatively recent historical phenomenon. For radical critics such as

Thomas Szasz, a psychiatrist himself, the very concept of mental illness is a myth, one that is used to control people who exhibit behaviours that we as a society cannot understand or tolerate (Szasz, 1961). The mind, like the economy, can only be sick in a metaphorical, not a literal, sense.

Once so labelled, it is also the case that people's statuses can change in ways that can undermine their humanity. Others may cease to see them as people, with histories, desires and aspirations, but as 'the schizophrenic', the mad, as object rather than subject. The person becomes the patient and is liable to lose many of the rights of citizenship that most people take for granted, such as the right to liberty unless convicted of a crime and the right to refuse medical treatment even if doctors deem it to be in their best interest. Once given a psychiatric diagnosis, the now patient, subject to certain conditions being met, can be detained indefinitely under mental health legislation and given medical treatment against their will. To address some of these concerns, several strategies have been proposed to alleviate discrimination and stigma and improve the rights of citizenship of those labelled as mentally ill or learning disabled.

Challenging stigma

Within the arena of mental health, four broad models of anti-discrimination have been identified: the brain disease model; the libertarian model; the disability inclusion model and the 'continuum', or individual growth model (Sayce, 2000).

The brain disease model sees mental illnesses as similar to other bodily diseases, with their roots in genetic or biochemical malfunction. Suffering from a mental illness is not due to moral weakness, problematic family relationships or environmental factors, but is located within the individual sufferer's biological make-up. Many families favour this perspective, in part because it absolves the family of responsibility for the sufferer's problems. However, this has to be seen in context as not only a rejection of familial influence and of the embracement of biomedical psychiatry, but also as a response to the Laingian notion that family upbringing plays a large part in the development of future mental illness. Such was the strength of this idea in the 1970s that carers could find themselves castigated for 'causing' the schizophrenia of their offspring (Sedgwick, 1982).

The anti-stigma rationale of this approach is that if mental illness is a disease just like other bodily disease, no stigma should be attached to it. Sufferers are not to blame for their behaviour so should not be assigned any responsibility. If individuals are seen, however, as not being in control of their actions, it follows that they need monitoring and controlling on the presumption that they lack judgement. The less responsibility you have, the fewer rights of citizenship you possess. However, as Sayce points out, 'A non-discriminatory position is one which recognises that mental disorder *per se* does not invalidate judgement. Many citizens make unwise decisions. User/survivors should not be expected to be any wiser than anyone else. Overruling someone's decision – even when it seems, to well-motivated professionals, to be an unwise decision – must be heavily constrained. And if users commit crimes, it should not be assumed that it is not their fault' (p. 95). She goes on: 'The "no-fault" brain disease model removes the moral taint of mental illness but raises new difficulties on numerous fronts. Allocating no fault, and no responsibility, is fundamentally problematic in terms of the sharing of rights and responsibilities necessary to citizenship' (p. 99).

Advocates of the libertarian model demand equal civil rights and in return are willing to accept equal criminal responsibility. Mental health law allows people diagnosed as suffering from a mental disorder to be detained against their will, not necessarily on account of what they have done but of what professionals think they might do in the future, a form of 'pre-emptive strike'. Influenced by the writings of those such as Szasz (1961), libertarian activists argue that they should be locked up for what they do, not what professionals think they may do. The libertarian movement has had a valuable role in highlighting the often-coercive nature of mental health legislation, but it also leads to situations where people, who are clearly ill or incapacitated without full responsibility for their actions, are treated within a punitive prison system rather than receiving the care that they require. Sayce (2000) gives the example of some libertarian extremists in the US who refused to campaign to save a man with learning disabilities from execution on the grounds that he should accept full responsibility for his actions. For them, whilst his potential execution was a tragedy, it was nothing compared to the deaths and forced incarceration of tens of thousands of psychiatric patients annually.

The disability inclusion model is the one that Sayce sees as having the most potential in realizing increased citizenship rights for mental health users by challenging discrimination 'wherever it occurs, from the government committee report to the conversation in a bar' (p. 143). She views this model as highly inclusive as 'it can accommodate people seeking healing or cure, through any means from chanting to Prozac, but being "healed" or "in recovery" is quite unnecessary to be in this change movement, which explicitly values people whether they "recover" or not' (p. 143). It argues against attaching shame to mental health problems whilst simultaneously seeking to change attitudes and practices by use of such things as legislative changes and public awareness campaigns.

All such perspectives have their strengths and weaknesses. From a theoretical and philosophical stance, however, it is arguably the idea of the 'continuum' that has the most advocates today. From this perspective, mental health or distress must be understood as a continuum, with mental health at one end and mental distress at the other. We are all placed somewhere on the continuum, and we will all, at some point, move along it, for better or worse, in one direction or another. There is no rigid divide between mental health and mental illness; therefore, to classify some people as mentally ill sets up an 'us and them' situation, with 'them' being stigmatized and oppressed. The influence of postmodernism and post-structuralism is clear here, because these arguments do much more than merely disrupt the binaries of disabled/able-bodied, illness/ health; they question the legitimacy of attempts at classification, the objects classified being seen as merely the effect of language.

Such insights make us aware of the dangers of medicalizing human experience; nevertheless, there are many problems with the notion of mental health and illness as a continuum. First, the continuum argument may be valid in seeing that all mental experiences involve the emotions and that there is no rigid, ahistorical or apolitical dividing line between what is classed as normal or abnormal: yesterday's naughty child is today's ADHD sufferer; the shy adult now has 'avoidant personality disorder'. To conflate all emotional states as belonging on the same continuum – for example, severe depression with life's ups and downs – is, however, as absurd as conflating a child's sandpit with the Sahara desert; both contain sand, but the similarity ends there.

Another weakness in the continuum case is that, in reality, there has to be a boundary, however unstable and subject to change, between those who require professional intervention and those who do not. For example:

> even the most radical and progressive mental-health resource programmes, such as therapeutic communities and user/survivor asylum and support interventions, make assessments as to who should and who should not access their services. In other words, they operate eligibility criteria, making a distinction between people on the basis of their mental state. They may reject the medical model of classification and treatment, but they themselves classify and differentiate. Whatever model of mind is used to make the distinction, the end result is the same: the continuum is broken.
>
> *(McLaughlin, 2011, n.p.)*

313

There is also within this model a presumption of vulnerability within each of us. Whilst this is obviously true, it fails to see the political and historical specificity of the concept of vulnerability, which when viewed from a critical perspective casts doubt on the political gains to be made from the embracement of vulnerability.

Uniting critical perspectives: radical vulnerability

The concept of vulnerability is ubiquitous within UK social services and disciplinary systems of assessment for, and provision of, services. Examples are allocating social housing and protection of children, young people and many adults; it also plays a part within the criminal justice system. Such ubiquity can give the impression of a natural ahistoric concept, rather than a relatively recent framework for understanding individual problems and social relations. It is a term whose use has expanded in recent years to encompass ever more people within its reach.

For some, 'vulnerability' can be harnessed for progressive social and political purposes, becoming a platform for collective forms of action to achieve social justice. From this perspective, it offers opportunities for reconceptualizing human relations in general (Brown, 2010) and for specific groups such as people with physical or learning disabilities (e.g. Goodley & Runswick Cole, 2016). For Goodley, taking an affirmative approach to vulnerability

> shifts us away from a humanist reliance on the independent sovereign self to a post-human celebration of interdependence. The vulnerable self depends upon others to live. Numerous disabled selves that are normatively understood as dependent are now recast as sources of interdependence. Disability, we might suggest, demands interdependency, thus inviting new ways of thinking about what it means to be a (post) human subject.
>
> *(Ecclestone & Goodley, 2016, p. 180)*

Others have seen the operation of the vulnerability discourse as paving the way to state paternalism (Furedi, 2004), reducing socio-political problems to psychoemotional ones (Wainwright & Calnan, 2002; Frawley, 2015) and representing a process of political stagnation and the decline of belief in wider social change (McLaughlin, 2012). The concept has also been critiqued in areas such as education (Ecclestone & Hayes, 2008) and groups such as young people (Brown, 2015), disabled people (Oliver, 1990) and people with learning difficulties (Hollomotz, 2009). Vulnerability, then, has become a key component of contemporary sociological and political discourse, leading Brown (2015) to argue that we are living within a 'vulnerability zeitgeist'.

A belief in the innate vulnerability of certain people or groups can also lead to a patronizing, protective attitude towards them that can undermine their rights and deny them agency. Such a discourse acts to single out and 'other' certain groups in ways that can be controlling, stigmatizing and oppressive (Brown, 2015).

Recognizing this, many disability theorists and activists choose not to challenge the presumption of vulnerability, but to embrace and seek to expand the category by emphasizing that vulnerability is an inevitable part of the human condition (e.g. Oliver & Sapey, 2006; Fineman, 2010). The intention is to highlight the ways in which we are all vulnerable, some more so than others, some for longer than others, but nevertheless, vulnerability is a human universal. In addition, it is pointed out that to cope with life, we all require the help and support of others, in the form of such things as social organization, emotional connection or healthcare. From this perspective, acknowledging, embracing, even celebrating, our common vulnerability, can play a part in fostering a more tolerant and inclusive society, as well as a more socially just welfare state as a counter to the current neoliberal one.

Such writers aim to:

> depathologise official categories by recasting vulnerability as a progressive attribute of a relational citizenship, integral to the 'fragile and contingent nature of personhood' where we are all 'potentially vulnerable' and where vulnerability is a 'universal ontological dimension of human experience and identity'.
>
> *(Ecclestone & Goodley, 2016, p. 177)*

They hope such approaches protect people from any detrimental effects of potential vulnerabilities and also from pathologizing and intrusive state-sponsored interventions, while simultaneously allowing those with current vulnerabilities to be supported according to their specific situation and associated needs.

These perspectives present collective and specific vulnerabilities as potential sources of political mobilization: for example by highlighting suffering caused by contemporary social, economic and political relations. Vulnerability is here used for anti-capitalist and social reformist purposes. For example, Butler links notions of vulnerability to precarity as a vehicle to combat oppression: 'Precariousness [is] a function of our social vulnerability and exposure that is always given some political form, and precarity as differentially distributed [is] one important dimension of the unequal distribution of conditions required for continued life' (quoted in Ecclestone & Goodley, 2016, p. 178). In a similar vein to standpoint theory, where the oppressed are said to have a better understanding of the reality of social conditions than the rulers, precarity and vulnerability can awaken us to the problems of the age.

Analyses of vulnerability often acknowledge that, like risk and fear, it is primarily a subjective, not objective, phenomenon. However, for Ahmed (2014), what is relatively unconsidered is the question of 'why some bodies are more afraid than others? How do feelings of vulnerability take shape?' (p. 68). Ahmed notes that, while fear may be experienced individually, it is 'structural and mediated, rather than an immediate bodily response to an objective danger' (p. 69). Hence, such feelings of vulnerability 'shape women's bodies as well as how those bodies inhabit space' (p. 70).

If feelings of vulnerability are structured and mediated, however, they are also historically specific in how they are experienced, conceptualized and strategized, both in how to improve individual feelings and in the social conditions from within which they arise. For example, the rise of 'work stress' resulted largely from trade unions recasting problematic workplace relations in the language of individual vulnerability because older, more collective responses to such issues, such as industrial action, had become weakened (Wainwright & Calnan, 2002). The rise of the 'survivor identity' in recent years has also been influenced by the changing nature of both individual and group demands for recognition of individual vulnerability rather than collective strength (McLaughlin, 2012).

The main contribution of the continuum model's advocates is the way in which they highlight the historical construction of contemporary psychiatric and disability theory, diagnosis and practice, including the role of politics and social change in our understanding of the causes of, and attempts to alleviate, mental distress. Their main weakness is a failure fully to appreciate the impact of such factors on current mental health debate. If the traditional concept of mental illness arose due to the interplay of wider social phenomena, so too did the current trend to view us all as on a continuum and in need of therapeutic help to maintain our equilibrium. In other words, their historical analyses fail to adequately analyze the present historical epoch.

Conclusion: considerations for critical social work

Within social work, the term 'critical theory' is used to cover different perspectives. For example, Healy (2001: online) uses the term 'critical social work' to refer to a broad range of practice theories that share the following orientations:

> recognition that large scale social processes, particularly those associated with class, race and gender, contribute fundamentally to the personal and social issues social workers encounter in their practice; the adoption of a self-reflexive and critical stance to the often contradictory effects of social work practice and social policies; a commitment to co-participatory rather than authoritarian practice relations. This involves workers and service users, as well as academic, practitioners and service users as co-participants engaged with, but still distinct from, one another; working with and for oppressed populations to achieve social transformation.

I have discussed in this chapter aspects of such definitions in relation to some popular trends within critical intellectual thought. In conclusion, I wish to detail some of the implications for social work that might generate views from practitioners about how these are wrestled with in the intensity of frontline practice.

The anti-stigma models discussed above need to be considered by social work practitioners. At times, a flexible approach will be necessary. For example, the libertarian approach is commendable in allowing clients the freedom to make their own mistakes and alerts us to the dangers of an authoritarian, risk-averse form of practice. We may see this in the overuse of community treatment orders which, it has been argued, are more about protecting professionals, in case something goes wrong post discharge, than patients (McLaughlin & Cordell, 2013). At times, however, intervention is necessary against the wishes of the patient. Social workers have to balance this predicament. That it is not easy is a good thing. We should never lose sight of the importance of the power we have over many people suffering hardship or distress, and any such decision should not be taken without careful consideration of all relevant factors. The brain disease model, whilst often criticized as medicalization, also needs to be considered because we will often be arguing that, for reasons such as mental or intellectual incapacity, individuals are not *fully* responsible for their actions. We do not want to go to the extreme of prosecuting or imprisoning those who are not, or were not at the time, in full control of their faculties. The disability inclusion model can allow the law and campaigns to address instances of discrimination. Social workers are well placed here given their statutory powers.

Debates over what we mean by 'inclusion' are important, however, as it is possible that it becomes tokenism. The continuum and vulnerability models alert us to the fluid nature of the human condition and the dangers of objectifying others. We should not be afraid, however, to differentiate between those who need help and those who do not. Viewing everyone as vulnerable and mental health as a continuum does not help those who do require professional intervention. Also, for those who see state oppression as problematic, emphasizing our vulnerability and mental weakness will not change wider social structures and power bases.

In this chapter, I have sought to introduce readers to some common critical perspectives and to highlight the overlaps and tensions between them. For social workers, the contradictions and tensions within the role will have already become all too clear to them as they go about their daily work. I hope I have helped to give them some more context to the dilemmas they have to consider as they attempt what is at times a careful balancing act between various political and philosophical perspectives.

Further reading

How, A. (2003). *Critical theory*. Basingstoke: Palgrave Macmillan.
This book provides a good introduction to critical theory. There are also good online resources, such as https://plato.stanford.edu/entries/critical-theory/.

McLaughlin, K. (2017). Disabling the subject: From radical vulnerability to vulnerable radicals. *Annual Review of Critical Psychology, 3,* 1–15 Retrieved from https://thediscourseunit.files.wordpress.com/2017/08/arcpkenm.pdf
A further discussion of issues concerned with critical vulnerability.

References

Ahmed, S. (2014). *The cultural politics of emotion* (2nd ed.). Edinburgh: Edinburgh University Press.
Arendt, H. (1958). *The human condition*. Chicago: University of Chicago Press.
Brown, B. (2010). The power of vulnerability. *TED Talks*. Retrieved from www.ted.com/talks/brene_brown_on_vulnerability
Brown, K. (2015). *Vulnerability and young people: Care and social control in policy and practice*. Bristol: Policy Press.
Community Care. (2002). *Full text of Jacqui Smith's speech to Community Care Live*. Retrieved from www.communitycare.co.uk/2002/05/22/full-text-of-jacqui-smiths-speech-to-community-care-live-2002/
Derrida, J. (1978). *Cogito and the history of madness in writing and difference* (A. Bass, Trans., pp. 36–76). London and New York: Routledge.
Ecclestone, K., & Goodley, D. (2016). Political and educational springboard or straitjacket? Theorising post/human subjects in an age of vulnerability. *Discourse: Studies in the Cultural Politics of Education, 37,* 175–188.
Ecclestone, K., & Hayes, D. (2008). *The dangerous rise of therapeutic education*. Abingdon: Routledge.
Fineman, M. (2010). The vulnerable subject and the responsive state. *Emory Law Journal, 60,* 251–275.
Frawley, A. (2015). *Semiotics of happiness: Rhetorical beginnings of a public problem*. London: Bloomsbury.
Friere, P. (1970). *Pedagogy of the oppressed*. New York: Continuum.
Furedi, F. (2004). *Therapy culture: Cultivating vulnerability in an anxious age*. London: Routledge.
Goodley, D. (2007). Becoming rhizomatic parents: Deleuze, Guattari and disabled babies. *Disability and Society, 22,* 145–160.
Goodley, D., & Runswick Cole, K. (2016). Becoming dishuman: Thinking about the human through dis/ability. *Discourse: Cultural politics of Education, 37,* 1–15.
Hall, S. (2016). *Cultural studies 1983: A theoretical history* (J. D. Slack & L. Grossberg, Eds.). London: Duke University Press.
Hall, S., Critcher, C., Jefferson, T., Clarke, J., & Roberts, B. (1978). *Policing the crisis: Mugging, the state and law and order*. London: Palgrave Macmillan.
Healy, K. (2001). Reinventing critical social work: Challenges from practice, context and postmodernism. *Critical Social Work, 2*(1). Retrieved from http://www1.uwindsor.ca/criticalsocialwork/reinventing-critical-social-work-challenges-from-practice-context-and-postmodernism
Hollomotz, A. (2009). Beyond 'vulnerability': An ecological model approach to conceptualizing risk of sexual violence against people with learning difficulties. *British Journal of Social Work, 39,* 99–112.
Horkheimer, M. (1941). The end of reason. In A. Arato & E. Gebhardt (Eds.), *The essential Frankfurt school reader* (pp. 26–48). Oxford: Blackwell.
Horkheimer, M. (1972). *Critical theory: Selected essays*. New York: Continuum.
Horkheimer, M. (1993). *Between philosophy and social sciences: Selected early writings*. Cambridge, MA: MIT Press.
How, A. (2003). *Critical theory*. Basingstoke: Palgrave Macmillan.
Johnstone, L. (2000). *Users and abusers of psychiatry* (2nd ed.). London: Routledge.
Jones, C., Ferguson, I., Lavalette, M., & Penketh, L. (2004). *Social work and social justice: A manifesto for a new engaged practice*. Retrieved from www.socialworkfuture.org/articles-resources/uk-articles/103-social-work-and-social-justice-a-manifesto-for-a-new-engaged-practice
London Edinburgh Weekend Return Group. (1980). *In and against the state*. London: Pluto.
Marx, K. (1845). *Theses on Feuerbach*. Retrieved from www.marxists.org/archive/marx/works/1845/theses/theses.htm
McLaughlin, K. (2011). The unhelpful myth that we're all a bit mad. *Spiked*. Retrieved from www.spiked-online.com/newsite/article/10599#.WTWIGE2GOM8

McLaughlin, K. (2012). *Surviving identity: Vulnerability and the psychology of recognition.* London: Routledge.

McLaughlin, K., & Cordell, S. (2013). Doing what's best, but best for whom? Ethics and the mental health social worker. In L. Green & M. Carey (Eds.), *Practical social work ethics: Complex dilemmas within applied social care* (pp. 111–130). London: Routledge.

Oliver, M. (1990). *The politics of disablement.* London: Palgrave Macmillan.

Oliver, M., & Sapey, B. (2006). Social work with disabled people (3rd ed.). Basingstoke: Palgrave Macmillan.

Parker, I. (2007). *Revolution in psychology: Alienation to emancipation.* London: Pluto.

Ramsey, A. (2000). The Frankfurt school. In H. Andersen & L. B. Kaspersen (Eds.), *Classical and modern social theory* (pp. 142–159). Oxford: Blackwell.

Rice, C., Chandler, E., Liddiard, K., Rinaldi, J., & Harrison, E. (2016). Pedagogical possibilities for unruly bodies. *Gender and Education,* 1–13. Advance online publication. Retrieved from http://dx.doi.org/10.1080/09540253.2016.1247947

Sayce, L. (2000). *From psychiatric patient to citizen: Overcoming discrimination and social exclusion.* Basingstoke: Palgrave Macmillan.

Sedgwick, P. (1982). *Psycho politics.* London: Pluto.

Szasz, T. S. (1961). *The myth of mental illness: Foundations of a theory of personal conduct.* New York: Dell.

Thomas, P. (1997). *The dialectics of schizophrenia.* London: Free Association.

Wainwright, D., & Calnan, M. (2002). *Work stress: The making of a modern epidemic.* Buckingham: Open University Press.

27

The return of macro approaches in social work

Iain Ferguson

Introduction: the client speaks

> I think that if you are going to have someone interview you and you need help like that, they should send someone who has a family and has gone through this and knows much more about it. Now this lady, I suppose, has been to college and had a good upbringing and was never short of money . . . but they don't know what it is to be short of money . . . I think they should go through a course of being in a family and see what happens. They just don't understand.
>
> *(Mrs Adam, social work client, quoted in Mayer & Timms, 1970, p. 121)*

Such pleas for understanding from social work clients in Mayer and Timms's classic 1970s text *The Client Speaks: Working-class impressions of casework* were one factor in highlighting the limitations of a then dominant psychosocial approach within professional social work which located clients' difficulties primarily in their early life experience and relationships (Mayer & Timms, 1970). Three issues were raised. Firstly, concern about the neglect of poverty highlighted the need for social workers in their assessments to address the material factors, such as lack of money, debt and housing issues, which often lay behind the difficulties which clients were experiencing. It also highlighted the need to be aware of the danger of seeing these difficulties solely as 'presenting problems' which masked the 'real', underlying (and usually psychosocial) problem. Secondly, the book pointed to the need for social workers to find new ways, including community work responses, of addressing the structural factors which were creating, or at least contributing to, the problems which their clients were experiencing. And thirdly, it provided early evidence of the importance of listening to service users and taking their views seriously.

In response to that critique of casework, practitioners and academics in the early 1970s began to develop new models of social work which sought to move beyond the level of the individual client while still incorporating it to a greater or lesser degree and to engage with the wider structural issues which Mayer and Timms and others had highlighted. One outcome was the radical social work movement which emerged at this time, principally in Britain and other English-speaking countries, such as Australia, Canada and the US. This movement, which was influenced by Marxism, located clients' problems in the operation of capitalism and encouraged more collective responses to these problems (Bailey & Brake, 1975). Another was the systems or ecological model developed in books such as Pincus and Minahan's *Social Work: Model and Method*, probably the most widely used textbook in British social work courses in the 1970s (Pincus & Minahan, 1973). Systems approaches shared features with radical approaches, especially in directing practitioners away from an exclusive focus on the individual client towards wider systems, such as the family, the school or the housing agency, that might be contributing to his or her problems and which would then be seen as the target for intervention. For that reason, they were seen by some on the social work left as possessing a radical potential (Leonard, 1975; see also Chapter 15). Unlike radical social work, however, they offered no wider political or economic analysis of 'the system' as a whole. They were open to the critique of systems approaches more generally, that they relied on a consensus model of society in which the different sub-systems could, through a judicious intervention if necessary, harmoniously work together (Harris & White, 2013, pp. 448–449).

'Macro' approaches in social work, the main topic of this chapter, have features in common with both radical and systems approaches. Along with *micro* and *mezzo* approaches, they formed one element of a framework which also sought to steer social workers towards the most appropriate level of intervention (Lymbery & Butler, 2004). Like the former, they point to ways in which wider structural factors such as poverty, racism and sexism can shape the lives of social work service users and so encourage practitioners to address these factors in their assessments and consider how they can respond most effectively in terms of the methods they adopt. Like the latter, they explicitly acknowledge the need for social workers to intervene at different levels, including the level of the individual client. They do not, however, carry the ideological baggage associated with systems theories.

Later in this chapter, I will explore the forms that macro approaches in social work take in different parts of the world today. The world of the 21st century, however, is in important respects very different from that of the 1970s when these debates took place. Above all, the transition to a neoliberal model of capitalism in the 1970s and 1980s, consequent on the global economic crisis of 1973, has had profound implications for every aspect of life and society – political, economic, social and cultural – and not surprisingly, has also transformed social work (Harvey, 2005; Ferguson, 2008). That means the debates of today concerning the meaning and relevance of micro, mezzo and macro approaches cannot simply take up where the debates of the 1970s left off. The next part of this chapter, therefore, explores the ways in which that transition, as well as other major political, economic and cultural changes of the past few decades, have changed the terms of the debate and the usefulness or otherwise of micro/mezzo/macro framework as a way of addressing these changes. This will involve a discussion, firstly, of micro approaches, followed by a necessarily brief discussion of mezzo approaches. The final part of the chapter will consider the forms that macro approaches are taking today, based on the experiences and activities of groups of social workers across the globe involved in challenging oppressive practices and policies.

The micro level

In considering the three approaches discussed above (radical, systems and micro/mezzo/macro), it is important to remember that all three were *models* or *approaches* to social work. That is, they did not prescribe a particular method, such as task-centred work or group work or community work. Bailey and Brake (1975, p. 9), for example, defined radical social work as 'essentially understanding the position of the oppressed in the context of the social and economic structure they live in'. Nor did they or supporters of systems approaches reject all individual or casework approaches: 'Our aim is not . . . to eliminate casework but to eliminate casework that supports ruling-class hegemony'.

Rather, the critique of casework was based on three main arguments. Firstly, advocates of all three approaches criticized what they saw as an over-reliance on casework or individual approaches as the method of choice, regardless of the problem which the client was experiencing.

The second element of the critique was more specific in targeting the dominant casework approach of the time, the psychosocial model. The particular version of psychoanalysis which prevailed in the West in the 1950s and 1960s, driven by US-based psychiatry and adopted in a diluted form into social work, was often politically conformist, highly individualistic and, at least as far as women and gays were concerned, frequently oppressive and pathologizing. For example, as Herzog notes, before the early 1980s, some 500 psychoanalytic essays and books had been written on the topic of homosexuality. Of these, 'less than half a dozen clamed homosexuality might be part of a satisfactory psychic organization' (Herzog, 2017, p. 84). It took a concerted and militant campaign by US-based gay and lesbian organizations to convince the American Psychiatric Association in 1973 that homosexuality was not a mental illness.

The third strand of the critique of casework came above all from the emerging radical social work movement. For radical social workers, a central issue was the *ideological* role of casework in a society divided by class. Reflecting four decades later on the edited collection *Radical Social Work* which appeared in 1975, Bailey, with Mike Brake, one of the two editors, argued:

> What we did was to legitimize the notion that we could criticise the psychodynamic model or framework that dominated social work theory and practice. Mike and I were concerned to locate that theory and practice within the wider context of a political economy. We raised the idea that it was possible to resist being stigmatised, and to resist poverty being blamed on poor people. We hoped that social work in its understanding and practice might provide assistance to the victims of the worst excesses of a capitalist economy.
>
> *(Bailey, 2011, p. x)*

Revisiting the debates of the 1970s

How relevant, then, is that 1970s critique to our current situation? The starting point for any discussion of contemporary social work, where practice has been transformed by neoliberal ideology and policies, must be the widespread dissatisfaction felt by practitioners about the limited opportunities for what they often describe as 'real' social work. Early evidence of that dissatisfaction came from Jones's (2001) influential study of the views of experienced workers in the UK, and later evidence came from more official sources (for example, Scottish Executive, 2006; Department of Education, 2011). Lymbery and Butler summed up the prevailing mood:

> [M]any social workers practitioners and students in the United Kingdom experience a gap between the ideals that informed their entry into the profession – for example, a commitment to social justice and to making a difference in people's lives – and the realities of practice with which they are confronted. Practitioners are struggling to survive (let alone thrive) as they experience externally imposed changes to their work that move them away from their professional values.
>
> *(Lymbery & Butler, 2004, p. 1)*

In the same year that their book was published, a well-attended meeting of social workers, students and academics in Glasgow that was the launchpad of the Social Work Action Network (www.socialworkfuture.org) took place under the title 'I didn't come into social work for this!'

While different factors contributed to that dissatisfaction, by far the most important were the 'externally imposed changes' referred to by Lymbery and Butler. In particular, the implementation by a Conservative government in the early 1990s of a care management model in the context of a market in social care transformed the social work role and vastly reduced the opportunities for social workers to engage in direct work with clients (or service users, as they were now more often described) (Harris, 2002).

Relationship-based individual work (see Chapter 12) was undoubtedly one major casualty of the dominance of care management approaches. So, too, were collective approaches in any form, including group work and community development. Hence the insistence by the authors of the 2004 *Social Work and Social Justice: A Manifesto for a New Engaged Practice* on the need to defend a range of social work methods and, more importantly, the values which underpinned them:

> So in opposition to those who would be happy to see a defeated and silenced social work occupation, we are seeking a social work that has prevention at its heart and recognises the value of collective approaches. At the same time we also recognise that good casework has also suffered as a result of the trends referred to above. We are looking to a social work that can contribute to shaping a different kind of social policy agenda, based on our understanding of the struggles experienced by clients in addressing a range of emotional, social and material problems and the strengths they bring to these struggles.
>
> (Jones, Ferguson, Lavalette, & Penketh, 2004)

Relationship-based, one-to-one work, then, and more generally, the importance of relationship was recognized in the manifesto as one component of good social work practice. And while the potential contribution of psychoanalytic theory to such practice remains a matter of debate (with some arguing that the radical critique threw out the baby with the bathwater: Pearson, Tresseder, & Yelloly, 1988), few would dispute as a minimum the need for practitioners to have an awareness of the place of emotions in their work. In a paper directed primarily at probation officers but with obvious relevance to social workers, the criminologist David Smith suggests the following:

> [R]emember that clients see you in your capacity as a member of an agency, and that this shapes the way they present their problems, as well as your response to them; attend closely to what clients say, how they say it, and what they do not say; be aware of the emotional as well as the rational, cognitive content of communication; be sensitive to the emotional effects clients have on you, the worker (because your relationship with the client may be shaped by feelings of which neither of you is fully aware); try to see clients in the context of their relationships, past as well as present; have respect for the complexity and ambiguity of clients' emotions, just as you have respect for the complexity and ambiguity of your own emotions, and the emotions of those who are close to you; and remain aware that emotions, which may be unconscious or unacknowledged, can be as important in shaping action as conscious, rational thinking.
>
> (Smith, 2006, p. 369)

Such individual, relationship-based work can be viewed as one element of a radical approach, especially if it also addresses service users' material needs, challenges internalized stigma and stereotypes (what Bailey and Brake called 'ruling-class hegemony') and promotes their strengths and agency. There is now a very considerable body of literature from service users and their allies regarding what qualities and skills they find helpful in workers and which should underpin all such work (Beresford et al., 2011).

However, such individual, or micro, work also needs to carry a health warning. Governments frequently deploy the rhetoric of individual responsibility and 'independence' as a cover for draconian cuts to the welfare state. In this political context, even progressive approaches which highlight personal agency, such as strengths-based models or recovery approaches in mental health, can easily be subverted by right-wing politicians to suggest that poor or disabled people should 'pull themselves up by their own bootstraps'. As an example, consider the following excerpt from a speech by the British Conservative politician Michael Gove in 2014 on the need for 'reform' in social work education:

> In too many cases, social work training [sic] involves idealistic students being told that the individuals with whom they will work have been disempowered by society. They will be encouraged to see these individuals as victims of social injustice whose fate is overwhelmingly decreed by the economic forces and inherent inequalities which scar our society. This analysis is, sadly, as widespread as it is pernicious. It robs individuals of the power of agency and breaks the link between an individual's actions and the consequences ... Instead of working with individuals to get them to recognise harmful patterns of behaviour, and improve their own lives, some social workers acquiesce in or make excuses for these wrong choices.
>
> *(Gove, 2013)*

In this context, a stress on 'the power of agency' means ignoring or even denying the role played by poverty, inequality and oppression in shaping people's lives and instead seeing their problems as the result of 'wrong choices'. It is not hard to see how politically convenient that view is for governments, including the one of which Gove was a member, committed to a politics of austerity and shrinking and privatizing the post-war welfare state.

Similarly, the disability activist and writer Morris has pointed to the ways some strategies of the disability movement have been exploited by both Conservative and New Labour governments in the UK as a means of undermining the universalist provisions of the welfare state (Morris, 2011). This includes, for example, the legitimate demand for individual payments to enable disabled people to gain increased independence and control over their lives.

Finally, while recognizing the radical potential within micro approaches, we still need to remind ourselves of their limitations, the most obvious one being that they are 'downstream' approaches which rarely tackle the *causes* of service users' problems: hence the need also to develop more for more preventative, 'upstream' approaches (Ferguson & Woodward, 2009). In the final section of this chapter, some of the ways in which social workers are currently challenging macro social problems such as the current refugee crisis will be considered. Here we will consider one contemporary example: loneliness and social isolation.

It is now clear that three decades of neoliberal policies based on Margaret Thatcher's dictum that 'there is no such thing as society, only individuals and families' has contributed to an epidemic of loneliness which is severely damaging the mental and physical health of millions of people, especially older people (Cox Commission, 2017). A social work response based on micro approaches would at best help a small number of individuals, even leaving aside the reality of rising eligibility criteria that mean that many people would not receive a service. By contrast, a social networking or community development approach of the type which might well have been employed in the 1970s or early 1980s could make connections between people. This includes bringing them together in a range of different forums, from social clubs and activity groups to discussion forums and campaigning groups (see Chapter 25). In themselves such responses may not sound very radical. However, they challenge the dominant individualism and reassert the importance of 'the social' (see Chapter 5). As Monbiot has argued, the current crisis of loneliness raises questions about the impact of neo-liberalism on our society and our social relationships and highlights the need for fundamental change:

> This does not require a policy response. It requires something much bigger: the reappraisal of an entire worldview. Of all the fantasies human beings entertain, the idea that we can go it alone is the most absurd and perhaps the most dangerous. We stand together or we fall apart.

> *(Monbiot, 2016)*

Mezzo approaches

The mezzo level, Lymbery and Butler suggest, refers to

> The organizational location of social work, and explores the way in which organisations have sought to manage their roles given the impact of social forces and government policies.
> *(Lymbery & Butler, 2004, p. 6)*

Recognition of the ways agency structure and function shape, enable or, conversely, constrain social work practice is not a new development. It was a central concern of the functional approach to social work developed by two academics, Taft and Robinson, at the University of Pennsylvania in the 1930s. While not explicitly radical, the political significance of their findings was quickly grasped by US-based social work radicals of the period, organized in the Rank and File Movement. According to Reisch and Andrews, in contrast to traditional models of practice, their model

> Provided radical social workers, especially those in the public services, with a practice paradigm that justified social action and the recognition of the mutuality of the worker-client relationship.
> *(Reisch & Andrews, 2002, p. 77)*

The mezzo level is not the focus of this chapter, so its implications for practice can only be touched on. Despite that, an understanding of the organizational context of social work and the ways in which that context has been transformed by the managerialist policies of the past three decades is an essential starting point for assessing the possibilities for progressive practice.

The implications of that transformation for practice have been the subject of debate in the literature in recent years, often framed around the issue of professional 'discretion', drawing on Lipsky's classic text, *Street Level Bureaucracy* (Lipsky, 1980). Without re-entering that debate, few would dispute that the combination of the organizational changes to which social work has been subjected since the early 1990s have significantly constrained the practice of even the most creative and committed workers. Examples include the relocation of social workers in many areas into call centres far removed from the communities they serve and ever-higher eligibility criteria which reinforce the prioritization of risk over need. Also, the overall impact since 2010 of austerity policies have increased demand on services while hugely reducing the resources of both local authorities and voluntary organizations. In her preface to the 2014–2015 *Survey of Social Work in the UK*, for example, which was conducted by the recruitment consultancy Liquid Personnel and based on responses from around 1,500 social workers at all levels, Munro writes:

> There are a few positive findings: despite all the difficulties, a quarter of respondents rate their morale as high or very high and only a third rate it as low or very low; many newly qualified workers appear to be given the extra support they need as they start their career. However, there is plenty here to depress the reader. While direct cuts to front line social work have been limited, there have been significant cuts that hamper social workers' ability to provide a good service. Cuts to managers reduce the capacity of the organisation to provide a good level of supervision. Cuts to administrative staff increase the bureaucratic demands on social workers. Despite the removal of many nationally prescribed timescales and targets allowing more local flexibility, time with families still seems a low priority in many offices.

Her conclusion is that:

> Priorities need to shift away from processes and towards actively helping individuals and families who need a social worker. One major under-used resource at present is the expertise in the workforce that cannot be fully utilised because of the dysfunctional conditions in which practitioners are working. Rectifying this will be the most productive line of action.
>
> *(Liquid Personnel, 2015, p. 2)*

While the survey usefully highlights the pressures on practitioners, noticeably absent from the discussion section is any consideration of the possibility of *collective* responses to these pressures, above all in the form of trade union responses but also through coalitions of workers and service users or through professional organizations. While few would dispute that the record of public sector unions in defending either services or their members' conditions in recent years has often been uninspiring and ineffective, there have nevertheless been examples of successful campaigns and industrial action. Also significant is the change that has taken place in the political climate in recent years. We will now turn to a consideration of that change, and to the possibility of social workers being able to influence the macro level.

Macro approaches today

Writing in 2005, the president of the American Psychiatric Association expressed his concern about the domination of biomedical psychiatry by the major drug companies (see also Chapters 6, 26 and 36), arguing that:

> If we are seen as mere pill-pushers and employees of the pharmaceutical industry, our credibility as a profession is destroyed. As we address these Big Pharma issues, we must examine the fact that as a profession, we have allowed the bio-psychosocial model to become the bio-bio-bio model.
>
> *(Scharfstein, cited in Mosher et al., 2013, pp. 134–135)*

In a similar fashion, if for different reasons, the micro/mezzo/macro model of social work has also in reality become the micro/micro/micro model. For example, it would be interesting to know just how little room is currently made available within social work education course curricula for the consideration of collective approaches such as community development, political action or even group work.

One of the reasons for that narrowing of the social work role, in the UK in particular, has already been discussed. A key feature of the neoliberal agenda as applied to social work and social policy in the early 1990s was the imposition of a care management model imported from the US and aimed at promoting a value-light social work capable of operating within the framework of a developing social care market. Unsurprisingly, advocates of that model had little tolerance for critical or structural social work arguments which suggested that the operation of these same market forces at a societal and global level was responsible for most of the poverty and inequality that led people to seek social work help in the first place.

In addition, radical social movements of the 1970s retreated into a narrow identity politics in the following decade. This led to the ascendancy of a neoliberal individualism which denigrated not only such collective struggles, but also the very notion of 'the social' and any form of concern for the other.

Since the late 1990s, however, continuing to the present day, there have been repeated challenges to the suffocating grip of neoliberal capitalism and to the economic and military competition which it fosters. The anti-capitalist or global justice movement which grew out of the protests against the World Trade Organisation in Seattle in 1999, for example, was followed soon after by a worldwide movement against the invasion of and war in Iraq. While this failed to stop the invasion, it politicized millions and made such future invasions and wars more difficult (Callinicos, 2010). The emergence of Occupy Wall Street in 2012 as a protest initially against growing levels of inequality in the US quickly went global. The Indignados movement in Spain also emerged in 2012, with huge occupations of city squares by hundreds of thousands of mainly young people protesting a housing crisis and extremely high levels of youth unemployment. The austerity policies consequent on the global economic crash of 2008 have also given rise to resistance, most notably in Greece where their effects have been most brutally felt (Ioakimidis & Teloni, 2013; Ovenden, 2015).

These movements, coming on top of the dissatisfaction of many social workers about what their profession has become, have impacted on social work at a national and global level. They have contributed to a revival of interest in radical social work and to the search for macro responses to problems of poverty, inequality, racism and environmental destruction. 'Macro' responses in social work can, of course, take many different forms. These move from working to ensure the election of a candidate or political party sympathetic to social work goals and values to the involvement of national and international social work bodies with global campaigns and in developing policy responses.

All these approaches have their place. Here, however, the focus will be on macro approaches 'from below', on the activities and organization of practitioners seeking to change government or business policies or ideologies or at least to challenge their effects. The period since the beginning of the 21st century has seen the emergence of groups of social workers, students and academics in several different countries committed to exploring and developing new forms of social work practice which challenge oppressive policies and the effects of these policies. To name just a few, they include the Boston Health Liberation Group in the US; the Orange Tide in Spain; the New Approach group in Hungary; the Progressive Social Work Network in Hong Kong; the Radical and Critical Social Work Groups in Germany; Rebel Social Work in New Zealand and the Social Work Action Network with groups or affiliates in the UK, Ireland, Greece, Japan and Denmark. Social workers are also involved with a range of radical social movements in much of the Global South: for example, in Brazil and South Africa (for more details, see Ferguson, Lavalette, & Ioakimides, 2018 and Chapter 10). The activities of these groups differ from country to country depending on the local issues. Most are characterized by an overall orientation that is well summed up on the website statement of the New Approach group in Hungary:

> The New Approach to community work and radical social work is based on the idea of combining workshops and action groups, and also the renewal of social work codes of ethics. This dual function is located in a long-term goal:
>
> Workshops: we want to provide space for discussing issues concerning the social sphere, development of action strategies.
>
> As an action group we are committed to the profession and the public's attention is drawn to the situation of those excluded. We seek to be a professional community that is not afraid to stand up for those in need.
>
> *(New Approach, 2011)*

The first point requires creating safe spaces for critical and collective discussions, both theoretical and practical, on social work practice and strategy. Such forums are essential for four reasons:

1   The dominance of managerialism (see Chapter 4) has not only shaped the way in which social workers respond to those who need help. It has also undermined collective forms of workplace organization and discussion, whether in the form of trade unions or team meetings, and left many workers feeling atomized and isolated. Bringing practitioners together, then, is a way of breaking down that sense of isolation.
2   Across much of the public sector, in health services and higher education as well as in social work and social care, that dominance of managers whose values and priorities are often very different from those whom they manage has led to what workers often refer to as 'a climate of fear', an inability to speak out or criticize policy or management decisions for fear of being punished. Creating safe spaces, therefore, where workers can speak openly and critically about their practice experience without fear of victimization is a crucial part of developing a new engaged social work practice.
3   To a degree, such collective gatherings can embody 'the change we wish to see' in prefiguring new ways of working, both in the sense of modelling anti-oppressive practice and also in actively involving service users at every level.
4   By bringing together academics, practitioners and service users, they provide opportunities for developing social work theory in close connection with practice and not in ivory-tower isolation and abstraction.

The second function identified by Hungarian colleagues is no less important. In almost every case, the groups referred to are actively involved in one or more forms of social action. Most commonly, this has involved highlighting and challenging the effects of specific government policies, whether national or international. Perhaps not surprisingly, work with asylum seekers and refugees has been a central activity for many of these groups, given the refugee crisis of recent years, which has seen people forced to abandon their homes and countries and seek a new life elsewhere. Thus, social workers in Greece have been actively involved in supporting the tens of thousands of refugees arriving on the Greek islands (Teloni, 2011; Chalalet & Jones, 2015). In the UK, organizations such as Social Workers without Borders, the Social Work Action Network and the British Association of Social Workers have been involved in different ways in showing solidarity with asylum seekers and refugees, especially those languishing in makeshift camps in the north of France who are trying to reach Britain. In 2016, two social workers in Kent set up Social Work First. In an article in the *Guardian* newspaper describing their project, they discussed the challenges faced and, in the process, pointed to what macro approaches mean today:

> The SWF project is in its early days, but so far we have faced numerous barriers. In working alongside migrants and asylum seekers we are up against a dominant political narrative that dehumanises and blames. It is not possible to talk about empowerment without addressing the socio-political onslaught that refugees are facing from the British and French states, which knowingly demonise and marginalise them.
>
> To acknowledge this, we are trying to tackle the crisis on both the political and the social fronts by providing a social work presence in the camp to assess, support and safeguard vulnerable people, while campaigning for Britain and France to uphold the human rights of the camp's inhabitants. . . . This is an opportunity to use the unique skills and wisdom of the social work profession to defend the rights of some of the most marginalised people in the world today, right here on our doorstep. This is our chance to reclaim the profession from state administration and practise international social work.
>
> *(Social Work First, 2016)*

Social workers in Hungary have campaigned against the brutal homelessness policies of their government; social workers in the US have been actively involved in the Black Lives Matter campaign; and the Palestine -UK Social Work Network has continued to highlight the plight of Palestinian child prisoners in Israeli jails (Shennan, 2015).

Conclusions: whither macro approaches in social work?

The above examples show that growing numbers of social workers are attempting to raise their eyes above the immediacy of their day-to-day practice and to challenge oppressive policies and ideologies that are causing so much misery and hardship to human beings both at home and abroad. Not surprisingly, given the hegemonic grip of neoliberal ideology and policies in recent decades, they are still far from being the norm. However, the spread of these groups to almost every part of the globe and the evident desire among increasing numbers of practitioners for a social work rooted in social justice (see also Chapter 10), show the possibilities for the development of new macro approaches capable of addressing the challenges of the 21st century. This is reflected, for example, in well-attended conferences on critical and radical social work from Britain to Hong Kong.

In conclusion, two questions face those who wish to develop such approaches. Firstly, how can they incorporate macro approaches into their day-to-day practice, as opposed to their being activities in which they are involved outside the working day, as is often the case at present? Secondly, how can action groups or professional organizations engage in policy change and development without being incorporated into and neutralized by much more powerful players? These are serious issues with no easy solutions. What is important and positive, however, is that for the first time in many years, recognition of the need for macro approaches, often linked to a desire for a more radical social work, is back on the social work agenda. Given the global challenges that we face, that can only be a good thing.

Further reading

Fenton, J. (2017). *Values in social work: Reconnecting with social justice*. London: Palgrave Macmillan.
Martinez, D. B., & Fleck-Henderson, A. (Eds.). (2014). *Social justice in clinical practice: A liberation health framework for social work*. London: Routledge.
Lavalette, M., & Penketh, L. (Eds.). (2014). *Race, racism and social work: Contemporary issues and debates*. Bristol: Policy Press.

References

Bailey, R. (2011). Foreword. In M. Lavalette (Ed.), *Radical social work today: Social work at the crossroads*. Bristol: Policy Press.
Bailey, R., & Brake, M. (Eds.). (1975). *Radical social work*. London: Arnold.
Beresford, P., Fleming, J., Glynn, M., Bewley, C., Croft, S., Branfield, F., & Postle, K. (2011). *Supporting people: Towards a person-centred approach*. Bristol: Policy Press.
Callinicos, A. (2010). *Bonfire of illusions: The twin crises of the liberal world*. London: Polity.
Chalalet, S. A., & Jones, C. (2015). The refugee crisis in Samos, Greece. *Critical and Radical Social Work*, *3*(3), 445–453.
Cox Commission. (2017). *Combatting loneliness one conversation at a time*. Retrieved from www.jocoxloneli ness.org/pdf/a_call_to_action.pdf
Department of Education. (2011). *The Munro review of child protection: Final report*. London: HMSO.
Ferguson, I. (2008). *Reclaiming social work: Challenging neoliberalism and promoting social justice*. London: Sage.
Ferguson, I., & Woodward, R. (2009). *Radical social work in practice*. Bristol: Policy Press.
Ferguson, I., Ioakimidis, V., & Lavalette, M. (2018). *Global social work in a political context: Radical perspectives*. Bristol: Policy Press.
Gove, M. (2013). Speech to the NSPCC. Retrieved from www.gov.uk/government/speeches/getting-it-right-for-children-in-need-speech-to-the-nspcc
Harris, J. (2002). *The social work business*. London: Routledge.
Harris, J., & White, V. (2013). *Oxford dictionary of social work and social care*. Oxford: Oxford University Press.
Harvey, D. (2005). *A short history of neoliberalism*. Oxford: Oxford University Press.
Herzog, D. (2017). *Cold war Freud: Psychoanalysis in an age of catastrophes*. Cambridge, UK: Cambridge University Press.
Ioakimidis, V., & Teloni, D. D. (2013). Greek social work and the never-ending crisis of the welfare state. *Critical and Radical Social Work*, *1*(1), 31–49.
Jones, C. (2001). Voices from the front line: State social work under New Labour. *British Journal of Social Work*, *31*, 547–562.
Jones, C., Ferguson, I., Lavalette, M., & Penketh, L. (2004). *Social work and social justice: A manifesto for a new engaged practice*. Retrieved from www.socialworkfuture.org/articles-resources/uk-articles/103-social-work-and-social-justice-a-manifesto-for-a-new-engaged-practice
Leonard, P. (1975). Towards a paradigm for radical practice. In R. Bailey & M. Brake (Eds.), *Radical social work* (pp. 46–61). London: Arnold.
Lipsky, M. ([1980] 2010). *Street-level bureaucracy: Dilemmas of the individual in public services* (2nd ed.). New York: Russell Sage Foundation.
Liquid Personnel. (2015). *The social work survey 2014/2015*. Manchester: Liquid Personnel. Retrieved from http://cdn.basw.co.uk/upload/basw_40843-5.pdf
Lymbery, M., & Butler, S. (Eds.). (2004). *Social work: Ideals and practice realities*. Basingstoke: Palgrave Macmillan.
Mayer, J. E., & Timms, N. (1970). *The client speaks; Working-class impressions of casework*. London: Routledge & Kegan Paul.
Monbiot, G. (2016, October 12). Neoliberalism is creating loneliness: That's what wrenching society apart. *Guardian*. Retrieved from www.theguardian.com/commentisfree/2016/oct/12/neoliberalism-creating-loneliness-wrenching-society-apart
Morris, J. (2011). *Rethinking disability policy*. New York: Joseph Rowntree Foundation. Retrieved from www.jrf.org.uk/report/rethinking-disability-polic
Mosher, L., Goseden, R., & Beder, S. (2013). Drug companies and schizophrenia. In J. Read & J. Dillon (Eds.), *Models of madness* (2nd ed.). London: Routledge.

New Approach. (2011). *Uj szemlelet a radikalis szocialis munka megjelenese magyarorszagon*. Retrieved from http://annyit.blog.hu/2011/03/12/uj_szemlelet_a_radikalis_szocialis_munka_megjelenese_magyarorszagon

Ovenden, K. (2015). *Syriza: Inside the labyrinth*. London: Pluto.

Pearson, G., Tresseder, J., & Yelloly, M. (Eds.). (1988). *Social work and the legacy of Freud*. Basingstoke: Palgrave Macmillan.

Pincus, A., & Minahan, A. (1973). *Social work practice: Model and method*. Itasca, IL: Peacock.

Reisch, M., & Andrews, J. (2002). *The road not taken: A history of radical social work in the United States*. New York: Brunner-Routledge.

Scottish Executive. (2006). *Changing lives: Report of the 21st century social work review*. Edinburgh: Scottish Executive.

Shennan, G. (2015). The Palestine-UK social work network: Taking collective responsibility for social justice and human rights. *Critical and Radical Social Work, 3*(1), 125–130.

Smith, D. (2006). Making sense of psychoanalysis in criminological theory and probation practice. *Probation Journal, 53*(4), 361–376.

Social Work First. (2016, 22 June). Children in the refugee camp in Calais are at risk: Social workers must act. *Guardian*. Retrieved from www.theguardian.com/social-care-network/social-life-blog/2016/jun/22/calais-refugee-camp-abuse-social-work-silent

Teloni, D. (2011). Grassroots community social work with the 'unwanted': The case of Kinisi and the rights of refugees and migrants in Patras, Greece. In M. Lavalette & V. Ioakimidis (Eds.), *Social work in extremis* (pp. 65–80). Bristol: Policy Press.

28

Empowerment ideas in social work

Paul Stepney

I have a dream ... that all men are created equal and that one day my four little children will live in a nation where they will be judged by the content of their character not by the colour of their skin.
— *(Martin Luther King, Washington, 28 August 1963)*

Introduction

I am standing in a small gallery of contemporary art in a village just south of Virrat in central Finland, attracted by an exhibition to celebrate the work of the Finnish artist Lars Holmström. He is considered to be one of Finland's most important constructivist artists, whose abstract style very much reflects his avant garde thinking. I ask Olli, the gallery owner, to tell me what *Toivo vastoinkäymisten keskellä*, the theme of one set of particularly engaging prints (www.larsholm strom.fi) that appear to have a subtle social message, means. He smiles, shrugs his shoulders and says, 'It is difficult to give an exact translation, but this theme has something to do with finding hope amidst adversity or what we might call empowerment'. Although contemporary art is clearly capable of many different interpretations, it would seem that these Holmström prints capture something rather important in social work – a concept that we have been striving to define and are inclined to refer to rather loosely and over enthusiastically in our practice. In this chapter, I want to look more closely and critically at this concept and explore the development of empowerment ideas in social work.

Empowerment has become something of a popular slogan which people across the political spectrum find irresistible, thus making it an 'intellectually messy' concept (Dominelli, 2012, p. 214). It follows that empowerment is a highly contested term concerned at one level with societal transformation (Rees, 1991) and 'changing the relationship between rich and poor' (Berner & Phillips, 2005, p 26), whilst at another level, it is concerned with the psychology of liberation and personal change (Riger, 1993). It can of course be used to connect both levels and argue for a more holistic community-based approach that situates people's exclusion and oppression within an analysis of global social and economic development (Lee, 2001) and the wider socio-economic structure (Fook, 2012).

In mainstream political debate, empowerment is a concept that appears to have considerable utility and resonance, such that everyone appears to be in favour of it. For example, those on the political right use it to argue for greater individual responsibility and extending consumer choice in the market – a view criticized by Leonardsen (2007, p. 8) for advocating 'responsibility without power', while those on the left see it as a means of developing a collective identity among marginalized groups to achieve greater equality and social justice. In social policy empowerment is said to be a core aim of modernization and the restructuring of public services (Stepney, 2017a), while conversely, it may well be deployed as a means of resistance by those who oppose such change. As a multilevel construct, it is concerned with individual development and group processes as well as wider organizational and social change (Forrest, 1999), thus making it a rather slippery term to define.

Towards a definition of empowerment

Empowerment is a concept that has come to occupy an important place in the social work literature (Adams, 2008; Smith, 2008; Thompson, 2006), but it has been defined in several ways. Payne (2014) argues that empowerment 'seeks to help clients gain powers of decision and action over their own lives' (p. 294). It does this in three main ways: by removing social and personal barriers, increasing people's capability and self-confidence, and shifting power to the powerless. Similarly, it is seen as a 'multi-dimensional social process that helps people gain control over their lives' (Page & Czuba, 1999, p. 2), and it achieves this by drawing on the seminal work of Freire (1972) and Gutiérrez et al. (2003) by emphasizing 'the need to increase the personal, interpersonal and political power of oppressed and marginalised people' (Turner & Maschi, 2015, p. 152). This connects with the International Federation of Social Workers (IFSW) definition, which locates empowerment within a framework informed by the principles of human rights and social justice (IFSW, 2013).

One of the issues that emerges from these various definitions is whether empowerment is a theory or a process or even something broader that connects the two? Many writers clearly see it as a complex process informed by a range of theoretical ideas. The process may be like a journey that develops and expands as we experience it. Combining theory with an appreciation of the empowerment process can help us to make sense of our experience in three interconnected stages:

- First, it begins with recognition and awareness.
- Then, with skilled intervention and support awareness, it can develop into what Freire (1972) called 'critical consciousness', which opens up new choices and opportunities.
- Finally, it reaches the stage of 'transforming choices into action'.

(Albuquerque, Santos, & Almeida, 2017, p. 90)

In the context of social work, Lee (2001) suggests that empowerment is neither a theory nor a process but more a 'variety of conceptually coherent social work approaches and frameworks for practice' (p. 31). Consequently, for the social worker, seeing it as an overarching theoretical framework for practice may be a more helpful formulation and one that potentially can be applied to work with any client group. An empowerment framework can be used in mental health settings to challenge the medicalization of services and stigma and to shift the lens towards client interaction with their social environment.

Focusing on empowerment often exposes a deeper crisis of meaning in modern industrial societies, which reveals itself in the problems reported by clients in the practice focus above, associated with social isolation, stigma and stress (Leonardsen, 2007). Seeing empowerment as a theoretical framework can offer an enabling context for practice: specifically, to enable clients to exercise more control and feel, perhaps for the first time in many years, that they are not powerless but have some power to change their lives. It follows that adopting this approach inevitably raises questions about social justice, diversity and equality that must be addressed. In this we are indebted to the legacy of Barbara Solomon (1976) and her work with the African American community in the United States, as well as, of course, the vision of Martin Luther King in the 1960s.

Black empowerment

In many important respects, the work of Barbara Solomon (1976) on black empowerment has provided a benchmark for subsequent theorizing and analysis about working with all oppressed groups and communities. In analyzing the oppression and stigmatization of black people, Solomon argues that we must work for the collective empowerment of all by concerted community action. Historically, social work has found it difficult to transcend the individual or family level to tackle oppression at the institutional, policy and societal levels. But going beyond the personal and interpersonal dimensions of oppression is frequently necessary. Hence, building on the iconic work of Solomon, a model of practice is proposed that overcomes negative stereotypes, builds self-confidence and seeks to find ways through problem-solving to remove power blocks in people's lives (see also Chapter 29). According to Solomon (1976), this can be done at individual, group and community levels by:

- Redefining the issues to be addressed with oppressed groups so they become change agents.
- Harnessing knowledge and skills to construct an agenda for change with appropriate goals.
- Participating in community action for the collective good of the community, using their perceived 'difference' from accepted norms as a source of strength rather than an adjunct of powerlessness.

By definition, empowerment implies a sharing of power, but this may be problematic unless it is supported by other changes that facilitate and support power-sharing initiatives. We must therefore examine the concept of power in empowerment more closely, drawing on the work of theorists, including Foucault, Habermas, Freire and Lukes.

Foucault: reconceptualizing power, freedom and 'self'

There has been a strong belief in traditional thought about freedom and power, that our individual 'self' is separate and ontologically distinct from political, economic and social power. Power was seen as an external force acting on and shaping the 'self'. However, the ideas of Foucault (1978) changed all this by suggesting that the 'self' could be a site of power struggle and conflict. This relates well to the life experience of mental health clients and the tensions associated with the construction of 'normal' everyday life events. Whilst the term 'normal' is used to account for a range of acceptable behaviours, customs and appearance, those who do not or cannot conform may be labelled 'abnormal' and experience discrimination and stigma. Hence, the self is formed through 'discourses of normalisation' which are likely to be reinforced by society's norms, which welfare practice and the expert power of professionals may uphold.

Foucault's ideas challenge conventional modernist notions of power and suggest that power is 'neither something that can be possessed, nor is it strictly an oppressive force' (Rivest & Moreau, 2015, p. 1860) but is found in power relationships. Such relationships are informed by knowledge and . . . as the saying goes 'knowledge is power' (sometimes attributed to Francis Bacon, 1597). Power for Foucault operates within a system of governmentality – ultimately, how we manage ourselves and are governed by the knowledge and power of the state (Pease, 2002). Managers, officials and professionals like psychiatrists, who Foucault (2003) called *normalizing experts*, make judgements often supported by binary labels – normal/deviant, sane/mad, deserving/undeserving and so on. The social standing of *normalizing experts* is reinforced by their use of a professional language or discourse underpinned by scientific knowledge that confers privilege particularly on themselves. It also confers a presumption of truth, which in turn confers power.

According to Pease (2002), the implications of Foucault's micro analysis of power is that small-scale action and struggles have the potential for challenging self-regulatory processes and bringing about emancipatory change. He suggests that the social value conferred on scientific knowledge tends to marginalize other forms of knowledge which become devalued, downgraded and subjugated – so for Pease (2002), one of the key aims of empowerment is 'the insurrection of subjugated knowledge' (p 141). This is the local 'common sense' knowledge derived from experience, and is often viewed as the working-class knowledge of the client that finds its way into what social workers call 'practice wisdom' (Stepney, 2012, p. 24). This connects Foucault with what Habermas (1984) referred to as *communicative action*, which takes place when people reach mutual understanding and form identities that promote social integration and solidarity. It follows that *communicative action* is a good example of empowerment, to counteract the *strategic action* of normalizing experts and their use of scientific knowledge (Habermas, 1987). Empowerment through strategies that enhance social solidarity can also contribute to personal freedom and liberty – freedom from isolation and oppression (see also Chapters 5 and 10).

Freedom and power cannot be easily separated, and according to Rose (1999), freedom is a consequence of power, and power is a product of freedom. One consequence of this is that social work contributes most to individual freedom when it confers power on the self of the client as 'part of a productive network which runs through the whole social body' (Foucault, 1984, p. 61). This is very much what Freire and Gramsci had in mind to promote change.

The influence of Freire and Gramsci

The ideas of Freire and Gramsci are relevant to the empowerment debate in social work. Freire developed his pedagogic approach working as an adult educator to problematize the situation of oppressed groups in Brazil, but his ideas remain relevant to practitioners in advanced Western societies. Freire (1972) suggests that people are effectively disfranchised by the dominant ideology and divisive social relationships that exploit them, and that developing a 'critical consciousness' of their oppression can sow the seeds of liberation. This is a theme which connects with Gramsci's (1986) notion of hegemony and the power of ideas that permeate all relationships and shapes reality to achieve consent. However, as Payne (2014) notes, developing a person's awareness and consciousness of oppression does not necessarily lead to transformative action, but it is an important first step, a view supported by research with women and ethnic minority groups in the United States (Gutiérrez, 1995). An understanding of the contingencies concerning the use of power is required and, for this, we turn to the important work of Stephen Lukes.

Power: a radical view: the contribution of Lukes and Rees

Power has also been described by Lukes (2005) as the capacity to change one's environment, with three possible ways of doing this: first, through exerting direct influence on decisions;

second, exerting direct influence that leads to no decision being made (non–decision making) and finally, through indirect influence that shapes which issues come before decision makers, as revealed in the work of lobbyists and media professionals. For Lukes (2005), power may be categorized in three ways:

- Pluralist, where power is diversely distributed and potentially available to everyone, as evidenced by the growing influence of online blogs.
- Elitist, where power is the preserve of a social and economic elite, often buttressed by convention, ideology and social norms.
- Radical, a multidimensional view of power operating within and beyond various structural and institutional constraints.

The first and third views of power are likely to be most applicable to social work. Hence, it is time to look at how empowerment ideas may be applied to practice.

Application to practice

One of the contemporary problems we now face is that the term 'empowerment' may induce a degree of scepticism from the hard-pressed streetwise practitioner when it is introduced on training programmes (Thompson, 2012). I have encountered this myself in both the UK and on SOSNET (in-service) training courses in Finland when I introduced the term. Some practitioners raise their eyebrows, roll their eyes and say, 'Yes, yes, empowerment again . . . it's a nice idea, but is it really going to solve anything?' Clearly, they have heard it all before. However, the antidote to complacency and scepticism is the many examples of good empowering practice that can be cited (Thompson, 2006; Smith, 2008), which illustrate what can be achieved, particularly in promoting prevention alongside protection in high-risk cases (Stepney, 2014). The key to effectiveness can often be found in two important factors: first, the value of a sound partnership between practitioner and client and second, the need for shared ownership of the nature of the problems and, importantly, what should be done about them. According to Thompson (2012, online), 'shared ownership . . . provides the foundation for empowerment'.

Practitioners are frequently caught between encouraging a greater sense of personal responsibility and self-discipline in their clients and promoting empowering practice (Rivest & Moreau, 2015). What is required is practice that not only promotes individual empowerment but also operates at the interpersonal, community and wider policy levels in favour of marginalized groups. In so doing, it aims to 'give choices to tackle inequalities . . . and transform choices into effective action' (Albuquerque et al., 2017, p. 89). This is consistent with the original vision of empowerment proposed by Rees (1991), which has five essential elements:

- Biography as a way of analyzing experience and listening to the victim.
- Power as potentially liberating in all political processes.
- Political understanding to ensure practice is politically informed.
- Skills and knowledge that reflect power (Freire, 1972), which are necessary for liberation.
- Praxis – the connecting of policy and practice, as a necessary requirement for empowerment.

(Rees, 1991)

This accords well with Thompson's (2012) plans for empowerment through partnership – to help identify the source of clients' problems, boost confidence, address long-standing difficulties and agree on a way forward. The effectiveness of empowerment strategies has been supported by many research studies from the international literature. For example, Li-yu Song (2015) studied the impact of empowerment strategies used by social workers to protect victims of intimate partner abuse in Taiwan. She found that, of the five groups of contextual variables present, empowerment strategies were by far the most important for producing change. Given that the majority of victims stayed with the perpetrators, empowerment proved to be the most effective strategy to prevent reoccurrence of violence, improve victims' mental health and ensure their safety through better decision-making.

Searching for better ways to measure the effectiveness of social work practice, Depauw and Driessens (2016) developed a scale to measure client empowerment which was tested, in consultation with social workers and people in poverty, in two public welfare centres in Belgium. They found that the dimensions of psychological empowerment can be translated into concrete practice and measured. The results provided helpful translation of internal clients' perspectives, emphasizing client strengths, improved dialogue and provided additional data on clients support networks directly relevant to practice outcomes.

Using empowerment as a framework for practice is particularly relevant for social workers in the fields of mental health, adult services and community social work, but also child protection.

Social workers in children's services have many cases where the child protection role is paramount but soon gives way to the need for client empowerment and family support. A community social work approach can therefore be deployed with the aim of community empowerment and creating new informal networks of care. The need for a wide range of empowering community and family support services for clients has never been greater, given the way children's services in the UK increasingly concentrate on early intervention, child protection and risk management (Featherstone, Morris, & White, 2014).

Community empowerment

Community social work is primarily concerned with working alongside clients and community members to develop more preventative local services, reflecting its commitment to empowerment, social justice and establishing new and more inclusive local services (Stepney, 2017b; see also Chapter 25). Lee (2001) proposes an approach to empowerment very much within this tradition by locating clients' problems within an understanding of the way the global market impinges on the quality of life in local communities. Drawing on her experience of working with women and children in poverty, she suggests practitioners should work with clients to:

- Develop a positive sense of self.
- Help construct a critical conception of their life circumstances and problems.
- Mobilize resources and develop strategies to achieve both personal and collective goals.

(p. 34)

A community social work approach aims to achieve both personal, interpersonal and community empowerment. Yoo et al. (2004) provide a good example of community empowerment in the field of health promotion designed to empower individuals to improve the well-being of one community in New Orleans. The project was effective in creating a framework for group facilitation and inclusion. In their evaluation, several factors were identified which reinforced community empowerment, and these can be contrasted with those that challenged or restricted it, as shown in Table 28.1.

A second example comes from Mitchell (2001) in the south west of England, concerning the establishment of a dementia service for older people. The project involved the systematic

Table 28.1 Factors reinforcing and challenging community empowerment

Reinforcing Factors	Challenging Factors
Sound conceptual empowerment framework and vision	Unclear vision and limited resources
Clear understanding by participants of framework	Slow process with limited progress
Consistency at community meetings	Attracting wider participation
Supporting staff and community leaders	Safety concerns
Open communication	Uncertainty about how to promote the project in the community
Staying focused and on task	Ability to respond to situational factors mid-course
Good community support networks	Inadequate or non-existent support networks
Regular debriefing meetings among all staff and community facilitators	Staff working in isolation

Source: Adapted from Yoo et al., 2004, p 263.

mapping of clients' life domains to counteract the pessimism associated with much conventional care. The medical model of 'warehousing' older people with mental health needs was rejected in favour of early intervention with a person-centred approach. Acknowledging the influence of Kitwood (1997), Mitchell worked with carers to produce a 'dementia voice' magazine, outreach service, daycare without walls, a respite care programme, group reminiscence therapy and a support and action group for carers. The group began as a support group but, as a result of individual members' experience and the influence of social workers, soon began to influence service planning and policy. This resulted in a paradigm shift from passive recipient to active partnership in the planning and provision of care. Today there is a 'memory cafe' in many UK doctors' surgeries.

These findings are consistent with those in the wider literature (Ohmer & Korr, 2006) and provide a useful checklist against which practice within a framework of community empowerment can be evaluated.

Conclusion

One of the crucial questions underpinning the empowerment debate is whether it is about helping individual clients take more control of their lives to achieve greater well-being or concerned with wider social change. The position adopted here is that it is about both. In the messy field of practice, these two positions are not just closely related but, with skilled and committed inputs from the practitioner, 'liberation for wellbeing' can lead to wider policy change (Mitchell, 2001). This is why empowerment is such an influential and all-encompassing concept.

From the extensive international literature, it is noted that critiques of empowerment (Pease, 2002; Fook, 2012) suggest that many of the problems clients face are structural in origin. Consequently, restricting empowering practice to improving individual well-being may reduce it to 'palliative practice' (Albuquerque et al. (2017). This is one of many challenges facing the practitioner, and it is worth remembering that 'social workers can never become neutral benefactors in a society of inequalities' (Leonardsen, 2007, p. 10). Also, attention to the process of change (Freire, 1972) brings out the folly of thinking that empowerment ideas can ever be imposed as vehicles for structural change.

Empowerment is a broad, highly persuasive and positive concept that continues to have a major influence on social work practice. The growth of the client or service user involvement and advocacy movement (see Chapter 30) owes much to empowerment ideas translated into practice. Empowerment has developed both as an overarching and 'conceptually coherent framework for practice' (Lee, 2001, p 32), as well as one important aspect of practice that informs a range of social work methods – from CBT to crisis intervention and task-centred practice and from psychotherapeutic approaches to ecological systems theory. However, it exerts a decisive influence without fully embracing the underpinning theory (Payne, 2014).

Empowerment helps practitioners hold on to the possibility of achieving positive change even in the most discouraging situations when all seems lost. Clients generally respond well to this, and so the real challenge is to support the client to do it for themselves and then try to build upon this within the local community. Empowering ideas can clearly make a critical difference to clients' lives and are an important dimension in developing critically reflective practice.

Further reading

Lee, J. A. B. (2001). *The empowerment approach to social work practice: Building the beloved community* (2nd ed.). New York: Columbia University Press.
A comprehensive American text which combines criticality with a multiple focus that locates progressive practice within its appropriate community context.

Leonardsen, D. (2007). Empowerment in social work: An individual vs. a relational perspective. *International Journal of Social Welfare, 16*, 3–11.
A thoughtful Nordic account of empowerment with an important discussion about the implications for the education of social workers.

Rivest, M-P., & Moreau, N. (2015). Between emancipatory practice and disciplinary interventions: Empowerment and contemporary social normativity. *British Journal of Social Work, 45*, 1855–1870.
An important article by two Canadian academics that offers a Foucauldian critique of empowerment as practitioners tread the thin line between promoting emancipatory practice and enforcing social discipline.

References

Adams, R. (2008). *Empowerment, participation and social work* (4th ed.). Basingstoke: Palgrave Macmillan.
Albuquerque, C. P., Santos, C. C., & Almeida, H. (2017). Assessing 'empowerment' as social development: Goal and process. *European Journal of Social Work, 20*(1), 88–110.
Berner, E., & Phillips, B. (2005). Left to their own devices? Community self-help between alternative development and neo-liberalism. *Community Development Journal, 40*(1), 17–29.
Depauw, J., & Driessens, K. (2016). Taking the measure: A participatory approach to measuring and monitoring psychological empowerment in social work practices. *European Journal of Social Work*. Retrieved from http://dx.doi.org/10.1080/13691457.2016.1255878
Dominelli, L. (2012). Empowerment: Help or hindrance in professional relationships. In P. Stepney & D. Ford (Eds.), *Social work models, methods and theories: A framework for practice* (2nd ed., pp. 214–235). Lyme Regis: Russell House Publishing.
Featherstone, B., Morris, K., & White, S. (2014). A marriage made in Hell: Early intervention meets child protection. *British Journal of Social Work, 44*, 1735–1749.
Fook, J. (2012). *Social work: A critical approach to practice* (2nd ed.). Los Angeles: Sage.
Forrest, D. (1999). Education and empowerment: Towards untested feasibility. *Community Development Journal, 34*(2), 93–107.
Foucault, M. (1978). *The history of sexuality, Volume one: An introduction*. New York: Vintage Books.
Foucault, M. (1984). *The Foucault reader* (Paul Rabinow, Ed.). Harmondsworth: Penguin.
Foucault, M. (2003). *Abnormal: Lectures at the college de France, 1974–1975* (G. Burchell, Trans.). London: Verso.
Freire, P. (1972). *Pedagogy of the oppressed*. Harmondsworth: Penguin.
Gramsci, A. (1986). *Selections from prison notebooks*. London: Lawrence & Wishart.

Gutiérrez, L. M. (1995). Understanding the empowerment process: Does consciousness make a difference? *Social Work Research, 19*(4), 229–237.

Gutiérrez, L. M., Parsons, R. J., & Cox, E. O. (2003). *Empowerment in social work practice: A sourcebook* (2nd ed.). Pacific Grove, CA: Brooks/Cole.

Habermas, J. (1984). *Theory of communicative action, Volume one.* Boston: Beacon.

Habermas, J. (1987). *Theory of communicative action, Volume two.* Cambridge, UK: Polity Press.

International Federation of Social Workers. (2013). *Global definition of social work.* Retrieved from http://ifsw.org/get-involved/global-definition-of-social-work/

Kitwood, T. (1997). *Dementia reconsidered.* Buckingham: Open University Press.

Lee, J. A. B. (2001). *The empowerment approach to social work practice: Building the beloved community* (2nd ed.). New York: Columbia University Press.

Leonardsen, D. (2007). Empowerment in social work: An individual vs. a relational perspective. *International Journal of Social Welfare, 16,* 3–11.

Lukes, S. ([1974] 2005). *Power: A radical view* (2nd ed.). Basingstoke: Palgrave Macmillan.

Mitchell, J. (2001). Creating a comprehensive system of community services for people with dementia. *Managing Community Care, 9*(3), 7–17.

Ohmer, M., & Korr, W. (2006). The effectiveness of community practice interventions: A review of the literature. *Research on Social Work Practice, 16*(2), 132–145.

Page, N., & Czuba, C. (1999). Empowerment: What is it? *Journal of Extension, 37*(5), 1–4.

Payne, M. (2014). *Modern social work theory* (4th ed.). Basingstoke: Palgrave Macmillan.

Pease, B. (2002). Rethinking empowerment: A postmodern reappraisal for emancipatory practice. *British Journal of Social Work, 32,* 135–147.

Rees, S. (1991). *Achieving power.* London: Allen & Unwin.

Riger, S. (1993). What's wrong with empowerment? *American Journal of Psychology, 21*(3), 279–292.

Rivest, M-P., And Moreau, N. (2015). Between emancipatory practice and disciplinary interventions: Empowerment and contemporary social normativity. *British Journal of Social Work, 45,* 1855–1870.

Rose, N. (1999). *Powers of freedom.* Cambridge, UK: Cambridge University Press.

Smith, R. (2008). *Social work and power.* Basingstoke: Palgrave Macmillan.

Solomon, B. (1976). *Black empowerment: Social work in oppressed communities.* New York: Columbia University Press.

Song, L. (2015). The association between the utilisation of empowerment strategies and clients' changes of self in the field of intimate partner abuse: From the perspective of social workers. *British Journal of Social Work, 45,* 527–548.

Stepney, P. (2012). An introduction to social work theory, practice and research. In P. Stepney & D. Ford (Eds.), *Social work models, methods and theories* (2nd ed., pp. 20–35). Lyme Regis: Russell House.

Stepney, P. (2014). Prevention in social work: The final frontier? *Critical and Radical Social Work, 2*(3), 305–320.

Stepney, P. (2017a). Theory and methods in an international context: Policy and organizational factors. In N. Thompson & P. Stepney (Eds.), *Social work theory and methods: The essentials* (pp. 44–62). New York: Routledge.

Stepney, P. (2017b). Community social work. In N. Thompson & P. Stepney (Eds.), *Social work theory and methods: The essentials* (pp. 227–139). New York: Routledge.

Thompson, N. (2006). *Power and empowerment.* Lyme Regis: Russell House.

Thompson, N. (2012). *Partnership and empowerment.* Blog post. Retrieved from https://swscmedia.word press.com/2012/12/10/partnership-and-empowerment-by-dr-neil-thompson/

Turner, S. G., & Maschi, T. M. (2015). Feminist and empowerment theory and social work practice. *Journal of Social Work Practice, 29*(2), 151–162.

Yoo, S., Weed, N., Lempa, M., Mbondo, M., Shada, R., & Goodman, R. (2004). Collaborative community empowerment: An illustration of a six-step process. *Health Promotion Practice, 5*(3), 256–265.

29

Anti-oppressive practice

Jane Dalrymple and Beverley Burke

Introduction

It is important to note that 'historically, some of the most progressive developments in social work have not been generated 'internally' from within the profession, but have come about through engagement with social movements' (Moran & Lavalette, 2016, p. 109). The collective experiences of marginalized, disadvantaged and oppressed individuals, groups and communities continually inform academic debates and scholarship, as well as shaping practice responses which do not further compound situations of inequality and social injustice. Anti-oppressive practice, described as 'a key methodological and theoretical paradigm in social work' (Danso, 2015, p. 573) and 'a dominant theory of critical social work practice' (Healy, 2014, p. 192), developed as professionals found methods of working with users of welfare services which took into account the oppression and inequality people experienced in their daily lives (Davis & Garrett, 2004, p. 14). Anti-oppressive practice, drawing on critical social science theories and informed by humanistic and social justice values, is acknowledged as 'one of the main forms of social justice oriented social work theory and practice today' (Baines, 2006, p. 4).

A commitment to socially just social work theory and practice is reflected in the international definition of social work, which states that 'Principles of social justice, human rights, collective responsibility and respect for diversities are central to social work' (IASSW, 2014). Putting these principles into practice can be demanding since the struggles of welfare services to meet the needs of service users within a globalized world is a complex political and moral issue requiring significant structural change in society. Unequal power relations between people using services, social workers and their employers, and between public services and the state, shape how services are provided (Pollack, 2010). Anti-oppressive social work practice, therefore, has to take into account the broader framework of political, social and economic factors and policies that shape the context of welfare service delivery (Strier & Binyamin, 2014). For many practitioners, commitment to social justice within this context is a useful starting point to considering and developing anti-oppressive theory and practice (Baines, 2006; see Chapter 10).

In a case study evaluation over a ten-year period, Strier and Binyamin found that people using services did not feel that their life situation could improve, despite underpinning anti-oppressive principles and changes in professional rhetoric from 'an individualized pathological discourse on poverty to a more collective, emancipatory, social change oriented professional approach' (2014, p. 2). Service users in the study believed they would remain in poverty despite the distinct anti-oppressive approach of their social workers. For the researchers this was a reminder that oppression cannot be challenged solely by the efforts of public sector social workers – it also requires political will and structural change. Baines suggests, however, that rather than accept that social workers are impotent to change the state apparatus, consideration of the state 'as a constantly changing, unstable equilibrium of struggles and counter-struggles' (2007, p. 17) enables social workers to find possibilities in that instability to challenge oppression and develop new ways of working. Social workers hold a privileged and powerful position in relation to the people they are working with, and research has shown that anti-oppressive practice can be a 'powerful instrument of resistance' (Danso, 2009, p. 550). Despite the difficulties of restructuring and dominant neoliberal policies, it is possible to maintain a positive outlook on the future of social work. While the impact of social workers committed to anti-oppressive practice may be limited, research suggests that such an approach is important in providing social care services 'in an era characterized by growing polarization of rich and poor and the uniculture prompted by corporatism and consumerism'. (Baines, 2006, p. 45).

Clifford (2016, p. 4) observes that supporters and critics of anti-oppressive practice do not necessarily understand the ethical commitment of social professionals whose work is led by such an approach. He argues that, while a concept of ethics which relates to the changing inequalities of the concrete social world must itself expect to develop and change, an awareness of oppression and the 'underlying "ethical demandingness" of human needs, vulnerability and caring in societies characterized by enduring structures of inequality' (2016, p. 16) must remain. Baines (2006) also recognizes the need for anti-oppressive practice to refine its theory and practice to address changing social conditions and notes that it has never set out to be a model with answers to all social problems. In this chapter, we consider these debates, examine some of the strengths and difficulties of an anti-oppressive practice approach and indicate how it can be used to inform current practice.

The critical tradition of social work

From the 1970s through to the 1990s, anti-oppressive theories developed from radical approaches (reviewed in Chapters 26–28), through feminist writing (see Chapter 31), poststructural and postmodernist writers (see Chapters 5 and 28) and, since the beginning of this century, what has been described as 'a blending of critical postmodernism and intersectionist class analysis' (Baines, 2006, p. 9). Baines (2006) suggests that despite the debates inevitably engendered by such a combination of theories (McDonald, 2006; Dominelli, 2002, 2004; Allan, 2003; Fook 2002; Fook & Pease, 1999), it has provided the foundation for practitioners and academics to develop anti-oppressive practice theory and consider a social justice–oriented approach to practice in the 21st century.

Adams, Dominelli, and Payne (2002) take three points from such ideas to demonstrate their use for critical practice. First is an emphasis on *social change* and the need to develop collective action to achieve it. This means, for example, that individual action is always part of wider action and, as such, is a form of political agency. The critical professional 'is engaged in collective action, working across differences with clients and colleagues in specific local issues towards a common goal of ending injustice' (Batsleer & Humphries, 2000, p. 13). Second is the focus of critical theory on *intentionality* – the conscious intention, through thinking critically, to create planned change. Finally, the implication of critical theories for social workers is that thinking and acting critically 'needs to be placed within analyses of how the *limitations of social divisions* such as class and gender and social assumptions about disability, sexuality and ethnic origin are created within social ideas that appear rational and that we take for granted, but are also changeable and changing' (Adams et al., 2002, p. 10).

Perspectives such as Marxism and feminism and newer theoretical schools such as critical postmodernism and post-structuralism all argue for ongoing refinement of theory in response to changing social conditions. Hick and Pozzuto (2005) note that the mingling of postmodern and critical theories is a necessary aspect of theorizing social work today. Indeed, theories change in response to historical, social, political and economic factors. Global capitalism, neo-liberalism and managerialism create challenges for social workers which lead to contradictions and tensions (Payne, 2000) and the need to work with people using services to understand their lived experiences of oppressions and exclusion to be able to challenge them (Stepney & Ford, 2000). The development of anti-oppressive practice is, however, more than theoretical progression. Baines argues that an approach that incorporates the strengths of different critical perspectives provides 'the greatest potential for ongoing development and refinement of theory and practice' (2007, p. 8).

Anti-oppressive practice, power and oppression

Since practitioners hold positions of power and influence through the institutional structures in which they are located, the potential for discrimination and oppression is inevitably present. Williams and Graham (2016) suggest that to practice anti-oppressively requires the practitioner to engage in constant critical examination and be more aware of how their identity and social status impacts their practice. A crucial element of such critical examination is to take seriously 'the complex memberships of major social divisions that affect individuals' perspectives and actions, and to which they respond in different ways' (Clifford, 1998, p. xiii). This theoretically based approach to practice provides a much-needed oppositional perspective to neoliberal ideas and practices which fail to contribute to social justice principles.

The concepts of power and oppression are key elements of anti-oppressive practice theory. They are contested, socially constructed, complex and value-laden concepts. An anti-oppressive understanding of power and oppression draws our attention to the fact that as social processes they are contradictory and multi-layered. An anti-oppressive analysis of power should also account for the fact that there is structural inequity in the distribution of power within social relationships where the 'interests' of some individuals and groups, supported by political, economic and cultural systems, are prioritized over other competing interests and needs of others. (Clifford, 1998; Mullaly, 2018; Clifford & Burke, 2009). An understanding of power, which draws on the 'grand narrative' of structural theories, provides cogent arguments of how social structures generate, maintain and sustain inequalities and is also simultaneously appreciative of postmodernist understandings of power as omnipresent, fluid, relational and interactive (Foucault, 1980; Clifford, 2016). Power is *relational* as well as *structural* in its nature. Understanding and working with the outcome of this complex interrelationship provides anti-oppressive practice with a particular and unique position. An appreciation of this dynamic leads to a more complex understanding of power relations within social situations and indicates the nature of practice and action which is needed in relation to practising ethically and anti-oppressively (Dalrymple & Burke, 2006).

Clifford urges practitioners to consider the implications of taking oppression 'seriously' (2016, p. 5). He argues that inequalities and injustices originate from both individual differences and systemic actions that come from the concentration of power within some social groups. These are enduring differences that impact people's lives both materially and psychologically. He suggests that whether people oppose, collude with or strengthen these differences, they become resistant to change because they are incorporated in structural, institutional and psychological realities. Mattson (2014, p. 9) adds to this point, stating that 'unreflective, everyday practice', where beliefs, assumptions and actions are not scrutinized in relation to possible harmful outcomes, contributes to maintaining and sustaining oppression and injustice, even though this was not what was intended.

Social workers are afforded a position of power not only by virtue of the social divisions to which they belong but also by their professional position as social workers. Given this, social workers should critically analyze their decision-making processes and actions by asking critically reflective, reflexive, ethical and evaluative questions about their role in contributing to inequality and oppression in their individual or collective practices. The concept of intersectionality, (Crenshaw, 1991; Hill-Collins, 2000), resonates with and contributes to understanding anti-oppressive practice and its underpinning theory and, in a similar way to anti-oppressive practice theory, it too is constantly debated and developed (Walby, Armstrong, & Strid, 2012). An intersectional framework enables understanding of power relations as being generated by the interactions and interconnections between various social divisions (Hill-Collins & Bilge, 2016). By focusing on the lived experiences of marginalized individuals, groups and communities, the multidimensional nature of people's identity and experiences are brought into sharp relief, providing a fuller picture of the relationship between how the very concrete, and not so concrete, differences between people are played out and are connected to social structures (Mehrotra, 2010). An intersectional analysis makes it possible to understand and problematize the unequal power relationship between practitioner and service user (Mattsson, 2014), by enabling practitioners to analyze the complex ways 'social structures produce and entrench power and marginalization and by drawing attention to the ways that existing paradigms that produce knowledge and politics often function to normalise these dynamics' (Carbado, Crenshaw, Mays, & Tomlinson, 2013, p. 312).

Strengths and difficulties of anti-oppressive practice theory

The centrality of social justice within the model is recognized as a key strength (Healy, 2014). Commentators also identify how anti-oppressive practice has extended radical approaches to take account of the different bases for the oppression of various groups and inequalities and divisions in society (Ferguson & Woodward, 2009). Furthermore, the union of particular aspects of modernist and postmodernist ideas about the concept of power enables practitioners to make links intellectually between individual subjective intersectional experiences of oppression and broader social and political structures. It may well be difficult to manage the tension between structure and agency, and it can be difficult to translate structural analysis into action at the micro level and vice versa. An anti-oppressive perspective does not simplistically posit a view that individuals and groups are only determined by macro social and economic structures. It addresses the interplay between individual experience and action and the micro, mezzo and macro structures of social life (see Chapters 15 and 27 on systems ideas). Holding an anti-oppressive perspective supports practitioners in choosing practice methods and interventions which enable them to both work with specific subjective experiences of particular forms of oppression and take into account the complex power relations (Clifford, 2016). When agency is seen as in dynamic interaction with social structures, assessment and intervention strategies will acknowledge and work with the needs of individuals as well as making appropriate challenges to the social systems that structure and maintain the individual, family, group or community experiences of marginality and structural oppression. In short, anti-oppressive practice highlights the very political role of social work, a view of social work which has been criticized for being politically and morally idealistic (Jones, Cooper, & Ferguson, 2008).

An unpoliticized understanding of anti-oppressive values and principles can lead to practitioners engaging in practices which are complicit in sustaining and maintaining systems of oppression and inequality. Humphries (2004), using the case of the social work profession's involvement in internal immigration, evidences how the profession on the one hand is committed to anti-oppressive practice and values while on the other is engaging in practices which are in direct opposition to them. This point is picked up by Millar (2008), who, using a conservative functionalist sociological perspective, characterizes anti-oppressive values as a system of ideas that serves a function in relation to the way social workers perceive themselves (Clifford & Burke, 2009, p. 6). It can be argued, however, that 'any set of values, including anti-oppressive values, can be subverted in practice (and in theory) and may serve roles and functions for which they are not intended' (Clifford & Burke, 2009, p. 6), particularly within a society 'dedicated to individual self-interest' (Simey, 1996, p. 162). Values which are anti-oppressive are often viewed as morally idealistic and politically naive.

Like all theoretical and practice methodologies, however, anti-oppressive theorizing and practices are subject to development, academic scrutiny and critique. It has attracted criticism from a range of observers holding different political and ideological perspectives and values: for example Sinclair and Albert (2008), Harrison and Turner (2011) and Williams and Graham (2016). In fact, 'stereotypical assumptions are sometimes made about "anti-oppressive" practice which pigeon-hole the concept as an outdated structuralist position unsuitable for contemporary practice, and inconsistent with contemporary post-modern thinking' (Clifford & Burke, 2009, p. 15). This perceived singular focus on a structural analysis of people's difficulties, and its consequent failure to address the range of multiple factors which shape and constrain peoples' lives, is taken up by Sakamoto and Pitner (2005). They suggest that anti-oppressive practice is limited to structural concerns and its overarching modernist view fails to appreciate and hence work with the unique expressions of oppression which individuals experience. Healy (2014) also expresses concerns about applying anti-oppressive practice in situations such as safeguarding, mental health and criminal justice. She argues that the strong critique of 'psy' discourse that appears to underpin the theory of anti-oppressive practice, alongside the importance placed on structural issues, can mean that social workers fail to address psychological and personal factors that might contribute to higher risk in some situations.

Such a reading of anti-oppressive practice fails to recognize that the ideas and theoretical tension between modernist and postmodernist conceptions of power and oppression is taken into account within the theoretical pluralism which characterizes anti-oppressive frameworks. While understanding this, we are aware of the often-contradictory relationship between structural interlocking systems, the processes of oppression and the subjective experience(s) of oppression and social injustice. We have argued (Burke & Dalrymple, 2017, for example) that the controlling and restrictive elements of legislation have the potential to move social workers away from responding to need to a focus on managing risk. The difficulty then is that practitioners can be drawn into 'defensive and morally timid social work practice' (Stanford quoted in Whittaker & Havard, 2015).

In their critique of the intellectual ownership of anti-oppressive practice, Williams and Graham (2016, p. 11) support Wilson and Beresford's (2000) critique regarding the alleged failure of anti-oppressive theorizing and practice to take into account, and be informed by, the views and experiences of the very people it claims to be working with. The contention of this position is that by failing to engage critically with service user perspectives and movements in its development, anti-oppressive practice merely becomes an ideological tool which reproduces the oppression it wishes to diminish. This is a relevant point, and we wholeheartedly agree that an anti-oppressive justice-orientated approach to practice must include a clear and active commitment to service users' rights and involvement. Involvement means that service users should have a voice in decisions that concern their lives and that through their own systems and activism they are fully engaged in policy development and service design and delivery (Dalrymple & Boylan, 2013; Sheedy, 2013). Collaborative, partnership and co-production principles are part of the bedrock on which anti-oppressive practice and welfare services are built. The direct involvement of, and with, those who are living with the consequences of inequality and oppression inform and improve the provision of services. This can certainly be seen in the development of alternative, politically conscious service provision found outside the mainstream statutory social work sector which, in its response to particular forms of need, delivers practice that is anti-oppressive (Jones & Lavalette, 2013).

There is a reflexive and dynamic relationship between lived experiences of oppression, social work scholarship and practice. Many of those engaged in the anti-oppressive project have not just one identity but many identities and experiences, including that of 'service user' and 'belonging to marginalized or dominated groups'. These actual and developing identities and related experiences inform developments in anti-oppressive practice. The reflexive dimension of anti-oppressive thinking assists practitioners and academics to work from a perspective that is actively informed and transformed by knowledge generated by engagement in the realities of peoples' lived experiences as well as their own (Clifford & Burke, 2009).

The future of anti-oppressive practice

Contemporary anti-oppressive practice occurs within the context of globalization, the modernizing agenda of many governments and increasing privatization of the welfare state and, in Western industrialized nations, a widening gap between the rich and poor (Wilkinson & Pickett, 2009). Such approaches challenge all practitioners to reflect on how we contribute to the control and surveillance of people we are seeking to assist. The struggle to reconcile anti-oppressive practice and the elements of social control noted by Healy is a tension that requires ongoing critical reflection, particularly in contexts of practice where practitioners believe that professional discretion is being managed out of their role (Baldwin, 2004). This process enables practitioners to focus on how they 'construct and understand their place, position, purpose, role, practice and power within and in relation to the organisation' (Fook, 2004, p. 73). Making a case for a 'critical best practice', Ferguson (2008) contributes to this debate, noting that forms of theorizing are required that engage with what he calls 'life politics' (2001, title). That is, the politics of the personal is experienced through lived experiences. This includes recognizing power and the impact of structures on the problems of people needing support by locating them in the reality of people's lives.

The changing landscape of social work practice provides opportunities for social workers to appraise their role. The introduction of more personalized responsive social care is one mechanism for supporting this approach. This can be seen across services in the UK. For example, the Care Act 2014 requires local authorities to use a strengths-based approach in adult social care (Saleebey, 2006; see Chapter 18). Here the relationship between social worker and people needing support values the strengths that both bring to the process, and working in partnership means that people are not just consumers of services but can also be co-producers of services (Duncan & Miller, 2000; Morgan & Ziglio, 2007). The Mental Capacity Act 2005 is structured both to empower and protect people who might not have the capacity to make decisions for themselves with respect to particular situations. It places the wishes, feelings and needs of service users at the forefront of decision-making and has been described as an 'emancipatory' act (Graham & Cowley, 2015). However, they highlight the need for practitioners asked to undertake routine capacity assessments to continually question whether the assessment is needed since it could be argued that this routinization contributes to a wider process of discrimination.

In such complex areas it is necessary to reflect on the ethical dilemmas of practice and on how different ways of applying the law can affect people using services, particularly when it concerns capacity and consent (Johns, 2017). This can be illustrated by the following case example of an 84-year-old black woman who moved from Jamaica to Manchester in the 1950s, who has recently been bereaved and is living with a diagnosis of dementia and whose needs are being assessed (Care Act, 2014). There have been questions asked about whether she lacks capacity – based, it would appear, on the diagnosis of dementia. Power issues in social relationships need to be analyzed at different levels – both at the structural level (political, social and economic) and at the level of personal power, which comes from cultural, institutional and psychological factors (Clifford, 1998). The anti-oppressive practitioner will try to make a systematic power analysis of the situation which will support decision-making regarding the level of vulnerability the person has, as well as the potential strengths with respect to possible risk. This would include considering the nature of power that the service user has; whether that relates to her membership in various social divisions; the physical, material and financial resources of the person and the cultural and psychological strengths and vulnerabilities of the person.

In children's services, practitioners work jointly with people using services and other professionals to develop a culture of shared working. Approaches such as Family Group Decision Making (FGDM) are underpinned by social justice goals, although anti-oppressive practitioners are still mindful of the potential dilemmas. For example, research into FGDM found that the voices of participants in the participatory process were 'co-opted by the more forceful child protection discourse, itself shaped by legal, bureaucratized, and neoliberal discourses' (Ney, Stolz, & Maloney, 2013, p. 1).

Concluding comments

Increasing levels of inequality, poverty and the oppression of diverse groups within the UK and Europe have been exacerbated by neoliberal ideologically informed social, political and economic policies. At the same time we are witnessing the rise of nationalistic right-wing political parties, the emergence of grassroots social movements has provided counter ideological discourses to dominant pathologizing discourses. Mass movement of people between and within countries means that anti-oppressive practice has to meet the challenging demands of a globalized world and the complex needs of diverse communities. The lack of financial resources makes it difficult for many social, health and welfare organizations to meet the needs of those accessing their services. Care and caring, highly contested and politicized concepts, take on particular meanings within these changing times and contexts (see Chapter 7).

Adoption of an anti-oppressive approach to practice has implications for all concerned in the development of just welfare services. Social problems require the engagement of diverse humanitarian and emancipatory micro, mezzo and macro social, political and economic interventions. Practitioners can individually and collectively use their relative power to intervene in organizational and political structures which express and consolidate oppressive relations. Social action involves the development of both informal and formal strategies, from voicing concerns personally and collectively and working with service user and carer groups to making links with communities who are engaged in political activism. Facilitating the coming together of people to reframe personal concerns into wider collective issues necessitates action that moves beyond the boundaries of individual practice. Such action requires courage and preparedness to challenge, as well as making creative and sustainable alliances with individuals, groups, communities and organizations wishing to engage in the anti-oppressive project.

Further reading

Baines, D. (2017). *Doing anti oppressive practice: Building transformative, politicized social work* (3rd ed.). Nova Scotia: Fernwood.
This introduces readers to anti-oppressive social work, its historical and theoretical roots and the specific contexts of anti-oppressive social work practice.

Dalrymple, J., & Burke, B. (2006). *Anti-oppressive practice: Social care and the law* (2nd ed.). Maidenhead: Open University Press.
This explores the issues of power and oppression, demonstrating how the law can be used to inform the development of critical anti-oppressive practice.

Healy, K. (2014). *Social work theories in context: Creating frameworks for practice* (2nd ed.). Basingstoke: Palgrave Macmillan.
Chapter 9, 'Modern critical social work, from radical to anti-oppressive practice', presents a helpful analysis and critique of anti-oppressive practice.

Payne, M. (2014). *Modern social work theory* (4th ed.). Basingstoke: Palgrave Macmillan.
Chapter 14, 'Anti-oppressive and multicultural sensitivity approaches to practice', offers an accessible consideration of the theory and its application to practice.

References

Adams, R., Dominelli, L., & Payne, M. (Eds.). (2002). *Critical practice in social work*. Basingstoke: Palgrave Macmillan.
Allan, J. (2003). Theorising critical social work. In J. Allan, B. Pease, & L. Briskman (Eds.), *Critical social work: An introduction to theories and practices* (pp. 32–51). Crows Nest: Allen & Unwin.
Baines, D. (2006). *Doing anti oppressive practice: Building transformative, politicized social work*. Halifax, NS: Fernwood.
Baldwin, M. (2004). Critical reflection: Opportunities and threats to professional learning and service development in social work organizations. In N. Gould & M. Baldwin (Eds.), *Social work, critical reflection and the learning organisation* (pp. 41–56). Aldershot: Ashgate.
Batsleer, J., & Humphries, B. (2000). Welfare, exclusion and political agency. In J. Batsleer & B. Humphries (Eds.), *Welfare, exclusion and political agency* (pp. 1–21). London: Routledge.
Boylan, J., & Dalrymple, J. (2009). *Understanding advocacy for children and young people*. Maidenhead: Open University Press.
Burke, B., & Dalrymple, J. (2017). Anti-oppressive practice and the law. In A. Brammer & J. Boylan (Eds.), *Critical issues in social work law* (pp. 26–44). London: Palgrave Macmillan.
Carbado, D. W., Crenshaw, K. W., Mays, V. M., & Tomlinson, B. (2013). Intersectionality: Mapping the movements of a theory. *Du Bois Review: Social Science Research on Race, 10*(2), 303–312.
Clifford, D. (1998). *Social assessment theory and practice*. Aldershot: Ashgate.
Clifford, D. (2016). Oppression and professional ethics. *Ethics and Social Welfare, 10*(1), 4–18.
Clifford, D., & Burke, B. (2009). *Anti-oppressive ethics and values in social work*. Basingstoke: Palgrave Macmillan.
Crenshaw, K. (1991). Mapping the margins: Intersectionality, identity, and violence against women of color. *Stanford Law Review, 43*(6), 1241–1300.
Dalrymple, J., & Boylan, J. (2013). *Effective advocacy in social work*. London: Sage.
Dalrymple, J., & Burke, B. (2006). *Anti-oppressive practice: Social care and the law* (2nd ed.). Maidenhead: Open University Press.
Danso, R. (2009). Emancipating and empowering de-valued skilled immigrants: What hope does anti-oppressive social work practice offer? *British Journal of Social Work, 39*(3), 539–555.
Danso, R. (2015). An integrated framework of critical cultural competence and anti-oppressive practice for social justice social work research. *Qualitative Social Work, 14*(4), 572–588.

Davis, A., & Garrett, P. M. (2004). Progressive practice for tough times: Social work, poverty and division in the twenty-first century. In M. Lymbery & S. Butler (Eds.), *Social work: Ideals and practice realities* (pp. 13–33). Basingstoke: Palgrave Macmillan.

Dominelli, L. (2002). *Anti-oppressive social work theory and practice.* Basingstoke: Palgrave Macmillan.

Dominelli, L. (2004). *Social work: Theory and practice for a changing profession.* Cambridge, UK: Polity Press.

Duncan, B. L., & Miller, S. D. (2000). The client's theory of change: Consulting the client in the integrative process. *Journal of Psychotherapy Integration, 10*(2), 169–187. Retrieved from https://doi.org/10.1023/A:1009448200244

Ferguson, H. (2008). The theory and practice of critical best practice in social work. In K. Jones, B. Cooper, & H. Ferguson (Eds.), *Best practice in social work* (pp. 15–37). Basingstoke: Palgrave Macmillan.

Ferguson, I., & Woodward, R. (2009). *Radical social work in practice: Making a difference.* Bristol: Policy Press.

Fook, J. (2002). *Social work: Critical theory and practice.* London: Sage.

Fook, J. (2004). Critical reflection and organisational learning and change: A case study. In N. Gould & M. Baldwin (Eds.), *Social work, critical reflection and the learning organisation* (pp. 57–73). Aldershot: Ashgate.

Fook, J., & Pease, B. (1999). Emancipatory social work for a postmodern age. In B. Pease & J. Fook (Eds.), *Transforming social work practice: Postmodern critical perspectives* (pp. 224–249). London: Routledge.

Foucault, M. (1980). *Power/knowledge: Selected interviews and other writings by Michel Foucault 1972–1977.* (C. Gordon, ed.). New York: Pantheon.

Graham, M., & Cowley, J. (2015). *A practical guide to the Mental Capacity Act 2005: Putting the principles of the act into practice.* London: Jessica Kingsley.

Harrison, G., & Turner, R. (2011). Being a 'culturally competent' social worker: Making sense of a murky concept in practice. *British Journal of Social Work, 41*(2), 333–350. Retrieved from https://doi.org/10.1093/bjsw/bcq101

Hick, S., & Pozzuto, R. (2005). Introduction: Towards 'becoming' a critical social worker. In S. Hick, J. Fook, & R. Pozzuto (Eds.), *Social work: A critical turn.* Toronto: Thompson.

Hill-Collins, P. (2000). *Black feminist thought: Knowledge, consciousness, and the politics of empowerment* (2nd ed.). New York: Routledge.

Hill-Collins, P., & Bilge, S. (2016). *Intersectionality.* Cambridge, UK: Polity Press.

Humphries, B. (2004). An unacceptable role for social work: Implementing immigration policy. *British Journal of Social Work, 34*, 93–107.

International Association of Schools of Social Work. (2014). *Global definition of social work.* Retrieved from www.iassw-aiets.org/global-definition-of-social-work-review-of-the-global-definition/

Johns, R. (2017). Coercion in social care. In A. Brammer & J. Boylan (Eds.), *Critical issues in social work law* (pp. 59–72). London: Palgrave Macmillan.

Jones, C., & Lavalette, M. (2013). The two souls of social work: Exploring the roots of 'popular social work'. *Critical and Radical Social Work, 1*(2), 147–165.

Jones, K., Cooper, B., & Ferguson, H. (2008). *Best practice in social work.* Basingstoke: Palgrave Macmillan.

Mattsson, T. (2014). Intersectionality as a useful tool: Anti-oppressive social work and critical reflection. *Affilia, 29*(1), 8–17.

Mehrotra, G. (2010). Toward a continuum of intersectionality theorizing for feminist social work. *Affilia, 25*(4), 417–430. Retrieved from https://doi.org/10.1177/0886109910384190

McDonald, C. (2006). *Challenging social work: The institutional context of practice.* Basingstoke: Palgrave Macmillan.

Millar, M. (2008). 'Anti-oppressiveness': Critical comments on a discourse and its context. *British Journal of Social Work, 38*(2), 362–375.

Moran, R., & Lavalette, M. (2016). Co-production: Workers, volunteers and people seeking asylum – 'popular social work' in action in Britain. In C. Williams & M. J. Graham (Eds.), *Social work in diverse society* (pp. 109–126). Bristol: Policy Press.

Morgan, A., & Ziglio, E. (2007). Revitalising the evidence base for public health: An assets model. *Promotion and Education, 14*(Sup2), 17–22.

Mullaly, B. & Dupré, M. (2018). *The new structural social work: Ideology, theory and practice* (4th ed.). Don Mills: Oxford University Press.

Ney, T., Stolz, J., & Maloney, M. (2013). Voice, power and discourse: Experiences of participants in family group conferences in the context of child protection. *Journal of Social Work, 13*(2), 184–202. Retrieved from https://doi.org/10.1177/1468017311410514

Payne, M. (2000). *Anti-bureaucratic social work.* Birmingham: Venture.

Pollack, S. (2010). Labelling clients 'risky': Social work and the neo-liberal welfare state. *British Journal of Social Work*, *40*(4), 1263–1278.

Sakamoto, I., & Pitner, R. (2005). Use of critical consciousness in anti-oppressive social work practice: Disentangling power dynamics at personal and structural levels. *British Journal of Social Work*, *35*(4), 435–452. Retrieved from https://doi.org/10.1093/bjsw/bch190

Saleebey, D. (2006). *The strengths perspective in social work practice* (4th ed.). Boston: Allyn & Bacon.

Sheedy, M. (2013). *Core themes in social work: Power, poverty, politics and values.* Maidenhead: Open University Press.

Simey, M. (1996). *The disinherited society: A personal view of social responsibility in Liverpool in the twentieth century.* Liverpool: Liverpool University Press.

Sinclair, R., & Albert, J. (2008). Social work and the anti-oppressive stance: Does the emperor really have new clothes? *Critical Social Work*, *9*(1). Retrieved from http://www1.uwindsor.ca/criticalsocialwork/social-work-and-the-anti-oppressive-stance-does-the-emperor-really-have-new-clothes

Stepney, P., & Ford, D. (2000). *Social work models, methods and theories: A framework for practice.* Lyme Regis: Russell House.

Strier, R., & Binyamin, S. (2014). Introducing anti-oppressive social work practices in public services: Rhetoric to practice. *British Journal of Social Work*, *44*(8), 2095–2112.

Walby, S., Armstrong, J., & Strid, S. (2012). Intersectionality: Multiple inequalities in social theory. *Sociology*, *46*(2), 224–240.

Whittaker, A., & Havard, T. (2015). Defensive practice as 'fear-based' practice: Social work's open secret? *The British Journal of Social Work, 46*(5), 1158–1174.

Wilkinson, R., & Pickett, K. (2009). *The spirit level.* London: Penguin.

Williams, C., & Graham, M. J. (2016). *Social work in a diverse society.* Bristol: Policy Press.

Wilson, A., & Beresford, P. (2000). 'Anti-oppressive practice': Emancipation or appropriation. *British Journal of Social Work*, *30*(5), 553–573.

30
Advocacy ideas in social work

Tom Wilks

Introduction

Advocacy is a diverse and growing area of social work practice. It is highly pragmatic, providing a straightforward response to service user need and challenging powerful vested interests. At the same time, it draws upon quite a complex and eclectic theory base. One of the most striking things about advocacy is the diversity of different approaches it encompasses, ranging in scope from addressing individual need to working with groups around collective concerns, and in purpose from quasi-legal representation to emotional support within citizen advocacy. There are, however, common threads running through advocacy binding these disparate approaches together. The first is a common value base and commitment to empowerment. A shared concern with and commitment to principled negotiation is also something many advocates have in common. Another important feature of advocacy is that it shares common ground with other approaches to social work, something we will explore in discussing cause advocacy's relationship to radical social work and to international development. Advocacy is also a contested area of practice, and there are important debates around the place of advocacy in statutory services and around promotional as against enabling advocacy.

The landscape of advocacy

A good starting place for any attempt to map out the place of advocacy in social work is Jordan's (1987, p. 135) argument that social work is archetypically characterized by two paradigms. The first of these is social worker as counsellor, 'skilful', 'attentive' and 'accurately empathetic'. The second is the social worker as advocate, championing the oppressed and fighting injustice and exploitation. One way of understanding these two paradigms is to see social worker as advocate and social worker as counsellor sitting at two ends of a continuum. Where social workers are positioned within this continuum is shaped by their own conceptions of their professional selves and the practice orientations of the organizations within which they work. The virtue of this linear presentation of where advocacy sits within social work and social work theory is its simplicity. However, it does not adequately represent the complexity of the relationship between these two poles of practice, the individual practitioner and the wider context of practice. There is an argument, which we will explore in more detail later, that advocacy is not social work and that the conflicts of interest between the statutory functions and organizational context of social work within the local state can make advocacy problematic for what Jones terms 'state social workers' (Jones, 1983, 2001). Another complexity of advocacy is its eclectic use of a range of mainstream social work theory and its engagement with ideas and frameworks from the periphery of social work practice: negotiation theory, community action and international development, for example.

Advocacy and empowerment

What is the significance of what appears a contradictory state of affairs: advocacy's close relationship with a range of activities that are peripheral to social work, yet its identification as a paradigmatic example of what social work is? One of the first and most significant things that social work practice teaches us is the significance of values in our work (Bisman, 2004; Reamer, 2006). As Banks (2012, p. 2) points out, 'Some argue it is the values of social work that hold it together'. It is to a cluster of values around empowerment that we must turn to begin to understand advocacy's significance for social work.

Pullen-Sansfacon and Cowden (2012) argue that empowerment has become the 'raison d'etre of contemporary social work' (p. 69) and that it is empowerment that renders social work practice – to use Adams's (2003, p. 3) term – 'transformational': able to extend its influence beyond the individual to shape change at a wider level. The International Federation of Social Workers (IFSW, 2014) definition of social work juxtaposes 'empowerment' and 'liberation', underlining the importance of empowerment in pursuing the transformational agenda within social work. If social work is to become this empowering transformational profession, many have argued that this can be achieved through embracing advocacy (Braye and Preston-Shoot, 1995; Brandon, 1995). Parrot (2010, p. 104) goes so far as to describe advocacy as 'inextricably linked with empowerment'.

What we have just looked at is empowerment as an aspiration for social work. Something that the profession, whose work is predominantly with the powerless, should embrace as a goal that is consistent with its value base. This is one way of understanding empowerment. We can also see empowerment, however, not as an endpoint, but rather as a process (Fook, 2002), where particular social work approaches are adopted to help service users gain power within their own lives. An important distinction in understanding this process of empowerment in relation to advocacy is that between the related concepts of structural and psychological empowerment.

Structural empowerment is about access to material goods and benefits. Psychological empowerment relates to our having a stronger sense of our own capacity to manage within the world to feel more psychologically powerful. An example of a very typical piece of advocacy-orientated social work practice will help elicit the differences between these two aspects of empowerment. If a social worker is working with a service user with a disability who lives in accommodation that is so damp that it is having an impact on the service user's physical well-being, they may use approaches to social work based on advocacy, to find alternative accommodation. This intervention makes a real material impact on the service user's life. It enables access to improved accommodation and has tangible benefits for the health of the service user. This is what we would call structural empowerment. This intervention may also, however, have a psychological impact and may help empower a service user by enhancing their self-esteem, and giving them a stronger sense of autonomy, all of which will increase their resilience and self-confidence when faced with similar challenges in the future.

For social workers the barriers to psychological empowerment may be manyfold. Barber (1991) and Adams (2008) draw upon Seligman's (1975) concept of learned helplessness to explore some of the main psychological barriers to empowerment. This is an idea echoed in Solomon's (1976) understanding of powerlessness within the context of anti-discriminatory practice. She sees powerlessness within black and minority ethnic communities as a product of the individual and their wider environment, where an individual's negative valuation of themselves drawn from the wider social environment contributes to their sense of powerlessness.

Returning to our earlier discussion of empowerment as an aspiration and empowerment as a process, a central message is that we need to adopt an approach to the advocacy process that attends to issues of empowerment in the way that it addresses the interaction between individual and environment. Process models are a common feature of social work approaches to advocacy. Most describe what is essentially a three-stage process of problem analysis and exploration, the gathering of information and action planning and the presentation of a case and negotiation (Brandon & Brandon, 2001; Bateman, 2000). To ensure that empowerment is addressed within the advocacy process, however, we also need an approach to process that is attuned to service user participation and control.

To achieve this, an advocacy process ought to address the following key aspects of empowerment (Wilks, 2012), as part of a process of increasing participation and control, where service users move from being passive recipients of help to, with others' assistance, actively addressing their problems and difficulties themselves.

Developing self-confidence and skills

There are a range of ways in which a social worker undertaking advocacy might achieve this: identifying previous strengths, affirmation of progress made, helping develop skills using preparation rehearsal and assertiveness techniques. The primary focus here is on the personal and psychological.

Linking with networks and support

As social workers, when we look at developing confidence and skills, we can often focus on the individual level. To sustain greater confidence successfully, however, a practitioner needs to consider wider networks of support and how service users can engage with these to help this process. This support might come from informal family or social networks. Over and above this, social workers undertaking advocacy roles need to encourage supported self-help and peer support as part of a wider approach to advocacy, helping service users share their experiences with others, drawing on this process to garner ideas and to embed confidence. Atkinson argues that self-advocacy 'should be the goal of all other forms of advocacy' (Atkinson, 1999, p. 6). Linking to peer advocacy support networks can help in this process. Engaging with those who have had similar experiences can act as a bulwark against fragile self-confidence, enabling service users to take a much more active role in the advocacy process. Peer networks are important therefore on an individual level. They can offer more than this, however, and act as a springboard to campaigning and wider social action.

Engaging with bigger issues

Social work is a profession which hopes to change the world (IFSW, 2014). Advocacy is often seen as the vehicle through which this aspiration is made manifest. As Goldberg Wood and Tully (2006, p. 139) put it, 'without advocacy social work would be like a deodorised skunk – never really able to make a stink about individual victims or classes of victims who are unable to obtain access to basic human needs or rights'.

The endpoint of the advocacy process, therefore, ought to be engagement with wider issues. The distinction drawn by Schneider and Lester (2001) between case and cause advocacy is very useful here. In case advocacy, the social worker's role is to work on a one-to-one basis to help secure a service user's rights. Cause advocacy extends and widens the role, involving a collective response to a social issue which impacts many people, raising awareness of an issue and seeking changes in the way it is dealt with. This interrelation between policy and practice, something emphasized by Rees (1991) in his work on empowerment, is what characterizes this dimension of the advocacy process.

These three aspects of empowering practice in advocacy – supporting self-confidence at the individual level, encouraging support within an immediate peer network and pursing wider social change through cause advocacy – resonate with structural models of discrimination (Keating, 1997; Thompson, 2016) describing discrimination occurring at the individual, community and societal levels and can provide a structured approach to advocacy that engages effectively with theoretical models of discrimination and oppression.

I have looked at how advocacy marks a boundary of social work yet is essential to the profession's aspirations to empowerment. We can see from our discussion so far that advocacy has the potential to support empowerment, particularly if we use a structured process model of advocacy in a way that is attentive to it. However, advocacy is more complex than the application of rather simple process-driven models. At this point, it is important to explore some of the principal debates within advocacy about the approaches that advocates adopt to their work and the shared space that exists between advocacy and other models of practice. This will help us understand more about the general significance of advocacy within a social work context. It will also help focus our attention on some of the tensions for advocacy within social work and on skills social workers need to possess to advocate effectively alongside the service users with whom they are working.

Enabling and promotional advocacy

A key distinction in advocacy is between advocacy that aims to enable the voice of others to be heard and advocacy that seeks to engage with those who have power by arguing a case, sometimes called promotional advocacy. One source of our models of advocacy is what we might term the legal archetype, involving expert representation within a formal forum, a court or tribunal: an essentially adversarial understanding of what it is to advocate. The word 'advocate' has its origins in legal representation (Ayto, 2005). Freddolino, Moxley, and Hyduk (2004, p. 121) describe social work advocates as engaging in 'the most adversarial forms of advocacy and adopting "quasi legal roles"'. If we understand advocacy in this way, the advocate's role is to make the most effective representations they can on behalf of their client to influence decisions or access to resources. This model does influence the way social workers work. For example, social workers might try and present service users' situations as positively as possible in a way which foregrounds strengths, whilst acknowledging difficulties, seeking help from a provider of social housing or attending a resource panel. This presentation of a case is not just something social workers do on behalf of service users. Where, for example, a service user seeks supported housing, a social worker might work with them to ensure that they present themselves as positively as possible for an interview with a housing provider.

In contrast to promotional advocacy, we have advocacy based on voice. A good example of this would be the statutory independent mental health advocate (IMHA) role in the UK. The focus of the IMHA role is on voice. IMHAs provide advocacy for patients with mental health problems who are detained against their will in psychiatric hospitals under the Mental Health Act 1983, which provides the legal framework for mental health in the UK. The advocacy they provide can be broken down into the following elements. The first is listening, with the IMHA taking the time they need to understand the service user's story using skills in empathetic communication. The next stage involves the IMHA providing information about the law and the service user's rights and options and checking the service user's understanding of their detention. As part of this process, the IMHA might help the service user find out more about their treatment, accessing information on aspects of medication or helping look at medical records, for example. All this helps the service user understand what is happening to them and make informed choices about their treatment. Finally, and most importantly, the IMHA will endeavour to ensure that the service user's voice is heard in the process of planning treatment and is addressed in that plan. This might mean speaking on behalf of the service user or helping the service users themselves put across their own perspectives. See also the discussion of 'decision support' in Chapter 39.

In practice these approaches to advocacy are perhaps more closely aligned than I have described. An IMHA with a voice-orientated approach might well, for example, discuss with a service user the most effective way to ensure their perspective was listened to in meetings with a psychiatrist. An advocate adopting a more promotional approach would certainly try to ensure that the service user's voice was heard and that they, where possible, would present their own case. This contrast does, however, capture something important about how advocates focus their work.

This distinction between enabling and promotional advocacy illustrates the diversity of activity and approach which falls under the rubric of advocacy. Bateman (2000) argues that a key thread running through the diverse range of approaches we might characterize as advocacy is negotiation theory. Certainly, in the examples we have just looked at, an advocate would benefit from a knowledge of negotiation skills in order to discuss a service user's treatment plan with a mental health team or present a case to a social housing provider. Bateman's focus on negotiation is, however, not just motivated by pragmatic reasons. His view is that there are many ways to conduct negotiations and that, since advocacy is a value-based area of practice, an approach to negotiation as part of advocacy should be adopted that is consistent with these values.

Advocacy and negotiation

Bateman (2000) draws upon the work of Fisher and Ury (1991) and applies it to negotiation in health and social care. This approach, known as 'principled negotiation' can be applied in a range of contexts. Three interrelated aspects of Fisher and Ury's work make it particularly relevant to advocacy. Firstly, and perhaps most importantly, what Fisher and Ury attempt to construct is a values-based approach to negotiation. They argue that negotiation ought to be underpinned by an appreciation that it offers benefit to both parties rather than a win for one of the two sides, a good outcome being a wise decision rather than a victory. This is the core principle underlying the negotiation process.

Secondly, to achieve this, Fisher and Ury reject the traditional idea of positional negotiation with a soft or hard bargain being struck and draw instead upon a conceptual framework that has much in common with theories of assertiveness. If one side in a negotiation adopts a soft negotiating style, seeking early resolution by making early concessions, it will leave them feeling exploited and resentful. Contrastingly, hard negotiators can exhaust goodwill, damaging the other party and the relationship they have with them. Theories of assertiveness propose similar consequences in relation to passive and aggressive behaviour (McBride, 1998). Assertiveness, particularly as it applies to negotiation, is based on three core principles: clarity in the presentation of a negotiating position, flexibility and willingness to compromise and the maintenance of open communication (Back & Back, 2005). Finally, Fisher and Ury provide a framework for negotiation consistent with these underlying values.

Fisher and Ury (1991) propose four elements to principled negotiation:

- Separating the people from the problem.
- Focusing on interests not positions.
- Inventing options for mutual gain.
- Insisting on using objective criteria.

Thinking about how this framework would apply to advocacy in social work, it is useful to consider separating the people from the problem and focusing on interests not positions as relating primarily to the process of negotiation. Inventing options for mutual gain and insisting on using objective criteria relate more strongly to outcomes. Overall, one great strength of Fisher and Ury's work is its emphasis on problem-solving: a helpful focus when we think about social work and advocacy. Applying a problem-solving approach to principled negotiation gives us two simple elements in the negotiation: exploring the problem and seeking solutions. I am going to consider each of these in turn.

Negotiation – exploring the problem

Earlier, we identified that advocacy as a theory applied to social work draws upon ideas from mainstream practice adapted to provide a theoretical frame for advocacy. Our model of negotiation is no exception to this. When we look at exploring the problem, this aspect of advocacy is very evident. Fisher and Ury (1991) propose two elements to problem exploration. The first is separating the people from the problem. Every negotiation has two elements to it: the substance of the negotiation and the relationship between the negotiators. Fisher and Ury suggest that these can become entangled.

It is through empathetic engagement with the other party that we begin a process of disentangling these elements. Cournoyer's (2014) work on preparatory empathy is important here. To negotiate effectively, we need to understand the assumptions we bring to the negotiation and the motivation of the other parties involved. More broadly, we need to appreciate the emotional significance of the negotiation.

The second element of problem exploration is to focus on common interests, not positions. Within any negotiation, if we step back sufficiently, we will be able to identify commonality despite parties adopting what at first sight appear to be irreconcilable positions. Solution-focused approaches (see Chapter 19) provide tools that can be applied to this element of the process of negotiation. Exception-finding and challenging impossibility ideas (Turnell & Edwards, 1999; Parton & O'Byrne 2000; Myers, 2007 and Chapter 19) are particularly relevant to moving away from positional thinking in negotiation. A more specific example illustrates how problem exploration works in practice. Advocacy in relation to housing providers is a very common feature of the day-to-day experience of social workers in all sorts of contexts (Reamer, 1989; McCarty, 2008). How would this model of negotiation help shape this core social work activity? Firstly, a social worker approaching a housing agency would explore their own preconceptions about the agency: for example, that the agency sees tenants with social needs as problematic. They would also attempt to empathize with the agency's perspective, perhaps considering the boundaries of the support the agency might provide and the reasons for those boundaries. An early part of the negotiation process might be to engage in a discussion about preconceptions on both sides.

A common interest in this type of negotiation, if the parties were able to step back from more entrenched positions, would simply be a positive housing outcome for a vulnerable person. Mapping the routes to achieving this might involve exception-finding; identifying circumstances where tenants with social care needs have been successfully supported to show that there is no fixed rule of failure here. This approach also challenges the idea that a particular way of working will never be successful, what would be seen within a solution-focused approach as confronting fixed-impossibility ideas.

Negotiation – seeking solutions

The major goal of problem exploration in negotiation within advocacy is to move discussion towards a process of identifying potential solutions shared by all parties in the negotiations. Again, this involves engagement with social work theory. Part of this process of solution-finding involves generating different options to identify creative ways to meet service users' needs. Systems and ecological theories provide a potential framework to support these processes (see Chapter 15). Finally, as we seek solutions looking for some sort of external validation, using established criteria for the outcome of the negotiation can be important. For social work, these independent criteria might well be relevant research and guidance into what works, particularly in the promotion of resilience and autonomy. This is one part of making advocacy an evidence-based approach (Davies, Townsley, Ward, & Marriot, 2009). For example, evidence suggests that successfully supporting service users with complex needs in housing requires effective inter-professional working (Institute of Public Care, 2013). This might lead to an outcome of negotiation involving the establishment of a range of mechanisms to support and enable inter-professional working.

Advocacy and radical social work

I looked earlier at cause advocacy, the collective pursuit of an advocacy goal by a group sharing a common problem. Schneider and Lester's (2001) model of how cause advocacy proceeds is process-orientated. It explores strategy, tactics and leadership and how they might contribute to a campaign. It also begins to acknowledge when it comes to cause advocacy 'that everything is political' (Schneider & Lester, 2001, p. 233). The approaches and techniques of cause advocacy as described by Schneider and Lester share quite a lot with community development (see Chapters 25 and 27), particularly in the practical approaches both adopt to building a campaign (Henderson & Thomas, 2002). This interface between community work and cause advocacy provides a starting place for a wider analysis of the links between advocacy and radical social work.

Radical social work has its roots in the political and social movements of the 1960s and 1970s (see Chapter 29). Drawing upon the seminal writing from that period (Bailey & Brake, 1975), it embraces an approach to practice that addresses the political context of social work and pursues the goals of wider social change. There are two important ways in which advocacy might be relevant for radical practice. We have already touched on collective community-orientated approaches to practice, and I will return to these shortly. Before doing that, I want to look at advocacy with individuals as a possible framework for radical practice as it potentially offers 'a way in which oppressed people can secure choice, justice, support, protection, social development and a general sense of empowerment' (Ferguson & Woodward, 2009, p. 124). Ferguson and Woodward argue that advocacy has the potential to provide an element of the theoretical underpinning for radical practice. They also stress, however, the importance of advocates being independent and not advocating in relation to the organizations within which they work. This is a theme taken up by Hardwick (2014) in her research into an Advocacy Rights Hub, which underlines the importance advocates within voluntary sector organizations ascribe to independence. However, there are dissenting voices. Baldwin (2011, p. 198) argues that for social workers in statutory sector organizations, 'to advocate on behalf of service users with managers and decision-making panels is to make a political statement about . . . the gap between how decisions ought to be made and how they are made' and as such 'can be classed as radical practice'. With an increasingly sub-contracted and outsourced social care marketplace (Trades Union Congress [TUC], 2015), the distinction between statutory and voluntary bodies is more blurred. Social workers in statutory organizations, however, often do have multiple loyalties, whilst an independent advocate has a single primary loyalty to the service user (Gates, 1994). It is therefore crucial that social workers are aware of the limitations that their professional role may place on their acting as advocates. It is also important that advocates are aware of the importance of empowering service users, and working towards the goal of supporting service users through peer and self-advocacy as a 'truly empowering practice would be upsetting and radical and would come from forces outside social work – from citizen users, advocacy groups, community activists and social movements' (Gray & Webb, 2013, p. 12).

Individual advocacy, then, has some potential as a framework for radical practice. I now want to return to cause advocacy as a potential radical approach. The idea of community engagement within social work, the development of collective responses to social problems and support of community-controlled institutions has a long history in social work (Banks, 2011). There are many claimants on this territory. They range from the communitarian view that participation within society is in itself a social good of inherent value (Etzioni, 1995), via the Big Society agenda (Office of Civil Society, 2010, Woodhouse, 2015), through to the recent reinvigoration of radicalism in social work (Turbett, 2014)

Cause advocacy

For Schneider and Lester (2001) pursuing a cause is an important endpoint of advocacy. The cause advocacy process essentially involves three stages that mimic the stages of advocacy with individuals which we looked at earlier (Wilks, 2012). The starting point is the creation of a coalition of interest; bringing together people with a common difficulty. Secondly the process involves evidence-gathering and research, and then finally campaigning and achieving goals. There are two types of goals that cause advocacy can achieve. It has the potential to raise awareness of an issue. Feldman, Strier, and Schmid (2016) argue that Bourdieu's concept of symbolic capital is useful in helping us understand what happens in successful cause advocacy. Marginalized groups can, through campaigning, 'challenge the dominant constructions of social problems' (Feldman et al., 2016, p. 1763). The success of the carers' movement in the UK could be understood in these terms. Initially campaigning for recognition of the impacts of caring on women, who bore the brunt of this unpaid labour, it redefined caring as no longer a natural role for relatives to undertake, but as a potentially problematic social issue (see Chapter 7). Cause advocacy can also succeed in achieving changes in policy, practice and the law, something the carers' movement also achieved.

At first sight this looks like a process consistent with the aspirations of radical social work. Consideration of Banks's distinction between community development and community action, however, helps show what might give this type of cause advocacy a radical edge (Banks, 2011). For Banks, community development is a participatory approach encompassing 'social change orientated' work (Banks, 2011, p. 168). Community action embraces a more radical stance and seeks to challenge power structures and to set campaigning within a political context (see Chapters 25 and 27). This can mean the adoption of advocacy activities that confront the structures and ideologies of oppression. One way to achieve this is through engagement with processes of consciousness-raising, 'learning to perceive social, political, and economic contradictions and to take action against the oppressive elements of reality' (Freire, 1970). Rose and Black's (1985) work with a group of service users with mental health problems as part of a deinstitutionalization programme is a good example of this. Using an advocacy framework explicitly informed by Freire's work, the programme's focus was on helping service users move from dependence to independence through a process of critical debate and conscientization.

The global context of advocacy

Collective approaches to advocacy have also had an influential impact on social work internationally. Interestingly, an important feature of the re-emergence of radicalism within social work, a key way current theorists of radical social work distinguish themselves from their 1960s and 1970s forebears, is the adoption of an internationalist perspective and an attempt to contextualize the sometimes-parochial concerns of UK social work within a global context (Ioakimidis & Lavalette, 2011; Ferguson, Lavalette, & Whitmore, 2005).

However, the applicability of models of social work practice developed in the West in other global contexts can be limited (Midgley, 1990, 2001; Graham, 1999). Midgley argues that Western models of social work, with their individualistic and often therapeutic focus, have limited relevance to those who live in poverty, lack resources and face hunger, environmental degradation and violence (Harrison & Melville, 2010; see Chapters 14 and 25). In this context community-orientated approaches to practice are better able to address the material circumstances of people's lives (Dominelli, 2010).

In international development, advocacy has been co-opted as a framework for grassroots campaigning and activism (Cox & Pawar, 2013). Voluntary Service Overseas's (2009) approach to participatory advocacy is a good example. It focuses on issues important to and identified by local communities, and provides a structured framework through which policy change can be pursued. A key element of the approach is participatory research led by those affected by local policy issues and focused on ensuring their voice and perspective are heard. Building on this research, a coalition of interest can be constructed, much like cause advocacy as described by Schneider and Lester (2001), and through lobbying and negotiation, policy influenced or changed. A key aim of the process is to equip participants with the skills they need to advocate on their own behalf in future. The final element in this approach to advocacy is to build links from local to national to international in pursuit of wider change.

Conclusion

One of the most striking things any overview of advocacy reveals is the central place that values play in this area of practice. To some extent, our perspective on social work values will shape our views on advocacy. However, a common aspiration to empower relatively powerless people and to challenge the powerful lies at the heart of this approach to practice. Reflecting on the global context of social work and advocacy seems an apt point to end this discussion. Social work and social care operate in an increasingly globalized world within which the sources of power are increasingly diffuse and difficult to pin down. This is a challenge for advocacy but also a reason for it to remain an essential part of social work.

Further reading

Ferguson, I., & Woodward, R. (2009). *Radical social work in practice*. Bristol: Policy Press.

Schneider, R., & Lester, L. (2001). *Social work advocacy: A new framework for action*. Belmont, CA: Thomson/Brooks Cole.

Wilks, T. (2012). *Advocacy and social work practice*. Maidenhead: Open University Press.

References

Adams, R. (2003). *Social work and empowerment*. Basingstoke: Palgrave Macmillan.

Adams, R. (2008). *Empowerment, participation and social work* (4th ed.). Basingstoke: Palgrave Macmillan.

Atkinson, D. (1999). *Advocacy: A review*. Brighton: Pavilion.

Ayto, J. (2005). *Word origins* (2nd ed.). London: Black.

Back, K., & Back, K. (2005). *Assertiveness at work: A practical guide to handling awkward situations*. London: McGraw-Hill.

Bailey, R., & Brake, M. (Eds.). (1975). *Radical social work*. London: Arnold.

Baldwin, M. (2011). Resisting the easycare model. In M. Lavalette (Ed.), *Radical social work today*. Bristol: Policy Press.

Banks, S. (2011). Re-gilding the ghetto: Community work and community development in 21st century. In M. Lavalette (Ed.), *Radical social work today* (pp. 165–186). Bristol: Policy Press.

Banks, S. (2012). *Ethics and values in social work* (4th ed.). Basingstoke: Palgrave MacMillan.

Barber, J. G. (1991). *Beyond casework*. Basingstoke: Macmillan.

Bateman, N. (2000). *Advocacy skills for health and social care professionals*. London: Jessica Kingsley.

Bisman, C. (2004). Social work values: The moral core of the profession. *British Journal of Social Work, 34*, 109–123.

Brandon, D. (1995). *Advocacy: Power to people with disabilities*. Birmingham: Venture.

Brandon, D., & Brandon, T. (2001). *Advocacy in social work*. Birmingham: Venture.

Braye, S., & Preston-Shoot, M. (1995). *Empowering practice in social care*: Buckingham: Open University Press.

Cournoyer, B. (2014). *The social work skills workbook* (7th ed.). Belmont, CA: Thomson/Brooks Cole.

Cox, D., & Pawar, M. (2013). *International social work: Issues, strategies, and programmes*. London: Sage.

Davies, L., Townsley, R., Ward, L., & Marriot, A. (2009). *A framework for research on costs and benefits of independent advocacy*. (Report for the Office of Disability Issues). London: Office for Disability Issues.

Dominelli, L. (2010). *Social work in a globalizing world*. Cambridge, UK: Polity Press.

Etzioni, A. (1995). *The spirit of community: Rights, responsibilities and the communitarian agenda*. London: Fontana.

Feldman, G., Strier, R., & Schmid, H. (2016). The performative magic of advocacy organisations: The redistribution of symbolic capital. *British Journal of Social Work, 46*(6), 1759–1775.

Ferguson, I., Lavalette, M., & Whitmore, E. (2005). *Globalisation, global justice and social work*. London: Routledge.

Ferguson, I., & Woodward, R. (2009). *Radical social work in practice*. Bristol: Policy Press.

Fisher, R., & Ury, W. (1991). *Getting to 'yes': Negotiating an agreement without giving in*. London: Random Century.

Freire, P. (1970). *Pedagogy of the oppressed*. New York: Continuum.

Freddolino, P., Moxley, D., & Hyduk, C. (2004). A differential model of advocacy in social work practice. *Families in Society, 85*(1), 119–128.

Fook, J. (2002). *Social work: Critical theory and practice*. London: Sage.

Gates, B. (1994). *Advocacy: A nurse's guide*. Harrow: Scutari.

Goldberg Wood, G., & Tully, C. (2006). *The structural approach to direct practice in social work*. New York: Columbia University Press.

Graham, M. (1999). The African centred world view: Developing a paradigm for social work. *British Journal of Social Work, 29*(2), 251–267.

Gray, M., & Webb, S. A. (2013). Towards a new politics of social work. In M. Gray & S. A. Webb (Eds.), *The new politics of social work*. Basingstoke: Palgrave Macmillan.

Hardwick, L. (2014). Advocacy versus social work: What the setting-up of an advocacy rights hub reveals about social work's ability to promote social inclusion. *British Journal of Social Work, 44*(7), 1700–16.

Harrison, G., & Melville, R. (2010). *Rethinking social work in a global world*. Basingstoke: Palgrave Macmillan.

Henderson, P., & Thomas, D. (2002). *Skills in neighbourhood work* (3rd ed.). London: Routledge.

Institute of Public Care. (2013). *Evidence review: Housing and social care*. London: Skills for Care.

International Federation of Social Workers. (2014). *Global definition of social work*. Retrieved from http://ifsw.org/policies/definition-of-social-work

Ioakimidis, V., & Lavalette, M. (2011). *Social work in extremis: Lessons for social work internationally*. Bristol: Policy Press.

Jones, C. (1983). *State social work and the working class*. Basingstoke: Macmillan.

Jones, C. (2001). Voices from the front line: State social workers and New Labour. *British Journal of Social Work, 31*(4), 547–562.

Jordan, B. (1987). Counselling, advocacy and negotiation. *British Journal of Social Work, 17*(2), 135–146.

Keating, F. (1997). *Developing an integrated approach to oppression*. London: Central Council for Education and Training in Social Work.

McBride, P. (1998). *The assertive social worker*. Aldershot: Arena.

McCarty, D. (2008). The impact of public housing policy on family social work theory and practice. *Journal of Family Social Work, 11*(1), 74–88.

Midgley, J. (1990). International social work: Learning from the third world. *Social Work, 35*(4), 295–300.

Midgley, J. (2001). Issues in international social work: Resolving critical debates in the profession. *Journal of Social Work, 1*(1), 21–35.

Myers, S. (2007). *Solution-focused approaches*. Lyme Regis: Russell House.

Office of Civil Society. (2010). *Building a stronger civil society*. London: Cabinet Office.

Parrot, L. (2010). *Values and ethics in social work practice*. Exeter: Learning Matters.

Parton, N., & O'Byrne, P. (2000). *Constructive social work*. Basingstoke: Palgrave Macmillan.

Pullen-Sansfacon, A., & Cowden, S. (2012). *The ethical foundations of social work*. Abingdon: Taylor & Francis.

Reamer, F. G. (1989). The affordable housing crisis and social work. *Social Work, 34*(1), 5–9.

Reamer, F. G. (2006). *Social work values and ethics* (3rd ed.). New York: Columbia University Press.

Rees, S. (1991). *Achieving power*. Sydney: Allen & Unwin.

Rose, S., & Black, B. (1985). *Advocacy and empowerment: Mental health care in the community*. New York: Routledge.

Seligman, M. E. P. (1975). *Helplessness: On depression, development and death*. San Francisco: Freeman.

Schneider, R., & Lester, L. (2001). *Social work advocacy: A new framework for action*. Belmont, CA: Thomson/Brooks Cole.

Solomon, B. (1976). *Black empowerment*. New York: Columbia University Press.

Thompson, N. (2016). *Anti-discriminatory practice* (6th ed.). Basingstoke: Palgrave Macmillan.

Trades Union Congress. (2015). *Outsourcing public services*. London: TUC.

Turbett, C. (2014). *Doing radical social work*. Basingstoke: Palgrave Macmillan.

Turnell, A., & Edwards, S. (1999). *Signs of safety: A solution and safety oriented approach to child protection casework*. London: Norton.

Voluntary Service Overseas. (2009). *Participatory advocacy: A tool kit for VSO staff volunteers and partners*. London: VSO.

Wilks, T. (2012). *Advocacy and social work practice*. Maidenhead: Open University Press.

Woodhouse, J. (2015). *The voluntary sector and the big society* (Briefing Paper 5883). London: House of Commons.

31

Feminist ideas in social work

Sarah Wendt

Introduction

This chapter reviews the contribution of feminism to social work practice. It provides an overview of feminism's intellectual base and how feminist knowledge continues to contribute to the evidence base of social work. The chapter outlines the major ideas emerging from third wave feminism, and identifies practice principles from such ideas. It concludes by acknowledging the value and impact of feminism in social work.

Feminism draws on a range of philosophical and political approaches to problem definition and problem-solving through engagement with modernist and postmodernist orientations (Wendt, 2016; Saulnier, 2013). Feminism has also been grounded in social movements, described as 'waves', and has emerged through practices of academia and debate in a range of disciplines (Saulnier, 2013, p. 3). With this rich tapestry of practice and thought across time, one cannot simply say 'feminism is . . .'. Instead, feminism offers many diverse frameworks and perspectives, and it is from this productive platform of ideas that social work engages with feminism.

On the other hand, to identify or name commonality and answer why feminism features in social work, it is because feminism broadly focuses on explaining and responding to the oppressed position of women in many societies across the globe (see Chapter 29). Women's experiences, roles and positions in societies become the focus in social work through utilizing feminist ideas (Payne, 2014, p. 348).

A rich history of ideas

To understand the current theoretical influences of feminism on social work and into the future, third wave and fourth wave feminism become particularly relevant. However, this does not mean first and second wave feminism are not relevant or the learnings from such waves ignored. The metaphor of waves within feminism provides an important image of continual development and reflection of ideas. Waves present an image of fluidity and constant movement (Chamberlain, 2016). As Budgeon (2011, p. 6) states, waves suggest a relationship of both continuity and discontinuity with a greater whole.

Third wave feminism encompasses multiple meanings, nuances and complexities about women's experiences, roles and positions in societies. It has been described as advancing second wave feminism by being more inclusive, emphasizing difference, valuing personal narratives and being comfortable with uncertainty of knowledge (Zimmerman, McDermott, & Gould, 2009; see Chapters 4 and 21). The third wave has been represented as seeking out a range of different voices and experiences, in contrast to the second wave, which has been predominantly viewed as representing only educated, white, middle-class and heterosexual women (Zimmerman et al., 2009). However, writers also note that the exclusiveness criticism needs to be treated with caution because black writers greatly advanced thinking about race, class and culture throughout the second wave. The focus on interrelations of gender, race and class and the questioning of women as a homogenous group can be seen in the second wave and influenced the third wave (Zimmerman et al., 2009; Mann, 2013; Wendt, 2016).

Third wave feminism has also been expressed as dialogue across social and cultural contexts in an effort to challenge, transform and abolish material, political and social power structures and systems (Zimmerman et al., 2009). Some therefore argue that the agendas of the second wave, such as challenging discrimination and prevailing notions of women's role in the family and workplace, equal pay and educational opportunities, reproductive rights and women and children's safety, to name a few examples, have been extended into the third wave (Gray & Boddy, 2010). But the third wave is more about forming a solidarity through recognition of different local contexts and climates for it has become widely accepted that no account of oppression is true for all women in all situations all the time (Zimmerman et al., 2009; Gray & Boddy, 2010). The third wave is an exploration and examination of gender, with many different feminisms arguing gender is performed, culturally constructed and not innate and gender intersects with other areas of oppression including race, ethnicity, class and sexuality, but also disability and age (Phillips & Cree, 2014). The third wave has deconstructed essentiality conceptions of 'woman' and 'man' and has emerged in understanding experiences of gender, discrimination and oppression (Mann, 2013).

Third wave feminisms have broadly become known for (1) insisting on exploring the interrelation of gender, race, class, sexuality, age and disability and other social categories (2) emphasizing local, individual and personal narratives and connecting local and global activism (Mahoney, 2016; Zimmerman et al., 2009). Intersectionality theory and post-structural theory have been identified as the major ideas influencing third wave feminism (Mann, 2013). They both embrace a strong social constructionist view of knowledge; hence, they explore and examine the relationship between knowledge and power, as well as how people construct knowledge and social reality from different social locations (Mann, 2013).

It is this embracing of social constructionist ideas that has interested social work because such epistemologies provide tools to explore, identify and interpret subjugated knowledges. Social work as a discipline and profession focuses on marginalization and promotes social change, development and empowerment of people in a diverse social changing world (International Federation of Social Workers, 2014). Third wave feminism has specifically influenced social work research where knowledge generation is being viewed as being co-constructed with service users in an interactive, dialogic process. Interpretation of different understandings, environments, experiences, practices and ways of knowing are forming social works knowledge. Reflexivity of the profession and encouragement of self-reflexivity of social workers also represents influences of third wave feminism, and this reflection is often seen in feminist social work publications (Mann, 2013; Wendt, 2016; Howe, 1994). Some examples of feminism expressed in the third wave are outlined below.

Intersectional feminism

Intersectional feminism criticizes the essentialism of white-identity politics. It highlights the intersections of racial and gender oppressions as well as class oppressions (Zufferey, 2016). Intersectional feminism in social work has grown to focus on the simultaneous and intersecting forces of racism, sexism, classism, heterosexism, ageism and ableism in the lives of women (Mann, 2013). It has become a significant theoretical tool to frame social work advocacy efforts across policy, practice, research and teaching (Zufferey, 2016).

For example, Zufferey (2016) argues that intersectional feminism enables social workers to examine how unequal power relations related to gender, class, race, ethnicity and sexual orientation intersect to represent experiences of homelessness and social work responses. She argues critical exploration of social identity categories is necessary to understand how they shape the embodied experiences of men and women who are defined as homeless. Another example, Laing and Humphreys (2013, p. 21), argue a feminist intersectional approach to domestic violence enables consideration of the complex ways in which women's multiple social (dis)locations intersect to shape their experiences of victimization and their opportunities for achieving safety and autonomy.

Feminist social workers have embraced intersectional feminism because it reveals the ways in which structural arrangements impact on certain social groups and provides opportunity to examine power, privilege and oppression (Krumer-Nevo & Komem, 2015). Intersectional feminism provides social workers with structural analysis of power relations but also enables a focus on the lived experiences of groups of women. In short, feminist social workers are able to investigate relationships between structural arrangements and subjective experiences for different groups of women (Krumer-Nevo & Komem, 2015).

Poststructural feminism

Poststructural feminism has emerged in social work as a response to past feminist thinking, which tended to universalize the experiences of women. Universalizing experience is seen to be oppressive and marginalizes women who do not fit the dominant feminist categories of white and middle class (Morley & Macfarlane, 2012). Rather than focus on emancipation, structural change, and large-scale transformation for woman as one uniform category which informed second wave feminist thought and practice in social work, poststructural thinking has created opportunity for dialogue about many local constructions of knowledge and meaning making among women. A range of multiple views, women's individual experiences and changing and competing subjectivities have become a focus to understand power relations within society and how these are maintained through discourse and language (Wendt & Boylan, 2008; Morley & Macfarlane, 2012). Poststructural ideas have enabled feminist social workers to challenge dominant constructions of women's experiences and examine how dominant knowledge forms arise about women and how these may be opposed. Through deconstruction, feminist social workers are attempting to open space to explore silenced or alternative constructions of women's experiences; hence attempting to be more inclusive (Morley & Macfarlane, 2012).

For example, Wendt and Zannettino (2015) engaged with poststructural ideas of discourse and subjectivity to understand how gender is constructed across different communities of women. They explore how meaning making shapes local understanding and experiences of gender and domestic violence. By exposing the complexities and nuances of gendered positioning, they argue, this helps explain domestic violence but also enables feminists to advance arguments of why gender matters and must remain central in research and practice regarding domestic violence. Another example, Moulding (2016), through his writings, has engaged with feminist poststructural ideas to explore women's experiences of eating disorders, child sexual abuse and other forms of violence. She looks to discourses and practices that construct such experiences to show how discursive fields form gendered dimensions of mental health and illness. Disability is also another field in which feminist poststructural ideas are recognized. For example, the medicalization of disability and the impact of professional power is explored, while taking into account personal and social experiences of disability, therefore understanding disability as a socially and culturally constructed phenomenon (Hiranandani, 2005). Feminist poststructural ideas are used to foreground the operation of power and knowledge and to highlight difference in disability (Fawcett, 2016).

Feminist social workers have engaged with poststructural ideas to emphasize the importance of context and to investigate and expose universal and dominant constructions of women. The concepts of discourse and subjectivities are being applied to expose how dominant knowledges, understandings and meaning making arise but also to expose the consequences of this dominance. For example, feminist social workers using these ideas attempt to show how various forms of knowledges are silenced or marginalized, how differences have been constructed and how meanings can change according to contexts (Fawcett, 1998; Wendt & Boylan, 2008)

Transnational and postcolonial

Chakraborty (2007, p. 101–102) writes that feminists of colour argue that the very idea of waves in feminism, such as the third wave, is an ideological construct of the Eurocentric subject that seeks to subsume and consume the challenges posed to it through notions of 'inclusion' and 'solidarity'. Instead of waves, Chakraborty (2007) uses the term 'hegemonic feminism' as a way of historicizing white or Western feminism. She uses this term to make the point that 'at the feminist table not everyone is equal' and the hegemonic feminist project is 'refusing to insist on a cogent and embodied critique of the discourse of difference' (p. 108). She points out that difference has been ghettoized into global feminism or branched out into broader postcolonial categories such as third world feminism, postcolonial feminisms, feminisms of colour and others. She then writes, 'These categories would not have such nomenclatural power and meaning in contexts outside of white-dominated multicultural nations' (p. 108). Chakraborty (2007, p. 109) argues we cannot negate the essential fact of being racialized and embodied entities.

The critique outlined above by Chakraborty (2007) has important implications and resonance for social work. For example, Moosa-Mitha and Ross-Sheriff (2010) point out that international social work is dominated by the Global North through universalizing epistemological and practice-based assumptions when engaging with social issues. They too point out that the Global North does not acknowledge their participation in inequitable processes of globalization. Moosa-Mitha and Ross-Sheriff (2010) advocate for social work to engage with transnational feminism to address these critiques and argue international social work can learn from transnational feminism to grow inclusionary social work practice. Transnational feminism has been identified as a response to international feminism, which grew from the second wave. International feminism engaged with globalization, however, has been critiqued by feminisms from the Global South for being too preoccupied with commonalities and solidarity without recognizing specific differences that women in the South experience, based on race and as a result of colonization (Moosa-Mitha & Ross-Sheriff, 2010). In short, international feminism was critiqued for being universalistic.

Transnational feminism has been identified as engagement with social, economic and political struggles that relate to dominance and exploitation in terms of colonial and national contexts. It examines the specific nature of oppression as it occurs through the intersectionality of race, class and other social-identity locations within a particular local context (Moosa-Mitha & Ross-Sheriff, 2010, p. 107). Transnational feminism also critiques global processes that result in inequities and that cross the boundaries of nation-states. It also aims to examine colonizing patriarchal state practices (Moosa-Mitha & Ross-Sheriff, 2010). The deconstruction of patriarchal practices as part of the process of decolonization has also been named postcolonial feminism (Valkonen & Wallenius-Korkalo, 2016).

As Cook Heffron, Snyder, Wachter, Msonwu, and Busch-Armendariz (2016) state, transnational feminism has moved away from dualistic thinking and values the nuances and linkages between and across time and space; that is, it focuses on place, belonging, identity and the fluidity of such experiences. Transnational and postcolonial feminism come together to work on specific agenda and concrete issues (Moosa-Mitha & Ross-Sheriff, 2010) and, specifically, postcolonial feminists aim to expose paternalistic extensions of colonialism and historic and structural inequalities that impede global justice (Deepak, 2011).

For example, Moosa-Mitha and Ross-Sheriff (2010, p. 107) point out that indigenous women who cross the boundaries of nation-states work together against discrimination against women that is part of colonial histories (see Chapter 23). Women coming together from different nation-states to expose environmental damage because of global capitalist development is another example. Dialogue across social and cultural contexts is central to transnational feminism and has an emphasis on personal and individual experiences linking to social change; therefore, political activism as local has global connections and consequences (Zimmerman et al., 2009). The agency of third world women or non-Western women is emphasized in transnational and postcolonial feminist theory (Deepak, 2011).

Intersectional, poststructural, transnational and postcolonial are some examples or expressions of feminisms identified as being part of the third wave. Broadly, third wave feminism is about inclusiveness and valuing and emphasizing personal narratives, responsible choices and individual-level political activism. It is also about being comfortable with an uncertainty of knowledge (Zimmerman et al., 2009) and is an acceptance of diversity and fragmentation as the structure and meaning of gender relations continue to change in contemporary societies (Budgeon, 2011). Feminisms representative of the third wave have much to offer social work because they focus on 'the power of a marginalized standpoint' (Zimmerman et al., 2009, p. 88), are comfortable with differences and multiplicities of social identities and therefore break down universality and dichotomous binaries within and across social work (Moosa-Mitha & Ross-Sheriff, 2010).

Fourth wave feminism

In writing about feminist ideas in social work, it is also worth noting that the fourth wave has recently been articulated. Phillips and Cree (2014) state that the fourth wave of feminism has been articulated in the social sciences, but not yet in social work writings. This wave has been discussed as emerging through social media and using an array of platforms such as blogs, Twitter, Facebook and other online media to evolve the agendas of the third wave. The online environment has also enabled a rise in public commentaries about the need for feminism and who calls themselves a feminist. Social media and the internet, Munro (2013, p. 23) argues, have created a 'call-out' culture, in which sexism or misogyny can now be 'called out' and challenged almost immediately. Many of these debates have also revealed 'the extremes of polarisation between pro- and anti-feminist opinions' (Phillips & Cree, 2014, p. 938). The internet has enabled activism and a platform for individuals, groups and communities of women to discuss and advocate around shared ideas and social issues impacting them. In short, the fourth wave has been associated with how technology has changed ways in which feminists can communicate with another, often rapidly and efficiently. Two prominent examples often named as evidence for the fourth wave is the Slut Walk, now an international march because of personal experiences of sexism. Similarly, Everyday Sexism was established to document women's everyday experiences of harassment and has now become internationally known (Benn, 2013).

More and more examples of online activism and demonstration can now be seen across the internet whereby individual incidents can gain momentum and scope very quickly as more and more people are made aware of sexism, harassment, violence and abuse of women as well as other social issues (Benn, 2013). For example, in 2017 women in more than 50 countries went on strike from paid and unpaid labour now known as the International Women's Strike (IWS). It is a grassroots movement established by women from different parts of the world. It was created in late October 2016 as a response to the current social, legal, political, moral and verbal violence experienced by contemporary women at various latitudes (http://parodemu jeres.com/). Another example: millions of people from all over the world marched in opposition to the agenda and rhetoric of the American president Donald Trump. Such mass organization happened across the internet and live reporting and photographs could be shared quickly across the world. The pussy hat became a visual image of support and solidity for women's rights.

Perhaps the fourth wave is an opportunity for feminist social work to move writings beyond traditional academic, policy and practice platforms. The dialogue facilitated by the internet is a creative future space that will enable feminist social workers to engage with each other quickly. It is also a space that provides another representation of the 'personal is political'. Positional dialogues on gender and other social identities can grow engagement quickly and encourage socio-cultural-political analysis on personal issues (Krumer-Nevo & Komem, 2015). It can be argued that the fourth wave offers feminist social work a shared public and political collective to showcase its richness and diversity beyond traditional academic journals (Chamberlain, 2016). In another example, we see a wide range of topics and writings featured in The Conversation (http://theconversation.com/uk), which is an independent source of news and views, sourced from the academic and research community and delivered direct to the public. Margaret Alston used this platform in 2012 to discuss the importance of feminism, International Women's Day and human rights. Blogs, Twitter, Facebook and online news and media platforms are just a few examples of the energized, highly visible social media outlets that provide opportunity to discuss and debate a wide range of social issues relevant to social work, feminism and human rights.

Feminism is a rich history of ideas that is always developing. The valuing of intersectional and fluid identities, recognizing heterogeneity, affirming agency and analyzing power (Cook Heffron et al., 2016) are key features that have emerged across time. These features offer social work much in terms of practice with women, and their children, families, communities and countries. For example, Pandya's (2014) account of feminist social work in India addressing violence against women provides a wonderful example of engagement with multiple ideas and practice principles represented in the waves of feminism.

This chapter has outlined particular feminisms that feature in recent social work writings and reflections; however, it is also worth noting that feminism has influenced social work in such a way that we now see many social workers not stating a particular feminist school of thought in their writing or practice but emanating a feminist perspective generally. This perspective enables social workers to be reflective and enables broad gender analysis and awareness of power relations (Orme, 2013) when examining agendas of feminism: for example, equal rights in employment and education, alleviating poverty, eliminating violence against women, interrogating sexualization of women and girls and improving women's health and well-being (Wendt & Moulding, 2016). Yet, as we move into the future, writers such as Gringeri, Wahab, and Anderson-Nathe (2010) suggest that social work should move beyond broader discussions and applications of feminism and be more explicit about critical articulation and reflection of third wave feminism thought in research and practice. They argue this explicitly is a way to acknowledge and celebrate diversity. Furthermore, clearly articulated application of particular feminist theories pushes social work to move beyond universalistic and binary claims and provides tools of application for practice.

Value and impact

As Chenoweth and McAuliffe (2015) state, if self is our mechanism for practice in social work, then we must have a high level of awareness about who we are and how we behave. Furthermore, it is argued across social work education contexts that social workers have an ethical and professional responsibility to have knowledge of established research theories that are grounded in social work values (Teater, 2010). This chapter has shown that feminism provides social workers with ideas to form self-awareness and inform advocacy and practice. Feminism offers explicit guidance for practice and this guidance is evidence of the value and impact of feminism in social work. The evidence of third wave feminisms influencing social work can be seen in the identification of particular practice principles and analysis of power relations. Some practice principles are listed below.

Self-awareness, reflexivity

Feminist social workers attempt to acknowledge positions of power and privilege in research, writings and practice related to a diverse range of social positioning in addition to gender. This principle of practice encourages social workers to unpack assumptions in their own thinking and within policy and practice. Self-awareness and reflexivity can open up communication about diversity and complexities of power in multiple relationships (Dominelli, 2002; Zimmerman et al., 2009; Wendt & Moulding, 2016).

Local contexts

Feminist social workers aim to learn about local cultures and contexts, recognizing multiple ways women make sense of their experiences since no account of oppression is true for all women in all situations all the time (Gray & Boddy, 2010). The complexity and nuanced realities of women's lives become the focus, not universalism (Wendt & Boylan, 2008; (Gringeri et al., 2010; Wendt & Moulding, 2016; Zimmerman et al., 2009).

Intersectional and fluid identities

Feminist social workers are committed to a more inclusive approach to other social positioning that intersects with gender including race, class, ethnicity, age, sexuality, religion, disability and location. Gender is theorized as a social construct that is fluid and diverse; hence, social workers are interested in interpreting how gender is performed and culturally constructed and how these constructions impact on and influence women's everyday lives. These ideas have been used to challenge essentialism of white-identity politics and embrace diversity and differences among women (Phillips & Cree, 2014; Swigonski & Raheim, 2011; Wendt & Moulding, 2016).

Dialogue and agency

Feminist social workers recognize and stress that women who are oppressed exercise agency, resilience and courage amid the challenges they face. Women are not passive victims (Cook Heffron et al., 2016, p. 174). Inclusiveness is a theme of practice whereby feminist social workers are sensitive to dialogue and so seek to accept and know others as who they are instead of thinking that one group can put themselves in the place of the other and speak for them. Dialogue and agency offer theorizing through deeply personal offerings of experiences to analyze a range of power relations (Zimmerman et al., 2009).

Personal is political

Feminist social workers are able to investigate relationships between structural arrangements and subjective experiences for different groups of women (Krumer-Nevo & Komem, 2015). 'The personal is political' is a well-known phrase of the second wave that now has many meanings and interpretations in the third wave. The personal narratives and local contexts of women's lives are significant in the third wave, but they are also viewed as politically active: that is, they are used to generate personal and local action which is then an impetus for social-level change (Zimmerman et al., 2009). Furthermore, postcolonial ideas have exposed how local knowledges are exploited and oppressed in forces of globalization related to issues of colonialism (Zimmerman et al., 2009; Gray & Boddy, 2010).

Conclusion

Third wave feminisms and the flow into a possible fourth wave provide rich theoretical ideas and practice principles for social work. Feminism continues to provide a foundation for social work to celebrate social justice values but to also recognize local knowledges. The complexity, contradictions and fluidity of women's lives are embraced by feminism, and this provides social work with an avenue to recognize agency but also the multiplicity of power relations in all aspects of women's lives in local and global contexts.

Further reading

Affilia: Journal of Women and Social Work. http://journals.sagepub.com/home/aff
This journal is the only peer-reviewed, scholarly social work journal from feminists' points of view, offering a unique mix of research reports, new theory and other creative approaches.

Morley, C., & Macfarlane, S. (2012). The nexus between feminism and postmodernism: Still a central concern for critical social work. *British Journal of Social Work, 42,* 687–705.
This edited collection provides a comprehensive exploration of how feminism is being used in social work conceptually and in terms of day-to-day practice.

Wendt, S., & Moulding, N. (2016). *Contemporary feminisms in social work practice.* London: Routledge.
This article provides an excellent overview of the development of feminism and how social work can engage with such ideas.

References

Benn, M. (2013). After post-feminism: Pursuing material equality in a digital age. *Juncture, 20*(3), 223–227.
Budgeon, S. (2011). *Third wave feminism and the politics of gender in late modernity.* Basingstoke: Palgrave Macmillan.

Chakraborty, M. (2007). Wa(i)ving it all away: Producing subject and knowledge in feminisms of colour. In S. Gillis, G. Howie, & R. Munford (Eds.), *Third wave feminism: A critical exploration* (pp. 101–113). New York: Palgrave Macmillan.

Chamberlain, P. (2016). Affective temporality: Towards a fourth wave. *Gender and Education, 28*(3), 458–464.

Chenoweth, L., & McAuliffe, D. (2015). *The road to social work and human service practice* (4th ed.). South Melbourne: Cengage.

Cook Heffron, L., Snyder, S., Wachter, K., Msonwu, M., & Busch-Armendariz, N. (2016). 'Something is missing here': Weaving feminist theories into social work practice with refugees. In S. Wendt & N. Moulding (Eds.), *Contemporary feminisms in social work practice* (pp. 165–180). London and New York: Routledge.

Deepak, A. (2011). Globalisation, power and resistance: Postcolonial and transnational feminist perspectives for social work practice. *International Social Work, 55*(6), 779–793.

Dominelli, L. (2002). *Feminist social work theory and practice.* Basingstoke: Palgrave Macmillan.

Fawcett, B. (1998). Disability and social work: Applications from poststructuralism, postmodernism and feminism. *British Journal of Social Work, 28,* 268–277.

Fawcett, B. (2016). Feminism and disability. In S. Wendt & N. Moulding (Eds.), *Contemporary feminisms in social work practice* (pp. 275–286). London and New York: Routledge.

Gray, M., & Boddy, J. (2010). Making sense of the waves: Wipeout or still riding high? *Affilia: Journal of Women and Social Work, 25*(4), 368–389.

Gringeri, C., Wahab, S., & Anderson-Nathe, B. (2010). What makes it feminist? Mapping the landscape of feminist social work research. *Affilia, 25*(4), 390–405.

Hiranandani, V. (2005). Towards a critical theory of disability in social work. *Critical Social Work, 6*(1), Online.

Howe, D. (1994). Modernity, post modernity and social work. *British Journal of Social Work, 24,* 513–532.

International Federation of Social Workers. (2014). *Global definition of social work.* Retrieved from http://ifsw.org/get-involved/global-definition-of-social-work/

Krumer-Nevo, M., & Komem, M. (2015). Intersectionality and critical social work with girls: Theory and practice. *British Journal of Social Work, 45,* 1190–1206.

Laing, L., & Humphreys, C. (2013). *Social work and domestic violence: Developing critical and reflective practice.* London: Sage.

Mahoney, K. (2016). Historicising the 'third wave': Narratives of contemporary feminism. *Women's History Review, 25*(6), 1006–1013.

Mann, S. (2013). Third wave feminism's unhappy marriage of poststructuralism and intersectionality theory. *Journal of Feminist Scholarship, 4,* 54–73.

Moosa-Mitha, M., & Ross-Sheriff, F. (2010). Transnational social work and lessons learned from transnational feminism. *Affilia, 25*(2), 105–109.

Morley, C., & Macfarlane, S. (2012). The nexus between feminism and postmodernism: Still a central concern for critical social work. *British Journal of Social Work, 42,* 687–705.

Moulding, N. (2016). Putting gender in the frame: Feminist social work and mental health. In S. Wendt & N. Moulding (Eds.), *Contemporary feminisms in social work practice* (pp. 181–195). London and New York: Routledge.

Munro, E. (2013). Feminism: A fourth wave? *Political Insight,* 22–25.

Orme, J. (2013). Feminist social work. In M. Gray & S. Webb (Eds.), *Social work theories and methods* (2nd ed., pp. 87–98). London: Sage.

Pandya, S. (2014). Feminist social work: An Indian lens. *Affilia, 29*(4), 499–511.

Payne, M. (2014). *Modern social work theory* (4th ed.). Basingstoke: Palgrave Macmillan.

Phillips, R., & Cree, V. (2014). What does the 'fourth wave' mean for teaching feminism in twenty-first century social work? *Social Work Education, 33*(7), 930–943.

Saulnier, C. F. (2013). *Feminist theories and social work approaches and applications.* London: Routledge.

Swigonski, M., & Raheim, S. (2011). Feminist contributions to understanding women's lives and the social environment. *Affilia, 26*(1), 10–21.

Teater, B. (2010). *Applying social work theories and methods* (2nd ed.). Maidenhead: Open University Press.

Valkonen, S., & Wallenius-Korkalo, S. (2016). Practising postcolonial intersectionality: Gender, religion and indigeneity in Sami social work. *International Social Work, 59*(5), 614–626.

Wendt, S. (2016). Feminism and social work. In S. Wendt & N. Moulding (Eds.), *Contemporary feminisms in social work practice* (pp. 11–23). London: Routledge.

Wendt, S., & Boylan, J. (2008). Feminist social work research engaging with poststructural ideas. *International Social Work, 51*(5), 599–609.

Wendt, S., & Moulding, N. (2016). *Contemporary feminisms in social work practice*. London: Routledge.

Wendt, S., & Zannettino, L. (2015). *Domestic violence in diverse contexts: A re-examination of gender*. London: Routledge.

Zimmerman, A., McDermott, M., & Gould, C. (2009). The local is global: Third wave feminism, peace and social justice. *Contemporary Justice Review, 12*(1), 77–90.

Zufferey, C. (2016). Homelessness and intersectional feminist practice. In S. Wendt & N. Moulding (Eds.), *Contemporary feminisms in social work practice* (pp. 238–248). London: Routledge.

Part 4
Theory in practice

32

Family social work practice

Fiona Morrison, Viviene E. Cree and Polly Cowan

Introduction

> Intervening in families who are multiply deprived is wrought with dilemmas, which
> are profoundly moral and cannot be solely or simply understood through a language
> of expertise and technique.
>
> *(Featherstone, Morris, White, & White, 2014, p. 6)*

This chapter aims to build connections between the theoretical ideas that underpin, and the
practice of, family social work. In doing so, it supports Featherstone et al.'s assertion that there
are no easy answers or 'quick fixes'; on the contrary, family social work is characterized by contradiction and complexity, not least because, as we will argue, families can be the best and the
worst of things, sometimes at the same time. So in this chapter, we first examine what 'family'
is and make explicit the central role that families have in all endeavours to protect and promote
children's welfare and well-being. We argue that the social work task is intimately entwined
with the needs and interests of the family. Drawing from the experience of social work in Scotland, we analyze how child welfare law and policy conceptualizes children and their families
and the implications this has for social work practice. We reflect on an example of practice with
families and, in doing so, explore some of the tensions and dilemmas that undoubtedly arise
from family-orientated social work. We consider the challenge of promoting and balancing
the linked, but separate, needs and interests of family members in child and family social work
practice.

Family – a contested term and space

The structure of the family has changed drastically in the last 30 years or so. Traditional depic-
tions of a nuclear family where women stay at home rearing children and men work outside the
home, engaged in full-time employment, no longer reflect the reality of many families in the
UK. Instead, numerous forms of family patterns are evident – for instance, lone parents, childless
couples, same-sex couple families and blended families. New formations of family have emerged
for different, often connected, reasons: greater numbers of women are now participating in the

labour market, there are increased levels of divorce and separation and attitudes towards marriage and sexuality more generally are changing. These changes are reflected in the results of the UK household survey, which reported in 2016 that dependent children lived in 4.8 million families with adults who were married or civil partners, 1.3 million families with adults who were cohabiting couples and 1.9 families headed by adults who were lone parents (Office for National Statistics, 2016).

This poses the question 'What does the term "family" mean?'. Perhaps 'family' refers to those whom we live with? Whom we have biological or legal ties to? Or does family refer to the people who are important to us in our lives? Can friends be family? We suggest that the concept of family is a shifting one, its definition changing depending on the context and culture in which it is used. This is articulated by Murray and Barnes (2010, p. 535) in their conceptualization of family:

> The myriad of conceptualisations of family reflect socio-cultural, economic, political, temporal and spatial contexts. Family can be kin or non-kin, and is often about care and trust in the context of enduring relationships. It has been a key site for debates concerning private and public responsibilities and gender relations.

We can see from this that who or what constitutes family is not fixed; family is about *enduring relationships* and the *care and trust* within these relationships. This conceptualization of family and its significance in protecting children is evident in developments like family group conferencing and kinship care, where they aim to work with and alongside families both in decision-making and in supporting families in a broader sense to care for and protect children (Broad, 2007; Mitchell, 2015). But Murray and Barnes's conceptualization raises two additional issues: what role does and should social work play in sustaining and supporting these 'enduring relationships'? And under what circumstances does and should the state become involved in what is effectively the private lives of citizens? Gender, age, ethnicity, mental health, disability and sexuality all have an impact on how this plays out in the 'real world' of social work practice (Cree, 2010). These are issues that we return to later in this chapter.

We now turn to the law to consider how family is conceptualized. Legalization is of great importance to social work because it provides social workers with mandates to be involved and to intervene in families' lives. Article 8 of the European Convention on Human Rights defines the right to respect for private and family life. Interference by the state in family life must be lawful, '*necessary and proportionate*' (Bainham, 2003, p. 65). In its preamble, the UN Convention on the Rights of the Child (UNCRC) establishes the premise that a child's well-being is best served in a family environment. The importance of the child-parent relationship is developed further in several of the UNCRC's articles. Article 7(1) establishes the right of a child to form a relationship with both parents from birth. Article 18(1) continues the idea that it is a child's right to be cared for by both parents. In Scots law, the Children (Scotland) Act 1995 (CSA) demonstrates this principle; Sections 1 and 2 of the CSA focus specifically on an individual child and those with parental responsibilities and rights for that child, not on the family in a broader sense. However, Section 22 of the CSA also places a legal duty upon local authorities to provide support and services to 'children in need' to safeguard and promote their welfare. It is important to note these services are required to promote the upbringing of children by their *families* as far as is consistent with the duty placed on these services to safeguard and promote children's welfare.

Getting It Right for Every Child (GIRFEC) is the national policy framework and practice model that has as its key objective the improved well-being of children in Scotland. It aims to coordinate multi-agency practice and embed early intervention and prevention within everyday practices of all agencies and practitioners supporting children and young people, to ensure that 'children and families get the help they need when they need it' (Scottish Government, 2012). Underpinned by four key principles, GIRFEC aims to be child-focused, based on an understanding of the well-being of a child and based on tackling needs early, and it requires 'joined-up' working (amongst children, parents and services).

The framework sets out eight domains of well-being (known by the acronym SHANARRI) that become central to all practice with children – children must be safe, healthy, active, nurtured, achieving, respected, responsible and included (Scottish Executive, 2005). GIRFEC further offers three assessment tools (the SHANARRI indicators, the 'Resilience Matrix', and the 'My World Triangle'), each of which places the child and family at the centre of the assessment and planning process. GIRFEC is designed to put children's needs first by 'ensuring that children and families are listened to and that they understand decisions affecting them' (Scottish Government, 2012). Working in partnership with families is viewed as crucial; Robertson and Haight (2012) argue that GIRFEC has encouraged both a shift in emphasis toward actively engaging families in identifying their concerns and challenges and a more holistic view of the child. The Children and Young People (Scotland) Act 2014 has acted to take forward the GIRFEC approach. It provides a legal definition for children's well-being (based on the SHANARRI indicators), establishing a single planning process for children who may require it. The act also attempted to introduce a provision so that every child in Scotland had a 'named person'. This provision was found to be unlawful by the Supreme Court in 2016 as some of the proposals around information sharing breached the right to privacy and a family life under the European Convention on Human Rights. At the time of writing, new draft legislation about information sharing and the named person was being consulted on.

What is interesting here is that although partnership with families is viewed as 'crucial', the focus in GIRFEC is self-evidently on children. It is *children*'s well-being that is assessed, not families', although these are linked, and it is *children* who have plans, not families (see Scottish Government, 2018). This has some interesting implications for social work practice with families.

Why families matter in social work practice

Social workers work with families across a range of different settings. In adult social care, social workers work with a vulnerable adult's relatives when co-ordinating support. In criminal justice, for example in circumstances of domestic abuse, social workers offer support to both the abused person, usually women, and any children who may be affected by domestic abuse. Social workers may also work with perpetrators of abuse trying to change their behaviour. In a children's disability team, a social worker may work with a child's siblings and their parents to gather information about the child's needs and assess how the child's disability is impacting the family more broadly. In this chapter, our focus is on children and families' social work. Here the task of social work relates to concerns about the nature of relationships in families and the linked capacity of adults to care for and nurture their children. Whether concerns relate to poverty, neglect, parental mental health, domestic abuse, substance misuse or some combination of other circumstances that may lead to child maltreatment or neglect, the role of social work is to operate and mediate between the private sphere of the family and the public sphere of the state to ensure that children are protected (Parton, 1991). A key tension for social work is how to balance the need 'to protect children from dangerous individuals and while at the same time protecting the family from unwarrantable interventions' (Parton, 2012, p. 92). We will now consider this more fully.

Tensions within social work practice with families

As in other areas of practice, tensions inevitably arise in family social work. While these tensions may not be unique to family social work, they can be particularly potent in this area of practice.

Who is the client?

In recent years, criticisms have been levelled about how social work considers and engages with families. It has been argued that the gaze of social work has become too narrow and indeed too 'child-centric', to the detriment of the children themselves and the families that it seeks to support and protect. Melton (2009, p. xii), reflecting on child protection systems across English-speaking countries asserts:

> . . . the current child protection system objectifies the children whom it seeks to protect and the parents whom it accuses. The ostensible mission of the system is lost as children are treated as evidence and 'treatments' are designed to provide verification of parents' 'failures'. In effect, a culture of caring is replaced by a culture of surveillance.

This brings us back to our earlier discussion about whether it is the child or the family that is the focus in child and family social work practice. Certainly, the legal and policy context in Scotland and in the UK more broadly positions the child as the client, not the family. This is, in part, due to children's greater dependency and vulnerabilities, as well as the fact that it is often the actions of adults that endanger children. But in seeing children as individual units and not members of families, the importance of wider family relationships may become obscured, including most often relationships with grandparents, aunts and uncles and siblings. Jones and Henderson (2017) note that 70 to 80 percent of accommodated children have siblings also in care, and around 70 percent of these experience separation yet most of these children and young people express a strong desire to stay in contact with brothers and sisters. Just as importantly, the reality, as we will now consider further, is that social workers cannot protect or promote the welfare of children *unless* we work with and support families.

Poverty and the 'austerity agenda'

Featherstone et al. (2014), discussing the English approach to child welfare and protection, argue that the stark inequalities that exist in society are not given sufficient weight or consideration in current policy and practice responses to child maltreatment. They write:

> The experiences of those trying to parent in a profoundly unequal society are not inter-rogated rigorously enough in current responses, with causation and correlation confused in a highly abstract language that renders real people and their practices invisible and/or unintelligible. For example, mental health difficulties, substance misuse and domestic abuse are advanced as central risk indicators for child abuse. However, they are not explored in the context of living with poverty and shame in an unequal society'.
>
> *(Featherstone et al., 2014, p. 6)*

At the heart of these criticisms is the point that rearing children is hard, but it is especially so when living in poverty. Research on child welfare inequality confirms this, providing evidence that poor families are disproportionately represented in the child protection system (Bywaters et al., 2015). What this means for family support practice is that there is a need to focus not only on child maltreatment but also on addressing all the adversities, including the economic, that families experience. Failing to do this makes protecting the welfare of children much more difficult.

The constrained spending in public services since the financial crisis that accelerated in 2008 is connected to the issue of poverty. The so-called 'austerity' programme has led to a retraction of public services which has been keenly felt in areas like family support and had a disproportionate impact on the well-being of families living in poverty (see Gallagher, 2017).

How is 'the family' viewed?

A further challenge emerges from Morris's (2012) analysis. She argues that, in practice, the family may be framed as both a *risk* and a *resource*. Kinship carers, for instance, are seen to be a resourceful family that may offer a place of care and protection for children. Whereas families that that are poor and experiencing multiple social problems are constructed as risky. The tension is that families are often both resourceful and risky. This seemingly contradictory view of families is problematic, and there is little evidence to explain how families themselves navigate such labels.

Gender

As we discussed earlier, gender and changing gender norms and relations have dramatically changed the family patterns. In children and families social work practice, however, mothers remain overwhelmingly the adult whom social workers engage with. This is an issue for women, who may be doubly criticized for not adhering to gender-stereotypical ideas about 'good' mothering. But it is also an issue for fathers. The absence of fathers from social work practice means that only a partial image of a family can be presented. Both the resources and the risks that fathers may bring cannot be adequately explored, addressed or exploited if they are not included in practice (see Clapton, 2017). Furthermore, an exclusive focus on women's parenting often results in women's parenting being held to a higher standard than men's; women may be doubly blamed if they are found guilty of neglecting or abusing a child or if they have harmed an unborn child through their alcohol or drug use. The whole issue of pre-birth assessments is a highly contentious and complex area for child and family social workers today; research from the US suggests that we need as a society to take a much more compassionate and rounded approach to women in this situation (see Cherry, 2014).

What is family-based social work practice? The C-C-C model

Family-based approaches to social work take place across the spectrum of services that intend to promote child well-being and protection – universal services, early intervention, targeted services and statutory child protection services. And family-based practice is best understood as operating across a range of levels. Building from our findings on the ESRC-sponsored 'Talking and Listening to Children' UK-wide research project into how social workers communicate with children in child protection (see www.talkingandlisteningtochildren.co.uk), we have developed a model to explain this in practice. The 'child-case-context' model recognizes that individuals, interactions, relationships and environment all influence one another, and so they have an impact on how social workers and children communicate with one another. This is, of course, not a new idea. As long ago as 1920, Nora Milnes, then director of the Edinburgh

School of Social Study and Training, argued that 'a wise understanding of social influence is necessary for the solving of child health problems' (p. 20). Some 50 years later, Bronfenbrenner (1979) claimed that it is not enough to focus only on the child; we also need to pay close attention to environmental and societal influences on child development. His work connects sociological ideas of structure and environment with psychological ideas of personality and development; it has been influential across the world in informing policy and practice in children's services.

This perspective is closely aligned to that of relationship-based practice (see Chapter 12). Ruch (2009) urges us to see the individual in context, the psychological and the social, because 'neither makes sense without the other' (p. 350). The concept of relationship-based practice can be seen as a contemporary reworking of the earlier psychosocial model; as well as attending to the uniqueness of the interpersonal encounter, it also places particular emphasis on reflexivity, the use of self and the relationship through which communication is channelled.

Another pillar on which the model is built is that of the strengths' perspective (see Chapter 18). Saleebey (2011) coined this term, reminding us that individuals, adults and children alike must be seen as whole people with strengths and coping mechanisms that should be respected and valued. Even when the going gets tough, there are opportunities for connection and learning for us and for those with whom we are working; authentic communication may not always be easy, but it is worth striving for – as Saleebey (2011) insists, 'every environment is full of resources' (p. 191).

The model's fourth contention is that every child and each family member is unique. The idea of person-centred practice (see Rogers, 2012; and Chapter 3) is at the heart of UK policy and is demonstrated, for example, in the Scottish government's GIRFEC approach, which, as we have seen, is predicated on the assumption that each child should be helped to achieve their full potential. And if every person is different, we must be flexible in our approach – there can be no simple set of rules for 'best practice' with children and young people.

At first glance, the model looks simple, but exploring more deeply, shows how complex encounters and practice with children and young people can be. While the concepts are presented separately, there will always be a degree of overlap and relationship between them. A political context of austerity, for example, will have implications for levels of poverty, which, in turn, have consequences for child welfare. Similarly, it has been known for years now that issues such as domestic abuse or substance misuse have major implications for children's wellbeing and how a child and their family may respond or react to each other and to social work.

Child

Things to consider: the age and stage of the child or young person; any disability or health problems; their ethnicity; language (Is English their first language or not? Do they have any communication, educational or developmental difficulties?); their gender; the relationships they have with siblings, peers and parents; their previous relationship with you or with another social worker; how you think about children and childhood (Is the child seen as a competent being with capacity, or do they need protection? Or are both true?).

Case

Things to consider: the nature of the referral (statutory versus voluntary, early intervention or risk assessment, routine monitoring or crisis?), who made the referral and why, what else is going on in the family (with siblings, domestic abuse, substance misuse, mental or physical health problems, caring needs of other family members etc.), how long the family has been involved with social services, what kind of work the social worker is doing with the child, how the wider family feels about this.

Context

Things to consider: the individual social worker (their experience and skills; personality and personal and professional background; their gender, ethnicity and age; their values and attitudes etc.); the social work agency/organization and its institutional and organizational environment; what other agencies are involved (police, school, youth club etc.); the cultural and socio-political environment and other structural pressures on the child and family, including, for example, stresses related to poverty; poor housing; racism.

Working with whole families

We will now use the child-case-context model to look at a practice example in more depth.

The Miller family

Tara (seven) and Michael (six) are white, Scottish siblings who live in a council flat on a peripheral housing estate with their mother, Sheila, who is in her late 20s. The children's father, John, separated from their mother five years ago. He now lives in another town and sees the children infrequently. Sheila is currently unemployed; she lost her part-time job in a shop some weeks before.

The housing department called the social work department following a neighbour's complaint that the children were being neglected and that there was a lot of shouting and crying coming from the house. The housing officer reported that Sheila had been drinking heavily. The children were constantly late for school, and the school staff noted a recent deterioration in their physical appearance and confidence. The children had stopped going to a club run by a third-sector organization for children whose parents have problems with alcohol or drugs. They had told their teacher that they had not seen their grandparents for a long time and that they missed them. When asked about this, Sheila told the teacher that she 'cannot manage everything'. The housing officer is anxious about how Sheila will feel about being referred to social work; she said that she 'hates social workers'.

Child

Children living in homes where there is alcohol misuse can be exposed to worry, confusion and chaos (O'Connor, Forrester, Holland, & Williams, 2014; Kroll, 2004; see Chapter 37). Use of the SHANARRI well-being indicators is a good place to start in working out what is going on for each of the children. Beyond this, a strengths-based approach such as 'signs of safety' may be a useful tool to use with the whole family. This is an approach with child safety at its core which aims to involve everyone in the thinking process, 'from the "biggest" person (often someone like a director general, a judge or child psychiatrist) to the "smallest" person (the child)' (Turnell, 2012, p. 9). Sheila had a supportive extended family and was perceived by all professionals involved to have loving relationships with her children. Highlighting Sheila's parenting strengths helped build her confidence, which also boosted her motivation to engage with support for her alcohol misuse. The children enjoyed spending time with Sheila's parents, and signs of safety allow the family themselves to identify the support they can offer, helping the children without Sheila feeling it as an imposition.

Case

Research shows that positive relationships between social workers and families are crucial to improving outcomes (Mason, 2012), and yet social workers are often confrontational in their language (Forrester, 2008) and difficult clients are often avoided by professionals (Brandon et al., 2008; Ferguson, 2009; Laming, 2003). We know that Sheila struggled with authority, and this needed to be acknowledged from the outset. Strengths-based and relational approaches share similar goals and are often thought to be interdependent (Oliver & Charles, 2016); in this situation, they complement each other. So a strengths-based approach aims to elicit strengths from the service user (in family work contexts, generally the parent) and to focus on these strengths to address difficulties within the family (Rapp, Saleebey, & Sullivan, 2005). It involves partnership working with the aim of reducing risk to children (Oliver & Charles, 2016) and aims to build relationships between social workers, families and the community (Ornstein & Ganzer, 2005; Robertson & Haight, 2012). Good relationships are central to working with families for positive outcomes (Munro, 2011). The relationship between the worker and the family will thus be used to attempt to facilitate positive outcomes (Dunst & Trivette, 2009)

Context

Again, research has shown that parental alcohol misuse and depressive symptoms can lead to higher risk of neglect (Lloyd & Kepple, 2017). Building a relationship with Sheila was crucial in supporting the whole family. Families describe a good relationship with social workers when they feel they have been listened to or been supported with practical issues (Thoburn, Cooper, Brandon, & Connolly, 2013; Mason, 2012). In addressing alcohol and substance misuse, good communication, honesty and integrity, fundamental tenets of relational social work, are crucial (Robertson & Haight, 2012). Taking a calm, open and non-judgemental approach with Sheila was essential. Involving her in discussions with the school, addiction support, third sector and housing department helps her to trust that there is not a hidden agenda. It will also enable practical issues that she perceives to be heightening her anxiety, and therefore alcohol consumption, to be addressed, such as how the children physically get to the club that is provided by the third-sector organization, giving Sheila a break whilst providing a safe and nurturing environment for the children.

Conclusion

In this chapter, we have sought to build connections between the theoretical ideas that underpin, and the practice of, family social work. We have explored some of the key contradictions and complexities that are present in family support in children and families social work. By setting this in the Scottish policy and legal framework, we have examined how child welfare law and policy conceptualizes children and their families and the implications this has for family support work. In our discussion of the child-case-context model, we have offered a possible way forward for an engaged, supportive family-based practice in the future.

Further reading

Canavan, J., Pinkerton, J., & Dolan, P. (2016). *Understanding family support: Policy, practice and theory*. London: Jessica Kingsley.
Connolly, M. (Ed.). (2017). *Beyond the risk paradigm in child protection*. London: Palgrave Macmillan.
Featherstone, B., White, S., & Morris, K. (2014). *Reimagining child protection*. Bristol: Policy Press.

References

Bainham, A. (2003). *Children and their families: Contact, rights and welfare*. Oxford: Hart.
Brandon, M., Belderson, P., Warren, C., Gardner, R., Howe, D., Dodsworth, J., & Black, J. (2008). The preoccupation with thresholds in cases of child death or serious injury through abuse and neglect. *Child Abuse Review, 17*(5), 313–330.
Broad, B. (2007). Kinship care: What works? Who cares? *Social Work & Social Sciences Review, 13*(1), 59–74.
Bronfenbrenner, U. (1979). *The ecology of human development: Experiments by nature and design*. Cambridge, MA: Harvard University Press.
Bywaters, P., Brady, G., Sparks, T., Bos, E., Bunting, L., Daniel, B., . . . Scourfield, J. (2015). Exploring inequities in child welfare and child protection services: Explaining the 'inverse intervention law'. *Children and Youth Services Review, 57*, 98–105.
Cherry, A. (2014). Shifting our focus from retribution to compassion: An alternative vision for the treatment of pregnant women who harm their fetuses. *Journal of Law and Health, 28*(1) (2015 Forthcoming) Cleveland-Marshall Legal Studies Paper No. 14–276. Retrieved from https://ssrn.com/abstract=2501969
Clapton, G. (2017). *Good practice with fathers in children and family services*. IRISS Insight 38, Glasgow: IRISS. Retrieved from www.iriss.org.uk/sites/default/files/2017-06/insights-38.pdf
Cree, V. E. (2010). *Sociology for social workers and probation officers* (2nd ed., ch. 2). London: Routledge.
Dunst, C. J., & Trivette, C. M. (2009). Capacity-building family-systems intervention practices. *Journal of Family Social Work, 12*(2), 119–143.
Featherstone, B., Morris, K., White, S., & White, S. (2014). *Re-imagining child protection: Towards humane social work with families*. Bristol: Policy Press.
Ferguson, H. (2009). Performing child protection: Home visiting, movement and the struggle to reach the abused child. *Child and Family Social Work, 14*(4), 471–480.
Forrester, D. (2008). How do child and family social workers talk to parents about child welfare concerns? *Child Abuse Review, 17*, 23–35.
Gallagher, B. (2017). Fewer staff, dwindling services: How austerity has hit child protection. *The Guardian Social Care Network*. Retrieved from www.theguardian.com/social-care-network/2017/jul/17/impact-austerity-child-protection
Jones, C., & Henderson, G. (2017). *Supporting sibling relationships of children in permanent fostering and adoptive families*. Glasgow: School of Social Work and Social Policy Research Briefing, no. 1, University of Strathclyde.
Kroll, B. (2004). Living with an elephant: Growing up with parental substance misuse. *Child & Family Social Work, 9*(2), 129–140.
Laming, H. (2003). *The Victoria Climbié inquiry: Report of an inquiry by Lord Laming* (Cmnd 5730). Norwich: The Stationary Office.
Lloyd, M. H., & Kepple, N. J. (2017). Unpacking the parallel effects of parental alcohol misuse and low income on risk of supervisory neglect. *Child Abuse and Neglect, 69*, 72–84.
Mason, C. (2012). Social work the 'art of relationship': Parents' perspectives on an intensive family support project. *Child and Family Social Work, 17*(3), 368–377.
Melton, G. (2009). Preface. In B. Lonne, N. Parton, J. Thomson, & M. Harries (Eds.), *Reforming child protection*. London: Routledge.
Milnes, N. (1920). *Child welfare from the social point of view*. London: Dent.
Mitchell, M. (2015). *Family group conferences – What do they tell us about the importance of relationships?* (Unpublished paper). Presented at the Centre for Excellence for Looked After Children in Scotland (CELCIS) Annual Conference.
Morris, K. (2012). Thinking family? The complexities of family engagement in care and protection. *British Journal of Social Work, 42*(5), 906–920.
Munro, E. (2011). *The Munro review of child protection: Final report*. London: Department for Education.

Murray, L., & Barnes, M. (2010). Have families been rethought? Ethic of care, family and 'whole family' approaches. *Social Policy and Society, 9*(4), 533–544.

O'Connor, L., Forrester, D., Holland, S., & Williams, A. (2014). Perspectives on children's experiences in families with parental substance misuse and child protection interventions. *Children and Youth Services Review, 38,* 66–74.

Office for National Statistics. (2016). *Statistical Bulletin: Families and households in the UK: 2016.* Retrieved from www.ons.gov.uk/peoplepopulationandcommunity/birthsdeathsandmarriages/families/bulletins/familiesandhouseholds/2016

Oliver, C., & Charles, G. (2016). Enacting firm, fair and friendly practice: A model for strengths-based child protection relationships? *British Journal of Social Work, 46*(4), 1009–1026.

Ornstein, E. D., & Ganzer, C. (2005). Relational social work: A model for the future. *Families in Society, 86*(4), 565–572.

Parton, N. (1991). *Governing the family: Child care, child protection and the state.* London: Macmillan.

Parton, N. (2012). Reflections on 'governing the family': The close relationship between child protection and social work in advanced western societies – The example of England. *Families, Relationships and Societies, 1*(1), 87–101.

Rapp, C., Saleebey, D., & Sullivan, W. P. (2005). The future of strengths-based social work. *Advances in Social Work, 6*(1), 79–90.

Robertson, A., & Haight, W. (2012). Engaging child welfare-involved families impacted by substance misuse: Scottish policies and practices. *Children and Youth Services Review, 34*(10), 1992–2001.

Rogers, C. R. (2012). *Client-centred therapy* (New ed.). London: Constable & Robinson.

Ruch, G. (2009). Identifying the critical in a relationship-based model of reflection. *European Journal of Social Work, 12,* 349–362.

Saleebey, D. (2011). Power in the people. In V. E. Cree (Ed.), *Social work: A reader* (pp. 184–194). London: Routledge.

Scottish Government. (2012). *A guide to getting it right for every child.* Edinburgh: Scottish Government.

Scottish Government. (2018). Understanding wellbeing. Retrieved from https://www.gov.scot/publications/getting-right-child-understanding-wellbeing-leaflet/pages/1/

Thoburn, J., Cooper, N., Brandon, M., & Connolly, S. (2013). The place of 'think family' approaches in child and family social work: Message from a process evaluation of an English pathfinder service. *Children and Youth Services Review, 35*(2), 228–236.

Turnell, A. (2012). *Signs of safety briefing paper V2.3.* Perth: Perth Resolutions Consultancy Retrieved from www.aascf.com/pdf/Signs%20of%20Safety%20Breifing%20paper%20April%202012.pdf

33

Theory for social work with children

Kathleen Manion

Introduction

Social workers engage with children in a variety of settings. They often hold a significant amount of power over children and families. Much social work practice coalesces around decision-making and supporting processes (O'Connor & Leonard, 2014) and is therefore helped by theoretical foundations. How social workers make these decisions and choose to engage with clients is influenced by the theories that they are exposed to and choose to embed in their practice. Taking a pragmatic approach, this chapter borrows a broad definition of 'theory', as something we use 'in an attempt to make sense of the world and/or particular events' (Trevithick, 2011, p. 29). Theories help us predict what is likely to happen in each situation and explain why a given situation is happening.

Relevant theories can be used both as sense-making and predictive tools. Several theoretical frameworks underpin social work practice, both practice-based theories and theory-based practices. As Rogowski (2013, p. 18) states, 'social work is not, and cannot be, common sense, despite what parts of the media and some politicians would have us believe'. While social work embraces grassroots practice-based theories more than other professions, inductive theories have also gained academic acknowledgement (Fisher & Somerton, 2000).

Social work includes direct or indirect practice at the micro, mezzo and macro levels. This holds true for both general social work and social work with children. While there are several foci within this field of study and practice, common ones include the social change or social justice perspective, the problem-solving or solution-focused perspective, person-in-environment ecological models and empowerment perspectives. Focus on individual or structural components of practice and deductive or inductive foundation or practice theories also exist (Armitage, 2003). Another undervalued influence continues to be a Freirean grassroots praxis perspective (Freire, 1970; Reynaert, Bouverne-De Bie, & Vandevelde, 2010).

Not without critique (e.g. Keskin, 2013), social workers tend to draw on a multitude of theoretical perspectives and weave them into an eclectic framework at the individual or institutional level. This wide-ranging approach has caused some challenges for implementing a cohesive theoretical framework. However, barriers have also instigated creativity and innovation.

This chapter focuses on those areas of practice with children that have been influenced by theories and, conversely, the theories that have been influenced by practice since 2000. Ungar (2005) eloquently states that 'We must be content with a collage of competing truths, each a vibrant local account of what we have come to think we know about children's well-being. The more dialogue across social, cultural, and linguistic barriers, the more convinced I am of a plurality of possible ways to account for children's resilience' (p. xv).

This provides a relevant opening to this chapter, which represents a tapestry of the ways theory shows up in practice with children. We will examine the areas of child social work practice, including family support, early intervention, well-being in school, community work, aboriginal practice, youth work, youth justice and intersections between health and social work with children. The chapter predominantly focuses on practice in English-speaking countries including the UK, Ireland, Canada, the US, Australia and New Zealand.

Context

Social workers often have the training, skills and knowledge to conduct preventative work. However, funding and resources for social work have traditionally been geared towards reactive practice. Social work broadly continues to be a contested practice, in terms of what it does and what it should incorporate (Rogowski, 2013). Within the milieu of social work with children, child protection dominates social work literature and practice. There are many other areas of practice undertaken within a variety of settings, however, including not-for-profit agencies, government agencies working with families, schools, private practice, hospitals and other multi-agency contexts. Macro social workers also work within research, evaluation and policy-making arenas (see Chapter 27). Given the breadth of work, the skills needed are equally varied, including counselling skills, family work, interview and advocacy skills, assessment, play therapy and developmental knowledge and understanding, as well as macro skills of policy formation, evaluation and research skills. These utilize a myriad of theoretical foundations. Social workers may work with certain child populations, like children with disabilities, adopted or fostered children, indigenous children and refugee and immigrant children, again influenced by a variety of theories. This tapestry of perspectives is diverse and dynamic.

Some have criticized social work, as a relatively new field, of not having a strong theoretical basis in comparison to other disciplines. Instead, I would argue that social work has embraced a multitude of theoretical foundations. This is a benefit and a challenge. The profession has had to work harder to articulate the importance of weaving theory and practice together into a cohesive whole. This weaving can take place within an individual social worker, their place of work, the state or province or national, regional, or international social work bodies; all can influence and drive theoretical underpinnings that result in unique practice. As a good example, the International Federation of Social Workers (IFSW; 2014) has expanded its definition of social work by saying it

is a practice profession and an academic discipline that recognizes that interconnected historical, socio-economic, cultural, spatial, political and personal factors serve as opportunities and/or barriers to human wellbeing and development. Structural barriers contribute to the perpetuation of inequalities, discrimination, exploitation and oppression . . . In solidarity with those who are disadvantaged, the profession strives to alleviate poverty, liberate the vulnerable and oppressed, and promote social inclusion and social cohesion . . .

Social work is both interdisciplinary and transdisciplinary, and draws on a wide array of scientific theories and research . . . Social work draws on its own constantly developing theoretical foundation and research, as well as theories from other human sciences . . . [They are] applied and emancipatory. Much of social work research and theory is co-constructed with service users in an interactive, dialogic process and therefore informed by specific practice environments.

Adding to the fuzziness of theoretical underpinnings, Trevithick (2011) argues that social work relies on a set of values, often articulated by international, regional and national social work bodies and promulgated by academic institutes and their workplace setting, more than a theoretical basis. 'Although many practitioners see their practice-based knowledge as intuitive and personal, and therefore unworthy of acknowledgement in an academic environment, it does not have to lack the rigour, testability or validation and evaluation of it' (Rutter & Brown, 2015, p. 30). I argue that for a critically reflexive social worker, it is from the articulation and reflection of both their values and their theoretical perspectives that consistent and effective practice can emerge.

Sites of theory-practice integration and reflection

Social workers embed their theoretical and practice-based knowledge into a holistic or haphazard framework at the beginning of their academic careers. This is a critical component of their practice education or service learning. Practice educators influence ongoing practice. They can embed reflective practice that turns academic insights into practice, including theoretical components and understandings of social phenomena.

At the same time, institutional and community values and theoretical frameworks continue to influence whether social work has a holistic or haphazard framework. This happens during organizational processes such as supervision, planning and evaluation. Supervision may be grounded in larger organizations, like child protection agencies, although large caseloads may undermine the practicality of this support. Sadly, in smaller, poorly funded agencies, supervision may not be integrated into practice, leaving the social worker without a way to develop their ideas further. Kahneman (2011) proposes that there is a good adaptive reason for intuitive, fast decision-making, but it is insufficient. Slower deliberative logical thinking is also important. Supervision provides an imperative to engage in this more deliberative thinking.

Penna points out that theory can sometimes be underplayed in practice, and therefore field supervisors play a critical role in supporting social workers to bridge the gap between theory and practice (cited in Boisen & Koh, 2015). This is a change and an opportunity for supervision. Effective field supervisors suggest that to 'be able to conceptualise cases theoretically was paramount to effective practice' (Boisen & Koh, 2015, p. 66). Having said that, others question the importance of theory. Further, some challenge the inherent lack of clear or consistent definition of theory, a practice model, or a framework (Boisen & Koh, 2015). Here, the critique states that practice without theory becomes a 'rudderless vehicle' (p. 67). Interestingly, in their study, students rated their experience higher when their field instructors helped link theory and practice (Boisen & Koh, 2015).

Teaching social workers about theories and instilling a sense of inherent curiosity about how the world functions, as well as the ability to integrate, synthesize and draw on theoretical models reflexively to make sense of their own work experience, provides a good foundation for ongoing reflexive practice.

Prominent theoretical framings

Given the disparate nature of social work with children, it is unsurprising that it traverses several theoretical grounds. However, it is difficult, if not impossible, to separate the theories that have influenced practice since 2000 without providing some context for the influential theories that came before and continue to impact practice. One way to explore high level differences across theory was proposed by Payne (2005), who highlighted three views of social work: reflexive-therapeutic views see social workers supporting individuals, groups and communities to thrive; socialist-collectivist views see social workers supporting disadvantaged individuals and groups to emancipate and overhaul oppressive practices; and individualist-reformist views see social workers as working like a bridge between the individual and society in order to maintain welfare and social order. These three views offer insights into the variety of ways theories are promulgated by individual social workers.

Focusing more on the political persuasions of social work practice, both Rogowski (2013) and Armitage (2003) highlight the following classifications of social work: critical, radical, structural, aboriginal, community development and feminist or anti-oppressive practice (see Chapters 23, 25–31). Again, these political leanings represent or influence how practice and theory are intertwined.

Continuing the theme of variety, an impressive range of different perspectives and foci have emerged. Theoretical frameworks strongly influence practice with children. Given the diversity of countries where social work practice with children exists, this chapter does not provide a comprehensive list of all theories impacting practice in all countries, but rather it illustrates some of the most commonly referenced theories used in practice with children regardless of context. Spray and Jowett (2012) suggest that attachment theory (Bowlby and Ainsworth as cited in Erford, 2016; Ateah, Kail, & Cavanaugh, 2015; Boyd, Johnson, & Bee, 2015; see Chapter 13), ecological theory (as highlighted by Bronfenbrenner & Evans, 2000), systems theory and solutions focused theory are commonly referenced (see Chapters 14, 15 and 19). Munford and Sanders (2015) highlight integrated strengths-based practice (as Saleebey, 1992, first outlined) within a New Zealand context, particularly with social work involving children (see Chapter 18). Additional theories include social cognitive theory (Bandura, 1986), psychosocial development (Erikson & Piaget as cited in Erford, 2016; Ateah et al., 2015; Boyd et al., 2015); psychodynamic theory (Freud as cited in Erford, 2016; Ateah et al., 2015; Boyd et al., 2015; see Chapter 12) and a theory of an ethic of care (Gilligan, 1982; Kohlberg, 1984; see Chapter 7). These are long-standing theoretical frameworks, although some modifications have been suggested. Theories that are emerging in a broader range of practice since 2000 include rights-based frameworks, aboriginal social work, green social work (Dominelli, 2012; see Chapter 14) and resilience-based theories (Ungar, 2005), all of which have infiltrated social work practice. While some of these theories complement one another, others clash.

Social workers tend to blend theories into a holistic theoretical framework that makes sense to them. Hick (2010) suggests this happens in one of three ways: with an integrative approach (where a variety of compatible theories are integrated into a logical whole), an eclectic approach (where practitioners draw on theories like items in a toolbox, using the one that best fits the scenario) or a dialectical approach (where practitioners use multiple theories that do not necessarily fit well together and often hold differing world conceptions but that, held in tension, add to the understanding of a given situation). I suggest that reflexive practice is important to promote a social worker's ability to shift perspectives and gain empathy. Mills (1959) called this the sociological imagination. He suggested

> . . . a quality of mind that will help them to use information and to develop reason in order to achieve lucid summations of what is going on in the world and of what may be happening within themselves. It is this quality, I am going to contend, that journalists and scholars,

artists and publics, scientists and editors are coming to expect of what may be called the sociological imagination.

(p. 5)

In building eclectic, integrative or dialectical theoretical frameworks, a social worker needs the ability to adapt. Mills suggests this provides 'the ability to acquire new ways of thinking' (p. 5). He further states, 'This condition, of uneasiness and indifference . . . is the signal feature of our period and the key task of social scientists' (p. 12).

Putting this into a child-centred social work perspective, Connolly, Crichton-Hill, and Ward (2006, p. 106) suggest

> put simply, theories are cultural resources, cognitive tools for solving problems that inevitably confront us as we make our way in the world. We require a wide range of different theories, each performing their own tasks. The fact that we rely on a variety of theories and cultural resources to explain, predict and understand the different environments within which our lives unfold, means that taking the time to stop and explicitly think about theoretical matters is a valuable and practical thing to do.

Theory in practice today

The sites of social change are varied in social work with children because of the importance of its practice base (IFSW, 2014). This chapter cannot go into depth, but this next section provides some illustration of the impact of theory in practice in a few sample locations.

Child protection is dealt with in Chapter 34 but within child protection, the increased use of differential response models means that many child protection agencies refer families to support services in the community that are heavily influenced by theoretical models like strengths-based practice, ecological models and 'signs of safety' (Turnell & Edwards, 1999). Strengths-based practice has been highly influential across child protection and broader child-centred social work practice.

Family support

Family support programmes are a common work context for many social workers (see Chapter 32). McCubbin and McCubbin (2005) note that the most common explanatory mechanism for how families cope with adverse events has been resilience theory. This has also permeated much family-based practice. Window, Richards, and Vostanis (2004) found that parents and children noted the impact of solution-focused theory in support programmes.

Family support includes training, counselling, resource provision and home-visiting programmes. Examples of their purposes include support for children with special needs, including children with disabilities or with mental health challenges; adopted or fostered children and children going through familial change like divorce or loss.

Parenting programmes are common examples. In Ontario, Young, McKenzie, Orme, Schjelderup, and Walker (2014b) evaluated the efficacy of strengths-based practice in child welfare as well as the integration of signs of safety. They inherently base practice on ecological models and attachment models. Increasingly, they are also based on evidence-informed practice coming from neuroscience. One intriguing new area of research involves mindfulness (see Chapter 22). Trauma-informed mindfulness-based parenting (MBP) intervention is also founded on attachment-focused practice (Gannon, Mackenzie, Kaltenbach, & Abatemarco, 2017).

Within family work is work on supporting adoptive children and their families. Fallon and Goldsmith (2013, p. 23) suggest that 'psychological theories influence our current thinking on the adoption process, the child's healthy psychological development, and successful integration of the child into the family'.

Lastly, outreach is an important element of social work practice with children, as an ally to home visiting. Resilience has been part of many integrated therapeutic outreach programmes (Winkler, 2014).

Early years intervention

Focus on the first five years of life and ensuring strong, healthy development for longer-term success is a new approach. Halgunseth (2009) notes the integration of ecological and social exchange theory in both early years practice and family engagement. Page (2017) illustrates how attachment theory, ecological models and psychodynamic models show up in early years intervention (see Chapters 13–15). Developments in neuroscience have pushed this change.

Well-being in school

Social work practice is particularly focused on child development within school settings (see Chapter 35). This is influenced by biological and evolutionary theories and psychoanalytic theories based on Freud and Erikson. Similarly, learning theories are commonly used based on earlier work by Skinner. Cognitive theories like those by Piaget and Vygotsky are imbedded in practice as are broader ecological models like Bronfenbrenner's or biopsychosocial models. Concepts of social justice have also been integrated: for instance, in those theories laid down by Gilligan's concept of the ethics of care (Boyd et al., 2015; see Chapter 7).

Community social work

European and North American models of theory and practice have dominated community social work practice in the literature. These models tend to have a more individualistic approach and are deficit focused. Culturally, this runs counter to the prevalent world view of many populations, reflected in Southern theories and indigenous theories, which encourage models that are holistic and community-oriented (see Chapters 23 and 25). These differing views are having an impact on traditional European and North American practice. An example of this is a study in the United States that illustrates the relevance and positive impact of quality after-school care on a sense of belonging. This study shows the integration of eco-developmental framework into the practice (Smith, Witherspoon, & Wayne, 2017; see Chapter 14).

Aboriginal practice

One of the largest shifts in many colonized countries is an increasing recognition of indigenous perspectives (see Chapter 23). In New Zealand, an integrated Maori framework articulates a nested ecological system integrating theory into practice that weaves ecological, community development, strength-based and attachment attributes together (Nash, Munford, O'Donoghue, & Nash, 2005).

In Canada, Baikie (2009) suggests: 'Indigenous social workers can creatively engage with multiple social work ways-of-knowing, doing and being while maintaining an Indigenous-centred practice . . . we need to reconceptualise our unique local Indigenous social work perspectives and practices within a global collective Indigenous-centred social work paradigm' (pp. 46–47). Sterling-Collins (2009) shares the importance of the medicine wheel framework as an inclusive and holistic approach covering physical, emotional, intellectual and spiritual aspects with a goal of reaching individual harmony, balance, interconnectedness and interdependence (p. 71). Neckoway, Brownlee, and Castellan (2007) explore the relevance of attachment theory for indigenous families, specifically for children with multiple attachments (see Chapter 13).

Youth work

Like social work with children, youth work covers a myriad of practice contexts and services. Ecological models, strengths-based practice and psychodynamic models exist widely. While exploring youth work in America, Stevens (2005) suggests that ecological models make sense when implemented alongside strengths-based practice. Another pertinent theoretical framing is intersubjectivity. This is popping up in a broader range of practice contexts, but it provides a useful framing within youth work. As an example, this approach considers a broader recognition of gender and sexual fluidity.

Youth justice

Youth justice sits in a different category with more influence from political pressures (Rogowski, 2016). This is not a new trend, but it continues. While practice-based theory may lend itself to more social development and ecological models, the governmental focus is dominated by punitive and criminogenic interests. Doolan (2009) highlights the emergence of a 'justice perspective' (i.e. 'just desserts' or punitive and behavioural), which has emerged alongside a restorative and rehabilitative perspective. These two perspectives are at odds with one another.

Social work intersection with health

Where social work and healthcare meet, there has traditionally been a focus on the medical model, but this is changing. The influence of the social determinants of health critically influenced and broadened the theoretical context for social work practice with children in hospital, with disabilities and with mental health issues. Within the area of social work with children with disabilities, much has changed. One framework has attempted to integrate the medical model, the social model and the transactional model into a 'systems model' (Hick, 2010), whereby parents have increased access to information and support including theoretical and medical information. This has also opened the space for client-professional partnerships (Bricout, Porterfield, Tracey, & Howard, 2004).

While mental health services are broadly defined, but there is a trend toward community care. Services for children with mental health issues remain chronically underfunded, and many healthcare providers will not diagnose children with mental health issues, so this remains a challenging area of practice. Exploring more broadly, Pack (2011) suggests child sexual therapists use eclectic theories as a way of providing protective factors to support children's well-being. With an alternative reading, Keskin (2013) noted the deficiency in US-based studies on children that lack explicit theoretical foundations. Where they were stated, the most commonly cited theories were Barry's acculturation and Bronfenbrenner's ecological model. Similarly, a study of vulnerable children affected by parents with mental health issues found that 46 percent of those studies did not explicitly state their theoretical underpinnings (James, Fraser, & Talbot, 2007). However, one prominent theoretical concept explored in mental health and behaviour issues with children is attachment theory. While there are criticisms of this model, including that it promotes mother-blaming and infant determinacy, it still has offered promising insights into the well-being of children (Shemmings & Shemmings, 2011).

Practice frameworks

In the last two decades, several practice frameworks have tried to integrate theory and practice in a meaningful and easy-to-grasp way. Connolly (2007), as a chief social worker and academic in New Zealand/Aotearoa, created several practice frameworks that articulated the integration of theory and practice for Child, Youth and Family, the New Zealand statutory child protection, youth justice and adoption authority. These were first introduced in 2005. Based on Maori tradition, these frameworks built on the idea of weaving knowledge and practice in a *kete* (a Maori basket) to support strong and effective practice. 'The practice framework weaves together a set of driving principles that are threaded through the phases of the work and linked to our desired outcomes for children and families' (Connolly, 2007, p. 828). 'Three sets of philosophical perspectives provide the basis for the framework: the child-centred perspective; the family-led and culturally responsive perspective; and the strengths and evidence-based perspective' (p. 829).

Alongside the child protection framework, there were also developments in a youth justice framework, a family violence practice framework and an adoptions framework within New Zealand. The youth justice framework included 'the justice and accountability perspective, the offender-focused perspective, and the strengths and evidence-based perspective. Like the earlier framework, these three philosophical perspectives are considered at each of the three phases of intervention: engagement, assessment and planning, changing offender behaviour, and sustaining lifestyle changes following the completion of therapy' (Connolly & Ward, 2007, p. 155). Later work by Connolly has included a kinship care practice framework (Connolly, Kiraly, McCrae, & Mitchell, 2017). Other frameworks support integration of theory and practice, including child rights (Ife, 2008) and indigenous frameworks that appreciate aboriginal ways of knowing and being.

The concept of theory knitting was introduced by Connolly, Crichton-Hill, and Ward (2006) with the intent to 'blend together different theoretical cultures into an holistic framework [called] the culturally reflexive model (CRM)' (p. 107).

In the UK, the introduction of the assessment framework performed a similar function, albeit with a less specific target on integrating theory and practice. Other jurisdictions have played with ways of increasing the efficacy of decision-making processes with the introduction of practice frameworks. The results of a small British qualitative study found that practitioners reported things that were incongruent with anti-oppressive values, illustrating that the realities of practice can conflict with the expectations of theories and ethical frameworks (O'Connor & Leonard, 2014).

Argyris and Schon (1974) coined the term 'double loop learning' to explain professional critical reflection practice. They noted that there was often a gap between practitioners espousing theoretical framework and their practised theoretical framework which went unexplored in single loop learning. Eraut (2004) noted that the integration of theoretical frameworks in practitioners was more complex than espoused in Argyris and Schon's double loop learning model. He suggested that practitioners utilize theories, concepts and values and intermingle them with personal experiential learning without thought. He argued that without critical reflection, both individuals and institutions can blindly tie themselves to uncritical and unrecognized theoretical frameworks. Given that Eraut (2006) later suggests that intuitive decision-making is an important element of many professional decision-making processes, it is even more critical to include processes like supervision and practice frameworks that give space for critical reflection and theory knitting. The capacity to acknowledge and discuss emotional responses within their work may be indicative of greater reflexivity developed through experience. 'In acknowledging their lived experience, [social workers] demonstrate awareness of emotions which may at times be in conflict with professional values and anti-oppressive practice. Recognizing these and the potential triggers which can influence decision making is a crucial element in critical reflective practice' (Fook, 2002, cited in O'Connor & Leonard, 2014, p. 1817).

Impact on social work practice

Even when social workers are not attending to theory, they are influenced by it. This becomes evident in a variety of ways, such as how intake forms are constructed or how interview questions are structured, as well as the underlying structure of the services offered or the way the social workers go about building relationships with children and their families.

As an illustration, there are a few core dichotomies that exist which illustrate the choices individual social workers or their services make. The dichotomy between problem-focused or strengths-based approaches, risk or resilience, partnership or paternalism (see Turnell & Edwards, 1999) are deeply imbedded in the process. These have theoretical perspectives. They may have similarities, but in practice they are diametrically opposed. Young et al., (2014a) note that the problem-focused orientation borrowed from other disciplines has infiltrated social work practice with children, particularly child protection work. They call for the creation of more social work–centred and supportive theory or frameworks that use child rights, community development and strengths-based practice. They also encourage a broader embrace of complexity. In general, there has been a postmodernist rejection of working towards a unified single theory, favouring instead processes that ask children and their families to co-create effective strategies for social change. There are multiple intersecting and conflicting theories and social and political factors that influence how practice happens. This does not just happen within the individual social worker but also affects the supervisor, the organization and the client. The fact that this messy patchwork of theories and practices comes together in any kind of logical and cohesive whole is a miracle. The innovative and agile approach to theory provides a dynamic environment for social workers open to making this work, despite multiple papers bemoaning the lack of a theoretical basis (e.g. Donovan, Rose, & Connolly, 2017).

Failures of influence and barriers to theory in practice

Rogowski (2013) suggests the different classifications of social work may be lost in translation in the minds of many social workers working with children. He maintains that these views are often at odds with one another. As Rogowski suggests, they are influenced by the governmental fiscal context, which does bend to the theoretical wills of the political elite. New managerialism and neoliberal policies significantly curtail social work practice, particularly preventative practice, yet demand ever-more specific outcomes. The gulf between the promise of social work practice and reality is influenced by multiple and conflicting priorities and clashing ideological frameworks. New managerialism has failed social work and disintegrated practitioners from families (Young et al., 2014a). Further concerns are often raised that academics are not sufficiently making their work available and digestible to deepen their theoretical concepts into practice.

Social work with children is a complex and sometimes contradictory landscape of theory-practice threading. Common tensions like that between problem-focused approaches and strengths-based approaches persist. The former is insufficient (Greene & Lee, 2011), and there is a need for solution-focused orientations. Similarly, Baskin (2009) suggests that indigenous social work is more relationship focused, culture based and interested in positive identity. This sits in contrast with more individual transactional processes.

As has been noted, the breadth of practice with children has meant that the practice, excepting child protection, sometimes risks disciplinary tunnel vision. Embracing the complexity of the landscape offers rich insight as long as it is tethered to critical reflection through something like supervision. At a more systemic level, ongoing consideration of the importance of integrated practice –for instance, as seen in New Zealand and Australia – and ecological approach, community development, strengths-based perspective and attachment is needed (Nash et al., 2005). In addition, Lein, Uehara, Lightfoot, Lawlor, and Williams (2017) highlight the need for social workers to look beyond the limits of practice to intentionally built collaborations across allied disciplines and the need to focus on the dynamic context of contemporary practice. This is in keeping with Munro's (2011) calls to move from a blame culture to a continuous learning organization model, which requires a broadening of services to ensure children's safety (Spray & Jowett, 2012).

The future of theory and practice with children

'Social work is a discipline innately engaged in and influenced by the political and social context in which it is practised' (Donovan et al., 2017, p. 1). Given its historic development, whether in child welfare leagues, residential school models, women's rights movements or the discovery of child abuse, social work practice grew out of grassroots practice. Its evolution slowly brought psychological and social theories into its mix, particularly as the schools of social work started to spread. This afforded social work more opportunity to mix theoretical frameworks, given the disconnect between theory and practice. Many social work pioneers have championed ways to tie these together, ensuring that praxis is an ongoing challenge.

This chapter has explored a 'plurality of possible ways' children's well-being has been approached by practitioners with a myriad of theoretical underpinnings. In looking forward, it is important to recognize some broad themes in practice, but more important than what theory is at play is the availability of time and space for social workers and their agencies to critically reflect on the ongoing relevance of those theories and how well they provide insight into ensuring children's well-being.

Further reading

Bronfenbrenner, U., & Evans, G. (2000). Developmental science in the 21st century: Emerging questions, theoretical models, research designs and empirical findings. *Social Development, 9*(1), 115–125. doi:10.1111/1467-9507.00114

Connolly, M. (2007). Practice frameworks: Conceptual maps to guide intervention in child welfare. *British Journal of Social Work, 37*(5), 825–837.

Spray, C., & Jowett, B. (2012). *Social work practice with children and families* (Social work in action). Los Angeles, CA: Sage.

References

Argyris, C., & Schon, D. A. (1974). *Theory in practice: Increasing professional effectiveness*. San Francisco: Jossey-Bass.

Armitage, A. (2003). *Social welfare in Canada* (4th ed.). Don Mills: Oxford University Press.

Ateah, C., Kail, R., & Cavanaugh, J. C. (2015). *Human development: A life-span view* (3rd ed.). Toronto: Nelson.

Baikie, G. (2009). Indigenous-centred social work theorizing a social work way-of-being. In M. Hart, R. Sinclair, & G. Bruyere (Eds.), *Wícihitowin: Aboriginal social work in Canada* (pp. 42–61). Halifax, NS: Fernwood.

Bandura, A. (1986). *Social foundations of thought and action: A social cognitive theory*. Englewood Cliffs, NJ: Prentice-Hall.

Baskin, C. (2009). Evolution and revolution healing approaches with aboriginal adults. In M. Hart, R. Sinclair, & G. Bruyere (Eds.), *Wícihitowin: Aboriginal social work in Canada* (pp. 133–152). Halifax, NS: Fernwood.

Boisen, L., & Koh, B. (2015). Integrating theory and practice methods in field education. In L. Hensley (Ed.), *The social work field instructor's survival guide*. New York: Springer.

Boyd, D., Johnson, P., & Bee, H. (2015). *Lifespan development* (5th Canadian ed.). Toronto: Pearson.

Bricout, J. C, Porterfield, S. L., Tracey, C. M., & Howard, M. O. (2004). Linking models of disability for children with developmental disabilities. *Journal of Social Work in Disability & Rehabilitation, 3*(4), 45–67.

Bronfenbrenner, U., & Evans, G. (2000). Developmental science in the 21st century: Emerging questions, theoretical models, research designs and empirical findings. *Social Development, 9*(1), 115–125. doi:10.1111/1467–9507.00114

Connolly, M. (2007). Practice frameworks: Conceptual maps to guide intervention in child. *British Journal of Social Work, 37*(5), 825–837.

Connolly, M., Crichton-Hill, Y., & Ward, T. (2006). *Culture and child protection: Reflexive response*. London: Jessica Kingsley.

Connolly, M., Kiraly, M., McCrae, L., & Mitchell, G. (2017). A kinship care practice framework: Using a life course approach. *British Journal of Social Work, 47*(1), bcw041. doi:10.1093/bjsw/bcw041

Connolly, M., & Ward, T. (2007). *Morals, rights and practice in the human services: Effective and fair decision-making in health, social care and criminal justice*. London: Jessica Kingsley.

Dominelli, L. (2012). *Green social work: From environmental crises to environmental justice*. Cambridge, UK: Polity Press.

Donovan, J., Rose, D., & Connolly, M. (2017). A crisis of identity: Social work theorising at a time of change. *The British Journal of Social Work, 47*(1), 87–105 doi:10.1093/bjsw/bcw180

Doolan, M. (2009). Social work and youth justice. In M. Connolly & L. Harms (Eds.), *Social work: Contexts and practice* (2nd ed.). Oxford: Oxford University Press.

Eraut, M. (2004). The practice of reflection. *Learning in Health and Social Care, 3*(2), 47–52.

Eraut, M. (2006). Feedback. *Learning in Health and Social Care, 5*(3), 111–118.

Erford, B. T. (2016). *An advanced lifespan odyssey for counseling professionals*. Boston: Cengage Learning.

Fallon, A. E., & Goldsmith, B. L. (2013). Theoretical contributions to the understanding of parent-child bonding in adoption. In V. M. Brabender & A. E. Fallon (Eds.), *Working with adoptive parents: Research, theory, and therapeutic interventions* (pp. 23–44). Chichester: Wiley.

Fisher, T., & Somerton, J. (2000). Reflection on action: The process of helping social work amended accordingly students to develop their use of theory in practice. *Social Work Education, 19*(4), 387–401.

Freire, P. (1970). *Pedagogy of the oppressed*. New York: Continuum.

Gannon, M., Mackenzie, M., Kaltenbach, K., & Abatemarco, D. (2017). Impact of mindfulness-Based parenting on women in treatment for opioid use disorder. *Journal of Addiction Medicine, 11*(5), 368–376.

Gilligan, C. (1982). *In a different voice: Psychological theory and women's development*. Cambridge, MA: Harvard University Press.

Greene, G. J., & Lee, M. Y. (2011). *Solution-oriented social work practice*. New York: Oxford University Press.

Halgunseth, L. (2009). Family engagement, diverse families and early childhood education programmes: An integrated review of the literature. *YC Young Children, 64*(5), 56–58.

Hick, S. F. (2010). *Social work in Canada: An introduction* (3rd ed.). Toronto, ON: Thompson.

Ife, J. (2008). *Human rights and social work: Towards rights-based practice*. Cambridge, UK: Cambridge University Press.

International Federation of Social Workers. (2014). *Global definition of social work*. Retrieved from http://ifsw.org/get-involved/global-definition-of-social-work/

James, E., Fraser, C., & Talbot, L. (2007). Vulnerable children in families affected by parental mental illness: The role of theory in programme development. *Vulnerable Children and Youth Studies, 2*(2), 142–153. doi:10.1080/17450120701403144

Kahneman, D. (2011). *Thinking, fast and slow*. New York: Farrar, Straus and Giroux.

Keskin, B. (2013). The recent explicit use of theory in empirical studies on acculturation of children. *Early Child Development and Care, 183*(1), 163–169.

Kohlberg, L. (1984). *The psychology of moral development: The nature and validity of moral stages*. San Francisco: Harper & Row.

Lein, L., Uehara, E. S., Lightfoot, E., Lawlor, E. F., & Williams, J. H. (2017). A collaborative framework for envisioning the future of social work research and education. *Social Work Research, 41*(2), 67–71.

McCubbin, L., & McCubbin, H. (2005). Culture and ethnic identity in family resilience: Dynamic processes in trauma and transformation of indigenous people. In M. Ungar (Ed.), *Handbook for working with children and youth: Pathways to resilience across cultures and contexts.* Thousand Oaks, CA: Sage.

Mills, C. W. (1959). *The sociological imagination.* Oxford: Oxford University Press.

Munford, R., & Sanders, J. (2015). Working with families: Strengths-based approaches. In M. Nash, R. Munford, K. O'Donoghue, & M. Nash (Eds.). (2005). *Social work theories in action* (pp. 158–173). London: Jessica Kingsley.

Munro, E. (2011). *The Munro review of child protection: Final report, a child-centred system.* London: The Stationery Office.

Nash, M., Munford, R., O'Donoghue, K., & Nash, M. (Eds.). (2005). *Social work theories in action.* London: Jessica Kingsley.

Neckoway, R., Brownlee, K., & Castellan, B. (2007). Is attachment theory consistent with aboriginal parenting realities? *First Peoples Child & Family Review, 3*(2), 65–74.

O'Connor, L., & Leonard, K. (2014). Decision making in children and families social work: The practitioner's voice. *British Journal of Social Work, 44*(7), 1805–1822.

Pack, M. (2011). Discovering an integrated framework for practice: A qualitative investigation of theories used by social workers working as sexual abuse therapists. *Journal of Social Work Practice, 25*(1), 79–93. doi:10.1080/02650533.2010.530646

Page, T. (2017). Attachment theory and social work treatment. In F. Turner (Ed.), *Social work treatment: Interlocking theoretical approaches* (pp. 1–22). New York: Oxford University Press.

Payne, M. (2005). *Modern social work theory* (3rd ed.). Chicago: Lyceum.

Reynaert, D., Bouverne-De Bie, M., & Vandevelde, S. (2010). Children, rights and social work: Rethinking children's rights education. *Social Work & Society, 8*(1). Retrieved from www.socwork.net/sws/article/view/23/64

Rogowski, S. (2013). Critical social work: Theory and concepts. In *Critical social work with children and families: Theory, context and practice* (pp. 17–34). Bristol: Policy Press.

Rogowski, S. (2016). *Social work with children and families: Reflections of a critical practitioner.* London: Routledge.

Rutter, L., & Brown, K. (2015). *Critical thinking and professional judgement for social work* (4th ed.). London: Sage.

Saleebey, D. (Ed.). (1992). *The strengths perspective in social work practice.* New York: Longman.

Shemmings, D., & Shemmings, Y. (2011). *Understanding disorganized attachment: Theory and practice for working with children and adults.* London: Jessica Kingsley.

Smith, E. P., Witherspoon, D. P., & Wayne, O. D. (2017). Positive youth development among diverse racial-Ethnic children: Quality afterschool contexts as developmental assets. *Child Development, 88*(4), 1063–1078. doi:10.1111/cdev.12870

Spray, C., & Jowett, B. (2012). *Social work practice with children and families.* Los Angeles: Sage.

Sterling-Collins, R. (2009). A holistic approach to supporting children with special needs. In M. Hart, R. Sinclair, & G. Bruyere (Eds.), *Wicihitowin: Aboriginal social work in Canada.* Halifax, NS: Fernwood.

Stevens, J. (2005). Lessons learned from poor African American youth. In M. Ungar (Ed.), *Handbook for working with children and youth: Pathways to resilience across cultures and contexts.* Thousand Oaks, CA: Sage.

Trevithick, P. (2011). *Social work skills and knowledge: A practice handbook* (3rd ed.). Maidenhead: Open University Press.

Turnell, A., & Edwards, S. (1999). *Signs of safety: A safety and solution oriented approach to child protection casework.* New York: Norton.

Ungar, M. (2005). Introduction. In M. Ungar (Ed.), *Handbook for working with children and youth: Pathways to resilience across cultures and contexts* (pp. XV–XXXIX). Thousand Oaks, CA: Sage.

Window, S., Richards, M., & Vostanis, P. (2004). Parents' and children's perceptions of a family support intervention for child behavioural problems. *Journal of Social Work Practice, 18*(1), 113–131.

Winkler, A. (2014). Resilience as reflexivity: A new understanding for work with looked-after children. *Journal of Social Work Practice, 28*(4), 461–478. doi:10.1080/02650533.2014.896784

Young, S., McKenzie, M., Orme, C., Schjelderup, L., & Walker, S. (2014a). Practicing from Theory: Thinking and knowing to 'do' child protection work. *Social Science, 3*(4), 893–915. doi:10.3390/socsci3040893

Young, S., McKenzie, M., Orme, C., Schjelderup, L., & Walker, S. (2014b). What can we do to bring the sparkle back into this child's eyes? Child rights/community development principles: Key elements for a strengths based child protection practice. *Child Care in Practice, 20*, 135–154.

34

Safeguarding children and the use of theory in practice

Penelope Welbourne

Introduction: theory in context

Child abuse is unfortunately a common phenomenon: the 2016 *Crime Survey for England and Wales* found the following rates for self-reported experience of childhood abuse:

> . . . 9% of adults aged 16 to 59 had experienced psychological abuse, 7% physical abuse, 7% sexual assault and 8% witnessed domestic violence or abuse in the home. With the exception of physical abuse, women were significantly more likely to report that they had suffered any form of abuse during childhood than men. This was most marked with regard to any form of sexual assault, where women were 4 times as likely as men to be a survivor of such abuse during childhood (11% compared with 3%).
>
> *(Office for National Statistics, 2016, p 1)*

These high rates of self-reported abuse suggest that as many as one child in ten may experience some form of abuse during their childhood. Society has developed greater awareness of different types of harm and increased requirements on those in contact with children in a professional capacity to identify it. There are demanding expectations that specialist practitioners will 'diagnose and treat' abuse: progressing through assessment of level of risk and type of harm to finding solutions to keep children safe and providing or signposting helpful therapeutic interventions. Increasingly complex thinking about what constitutes abuse and what we should do about it is a feature of this area of work. Safeguarding children progressed from a primary focus on physical abuse in the 1960s (Kempe, Silverman, Steele, Droegemueller, & Silver, 1962; Helfer, Kempe, & Krugman, 1968) to include contemporary awareness of sexual abuse, neglect, and abuse linked to coercive and controlling behaviour towards children and young people. A contemporary working definition of child abuse will reflect our developing understanding of exploitative behaviour targeting children, forced marriage, female genital mutilation and fabricated illness (UK Government, 2017; Rights of Women (n.d.); NHS (n.d.); UK Government, 2008). Any definition is a working definition and must be viewed as provisional because no definitive and lasting definition is possible. 'Child abuse' is a socially constructed idea, albeit one based on very real hurt and harm, and changes in our use of the term reflect changes in society. Greater cultural diversity and globalization have also impacted on safeguarding children as children move between countries and cultures, sometimes under duress. Social work practitioners have to be aware of a wider range of indicators of harm than ever before and have a wider range of strategies for assessment, intervention and support.

All safeguarding activity is grounded in a theoretical position about what children need, what constitutes adequate parenting and why specific responses to harm are useful and appropriate. Using a particular theoretical position involves adopting a related explanatory framework for understanding the world and predictions about what will happen as a result of certain interventions or actions. Safeguarding social workers need to be able to use a range of different types of theory, with awareness of what sort of theory it is and how evidence underpins the decisions they make in working with children and families.

Safeguarding social work operates within specific legal, organizational and professional frameworks that determine how theory may be used. Theories guide safeguarding actions but cannot on their own determine how social workers intervene or interact with service users. Social work values and service user preferences also shape interventions, as do resources and agency remit, but all actions need an explanatory framework that justifies ideas about how to intervene and how to evaluate the success of interventions. Theories cannot exist in a vacuum: all need a supporting evidence base to show how they correspond with the real experience of children. None of this should, however, prevent responsible, theoretically informed innovative practice.

All interventions to safeguard children in England and Wales must be undertaken in accordance with the statutory guidance: Working Together to Safeguard Children (DFE, 2018). This guidance does not presuppose any particular theoretical approach to be taken by the practitioner, but it sets standards for organizational response to concerns about the well-being or safety of a child. Similar guidance is produced in many countries.

The constraints within which children's protective social work operates have positive, protective benefits and some drawbacks. Guidance and operational requirements aim for consistent quality of response for all children, setting minimum standards for service delivery. Payne (2011) draws attention to the extent to which bureaucratic and administrative constraints limit social work action. Guidance and operational rules protect both children and workers by defining as clearly as possible what needs to be done when children are at risk but are unable to say what exceptionally good social work looks like. They leave open the possibility of restrictive interpretation of duties to children and families (Lipsky, 1980; Broadhurst, Wastell, White, & Pithouse, 2010). Reflective theory and evidence-informed practice counterbalances this. In practice, theory shapes practitioners' pursuit of certain types of knowledge: theories tell us what sorts of 'facts' are likely to be helpful in understanding what is happening, so they direct our attention to certain kinds of information. They act at the same time as a filter and a compass in dealing with the mass of information present in most inquiries into a child's welfare.

Theories are generalized, abstract ideas about how the world works. They offer explanations and suggest causal relationships. They must be testable, and they must be falsifiable (Popper, 1959). Many theories of development link past events with the present, to explain or predict behaviour or mental state. Early theorists of human behaviour such as Freud, Thorndike, Pavlov, Vygotsky and Skinner (Greene, 2008; Parrish, 2014) and later developments based on them, explain behaviour in terms of prior experience and suggest strategies for the resolution of problem behaviour in accordance with their diverse theoretical standpoints. Ideas derived from systems theory place more emphasis on interactions in the present (Dallos & Draper, 2015).

Theories in use in child protection social work today incorporate ideas from biology, psychology, sociology and learning theory. All offer, in one way or another, a 'lens' through which to understand the internal world of the child and their relationship to the social and familial world in which they live and form the theoretical basis for evaluating signs of well-being and safety or distress and harm.

Different types of theories

The social world is complex, and causal links may be equally complex. Similar outcomes may be reached by a variety of different 'pathways', and people with apparently similar histories may have very different outcomes. Research in social work often describes co-occurrences and clusters of phenomena. Examples of this type of research include research into the impact on children of parental addiction (Department of Health, 2011), outcomes of different kinds of care (Selwyn & Quinton, 2004; Selwyn & Briheim-Crookall, 2017), and patterns of repeated pregnancy among women who have lost a child to 'care' (Broadhurst et al., 2015). Such research tells us a great deal about vulnerabilities and risk factors, although individual responses will be very diverse.

Qualitative research is valuable in providing a perspective on service users' perspectives, drawing attention to people's lived experience and what these perspectives can tell us about what is helpful and unhelpful. Robbins and Cook's (2017) qualitative research into the experiences of victims of domestic violence involved in the child protection system is an example of this approach.

Some research studies use large data sets or meta-analysis of a number of studies to use complex statistical techniques to identify 'latent factors' that on their own may not cause a problem but, in combination with other vulnerability-creating factors, may do so. Such quantitative research takes us closer to understanding cause and effect in complex situations through looking at the interaction of various risk or protective factors in contributing to a particular outcome, as with Spratt's (2012) analysis of the impact of 'multiple adverse childhood experiences'.

Theories used in social work may be said to be mostly *underdetermined*, which means there are often different theories that might be used to understand what is going on, and there are seldom instances when one can say that one theory is proved to be true and another false. Many social work theories are, therefore, better regarded as working hypotheses, which is why the choice of theoretical approach is a matter of personal preference and ethics, to an extent that appears unusual in other professions, such as nursing or dentistry.

Safeguarding children's social work draws on an increasingly wide range of ideas of disciplinary and geographic influences. Sources of theory have always been broad, reflecting its wide range of roles, and work with a range of other disciplines. Cross-disciplinary ideas such as systems theory and attachment theory have proved very powerful influences, as have approaches developed in different countries, such as family group conferences from New Zealand (Barn & Das, 2016) and settlement conferences from Canada (Ministry of Justice, 2017). The former is based on the combination of two very powerful ideas in social work: the importance of culturally appropriate interventions and the value to be placed on preservation of birth families. It is underpinned by beliefs about ethical practice and the value of culture, as well as 'responsibilization' of wider families and communities and a preference for negotiated over imposed agreements. Evidence about outcomes supports its continued use, but the theory underpinning its inception comes from values rather than empirical evidence of 'what works'. Settlement conferences also emphasize negotiation over imposition. Both reflect a shift away from the idea that the proper role of the child protection/juridical process is to assess adequacy of parenting and remove children when parents cannot provide adequate parental care towards using the child protection process to seek mediated alternatives to removal. Parents involved in child protection cases face a serious challenge to retaining care of their children once they enter the realm of the court (Welbourne, Macdonald, & Bates, 2017), but there is growing interest in finding more collaborative ways to avoid a final child/parent separation where there may be the potential to do so (see also Harwin et al., 2016).

Theory, ethics and social context all interact to influence the organizational structures within which social work operates, set the objectives for social work intervention and shape the process of social work assessment and intervention, down to the micro level of influencing the content of conversations with service users.

Reflexivity and the inescapability of theory

Social work professionalism is allied to reflexive practice (Sheppard, 1998). Reflexivity involves awareness of self and others in the real world, as well as making links to theoretical constructs. Use of theory is inescapable as we make choices at every moment in social work practice, and every choice is based on explicit or implicit (not articulated or examined) theories about how the world works. Reflexive practice entails an intellectual effort to explore the links between theory and practice and the social, organizational and personal factors which make a practitioner choose one course of action over another. Reflexivity may suggest different ways of working or even identify new challenges that may not have been recognized as problematic before, such as service users' negative self-perception (Butler, Ford, & Tregaskis, 2007).

Reflection is *constitutive* of the social world as well as descriptive: we create reality as we live it and think and talk about it (Houston, 2015; see Chapter 5). We need to be reflexive to understand this process, instead of seeing knowledge as representing some form of 'objective truth' (Houston, 2015, p. 245). Theorizing about social work involves considering ourselves in context as social actors, as well as linking abstract theory to our everyday world.

Social work is defined by the International Federation of Social Workers as embedded in a changing world and responsible for making change happen. It is:

> . . . a practice-based profession and an academic discipline that promotes social change and development, social cohesion, and the empowerment and liberation of people. Principles of social justice, human rights, collective responsibility and respect for diversities are central to social work. Underpinned by theories of social work, social sciences, humanities and indigenous knowledge, social work engages people and structures to address life challenges and enhance wellbeing.
>
> *(IFSW, 2014)*

Reflexivity can be a means to self-actualization and the pursuit of life projects: Beck's 'reflexive modernization' (Beck, 1992). We are all subject to the constant pressure of social and organizational change and affected by power relations in society. Without reflexivity, we have limited capacity to consider how structures that create and sustain power influence ourselves and others. Without theory as an underpinning, we have no defensible strategy nor valid mandate for seeking change. Without reflexivity, theory can only be applied mechanistically: which is to say without awareness of the social structures that create and sustain power and our own role in that socially complex environment.

The idea that what we do in everyday life is based on proto-theories or working hypotheses about how the world works is inherent in key theories underpinning social work. A basic premise of attachment theory (see Chapter 13) is the idea that everyone builds a framework of constructs about how the world works in terms of human interactions, especially intimate 'family' relationships, and how the individual fits into that social and emotional world. In essence, we all start to develop theories about the way the world works from our first days of life (Howe, 2011). Piaget also studied how children develop an understanding of the relationship between cause and effect and other 'natural laws', again from very early in life (Piaget, 1930). We cannot be 'atheoretical'; we can only use theories consciously and reflexively or with the risks of bias and unethical practice that accompany unreflective action.

In safeguarding children, many very powerful social structures converge to influence what we may do and how we can do it (Payne, 2011) and affects how our actions are judged by others, both inside and outside the profession. Parliament, courts, service managers, inspectorates and the media all influence practice. The defensibility of practice (especially when things go wrong) is an interesting and complex area, linked to both evaluation based on outcomes (a consequentialist approach to responsibility) and evaluation of actions taken based on the availability of a well-founded rationale for actions taken (a principle-based or deontological approach to evaluating practice).

Agencies need a theoretically informed approach to service evaluation and development that enables them to identify risks and put in place a robust service response to reduce the risk of re-occurrence (Department for Education, 2017, p. 3) when things go wrong, information gathering has failed or decisions have been made without taking due notice of that information or weighing it accurately (Department for Education, 2017).

The limits to theory: complexity and wicked problems

There are problems that are so complex that it is difficult to theorize about them, or theories seem inadequate to deal with the problem, sometimes referred to as 'wicked' problems. Child abuse is characterized as a 'wicked' problem ('wicked problems' on Wikipedia gives a brief definition and history of the idea of wicked problems and suggests further reading: https://en.wikipedia.org/wiki/Wicked_problems).

Successive approaches to tackling it at a policy level have arguably failed because it is a multi-factorial complex social problem with many contributing causes. At the level of society and the individual, its causes are contested, and as a result there are multiple possible ways of approaching it. More than one approach may be needed at the same time to deal with the multiple contributing causes, but this makes identification of causal mechanisms problematic. Linear solutions, trying one thing at a time, are unlikely to be successful and may make the problem worse. Young, McKenzie, More, Schjelderup, and Walker (2014) argue that since we have no authoritative solutions to child abuse, we should involve families more in seeking solutions to their own problems.

The same complexity exists in the child protection system: it is '. . . complex and it is not possible to predict or control it with precision. This should lead to the recognition that the unintended will happen' (Munro, 2010, p. 135). Linear thinking attempts to link cause and effect in a relatively simple linear way, while nonlinear 'complex causality' (see Chapter 15) takes account of variation through time and subtle differences between families, workers and cases to understand why accurate prediction is not possible. A more dynamic and flexible way of thinking is needed. Social workers must be able to work with high levels of uncertainty, look more widely than the family itself and, when assessing risk, consider the dynamic nature of risk, interacting influences on the child and family and what causes child safety to fluctuate or stabilize (Stevens & Hassett, 2007, 2012).

Theories and hypotheses: keeping an open mind in a dynamic world

Theories in social work provide an overarching structure for understanding the social world; evidence describes aspects of the world. One's theoretical perspective suggests which questions to ask, shaping inquiry, whether in a child protection investigation or research. Understanding what is happening in a family is achieved by gathering evidence, which the social worker makes sense of by imposing order on it: structuring it in accordance with existing theories about how the world and families, in particular, work (Sheppard & Ryan, 2003). This section considers how important it is for child safety and well-being that social workers are critical practitioners in testing their ideas against 'reality' as they observe the family.

Instead of being a dynamic reflexive process, assessment can become stuck and resistant to change (Munro, 2010). Without a reflexive, critical approach, practitioners may be vulnerable to 'confirmation bias': continuing to interpret evidence according to their initial ideas about a family and slow to re-evaluate initial perceptions. This is dangerous if the initial assessment (a provisional hypothesis based on partial evidence) was hopeful and positive, but later information challenges that view. Hypothesizing about what is happening in a family needs to be a dynamic process in which practitioners challenge their own thinking, and supervision should enhance this.

Optimism is a two-edged sword in social work: belief in the capacity of people to make positive change is an essential attribute of social workers as a core part of the role is to promote positive change; it becomes problematic when professionals retain an attachment to optimism once *reasonable* hope is past. This 'toxic optimism' (Duschinsky, Lampitt, & Bell, 2016, cited in Kettle & Jackson, 2017) can be distinguished from theory-informed work towards positive goals, grounded in a realistic assessment of family strengths and challenges.

Doing child protection work involves asking people to change. Change is stressful: it involves giving up established habits of behaviour and learning new ones. Those changes may be very difficult to make as they may involve giving up long-ingrained behaviour, possibly learned inter-generationally, which may have value for the person. It may be something that helps them cope with problems, including the stress of having responsibility for others. The fact that some parents seek ways not to engage with the process of change is not surprising.

The phrase 'disguised compliance' is sometimes used to describe parents who are not com-plying with services attempting to change the way they parent but pretend they are (NSPCC, 2010). An accurate term would be 'disguised noncompliance', since what is being disguised is clearly non-compliance, not compliance. Having clarified this, the concept is relevant to the use of theory in child protection since the underlying idea is that social workers should not take appearance of cooperation at face value, but maintain attention on indicators of safety and parental change. This must be informed by theories of child development and by empirical observation: 'hypothesis testing' around the direction of change, or lack of it. Past child death inquiries reflect the fact that parents who have the potential to seriously harm children may have the ability to hide their resistance to change (London Borough of Haringey, 2008) while deflecting attention from their children (Ferguson, 2017). Putting this in context, social work-ers engage with thousands of families a year (Bilson & Martin, 2017) and work with many of them over extended periods, during which time things improve enough that child protection plans are stepped down, cases are closed and while some children are re-referred to children's services, many are not. Intervention with them has, one can only assume, been at least partly, if not wholly, successful. Compliance, in terms of changing behaviour, has occurred.

Motivational interviewing (MI) is an approach which aims to help people find their own reasons for changing problem behaviour (see Chapter 20). MI is 'a collaborative, person-centered form of guiding to elicit and strengthen motivation for change' (Miller & Rollnick, 2009, p. 13W0). A more collaborative approach to practice may reduce resistance (Wilkins & Whittaker, 2017).

Parents may have been asked to do things they may want to do but do not believe they are capable of doing and are afraid to say so. There may be factors that make cooperation difficult, such as the influence of a dominant controlling partner, depression or addiction. Thinking about barriers to change is important in cases of non-compliance. Theory can help consider what the personal, social and structural barriers are to change. Persistent lack of change is, however, a signal that another approach is needed, whatever the reason for lack of change.

Both 'optimism' and poor reflection and re-appraisal may be linked to the sheer emotional intensity of doing child protection work, leading to unsafe assessments based on partial or biased observations (Ferguson, 2017). Maintaining professional curiosity and creativity requires commitment and energy, which are arguably more likely to be engaged when practitioners have good quality support themselves. Thinking about one's work analytically is an active, intellectually demanding process, and changing the way one thinks is demanding for professionals as well as families.

Trauma and resilience

Child protection work inevitably links to theories about trauma and loss. Abuse causes trauma: even in those cases in which a victim does not experience abuse as distressing at the time that it happens, later recognition that what was done to them was wrong may cause hurt and distress. Parents involved in child protection processes may have been victims of traumatic events themselves: if not in childhood, then as a victim of abuse as an adult. A high proportion of families in which children are abused are also families in which another adult is being abused, and that abuse is also a probable cause of harm to the child, as identified in law (Children Act, 1989, s. 31) and by research (Bowen, Heron, Waylen, & Wolke, 2005; Holt, Buckley, & Whelan, 2008; Women's Aid, 2012/2013).

Trauma is defined both by the events that cause it (situations that carry a high level of perceived threat) and the individual response to that situation:

> Individual trauma [results from] an event, series of events, or set of circumstances that is experienced by an individual as physically or emotionally harmful or life threatening and that has lasting adverse effects on the individual's functioning and mental, physical, social, emotional, or spiritual well-being.
>
> *(SAMHSA, 2018)*

Responses to trauma depend on the nature of the traumatic events, the circumstances under which they occurred, including the level of support available to the person experiencing the trauma, and the resilience of the person. The US Child Welfare Information Gateway (2015, p. 2) says: '. . . The field is still in the beginning stages of gathering evidence about what is required to implement a trauma informed approach to child welfare, and what the outcomes of such an approach may be'. The age of the child, the frequency and severity of trauma and the relationship between the child and the person responsible for the trauma (for example, carer, stranger, peer) will affect the individual response of the person. Abuse that takes place in a familiar place at the hands of people known to the child is likely to be qualitatively different from abuse by strangers or taking place in a strange place, even an unfamiliar country and culture in the case of some trafficked children and young people. Whatever the context, any event that causes a child to experience a high level of threat, especially when it is repeated, is likely to require support with recovery.

Single traumatic events may also trigger an acute trauma response, overwhelming the child's ability to cope for a period, which may be long lasting. Repeated traumatic events may lead to more complex trauma responses that affect emotional responses and relationships, including with carers.

Resilience factors can moderate the impact of the trauma. While safeguarding social workers need to be aware of theories to help them support families through the crises that may have brought them to need help or the crisis of a protection intervention, they also need to be aware of the impact of trauma in many such families, particularly when family members have experienced repeated trauma. Once a child is in a stable, supportive environment, recovery can begin. The aim becomes the healing of past trauma and the child's development of confidence in themselves and the world around them. Social workers need to be able to engage with another area of theory relating to resilience to do this. There is insufficient space in this chapter to do justice to this essential aspect of safeguarding practice. Useful introductory material is available at NCH (2007), Pearce (2011) and Hart et al. (2014).

Conclusion

The theories and theoretically derived approaches to working with children and families in safeguarding and child protection are varied, encompassing both overarching theories, such as attachment theory, and evidence and theory-based approaches linked to a specific methodology, such as crisis intervention theory. Evaluative, outcome-based research can tell practitioners how successful certain approaches and techniques are in bringing about positive change, keeping children safe or leading to positive outcomes. To be truly accountable, one has to be able to say not only what one did, but also why one did it and how the approach taken to keeping children safe fits with a theoretical understanding of the wider social world within which children live.

Further reading

Karpetis, G. (2017). Theories on child protection work with parents: A narrative review of the literature. *Journal of Policy, Practice and Program, 95*(2). Retrieved from https://www.researchgate.net/publication/320336169_Theories_on_Child_Protection_Work_with_Parents_A_Narrative_Review_of_the_Literature.

This article provides a narrative review of 85 articles relating to child protection to critically analyse their explicit and implicit theoretical perspectives.

House of Commons Education Committee. (2012). Children first: The child protection system in England, *Fourth report of Session 2012–13*. Retrieved from https://publications.parliament.uk/pa/cm201213/cmselect/cmeduc/137/137.pdf.

Now several years old, this report nevertheless provides a rounded snapshot of the child protection system from different professional perspectives and some children's views. Offers an underpinning analysis for considering ongoing development of the child protection system.

Young, S., McKenzie, M., More, C., Schjelderup, L., & Walker, S. (2014). Practicing from theory: Thinking and knowing to 'do' child protection work. *Social Sciences, 2014*(3): 893–915.

Presents a theoretical model for practice, and links it with ideas about co-constructing social work practice in a New Zealand context, with a focus on 'worldviews' as well as theories of explanation and intervention.

References

Barn, R., & Das, C. (2016). Family group conferences and cultural competence in social work. *British Journal of Social Work, 46*(4), 942–959.

Beck, U. (1992). *Risk society: Towards a new modernity.* London: Sage.

Bilson, A., & Martin, K. (2017). Referrals and child protection in England: One in five children referred to children's services and one in nineteen investigated before the age of five. *British Journal of Social Work, 47*(3), 793–811.

Bowen, E., Heron, J., Waylen, A., & Wolke, D. (2005). Domestic violence risk during and after pregnancy: Findings from a British longitudinal study. *British Journal of Obstetrics and* Gynaecology, *112*(8), 1083–1089.

Broadhurst, K., Shaw, M., Kershaw, S., Harwin, J., Alrough, B., Mason, C., & Pilling, M. (2015). Vulnerable birth mothers and repeat losses of infants to public care: Is targeted reproductive health care ethically defensible? *Journal of Social Welfare and Family Law, 37*(1), 84–98.

Broadhurst, K., Wastell, D., White, S., & Pithouse, A. (2010). Risk, instrumentalism and the human project in social work: Identifying the informal logic of risk management in children's statutory services. *British Journal of Social Work, 40*, 1046–1064.

Butler, A., Ford, D., & Tregaskis, C. (2007). Who do we think we are? Self and reflexivity in social work practice. *Qualitative Social Work, 6*(3), 281–299.

Child Welfare Information Gateway. (2015). *Developing a trauma-informed child welfare system.* Washington, DC: US Department of Health and Human Services, Children's Bureau. Retrieved from www.child welfare.gov/pubPDFs/trauma_informed.pdf#page=1&view=Introduction

Dallos, R., & Draper, R. (2015). *An introduction to family therapy: Systemic theory and practice* (4th ed.). Maidenhead: Open University Press.

Department for Education. (2017). *Child death reviews: Year ending 31st April 2017.* Retrieved from www. gov.uk/government/uploads/system/uploads/attachment_data/file/627206/SFR36_2017_Text.pdf

Department for Education. (2018). *Working together to safeguard children.* Retrieved from www.gov.uk/ government/publications/working-together-to-safeguard-children--2

Department of Health. (2011). *Hidden Harm.* London: Department of Health. Retrieved from www.gov. uk/government/publications/amcd-inquiry-hidden-harm-report-on-children-of-drug-users

Duschinsky, R., Lampitt, S., & Bell, S. (2016). *Sustaining social work: Between power and powerlessness.* London: Palgrave Macmillan.

Ferguson, H. (2017). How children become invisible in child protection work: Findings from research into day-to-day social work practice. *British Journal of Social Work, 47*(4), 1007–1023.

Greene, R. R. (Ed.) (2008). *Human behavior theory and social work practice* (3rd ed.). New Brunswick, NJ: Transaction.

Hart, A., Heaver, B., Brunnberg, E., Sandberg, E., Macpherson, H., Coombe, S., & Kourkoutas, E. (2014). Resilience building with disabled children and young people: A review and critique of the academic evidence. *International Journal of Child, Youth and Family Studies, 5*(3), 394–422.

Harwin, J., Alrouh, B., Ryan, M., McQuarrie, T., Golding, L., Broadhurst, K., Tunnard, J., & Swift, S. (2016). *After FDAC: Outcomes 5 years later.* Lancaster: Lancaster University. Retrieved from http://fdac. org.uk/wp-content/uploads/2016/09/FDAC-Report-final-1.pdf

Helfer, M., Kempe, R., & Krugman, R. (Eds.). (1968). *The battered child.* Chicago: University of Chicago Press.

Holt, S., Buckley, H., & Whelan, S. (2008). The impact of exposure to domestic violence on children and young people: A review of the literature. *Child Abuse and Neglect, 32*, 797–810.

Houston, S. (2015). Enabling others in social work: Reflexivity and the theory of social domains. *Critical and Radical Social Work, 3*(2), 245–260.

Howe, D. (2011). *Attachment across the lifecourse: A brief introduction.* London: Palgrave Macmillan.

International Federation of Social Workers. (2014). *Global definition of social work.* Retrieved from http:// ifsw.org/get-involved/global-definition-of-social-work/

Kempe, C., Silverman, F., Steele, B., Droegemueller, W., & Silver, H. (1962). The battered-child syndrome. *Journal of the American Medical Association, 181*, 7–24.

Kettle, M., & Jackson, S. (2017). Revisiting the rule of optimism. *British Journal of Social Work, 47*(6), 1624–1640.

Lipsky, M. (1980). *Street-level bureaucracy: Dilemmas of the individual in public services.* New York: Russell Sage Foundation.

Miller, W., & Rollnick, S. (2009). Ten things that motivational interviewing is not. *Behavioural and Cognitive Psychotherapy, 37*, 129–140.

Ministry of Justice. (2017). *Settlement conferences pilot and evaluation.* Retrieved from www.judiciary.gov.uk/ publications/settlement-conferences-pilot-and-evaluation/

Munro, E. (2010). *The Munro review of child protection: Final report: A child-centred system*. London: Department for Education. Retrieved from www.gov.uk/government/uploads/system/uploads/attachment_data/file/175391/Munro-Review.pdf

NCH. (2007). *Literature review: Resilience in children and young people*. Retrieved from www.actionforchildren.org.uk/media/3420/resilience_in_children_in_young_people.pdf

NHS. (no date). *Female Genital Mutilation (FGM)*. Retrieved from www.nhs.uk/conditions/female-genital-mutilation-fgm/

NSPCC. (2010). *Disguised compliance: An NSPCC Factsheet*. Retrieved from www.nspcc.org.uk/globalassets/documents/information-service/factsheet-disguised-compliance.pdf

Office for National Statistics. (2016). *Abuse during childhood: Findings from the crime survey for England and wales, year ending March 2016*. Retrieved from www.ons.gov.uk/peoplepopulationandcommunity/crimeandjustice/articles/abuseduringchildhood/findingsfromtheyearendingmarch2016crimesurveyforenglandandwales

Parrish, M. (2014). *Social work perspectives on human behaviour* (2nd ed.). Maidenhead: Open University Press.

Payne, M. (2011). *Humanistic social work: Core principles in practice*. Basingstoke: Palgrave Macmillan.

Pearce, C. (2011). *A short introduction to promoting resilience in children*. London: Jessica Kingsley.

Piaget, J. (1930). *The child's conception of physical causality*. London: Routledge & Kegan Paul.

Popper, K. (1959). *The logic of scientific discovery*. New York: Basic Books.

Rights of Women. (n.d.). *Forced marriage and the law*. Retrieved from http://rightsofwomen.org.uk/get-information/family-law/forced-marriage-law/

Robbins, R., & Cook, K. (2017). Don't get us started on social workers: Domestic violence, social work and trust – An anecdote from research. *British Journal of Social Work*. Advance online publication. Retrieved from https://doi.org/10.1093/bjsw/bcx125

SAMHSA. (2018). *Substance abuse and mental health services administration, trauma and justice strategic initiative*. Retrieved from www.samhsa.gov/trauma-violence

Selwyn, J., & Briheim-Crookall, L. (2017). *Bright spots: 'Your life, your care' surveys of looked after children and young people*. London: Coram Foundation. Retrieved from www.coramvoice.org.uk/sites/default/files/FULL%20REPORT.pdf

Selwyn, J., & Quinton, D. (2004). Stability, permanence, outcomes and support: Foster care and adoption compared. *Adoption and Fostering, 28*(4), 6–15.

Sheppard, M. (1998). Practice validity, reflexivity and knowledge for social work. *British Journal of Social Work, 28*, 763–781.

Sheppard, M., & Ryan, K. (2003). Practitioners as rule using analysts: A further development of process knowledge in social work. *British Journal of Social Work, 33*(2), 157–176.

Spratt, T. (2012). Why multiples matter: Reconceptualising the population referred to child and family social workers. *British Journal of Social Work, 42*(8), 1574–1591.

Stevens, I., & Hassett, P. (2007). Applying complexity theory to child protection practice. *Childhood, 14*(1), 128–144.

Stevens, I., & Hassett, P. (2012). Non-linear perspectives of risk in social care: Using complexity theory and social geography to move the focus from individual pathology to the complex human environment. *European Journal of Social Work, 15*(4), 503–513.

UK Government. (2008). *Safeguarding children in whom illness is fabricated or induced*. Retrieved from www.gov.uk/government/publications/safeguarding-children-in-whom-illness-is-fabricated-or-induced

UK Government. (2017). *Child sexual exploitation: Definition and guide for practitioners*. Retrieved from www.gov.uk/government/publications/child-sexual-exploitation-definition-and-guide-for-practitioners

Welbourne, P., Macdonald, P., & Bates, P. (2017). *Getting it right in time: Parents who lack litigation capacity in public law proceedings*. Plymouth: Plymouth University & London: Nuffield Foundation. Retrieved from www.nuffieldfoundation.org/getting-it-right-time-parents-who-lack-litigation-capacity-public-law

Wilkins, D., & Whittaker, C. (2017). Doing child-protection social work with parents: What are the barriers in practice? *British Journal of Social Work*. Advance online publication. Retrieved from https://doi.org/10.1093/bjsw/bcx139

Women's Aid. (2012/2013). *Written evidence submitted by the Women's Aid Federation of England to the education committee – Children first: The child protection system in England*. Retrieved from https://publications.parliament.uk/pa/cm201213/cmselect/cmeduc/137/137vw65.htm

Young, S., McKenzie, M., More, C., Schjelderup, L., & Walker, S. (2014). Practicing from theory: Thinking and knowing to do child protection work. *Social Sciences, 3*, 893–915.

35

Child and adolescent mental health

A psychosocial perspective

Emma Reith-Hall

Introduction

There is no consensus about what children's mental health actually means (Strong & Sesma-Vazquez, 2015). Even within the field of child and adolescent mental health (CAMH), mental health difficulties encompass a broad range of problems and are conceptualized in different ways. In spite of this confusion, it is estimated that between one in five and one in ten children and young people worldwide experience mental health problems, and it is generally accepted that approximately half of mental health problems experienced in adulthood have their origins in childhood. The impact on children's development, relationships, educational attainment and the potential to live productive and fulfilling lives means that child and adolescent mental health is not an issue we can afford to ignore. CAMH is increasingly being recognized as a global public health concern yet knowledge of how best to understand and support this client group is limited. Social work theories are under-utilized, reflecting the neglected role of social workers within CAMH practice, literature and research. Yet calls for 'high integrity' mental health services for children (Wolpert, Vostanis, Martin, Munk, & Norman, 2017) will open up opportunities for transforming current provision. After considering some key issues in CAMH practice, this chapter explores how a psychosocial perspective can help social workers and allied professionals support the mental health and well-being of children and young people worldwide.

The biomedical approach

Much CAMH literature and research is dominated by the taken-for-granted biomedical approach (see Chapter 6). The various classification systems used throughout the world identify symptoms and levels of impairment to categorize mental health problems into psychiatric disorders. In child and adolescent mental health, these include developmental disorders, internalizing (emotional) disorders, externalizing (behavioural) disorders and psychotic disorders. Through the diagnostic process, the thoughts, feelings and behaviours of children and young people become framed through this biomedical discourse whereby mental health difficulty is conceptualized in terms of pathology or illness.

For some children, young people and their families, a biomedical approach is a helpful way of understanding mental health problems, opening doors to life-changing treatments. Yet for others, the construct of children's 'mental illness' is problematic. Young people have objected to the medicalizing of emotional difficulties (Plaistow et al., 2014) and report having their experiences invalidated (Harper, Dickson, & Bramwell, 2013). Children and young people's thoughts, feelings and behaviours may have interpretable subjective meaning, requiring opportunities for sense-making; hence many young people would prefer to receive psychotherapy (Bradley, McGrath, Brannen, & Bagnell, 2010) or simply talk to someone, rather than be 'fobbed off' with medication (Plaistow et al., 2014).

The diagnostic process itself is also problematic. Current psychiatric diagnoses 'do not capture the complex variety of difficulties that most children and adolescents present' (Wilson, 2016, p. 6); hence some practitioners have indicated that classifying disorders has limited use, particularly given the high degree of co-morbidity found in clinical practice. Young people have reported frustrations around having to meet tightly defined criteria to access services (Smith & Leon, 2001), supporting Timimi's (2016, p. 27) view that 'psychiatric diagnosis does not provide a rational basis for organizing and delivering mental health services'. There can be consequences, too, for those children and young people who do receive a formal diagnosis. A focus on illness and deficits detracts from the strengths, interest, talents and resources that children, young people and families hold, impacting negatively on identity, self-esteem and self-efficacy. The stigmatizing and 'othering' effects of the diagnostic labelling process experienced by users of adult mental health services are also evident in child and adolescent mental health services (CAMHS). The 'us and them' dynamic identified in Harper et al.'s (2013) research found young people felt powerless and blamed for their mental health problems.

When applied to a CAMH context, the 'unhelpful tendency to individualise issues, with a primary focus on [the] internal mental "pathology" of one person' (Tew, 2011, p. 76), locates the problem within the child or young person. Difficulties operating within a family system can produce emotional and behavioural responses that become reframed as a psychiatric disorder identified within the child. Assessment, diagnosis and some of the treatments that stem from these processes can be experienced as mystifying, pathologizing, blaming and shaming to those subjected to them, actually exacerbating the child or young person's presenting difficulty. A strictly biomedical approach to CAMH also ignores the influence of the social world. Focusing on individuals' symptoms fails to account for the socially unjust circumstances in which mental distress arises. The role of poverty and social disadvantage was articulated by Ferguson (Chapter 27) and the influence of social determinants on children's mental health acknowledged by Manion (Chapter 33). Children and young people are situated in families, schools, communities and societies – systems which impact on the development and continuity of good mental health or, conversely, mental health difficulty.

Limitations of the current evidence base

It is often assumed that pharmacological and psychological answers exist for the wide range of mental health problems experienced by children and young people. Whilst there are some medications and therapies that have repeatedly been evaluated as effective, overall the evidence base for CAMH is surprisingly weak. Concerns have been raised about the research methodology used for acquiring the current evidence base. Randomized controlled trials (RCTs) can demonstrate the effectiveness (or not) of drug treatments, but their utility in establishing the impact of psychotherapy is questionable since, by design, they factor out contextual variables (e.g. a child's motivation or known family stressors), which impact on outcomes in practice. Moreover, some interventions are disadvantaged by the prevailing positivist research methodologies: strengths-based approaches do not align to treating psychiatric symptoms because attending to problems and deficits is not in keeping with the underpinning philosophy, whilst in psychodynamic therapy, change arises through relational processes rather than specific measurable techniques.

We need to acknowledge the limits of the existing evidence base and consider the extent to which even widely researched interventions actually work. Explicit acknowledgement of this would allow practitioners to instigate more honest conversations about what might help and consider what to do if no improvement is made (Wolpert et al., 2017). This would lower unrealistic expectations that the wide range of increasingly complex problems encountered in practice can be 'fixed'. As we continue searching for effective strategies and interventions, utilizing a wide range of theories and research methodologies will help open up the process of knowledge creation for this important area of practice.

Lessons from adult mental health

In adult mental health, user or survivor movements 'have rejected the notion that there is an objective, value-free continuum that moves clearly through a symptom – diagnosis – treatment – cure – continuum' (Fawcett, 2004, p. 201). Instead, those with lived experience and their supporters have been instrumental in bringing about change in the way that mental distress and madness are defined, understood and researched and the ways that helping and coping are explored (see Chapter 38). In the UK, 'social approaches' to understanding adult mental health are beginning to claim their rightful place in the practice and policy arenas. No parallel movement exists within CAMH; hence, practitioners, advocates and researchers will need to work with children and young people in age-appropriate ways to undertake research and build theories that take account of child and adolescent viewpoints.

A psychosocial perspective

A psychosocial perspective, encompassing a range of theories, can extend our understanding of child and adolescent mental health. Psychosocial practice takes place at the intersection of the individual's psychological/internal world and subjective states and their social/external world and objective statuses (Megele, 2015, p. 3). Advocating for the use of a psychosocial model in CAMH practice, Walker (2011, p. 18) suggests including the original characteristics of a psychosocial perspective:

> Understanding the person as well as the problems they are presenting; recognising the inner psychological experience of the individual and the external social world, which may be in conflict; and actively making use of the service user's relationship with the social worker.

In addition, Walker (2011, p. 18) suggests that a contemporary psychosocial model requires refinement to ensure that 'practitioners adopt a holistic perspective and employ personal relationship skills to work in partnership with families and engage with other professionals through culturally competent, community orientated practice'.

The objective status of the external world (Megele, 2015) of particular relevance to CAMH practice is age, impacting on understandings of childhood, adolescence and mental health. The importance of listening to children has been clearly articulated in child protection contexts, with calls for child-centred approaches reflecting the value placed on children's rights more widely. In adult mental health, an individual's sense of personal agency is increasingly being recognized as important for understanding mental distress and recovering from it (Tew, 2011). The rationale for involving children and young people in CAMH, then, is not only obvious, but further supported by evidence demonstrating that engagement facilitates therapeutic outcomes (Kim, Munson, & McKay, 2012) and mitigates against high drop-out rates (Oruche, Downs, Holloway, Draucker, & Aalsma, 2014). In practice however, young people continue to report being treated 'like a child' (Harper et al., 2013), suggesting practitioner and organizational responses to the issues of age and child status warrant further attention.

Few children and young people self-refer into CAMHS, so the help-seeking process tends to be initiated by a concerned adult, with children and young people frequently occupying the pre-contemplation stage of change (Prochaska & DiClemente, 1983). Presenting problems are first seen and heard through an adult lens, with control over identification, diagnosis and treatment situated within parental and professional systems. Research exploring initial conversations (where people and problems begin to be understood through an assessment process) found that some clinicians failed to seek children's accounts of their presentation to CAMHS, and among those children who were asked, many answered with 'don't know', a position that was maintained if the practice of deferring to adults for an explanation continued (Stafford, Hutchby, Karim, & O'Reilly, 2016). It appears that the processes through which we begin to engage with children and young people about their mental health might exclude them. To challenge the half-membership status (Hutchby & O'Reilly, 2010) experienced by children and adolescents, practitioners must involve them as active participants.

Shared decision-making can be challenging due to considerations about developmental stage and mental capacity (Wolpert et al., 2017). However, since 'power issues are closely implicated in the onset of mental distress' (Tew, 2011, p. 47), practitioners must consider the lack of control children and young people hold over access to and involvement with services. It is important to understand the impact of this position of powerlessness, at a time when, developmentally, many young people are striving for autonomy and independence from parents and carers. This issue is particularly pertinent for children with experiences of abuse or neglect, where interpersonal experiences may have further undermined their sense of control (Wolpert et al., 2017). A psychosocial perspective encourages practitioners to consider critically potential sources of conflict operating between the child's internal world (where lack of control may contribute to psychological difficulty and distress) and the social world (where age and child status can inhibit access to and engagement with support). Social workers, familiar with the idea of 'working with' rather than 'doing to', are in a strong position to ensure that psychosocial assessment processes 'underpinned by partnership practice and service user involvement' (Walker, 2011, p. 40) are fully embedded into CAMH practice. Champions of social justice and anti-oppressive practice, social workers have a role to play in developing practices and services that respect children and young people's rights and wishes to be 'kept well informed, included in the decision-making processes and encouraged to participate during consultations' (Coyne et al., 2015, p. 566).

A key principle of psychosocial practice is to understand the person as well as the problem they are presenting, which fits with the recurring research theme that children and young people experiencing mental health difficulty want to be listened to and understood (Bone, O'Reilly, Karim, & Vostanis, 2015; Plaistow et al., 2014). Humanistic counselling and person-centred approaches (see Chapter 3) provide a starting point for helping practitioners achieve this aim and are a good fit for current agendas in rights-based and therapeutic practice outlined above. Humanistic theory sees the wholeness of individuals, recognizing people as 'experts by experience', believing in their personal agency and capacity to effect change or build more fulfilling lives for themselves.

Humanistic theory facilitates psychosocial practice by encouraging practitioners to demonstrate effective personal relationship skills using the core conditions of empathy, genuineness and unconditional positive regard to build an effective therapeutic alliance. The way the practitioner *is* with children and young people matters far more than what they *do*. Research into CAMH services found that children and young people want practitioners to be approachable, friendly, warm and non-judgemental (Coyne et al., 2015). The knowledge, values and skills that social workers bring mean they are well placed to communicate effectively with children and young people experiencing mental distress and to model a Rogerian person centred/child-centred approach within their teams. It is through a supportive, warm and trusting relationship that the inner psychological experience of the child or young person can be explored and understood.

A range of interventions based on humanistic theory such as non-directive art and play therapy and school counselling are widely used in practice. Often delivered in mainstream settings and experienced as less stigmatizing, there are many benefits to such approaches. However, their effectiveness in CAMH is under-researched, possibly escaping rigorous evaluation because they are delivered in non-clinical populations. Alternatively, since humanistic approaches encapsulate a 'way of being' (Rogers, 1995), as opposed to techniques of doing, it is possible that they fail to be fully recognized within interventions literature and research.

Psychodynamic theories and therapies also aim to understand the person and share with humanistic approaches the position of being widely used in practice but under-researched and under-represented in CAMH literature. Methodological limitations such as including a mixture of conditions in empirical studies and a potential sleeper effect (McLaughlin, Holliday, Clarke, & Ilie, 2013) have been identified as particular challenges. At the heart of the original psychosocial model is a commitment to recognizing the inner psychological experience of the individual. Ideas such as transference, whereby intense emotions stemming from an earlier relationship are projected onto the practitioner by the client, and countertransference, a redirection of the practitioner's feelings toward the client, remain important for understanding relationships and can help young people process difficult experiences and make sense of the past.

A focus on defence mechanisms and relationship dynamics indicates the depth at which psychodynamic therapies operate, helping to explain why they are often used when other therapies have not worked or in highly complex situations: for example, where maltreatment or family trauma has occurred (Ghosh Ippen, Harris, Van Horn, & Lieberman, 2011). Psychodynamic practice encapsulates another important psychosocial tenet – to actively make use of the service user's relationship with the social worker. Some young people have not experienced a positive relationship with an adult, so the importance of offering a safe and containing relationship in which distress and difficulties can be explored should not be underestimated. Understanding attachment theory and the need to provide a secure base may be crucial to demonstrate that a different relationship template is possible. Relationships, the centrality of which is discussed by Winter (Chapter 12), form an essential component of contemporary psychosocial practice. Through containment, the capacities for reflexivity and mentalization can be developed, which arguably foster resilience.

Cognitive behavioural therapy (see Chapter 16) is often the treatment of choice for anxiety and depressive disorders in CAMH. Some CBT techniques have proved consistently effective for helping children and young people: graded exposure, for example, helps children and young people overcome fears, phobias and obsessive-compulsive behaviours, whilst modelling is helpful in anger management. Through enabling children and young people to make sense of the problems they experience within their current environments and challenge unhelpful thoughts and beliefs, CBT supports the psychosocial perspective of recognizing the inner psychological experience of the individual and the external social world, which may be in conflict. CBT teaches children and young people specific techniques to modify thoughts, feelings and behaviours, potentially enabling them to help themselves in future. Research suggests young people value interventions that foster self-reliance (Plaistow et al., 2014), so CBT might be particularly appealing for adolescents, especially computerized programmes. A range of CBT programmes has been developed for different age groups, and the specific disorders and conditions it aims to treat continues to grow – trauma-focused CBT is a recent addition.

Mindfulness (see Chapter 22) with children and young people is currently being researched, both as a stand-alone intervention and as a component of CBT. Group-based mindfulness programmes appear popular, their use in schools expanding. Amidst concerns about the sense of self developing in young people in Western countries, whereby identities are increasingly being shaped by consumerism, competition and social media, mindfulness has real potential. By encouraging a focus on being present in the here and now, mindfulness can intervene at the site of conflict between the inner psychological experience of the individual and their external social world. Promoting acceptance, effective response to stress, improved emotional regulation and sense of well-being, mindfulness offers a promising way forward in CAMH practice.

Psychosocial practice also fosters approaches that account for people's strengths and interests. A strengths perspective (see Chapter 18) applied to CAMH assumes that all children and young people (including those with severe emotional and behavioural difficulties) and their families have within them strengths, interests, abilities and characteristics that can be identified, encouraged and utilized to effect change, foster improvement, achieve goals and promote well-being. By shifting the focus of attention away from deficits and pathology, a strengths perspective can help overcome the stigma associated with traditional approaches and is therefore in keeping with the social work value base.

Some of the concepts associated with a strengths perspective are clearly evident in practice. Assessments routinely ask about goals and strengths, although this is usually an aside and does not mean strengths work has been fully embedded in practice. Originally developed for child protection work, *Signs of Safety* (Turnell & Edwards, 1999), which explicitly incorporates a strengths-based approach, has been used in CAMH to support, protect and safeguard young people who self-harm or engage in other high-risk behaviours. Strengths-based programmes are increasingly found within schools and community environments, suggesting that better use is being made of children and young people's external resources. Of the specific strengths-based programmes that have been implemented, rigorous evaluation using experimentally controlled outcomes studies are largely absent, and the programme content is not always made clear (Brownlee et al., 2013).

However, the influence of a strengths perspective is perhaps more evident as a component within other therapies, with a long tradition in family therapy and family-based approaches, for example. Solution-focused brief therapy (see Chapter 19), whereby goals for preferred futures are identified and strategies to achieve them are considered, also builds on strengths and resources. This intervention is gaining support from CAMH practitioners, perhaps because specific techniques such as scaling and the miracle question can be learnt, alongside a growing recognition that young people welcome positive practitioners, and because self-selected goals and solutions foster culturally sensitive and anti-oppressive practice. The evidence base for solution-focused therapy in CAMH is developing: tentative support now exists for children and young people experiencing internalizing and externalizing behavioural difficulties (Bond, Woods, Humphrey, Symes, & Green, 2013). Although the full-scale adoption of a strengths perspective has not yet materialized, it has an important role to play in the future of psychosocial CAMH practice.

Narrative therapies allow problems to be externalized, separating them from the child or young person. Counteracting the individualizing pathologizing processes discussed above, narrative approaches adopt key psychosocial principles and allow for more constructive helping processes to be developed, often using creative and playful approaches. Again, narrative approaches are hard to locate in the research literature but used frequently in CAMH practice.

Child and adolescent mental health and mental health difficulty develop within a complex web of family and environmental systems (see Chapter 15); hence, adopting a holistic perspective and working in partnership with families is fundamental to a psychosocial approach to CAMH practice. The meaning attached to children's emotions and behaviours must be understood within their relationships and environments, an issue addressed within family therapy. Sometimes parents themselves are the focus of the intervention. For example, parent training, including non-violence resistance (NVR) training, is used to manage a range of emotional and behavioural difficulties. Modifying parental responses or patterns of interaction and making adaptations to a child or young person's home environment can be key to effecting change. At other times, parents and carers are the child's closest allies, enlisted as co-therapists, and playing a major role in spotting their child's negative thoughts, reinforcing positive or desired behaviours or noticing strengths and exception times.

Exploring family dynamics and people's positions and roles within a family is an important part of CAMH family work and can be helpful to support families to manage conditions such as anorexia and bulimia or where children have experienced trauma, neglect or abuse. The role of relationships is increasingly being recognized; hence, some of the newer attachment-focused interventions (see Chapter 13) such as Theraplay and dyadic developmental psychotherapy comprise sessions with children or young people and their parents. The use of family-based approaches such as multi-systemic therapy has risen in recent years, seeking to effect change in the contexts within which children and young people operate. Evaluation of these interventions is in its infancy and has produced mixed results. Benefits of family and systematic approaches include allowing multiple perspectives and hypotheses to be considered, bridging social care and mental health provisions, allowing strengths and resources to be activated and helping change family discourses and narratives.

Caregiver involvement is thought to improve mental health outcomes for children and young people and has been identified as improving adolescents' treatment experience (Oruche et al., 2014). However, there is a balance to be struck because parental attendance may also inhibit disclosure (Day, Carey, & Surgenor, 2006). A flexible appointment structure combining separate and joint appointments has been suggested by young people and their parents as a means of facilitating honest conversations that promote understanding in CAMH (Coyne et al., 2015). The age of the child, family dynamics, nature and causes of the presenting problem and selected intervention and support strategies may affect the level of participation required by caregivers, but sensitive and careful negotiation on a case-by-case basis and subject to ongoing review is also important.

Some parents or carers are in fact the perpetrators or facilitators of abuse, neglect or trauma. Close liaison with safeguarding and child protection staff and multidisciplinary input is required to ensure that children and young people's needs are met and that safety and well-being are prioritized. Engaging with other professionals is another key principle of contemporary psychosocial practice. Social workers have a thorough knowledge of child development, a good understanding of how parental factors and behaviours affect child development and well-being and a sound understanding of child protection and safeguarding procedures. This puts them in a key position to intervene directly and offer support or consultation to other professionals.

Social disadvantage such as poor education and poverty is linked to the development and maintenance of mental health problems. Unfortunately, the impact of the external social world on children and young people's mental health is often ignored or side-lined in practice. Walker

(2011) urges us to bear in mind our own prejudices and assumptions, examining how common stereotypes – for example, the view that young black males are aggressive – might surreptitiously be influencing our own practice. He reminds practitioners to work in partnership with the child or young person and their family to understand their perspectives and belief systems in a bid to develop practice that is culturally competent.

The wider contexts in which children and young people operate are beginning to receive greater attention, giving rise to more community-orientated practice. A variety of social interventions exist, and whilst experimental research for these lags well behind psychological and pharmacological interventions, the value of prevention, early intervention and fostering resiliency is clear. The evidence for school-based interventions, which are socially inclusive and non-stigmatizing, has grown rapidly in recent years. Successful interventions focus on positive mental health, deliver a mix of universal and targeted approaches, start early with younger children and include parents and community involvement, as well as co-ordinating work with outside agencies (Weare & Nind, 2011).

Conclusion

A contemporary psychosocial model of social work for CAMH practice 'offers the optimum framework to take account of all the individual, child, family and environmental variables interacting to produce the identified difficulties' (Walker, 2011, p. 18). Presently, the social aspect of the psychosocial approach is under-utilized. Embedding a psychosocial perspective more fully into CAMH practice provides a promising way forward to engage in culturally and socially inclusive practice to promote and support the mental health of children and young people.

Further reading

Campbell, S., Morley, D., & Catchpole, R. (Eds.). (2016). *Critical issues in child and adolescent mental health.* London: Palgrave Macmillan.
Midgley, N., Hayes, J., & Cooper, M. (2017). *Essential research findings in child and adolescent counselling and psychotherapy.* London: Sage.
Walker, S. (2011). *The social worker's guide to child and adolescent mental health.* London: Jessica Kingsley.

References

Bond, C., Woods, K., Humphrey, N., Symes, W., & Green, L. (2013). Practitioner review: The effectiveness of solution focused brief therapy with children and families: A systematic and critical evaluation of the literature from 1990–2010. *Journal of Child Psychology and Psychiatry, 54*(7), 707–723.
Bone, C., O'Reilly, M., Karim, K., & Vostanis, P. (2015). 'They're not witches . . .' Young children and their parents' perceptions and experiences of child and adolescent mental health services. *Child: Care, Health and Development, 41*(3), 450–458.
Bradley, K., McGrath, P., Brannen, C., & Bagnell, A. (2010). Adolescents' attitudes and opinions about depression treatment. *Community Mental Health Journal, 46*, 242–251.
Brownlee, K., Rawana, J., Franks, J., Harper, J., Bajwa, J., O'Brien, E., & Clarkson, A. (2013). A systematic review of strengths and resilience outcome literature relevant to children and adolescents. *Child and Adolescent Social Work Journal, 30*(5), 435–459.
Coyne, I., McNamara, N., Healy, M., Gower, C., Sarkar, M., & McNicholas, F. (2015). Adolescents' and parents' views of child and adolescent mental health services (CAMHS) in Ireland. *Journal of Psychiatric Mental Health Nursing, 22*, 561–569.
Day, C., Carey, M., & Surgenor, T. (2006). Children's key concerns: Piloting a qualitative approach to understanding their experience of mental health care. *Clinical Child Psychology and Psychiatry, 11*, 139–155.
Fawcett, B. (2004). Mental health practice and children: Dogma, discourse, debate, and practice. *Social Work in Mental Health, 2*, 2–3.

Ghosh Ippen, C., Harris, W., Van Horn, P., & Lieberman, A. (2011). Traumatic and stressful events in early childhood: Can treatment help those at highest risk? *Child Abuse and Neglect, 35*, 504–513.

Harper, B., Dickson, J. M., & Bramwell, R. (2013). Experiences of young people in a 16–18 mental health service. *Child and Adolescent Mental Health, 19*, 90–96.

Hutchby, I., & O'Reilly, M. (2010). Children's participation and the familial moral order in family therapy. *Discourse Studies, 12*(1), 49–64.

Kim, H., Munson, M., & McKay, M. (2012). Engagement in mental health treatment among adolescents and young adults: A systematic review. *Child and Adolescent Social Work Journal, 29*, 241–266.

McLaughlin, C., Holliday, C., Clarke, B., & Ilie, S. (2013). *Research on counselling and psychotherapy with children and young people: A systematic scoping review of the evidence for its effectiveness from 2003–2011.* Lutterworth: BACP.

Megele, C. (2015). *Psychosocial and relationship-based practice.* Norwich: Critical Publishing.

Oruche, U. M., Downs, S., Holloway, E., Draucker, C., & Aalsma, M. (2014). Barriers and facilitators to treatment participation by adolescents in a community mental health clinic. *Journal of Psychiatric and Mental Health Nursing, 21*(3), 241–248.

Plaistow, J., Masson, K., Koch, D., Wilson, J., Stark, R., Jones, P., & Lennox, B. (2014). Young people's views of UK mental health services. *Early Intervention in Psychiatry, 8*, 12–23.

Prochaska, J., & DiClemente, C. (1983). Stages and processes of self-change in smoking: Toward an integrative model of change. *Journal of Consulting and Clinical Psychology, 5*, 390–395.

Rogers, C. (1995). *A way of being.* New York: Houghton Mifflin.

Smith, K., & Leon, L. (2001). *Turned upside down: Developing community-based crisis services for 16–25 year olds experiencing a mental health crisis.* London: Mental Health Foundation.

Stafford, V., Hutchby, I., Karim, K., & O'Reilly, M. (2016). 'Why are you here?' Seeking children's accounts of their presentation to child and adolescent mental health service (CAMHS). *Clinical Child Psychology and Psychiatry, 21*(1), 3–18.

Strong, T., & Sesma-Vazquez, M. (2015). Discourses on children's mental health: A critical review. In J. Lester & M. O'Reilly (Eds.), *The Palgrave handbook of child mental health* (pp. 99–116). London: Palgrave Macmillan.

Tew, J. (2011). *Social approaches to mental distress.* London: Palgrave Macmillan.

Timimi, S. (2016). Non-diagnostic practice in child and adolescent mental health. In S. Campbell, D. Morley, & R. Catchpole (Eds.), *Critical issues in child and adolescent mental health* (pp. 14–29). London: Palgrave Macmillan.

Turnell, A., & Edwards, S. (1999). *Signs of safety: A safety and solution orientated approach to child protection casework.* New York: Norton.

Walker, S. (2011). *The social worker's guide to child and adolescent mental health.* London: Jessica Kingsley.

Weare, K., & Nind, M. (2011). Mental health promotion and problem prevention in schools: What does the evidence say? *Health Promotion International, 26*(1), 29–69.

Wilson, P. (2016). What evidence works for whom? In S. Campbell, D. Morley, & R. Catchpole (Eds.), *Critical issues in child and adolescent mental health* (pp. 1–13). London: Palgrave Macmillan.

Wolpert, M., Vostanis, P., Martin, K., Munk, S., & Norman, R. (2017). High integrity mental health services for children: Focusing on the person, not the problem. *British Medical Journal, 357*, 1–5.

36
Theories of mental health

Peter Benbow and Paul Blakeman

No single discipline can lay claim to 'owning' the paradigm that is mental health. Attempts to do so have provoked resistance and debate for centuries. Cicero (106–43 BCE) rejected Hippocrates's earlier theories of imbalanced bodily fluids ('humours') to posit that low mood was related to emotions. Later, in the Middle Ages, monks displaced these ideas in favour of humour-rebalancing bloodletting, whilst using prayer and dogma to promote well-being. In fact, the way emotional distress is understood tends to evolve in line with the cultural ideas of the day. So as science became more influential in society, then a scientific understanding of mental ill health naturally followed.

The medical model

The biological model of mental ill health is often described as the 'medical model' (see Chapter 6). It is a mistake to consider this a single entity as within it live many dynamic traditions. The neurologist, for example, might have one conceptualization, whilst a geneticist would have another. What they share is the underlying positivistic view that mental illness is a phenomenon (that is, it is something real that can be observed) and that the cause – and therefore cure – lies in the biology of the human body. Since the 1950s, the dominant model of mental disease in industrialized states has been related to the action of chemicals that affect the central nervous system. The dysfunction of these 'neurotransmitter' systems is hypothesized to lead to specific and categorizable signs and symptoms that have been clustered into diagnostic categories, codified internationally in the *International Classification of Disease* (*ICD*; World Health Organization, 1993) and the *Diagnostic and Statistical Manual of Mental Disorders* (*DSM*; American Psychiatric Association, 2013). These publications have become hugely influential and have had far-reaching effects.

The cutting edge of this science is now moving beyond the neurochemical theory and is exploring novel fields, such as quantum biology. Here, researchers theorize that the components of individual cell elements (such as the microtubule cytoskeleton) affect the actions of individual molecules in ways that manifest on a gross level as the specific and observable symptoms of diagnostic taxonomies (see Gardiner, 2017, for further discussion).

The diagnostic tradition that guides psychiatric medicine has, however, proved problematic. There are many criticisms that can be made here, one of which is that unlike their colleagues in physical medicine, psychiatrists take for granted the phenomena they are observing but have little objective evidence that it independently exists (Szasz, 1961). Szasz, along with other critics such as Laing (1965), challenged the orthodoxy of psychiatry in an attempt to humanize its practice but, overall, have had little impact on the profession itself. They have, however, inspired indirect developments such as user movements and given rise to the legitimacy of criticism.

Making a diagnosis requires belief in the validity of a social construct that cites distress as a sign of pathology. The labelling of various symptoms into a disease is, at face value, attractive. It reduces complex behaviour into a single explanatory framework: mental illness. Critics of this approach disagree. They would argue that diagnoses are over-reliant on subjective symptoms, with no recourse to observable signs. This leads to unreliability, bias and misinterpretation. The bias introduced by sociocultural and political norms negates, on the whole, the social and psychological impacts of inequality, oppression and exploitation and has the side effect of making the individual somehow responsible for their condition (Rogers & Pilgrim, 2010).

There are also arguments about the self-referential nature of psychiatric medicine. In the latter part of the 20th century, the diagnostic tradition in psychiatry has been seen as tautological, in that it uses symptoms typically found in a patient group to diagnose a person as being part of that group, with no independent criteria for inferring the condition in the first place (Bentall, 1990). This reification of ideas is circular, and the notion of mental illness being an objectively verifiable disease process continues to be hotly debated.

Diagnoses are also not free of social value. They are generally stigmatizing and can remove hope and construct in the minds of professionals and the public alike notions of dangerous and manipulative individuals who are both untreatable and responsible for their condition (see Chapter 26). Such conceptualizations have been unhelpful and are part of the explanation for low levels of social recovery and inclusion for those labelled in such ways (Perkins & Repper, 2013).

Challenge is however being generated internally. Authors such as Bracken and Thomas (2005) critiqued the psychiatric profession as being unable to see past its institutional origins to view a future that is free of the unhelpful elements of its historical legacy. Their 'postpsychiatry' agenda cites a profession committed to moving to contextualized, ethical and less coercive practices. This emancipatory approach continues to be globally disseminated through international organizations such as the Critical Psychiatry Network and Hearing Voices Network.

The psychological model

The dominant position of medicine in the field of psychiatric care has also been challenged by the psychological movement. Sharing some of the positivistic characteristics of medicine, psychology has long posited a range of alternative theories of mental ill health, some of which are directly opposed to the dominant model. These models place at their core the primacy of perception and the processes of thinking. Several distinct traditions, such as cognitive behavioural therapy (see Chapter 16), have evolved, many of which have become the treatment of choice for a range of mental disorders and are often used in complex casework where often the evidence base for pharmaceutical interventions is lacking (National Institute for Health and Care Excellence [NICE], 2009).

Looking towards the future of psychology, the publication of *The Power Threat Meaning Framework* (Johnstone et al., 2018) has been set out as a viable alternative to psychiatric diagnosis. It is intended to address many of the single-paradigm issues addressed above. It is theorized within the model that this approach will bring together the social, biological and psychological elements of experience that together produce the phenomena of distress. One way in which it diverges from a medical approach is that it views biology as a mediating rather than causal factor.

Psychological approaches are, however, open to criticism. There are again tautological concerns that psychological explanations are often self-referential. Critics also believe psychological approaches define how people should present through their concordance with established models, which problematizes diversity (Grant, 2011). Some authors have also noted that these approaches do not contextualize the person into their ecosystem, and therefore, their symptoms have no context. This leads to what Smail (2004) calls 'interiorization'. This occurs when the effects of real-world problems, such as abuse or poverty, are turned into problems of internal perception or process. This form of neo-Cartesian thinking, where the mind is independent from the world it inhabits, leads to responsibilizing the individual for their distress. This raises issues for practitioners following the anti-oppressive base of social work.

Recovery in psychology is often measured by changes in scores on validated rating scales. This is problematic in that it is an arbitrary set of values that decides if someone has recovered or not and ignores the subjective experience. 'Recovery' and 'distress' are professionally defined and quantified. Rather than reflect the subjective reality of emotional distress, approaches using such methods construct distress and recovery in ways that become scientifically plausible and dominant. But, as Grant (2011, p. 38) reminds us: 'The textual portrayal of human suffering is never neutral, in that the politics of representation inform the struggle over the definition and experience of selfhood'. The power of psychiatric and psychological labels are both far-reaching and potentially harmful (see Goffman, 1963), especially when used in a reductionist manner to redefine well-being in terms of rating scale scores.

Social factors

Neither the psychological nor the medical approaches truly manage to incorporate the real worlds that people live in. Industrialized countries have struggled to value and provide appropriate care for those considered mentally ill. Within the field of physical health, there is a well-recorded phenomenon that people who experience mental health problems have worse outcomes in terms of physical health. Once help is sought, they also receive sub-standard levels of care for a range of common but serious medical conditions (Bressington et al., 2018). Many of these conditions are easily treatable, but due to sub-optimal service, a person with schizophrenia can expect to lose 14.5 years of life when compared to a peer without the condition (Hjorthøj, Stürup, McGrath, & Nordentoft, 2017). These numbers are very significant and clearly present as a matter of social justice. Within the UK, these issues are believed to arise in part from a lack of 'parity of esteem' between physical and mental health services. Such structural and cultural inequalities are not easily addressed, and within the UK, the Health and Social Care Act 2012 is being used as a legal remedy. The fact that legal avenues are needed, however, says a great deal about the social positioning within a society of those with mental health problems.

Authors such as Marmot (2010) and Wilkinson and Pickett (2009) have also established that adverse social conditions, such as poverty and poor housing, can have a deleterious effect on physical and mental health. There are also strong links between social disadvantage and exclusion. Labonte (2004) provides a useful formulation of exclusion as the result of social processes, which differs perhaps from a currently more dominant neoliberal perspective of exclusion relating to a failure of the individual to take advantage of the opportunities afforded by a market economy. Indeed, van der Wel, Saltkjel, Chen, Dahl, and Halvorsen (2018) show that the current wave of European 'austerity' policies increases health inequalities with an association that grows over time, which further undermines the neoliberal argument of personal or moral failure.

There is a general tendency for unequal social systems to become self-perpetuating, and in socio-economic terms, these can often be characterized by racial groupings (Galabuzi & Labonte,

2002). Unequal societies tend to have higher rates of social and emotional problems than those that are more equal (Marmot & Wilkinson, 2006), and inequalities are strongly linked to poor mental health (Allen, Balfour, Bell, & Marmot, 2014). For many social workers, their daily work involves either helping to change unjust systems or helping people live with the effects of them. Part of these roles may be to facilitate the inclusion of those excluded into areas of society that are currently closed to them. Such areas may include better housing, employment and social contacts. In this sense, social work in mental health is always a political activity as social inclusion is an act of political will on behalf of the dominant groups. Of course, this approach needs to be used with care as sometimes the opening of opportunities results in little more than further exploitation of citizens if driven by market rather than humanitarian concerns.

Risk

Concepts of risk assessment and management have become integral to mental health practice. Many authors have noted how the issue of risk has become more prominent in recent years, driven by discourses around society's perception and expectations of risk. Beck (1992), most notably, described the 'risk society' which reflected this growing trend more widely. In mental health practice, Tew (2011) refers to the emergence of those with mental health problems as objects of risk despite the lack of actuarial evidence to support this. He points to the pathology of the individual as a dominant narrative, whereby dangerousness, and consequently blame, are placed within the individual service user, whilst contributing social factors are ignored. This may help explain the international phenomena whereby people with mental health problems are more likely to be victims of violence than perpetrators (Sin, Hedges, Cook, Mguni, & Comber, 2009).

People with mental health problems have become particularly vulnerable to pejorative media representations, with disproportionate media coverage. The resultant focus on the risk of violence by those with mental health problems is a key theme underpinning the discrimination they face (Sayce, 2016). This in turn has influenced the practice discourse of professionals involved in mental health care, with growing emphasis on safeguarding and risk management rather than need (Kemshall, 2014).

The difficulty of risk prediction is widely recognized, particularly for the high profile, though statistically rare, incidents of homicide (Szmukler, Daw, & Dawson, 2010) and also for the more frequent incidents of suicide (Heller, 2017). The concepts of false positives and negatives (see Szmukler et al., 2010) provide a useful theoretical model for conceptualizing the arena of decision-making by mental health professionals, including the significant ethical implications inherent within this. Crawford (2000, p. 152) provides an example here, citing that to prevent a single homicide by someone diagnosed with schizophrenia would require the detention of approximately 5,000 similarly diagnosed individuals who would not have committed this crime.

Social work practitioners face the challenge of working within agency guidelines which no doubt have risk prevention and management at the forefront, whilst striving to challenge any unnecessary or discriminatory emphasis on risk. This is often done within a legal framework.

Legislation

A key feature, therefore, of mental health practice is the role legislation plays in shaping services and intervention. Mental health is differentiated from general medicine through its use of treatment enforced via legislation, a course of action used by the majority of developed countries, though their methods of implementation differ (Tew, 2011). It is instructive to examine the theoretical drivers which underpin such intervention, particularly for social workers where, as Johns points out, 'the very idea of coercion in social care seems contradictory, and, to many, even abhorrent' (Johns, in Boylan & Brammer, 2017, p. 59)

Authors such as Bean (1986) and Rogers and Pilgrim (2010) have pointed to the use of mental health law as a method of social control with roots in capitalism's desire to maintain stability and economic development. A libertarian model (Sayce, 2016) argues that the legal distinction between physical and mental health is unethical, illogical and driven largely by discriminatory and stigmatizing perspectives of the mentally unwell, as well as consequently perpetuating such perspectives. A model proposed by Szmukler (2010) is for the removal of separate mental health legislation, replacing it with a single statute based solely on capacity rather than diagnosis or notions of risk. This would apply to everyone, not just those with a diagnosed mental disorder or impairment.

In the UK, for example, the introduction of the Mental Capacity Act 2005 saw a strengthening of the trend toward rights-based legislation. It defines how capacity is assessed and aims to protect those people who lack capacity to make decisions for themselves. Whilst strengthening the right of a capacitous person to refuse treatment for physical health problems, treatment for mental disorders can still be imposed via the Mental Health Act, even where a person has the capacity to object.

Social workers increasingly find their work shaped by statutory roles in adults practice (Lilo & Vose, 2016). Within the Mental Health Act, approved mental health professionals, a role still predominantly undertaken by social workers in the UK, act as an important counterweight to the medical perspective at the point of assessment, with a duty to promote a social perspective and service user rights. The act is founded on a medical framework of mental disorder and treatment which has remained essentially unchanged for several decades. By its very nature, then, this is a challenging and potentially ethically compromising role (Kinney, 2009). Pilgrim (in Matthews, O'Hare, & Hemmington, 2014) draws on concepts from Bourdieu to offer practitioners a practice model through which to explore how they carry out such statutory roles, in particular questioning the accepted assumptions that operate throughout mental health provision (see also Chapters 5 and 12). Assumptions, or 'doxa', such as 'people with mental health problems need help' and that the provision of such help is in their 'interests' are, as noted earlier, open to theoretical challenge but remain embedded as accepted and integral elements of British mental health policy and legislation. Furthermore, social workers are influenced by a process of 'secondary socialization': for example, through their training, which frames their disposition more broadly and shapes what they perceive as 'good' practice. Social workers may be vulnerable to becoming assimilated into medical discourses as a result of their organizational arrangements (Nathan & Webber, 2010). The challenge for the mental health social worker is to maintain an independent, socially orientated perspective whilst working effectively alongside their medical colleagues.

A recent area of development has been how theories underpinning mental health legislation have been exported to the community setting through the introduction of involuntary treatment in the community, known as community treatment orders in the UK. Those in support of this development point to the high number of 'revolving door patients' who could be spared repeated compulsory detention through enforcing their treatment in the community. Enforced treatment at home is less draconian than that taking place in hospital and thus promoted the 'least restrictive' principle of the MHA. Subsequent studies in the UK and other countries have called into question the efficacy of these measures. Two issues emerge: community treatment orders have not reduced hospital admissions as anticipated (Burns et al., 2013; Maughan et al.,

2014; Rugkasa, 2016), and certain groups are disproportionately represented, the most clear example being 'Black or Black British' people who were almost nine times more likely to being made subject to them (NHS Digital, 2017).

Recovery

Although it can be argued that several traditions lay claim to the exclusive right to define and portray distress and recovery in their own terms, approaches based on more value-based methods attempt to avoid such difficulties.

Approaches using what are known as 'recovery values' are gaining increasing traction. Such approaches aim to deliver the lifestyle that is defined by the service user, not the service providers, and one that is not judged by compliance and rating scales. Models using recovery values have been postulated (e.g. Spaniol, Wewiorski, Gagne, & Anthony, 2002; Andresen, Oades, & Caputi, 2003), although it is stressed that every individual's journey will be unique to them. Such approaches share much in common with the social model of disability (Oliver, 1996; see Chapter 38), in that the societal response to symptoms can be more limiting than the symptoms themselves, so care is taken to challenge discrimination and provide education where needed.

The aim of the recovery values approach is to deliver a life that is self-defined, hopeful and meaningful. This approach also facilitates spiritual understandings of experience, which other models do not. The notion of 'cure' is somewhat a side issue as the focus is on developing a personally significant life rather than symptom reduction (Byrne, Schoeppe, & Bradshaw, 2018). The two are, of course, not mutually exclusive. Despite its popularity, there remains inconsistency in the use of the term 'recovery', and its definition has changed over time (Ellison, Belanger, Niles, Evans, & Bauer, 2018). Studies have looked to identify core elements (e.g. Slade et al., 2017; Ellison et al., 2018). Whilst it is recognized that there is considerable heterogeneity across these studies, themes of hope, identity, opportunity and empowerment frequently appear. The issue of risk appears with regularity, with the recovery model inherently linked to a more therapeutic approach to working with perceived risk, encouraging individuals to take a greater stake in the risks they are exposed to and developing capabilities to manage them rather than being protected from them (Morgan, Felton, Fulford, Kalathil, & Stacey, 2016).

A critique of the recovery model has, perhaps naturally, emerged as it has become more embedded in government policies. Approaches using recovery values have seemed to falter when encountering highly organized health and social care providers, where the dominance of the medical model, coupled with organizational responsibilities in terms of financial and legal constraints, appear to hamper the effective adoption (Miller, Stanhope, Restrepo-Toro, & Tondora, 2017). As noted above, lack of clarity over the underlying definition and philosophy of recovery mean it has risked becoming a 'catch-all' term, meaning different things to different people. It has come under criticism for its primarily individualistic focus, whereby the service user is expected to develop a new way of being to manage their condition. This reflects current neoliberal discourse, whereby the state passes responsibility for well-being and regulation of behaviour on to the individual (Morgan et al., 2016). This, of course, jars somewhat when 'risk' becomes pre-eminent, and the neoliberal model melts into a paternalistic model of practice, where statutory tools (such as involuntary detention) are often applied. Indeed, it would appear that reconciling risk management with recovery-based approaches is challenging, although authors such as Felton and Stickley (2018) believe that it can be done through narrative approaches. These provide a context in which risk can be understood and how individual strengths, control and collaboration can be used to mitigate harm.

Structural factors which may have contributed to the development of an individual's mental distress, or indeed may serve to aid their recovery from it, are thus relegated, and the link between mental distress and social injustice is lost (Harper & Speed, 2012). There are further challenges with low levels of staff and user knowledge regarding implementing the phases or stages of recovery and the difficulties in designing valid measurement tools to assess its effectiveness (Slade et al., 2017).

Conclusion: bringing it all together

For the practising social worker, the field of mental health is contested and complex, with many areas of intersectionality. Whilst the authors are not inherently opposed to psychiatric or psychological approaches to mental health, we would assert that the predominance of these two models in particular limits the opportunities for social approaches to be used in routine practice. This is further compounded by the emphasis on risk and risk management, which is codified in many legislative frameworks. This also reflects a wider societal preoccupation with the perceived threat posed by mental health service users and the need for agencies to demonstrate their accountability and effectiveness in addressing these concerns.

Interventions based on recovery values have established themselves as a credible and viable addition to the field of mental health. In this sense, recovery requires statutory agencies to personalize and democratize the therapeutic process. It also requires cultural as well as technical shifts in work patterns that challenge structural and power-related barriers. The reality of practice requires workers to be able to successfully navigate complex social, political and cultural – currents that are frequently antithetical to each other – a role well suited to social workers due to the breadth and depth of their professional knowledge.

Practitioners familiar with personalization and critical practice may find themselves drawn to recovery-based approaches, although they may also find them practically challenging to implement. That said, social workers remain the professional group most likely to embrace recovery-orientated practice with fidelity and have an opportunity to reshape the international landscape of mental healthcare to better reflect the needs of those experiencing distress.

Further reading

Bracken, P., & Thomas, P. (2005). *Postpsychiatry: Mental health in a postmodern world*. Oxford University Press.

Sayce, L. (2016). *From psychiatric patient to citizen revisited*. London and New York: Palgrave Macmillan.

Tew, J. (2011). *Social approaches to mental distress*. Houndmills, Basingstoke, Hampshire and New York: Palgrave Macmillan.

References

Allen, J., Balfour, R., Bell, R., & Marmot, M. (2014). Social determinants of mental health. *International Review of Psychiatry, 26*(4), 392–407.

American Psychiatric Association. (2013). *Diagnostic and statistical manual of mental disorders* (5th ed.). Arlington, VA: American Psychiatric Publishing.

Andresen, R., Oades, L., & Caputi, P. (2003). The experience of recovery from schizophrenia: Towards an empirically validated stage model. *Australian & New Zealand Journal of Psychiatry, 37*(5), 586–594.

Bean, P. (1986). *Mental disorder and legal control*. Cambridge, UK: Cambridge University Press.

Beck, U. (1992). *Risk society: Towards a new modernity*. London: Sage.

Bentall, R. P. (1990). *Reconstructing schizophrenia*. London: Routledge.

Bracken, P., & Thomas, P. (2005). *Postpsychiatry: Mental health in a postmodern world*. Oxford: Oxford University Press.

Bressington, D., Badnapurkar, A., Inoue, S., Ma, H. Y., Chien, W. T., Nelson, D., & Gray, R. (2018). Physical health care for people with severe mental illness: The attitudes, practices, and training needs of nurses in three Asian countries. *International Journal of Environmental Research and Public Health, 15*(2), 343–357.

Burns, T., Rugkåsa, J., Molodynski, A., Dawson, J., Yeeles, K., Vazquez-Montes, M., . . . Priebe, S. (2013). Community treatment orders for patients with psychosis (OCTET): A randomised controlled trial. *The Lancet, 381*(9878), 1627–1633.

Byrne, L., Schoeppe, S., & Bradshaw, J. (2018). Recovery without autonomy: Progress forward or more of the same for mental health service users? *International Journal of Mental Health Nursing*, Online. Retrieved from https://doi.org/10.1111/inm.12446

Crawford, M. (2000). Homicide is impossible to predict. *The Psychiatrist, 24*(4), 152.

Ellison, M. L., Belanger, L. K., Niles, B. L., Evans, L. C., & Bauer, M. S. (2018). Explication and definition of mental health recovery: A systematic review. *Administration and Policy in Mental Health and Mental Health Services Research, 45*(1), 91–102.

Felton, A., & Stickley, T. (2018). Rethinking risk: A narrative approach. *The Journal of Mental Health Training, Education and Practice, 13*(1), 54–62.

Galabuzi, G., & Labonte, R. (2002). Social inclusion as a determinant of health (pp. 1–6). Presented at the Social Determinants of Health across the Life-Span Conference, Toronto, ON. Retrieved from www.phac-aspc.gc.ca/ph-sp/oi-ar/pdf/03_inclusion_e.pdf

Gardiner, J. (2017). The depression/schizophrenia continuum: Does cytoskeletal tensegrity play a role? *NeuroQuantology, 15*(4), Online. Retrieved from https://doi.org/10.14704/nq.2017.15.4.1121

Goffman, E. (1963). *Stigma: Notes on the management of spoiled identity*. Englewood Cliffs, NJ: Prentice-Hall.

Grant, A. (2011). A critique of the representation of human suffering in the cognitive behavioural therapy literature with implications for mental health nursing practice. *Journal of Psychiatric and Mental Health Nursing, 18*(1), 35–40.

Harper, D., & Speed, E. (2012). Uncovering Recovery: The resistible rise of recovery and resilience. *Studies in Social Justice, 6*(1), 9–25.

Heller, N. R. (2017). The limits and possibilities of risk assessment: Lessons from suicide prevention. In S. Stanford, E. Sharland, N. R., Heller, & J. Warner (Eds.), *Beyond the risk paradigm in mental health policy and practice* (pp. 71–85). London: Palgrave.

Hjorthøj, C., Stürup, A. E., McGrath, J. J., & Nordentoft, M. (2017). Years of potential life lost and life expectancy in schizophrenia: A systematic review and meta-analysis. *Lancet Psychiatry, 4*(4), 295–301.

Johns, R. (2017). Coercion in social care. In A. Brammer & J. Boylan (Eds.), *Critical issues in social work law* (pp. 59–72). London: Macmillan.

Johnstone, L., Boyle, M., Cromby, M., Dillon, J., Harper, D., Kinderman, P., . . . Read, J. (2018). *The power threat meaning framework: Towards the identification of patterns in emotional distress, unusual experiences and troubled or troubling behaviour, as an alternative to functional psychiatric diagnosis*. Leicester: British Psychological Society. Retrieved from https://www1.bps.org.uk/system/files/user-files/Division%20of%20Clinical%20Psychology/public/INF299%20PTM%20Main%20web.pdf

Kemshall, H. (2014). Conflicting rationalities of risk: Disputing risk in social policy – Reflecting on 35 years of researching risk. *Health, Risk & Society, 16*(5), 398–416.

Kinney, M. (2009). Being assessed under the 1983 Mental health act: Can it ever be ethical? *Ethics and Social Welfare, 3*(3), 329–336.

Labonte, R. (2004). Social inclusion exclusion: Dancing the dialectic. *Health Promotion International, 19*(1), 115–121.

Laing, R. D. (1965). *The divided self: An existential study in sanity and madness*. Harmondsworth: Penguin.

Lilo, E., & Vose, C. (2016). *Mental health integration past, present and future: A report of national survey into mental health integration in England*. Liverpool: Merseycare NHS Trust.

Marmot, M. (2010). *Fair society, healthy lives: The Marmot review*. London: The Marmot Review.

Marmot, M. G., & Wilkinson, R. G. (2006). *Social determinants of health* (2nd ed.). Oxford: Oxford University Press.

Matthews, S., O'Hare, P., & Hemmington, J. (2014). *Approved mental health practice: Essential themes for students and practitioners*. Basingstoke: Palgrave Macmillan.

Maughan, D., Molodynski, A., Rugkåsa, J., & Burns, T. (2014). A systematic review of the effect of community treatment orders on service use. *Social Psychiatry and Psychiatric Epidemiology, 49*(4), 651–663.

Miller, E., Stanhope, V., Restrepo-Toro, M., & Tondora, J. (2017). Person-centered planning in mental health: A transatlantic collaboration to tackle implementation barriers. *American Journal of Psychiatric Rehabilitation, 20*(3), 251–267.

Morgan, A., Felton, A., Fulford, K. W. M., Kalathil, J., & Stacey, G. (2016). *Values and ethics in mental health.* London: Palgrave Macmillan.

Nathan, J., & Webber, M. (2010). Mental health social work and the bureau-medicalisation of mental health care: Identity in a changing world. *Journal of Social Work Practice, 24*(1), 15–28.

National Institute for Care and Health Excellence. (2009, May 14). *Borderline personality disorder (BPD).* Retrieved from www.nice.org.uk/guidance/CG78/Guidance/pdf/English

NHS Digital (2017). Mental health act statistics, annual figures 2016/17. Retrieved 16 April 2019, from https://files.digital.nhs.uk/pdf/b/t/ment-heal-act-stat-eng-2016-17-summ-rep.pdf

Oliver, M. (1996). *Understanding disability: From theory to practice.* London: Palgrave Macmillan.

Perkins, R., & Repper, J. (2013). Prejudice, discrimination and social exclusion: Reducing the barriers to recovery for people diagnosed with mental health problems in the UK. *Neuropsychiatry, 3*(4), 377–384.

Rogers, A., & Pilgrim, D. (2010). *A sociology of mental health and illness* (4th ed.). Maidenhead: Open University Press.

Rugkåsa, J., & Burns, T. (2017). Community treatment orders: Are they useful? *BJPsych Advances, 23*(4), 222–230. doi:10.1192/apt.bp.115.015743

Sayce, L. (2016). *From psychiatric patient to citizen revisited.* London: Palgrave Macmillan.

Sin, C. H., Hedges, A., Cook, C., Mguni, N., & Comber, N. (2009). *Disabled people's experiences of targeted violence and hostility.* Manchester: Equality and Human Rights Commission.

Slade, M., Bird, V., Chandler, R., Clarke, E., Craig, T., Larsen, J., . . . Leamy, M. (2017). *REFOCUS: Developing a recovery focus in mental health services in England.* Nottingham: Institute of Mental Health. Retrieved from www.researchintorecovery.com/files/REFOCUS%20Final%20report.pdf

Smail, D. (2004). Therapeutic psychology and the ideology of privilege. *Clinical Psychology, (38)*, 9–14.

Spaniol, L., Wewiorski, N. J., Gagne, C., & Anthony, W. A. (2002). The process of recovery from schizophrenia. *International Review of Psychiatry, 14*(4), 327–336.

Szasz, T. S. (1961). *The myth of mental illness: Foundations of a theory of personal conduct.* New York: Harper.

Szmukler, G., Daw, R., & Dawson, J. (2010). A model law fusing incapacity and mental health legislation. *Journal of Mental Health Law, 20*, 11–12.

Tew, J. (2011). *Social approaches to mental distress.* Basingstoke: Palgrave Macmillan.

van der Wel, K., Saltkjel, T., Chen, W., Dahl, E., & Halvorsen, K. (2018). European health inequality through the 'Great Recession': Social policy matters. *Sociology of Health & Illness*, Online. Retrieved from https://doi.org/10.1111/1467-9566.12723

Wilkinson, R., & Pickett, K. E. (2009). *The spirit level: Why more equal societies almost always do better.* London: Allen Lane.

World Health Organization. (1993). *International classification of disease: Tenth revision. (ICD-10).* Geneva: World Health Organization.

37

Social work and addiction

Hilda Loughran

Introduction

Social workers have an important part to play in working with individuals and families experiencing substance use–related harm. This role has not always been acknowledged or supported. Over the past 30 years or so, there has been a shift in thinking about how best to manage substance use problems. The shift is best described as a move from addiction as the domain of specialist addiction-trained to substance use problems being viewed as a mainstream or primary concern to be managed by frontline workers and specialists working collaboratively.

This chapter examines the values, knowledge base and skills required to engage effectively with substance use problems. It will look at understanding addiction by reviewing a range of theoretical approaches that have influenced current thinking about addiction. The theories considered are central to understanding human behaviour and, as such, are typically embedded in generic social work training and education.

The chapter will present the argument that social work values, knowledge base and skills are compatible with working with substance use. What may be missing are opportunities for students to integrate and apply specific substance use knowledge to case examples and practice learning, thus validating their role in working with substance use issues and embedding it in general social work education. Social work can no longer support a position that places substance use interventions in the domain of the specialist. What is perhaps less clear is whether social service agencies are prepared to provide support to social workers to play their part in the response to substance use problems. Such role support is critical to the development of a sense of role legitimacy and role adequacy in substance use work (Loughran, Hohman, & Finnegan, 2010).

Social workers' engagement with substance use issues

The place for social workers as part of this broader response to substance use was confirmed by the Advisory Council on the Misuse of Drugs (2003), which found that parental alcohol or drug use was a factor with 25 percent of children on child protection registers. The legitimacy of social workers being involved with substance use may have been verified (Loughran, Hohman, & Finnegan, 2010), but questions about the adequacy of social work training remain

(Galvani & Forrester, 2011). In a survey conducted in the US, only 38 percent of social work students had received training in alcohol and other drugs (AOD) work as a student (Smith et al., 2006). More recently, Galvani and Forrester (2011) reported a serious shortfall in the education of social workers in relation to substance use issues. While inclusion of specific information about substance use may need to be addressed, the generic knowledge base of social workers in understanding human behaviour is very much applicable to work with addiction. Before looking at how such grand theories of human behaviour have influenced our understanding of addiction, it is important to define the term.

Addiction: a disputed term

The term 'addiction' is used here, but in the context of this chapter it refers to all levels of engagement with substance use that may be problematic and not exclusively to dependence. Social workers encounter addiction-related issues in a variety of settings. Most people probably associate it with child welfare and protection. In this setting, social workers need to be able to identify, assess and manage drug and alcohol problems which may be associated with parental use or, indeed, use by other family members. However, alcohol and drug issues are also prevalent in other social work settings, such as working within a mental health setting, healthcare, disabilities and older people (Loughran & Livingston, 2016). What is clear is that social workers need to be prepared to deal with alcohol and drug-related issues across a range of service provision. Before looking at how theories might help inform social workers about these problems, it is useful to clarify a few points about definitions of terms.

Morgan (2017, p. 73) refers to some problematic behaviours as 'process addiction'. These include sex addiction, food addiction and pathological gambling. Additional behaviours such as computer gaming could be incorporated into this category. While accepting that other problematic behaviours are referred to as addictions, this chapter will focus on addiction that relates to substance use disorders (SUD) as classified in the diagnostic criteria for DSM-5 (American Psychiatric Association, 2013). This classification covers a range of substances including alcohol, cannabis, phencyclidine, other hallucinogens, inhalants, opioids, sedatives, stimulants, tobacco and other/unknown (Morgan, 2013, p. 56).

The use of the term 'addiction' in this chapter title may be misleading. Addiction implies that there is evidence of both a physical and psychological dependence sufficient to meet the diagnostic criteria set out by alcohol/drug dependence syndrome (ICD-10, World Health Organisation [WHO]). In the social work context, we meet service users who do not necessarily meet all these criteria but for whom their substance use is causing major difficulties. It is important, then, to recognize not just these later stages of SUD but to be able to identify even early stages of problems with alcohol and other drugs (AOD). To achieve this, social workers should be familiar with the impact of a range of substance use rather than focusing on the more severe end of a continuum of use.

A continuum or levels of engagement with substance use

Addiction may be seen to refer to a level of substance use that involves physical and psychological dependence on the drug. The WHO's (1992) classification reflected the disease concept of addiction which was popular at that time, although it has changed the terminology from 'addiction' to 'dependence syndrome'.

> The Tenth Revision of the International Classification of Diseases and Health Problems (ICD-10) defines the dependence syndrome as being a cluster of physiological, behavioural,

and cognitive phenomena in which the use of a substance or a class of substances takes on a much higher priority for a given individual than other behaviours that once had greater value. A central descriptive characteristic of the dependence syndrome is the desire (often strong, sometimes overpowering) to take the psychoactive drugs (which may or not have been medically prescribed), alcohol, or tobacco.

One of the complex aspects of working with substance use is that someone who is not necessarily exhibiting dependence may still be in very serious difficulties with their substance use. For example, someone who is typically a social drinker may on one or two occasions consume sufficient quantities of alcohol to endanger either themselves or their children. This level of use might be referred to as hazardous use. The English Department of Health in *Models of Care for Alcohol Misuse* (2006, p. 12) clarifies that:

> There is no single concise way of categorising individuals in need of alcohol treatment. The extent to which individuals would benefit from interventions depends on a number of factors. Key factors include: the level of consumption, the context in which alcohol is used, the seriousness of the alcohol-related problems and the severity of the dependence on alcohol. MoCAM identifies four main categories of alcohol misusers who may benefit from some kind of intervention or treatment: hazardous drinkers; harmful drinkers; moderately dependent drinkers and severely dependent drinkers . . . Individual drinkers may move in and out of different categories over the course of a lifetime.

WHO (2017a) clarifies the difference between harmful and hazardous substance use. Harmful use is defined as:

> a pattern of psychoactive substance use that is causing damage to health. The damage may be physical (e.g. hepatitis following injection of drugs) or mental (e.g. depressive episodes

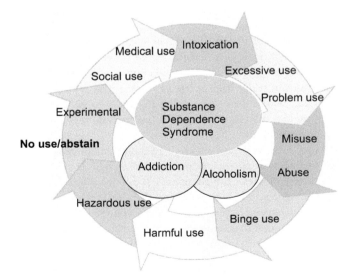

Figure 37.1 Levels of engagement with substance use: not using through experimental and social use to problematic levels of use to abstaining from use

secondary to heavy alcohol intake). Harmful use commonly, but not invariably, has adverse social consequences; social consequences in themselves, however, are not sufficient to justify a diagnosis of harmful use.

Hazardous use (WHO 2017b) is defined as:

> a pattern of substance use that increases the risk of harmful consequences for the user. Some would limit the consequences to physical and mental health (as in harmful use); some would also include social consequences. In contrast to harmful use, hazardous use refers to patterns of use that are of public health significance despite the absence of any current disorder in the individual user. The term is used currently by WHO but is not a diagnostic term in ICD-10.

Social workers need to understand the potential risks associated with different levels of use and different substances as this may impact individual users, their families and, more broadly, the community in which they live. This understanding or interpretation of what we see when we encounter substance use is influenced by a range of theories. These theories underpin the assessment of risk and resilience in cases where substance use is an issue. The chapter will now look at some of the 'grand theories' of human behaviour to consider what ideas they have contributed to social work understanding of addiction and the broader continuum of use. Concepts and ideas that have been particularly associated with substance use and how these have influenced the development of responses, interventions and treatment for substance users will be discussed.

Biopsychosocial theories

Theories of human behaviour span a range of disciplines. Typically, the grand theories are attributed to the physical and health sciences (bio), psychology (psycho) and sociological (social). Each of these purports to explain human behaviour from its different perspective. Social work does not have its own unique theoretical base but draws on and is influenced by the range of theories emanating from these grand theories.

It is useful for social workers to think about the ideas that shape how we understand and assess substance use. Some of these ideas seem to be pervasive in our society: for example, the idea that there is an addictive personality, that addiction is a disease and that only people in recovery from addiction can really help others in recovery. As professionals in the field, it is important to understand where these ideas come from and to consider how they influence assessment and responses to substance users. This understanding is then critical in planning appropriate actions or treatment.

Valentine (1998, pp. 23–35) reviewed a total of 16 theoretical positions that related to addiction. She included biochemical, biological and genetic as well as cultural and psychological theories. In an evaluation of these, Loughran (2002, p. 63) commented that this says more about what we do not understand about addiction than what we do. What is clear, however, is that there is an acknowledgement that addiction is a complex phenomenon and that many theoretical positions are required in an attempt to capture this complexity. This biopsychosocial approach to addiction fits well with social work's appreciation of many aspects of human behaviour. For the purposes of exploring what all this means for substance use and social work, this chapter will focus on a few of the most influential and probably best-known theoretical ideas. Some of these ideas continue to have a limited research base but have nonetheless retained their popularity as ways of discussing and managing substance use problems.

Biologically informed theories and addiction

Biologically informed theories encompass ideas that link problematic substance use to genetics. More recently these ideas have also been researched in conjunction with neuroscience (see Chapter 6). Genetics or neuroscience theories are sometimes criticized because they highlight the predetermined nature of addiction. For social work this is a challenging perspective because it focuses on genetically predetermined factors and therefore has implications for the conceptualization of change. This informs a debate about where a society places responsibility for addiction. In the biological orientation, the focus is less on individual responsibility and choice and more on predispositions. In contrast, psychological theories may emphasize choice and motivation, thereby placing responsibility on the individual without sufficient recognition of both biological and social factors. Social workers in practice need to see the role of possible predispositions but also acknowledge the role of the individual, society, culture and family. Carter and Hall (2013, p. 547), in considering the increased interest in the biological and neuroscience aspects of addiction, caution that although 'addiction has a genetic and neurobiological basis . . . attempts to translate these into treatment and social policies need careful ethical analysis'.

Addiction: a disease

The disease concept of addiction promotes the view of an illness with a genetic base involving individual predisposition. It has been very influential in the development of treatment responses to addiction, in particular a medical model approach. Jellinek (1952), who developed the disease concept in relation to alcohol, did focus on the biological but also recognized that other factors such as physiological and social influences might impact the illness and recovery. In his work Jellinek (1960) acknowledged that there were a number of different types or species of the disease. These species are very compatible with more modern ideas referred to as a continuum of problems associated with substance use. However, it was the 'species' of physical dependency that became most closely associated with his ideas. This species described alcoholism as a physical dependence involving craving, increased tolerance and loss of control.

A wide range of treatment responses can be attributed or connected to these theoretical influences. The medical model of addiction was very influential in the development of treatment. Treatment in this genre held the view that the only viable response to addiction was total abstinence from all addictive substances for life. This ideology informed such movements as therapeutic communities, the Minnesota Model of four to six weeks intensive inpatient treatment and the AA twelve-step self-help movement. These adopted a specialist approach to addiction so that addiction counsellors and often people in recovery themselves were seen to be the most appropriate to deliver treatment services. The treatment was then usually in a specialist unit, typically away from family and community. In treatment the individual was encouraged to take responsibility for their addiction and for the harmful consequences their addiction had for themselves and their families. Recently, the numbers of people in recovery working in such settings has diminished (White, 2000), and the emphasis has shifted to community-based services, including brief interventions by primary care professionals. White (2000) found that, despite the widely held views on the issue, there is no evidence that engaging professionals who are in recovery from substance use to provide treatment is a predictor of a better outcome.

Given the endurance of these biologically based theories of addiction and dependence, it may be easy to overlook some of the alternative interpretations or theories. Social workers, however, are familiar with the influence of the medical model approach and do consider viable alternative conceptualizations of problems.

Psychological theories

Psychoanalytic and psychodynamic theory

Arguably the most influential and enduring set of theories about human behaviour is the contribution of Freud and post-Freudians to thinking about human behaviour (see Chapters 3 and 12). This chapter will not attempt to provide a comprehensive account of this body of work but will highlight some of the key ideas in that theory and consider how these concepts have influenced thinking about addiction.

The concept of defence mechanisms refers to specific unconscious mechanisms that may form psychological barriers to working on life issues (Payne, 2005, p. 74). Addiction may be seen as a result of faulty defence mechanisms, which led the substance user to block out the reality of their drug use. Some of the defence mechanisms became attributed as traits of the substance user, such as users being viewed as defensive, being in denial and being resistant. More traditional treatment responses to these 'characteristics' included the use of confrontation to break down defences and the development of a position that substance users were manipulative, and so only people who had overcome such experiences could really understand the dynamics of this process. These views have been challenged by developments in treatment such as motivational interviewing (Miller & Rollnick, 2013) which takes an alternative view that being 'defensive' is a reaction to confrontation and not a characteristic of the substance user. In fact, Miller and Rollnick (2013) and Kim Berg and Reuss (1998) take the position that resistance and denial are unhelpful concepts in managing addiction.

The addictive personality

'Psychoanalytic personality theories assume that people are a complex of drives . . . the id pushes us to act to resolve our needs, but our actions do not always bring the desired results' (Payne, 2005, p. 75). This theoretical influence on understanding addiction underpins the widely held view of the addictive personality. It implies that the individual is prone to addictive behaviours and is likely to swap one addiction for another. From a treatment perspective, it informs the need for total abstinence from all substances, regardless of the drug of choice that has led to identification of the problems. While obviously the notion of having an addictive personality encompasses the biological predetermination principle, in practice this does not discount the individual's ability to manage their addictive behaviours. They will always have the addictive personality, however, so management is a lifelong commitment. The addictive personality theory has become a contested notion. Miller, Forcehimes, and Zweben's (2011, p. 19) found no evidence of a characteristic abnormal personality. There is no one personality type that displays or explains the impulsivity and lack of control typically associated with such an addictive personality type. This leaves us with the possibility that there is no such thing as an addictive personality, which is quite a challenge for such a widely influential view of addiction.

Cognitive behavioural theories

Key ideas associated with behaviour theory include those which attempt to explain why humans engage in behaviours or actions and why they replicate or repeat these behaviours. Included in this broad set of ideas are operant conditioning and social learning (Loughran, 2010). Put simply, humans repeat behaviours when there is a sufficient reward or positive consequence for that behaviour and do not repeat behaviours that result in negative consequences. Antecedents to the behaviour or the context in which the behaviour happens are also relevant. Behaviour can be explained by considering the context, the behaviour itself and the consequences of that behaviour. Social learning theory built on the earlier operant conditioning ideas and added the elements associated with interaction with others and our environment. Behaviour can be learned from observing or modelling the behaviour of others, especially peers and people of influence. Behaviour is learned and can be unlearned.

Cognitive theory then looks to understanding the role of our thinking capacity in influencing behaviours. Concepts such as rational and irrational thinking, self-efficacy and attribution can be aligned with cognitive theory. Self-efficacy refers to the belief in oneself and one's ability to change, while attribution refers to ideas about who is responsible for change and who gets the credit for change (Loughran, 2010). The importance of both understanding behaviour and our capacity to make sense of behaviour, thoughts and feelings contributed to the move to amalgamate these theories into a more comprehensive cognitive behavioural theory (see Chapter 18). This has been a very significant advance for the field of substance use interventions.

Behaviour and cognitive theories also inform ideas about addiction and substance dependence. Behaviour theories offer explanations of addiction which can be helpful in understanding problematic relationships with substances as well as with certain behaviours. Behaviour theories do not necessarily address the pharmacological aspects of the substance in question but look more to the psychological and even social context within which the substance use takes place (Heather & Robinson, 1998, p. 178). Behaviour theories offer alternative interpretations of addiction. Operant conditioning considers the contexts within which substance use happens, the actual behaviour around the use and the consequence experienced by the individual. It also looks at substance use as a learned behaviour influenced by peers and the social environment. These ideas support the development of a continuum of substance use: for example, the stage of experimental use. A young person who experiments with substances is likely to do this in a context where others of a similar age are also experimenting. Even with a socially more acceptable drug such as alcohol, young people tend to develop a relationship with alcohol with their peers. In addition, behavioural principles of learning and unlearning behaviours also inform the 'controlled use of substances' debate. This is a disputed view that people are capable of regaining control over their substance use. Given that loss of control is a central tenet of the disease concept of addiction, the idea that an individual could return to non-problematic levels of use was very controversial. Again, a shift in thinking from the two-world approach to addiction (Butler, 1996) that you are either alcoholic or you are not, an addict or not. With the continuum model, substance use may be anywhere along a continuum from use to misuse, abuse or dependence. This allows for movement along the continuum rather than the progressive route to dependence associated with the disease concept.

Cognitive behaviour theory has influenced attitudes toward abstinence and harm reduction and the place of brief interventions. These theories have informed interventions such as motivational interviewing and cognitive behavioural therapy and have produced strong evidence of effectiveness.

Associated treatment approaches

Application of behavioural and cognitive theory contributed to revolutionizing addiction treatment. The claims by Sobel and Sobel in the 1970s that alcohol-dependent drinking could be reversed and that someone could engage in social drinking met with outrage and is still a controversial topic in the field (Saladin & Santa Ana, 2004). Social learning theory, which espouses the view that behaviour is learned and therefore may be unlearned, underpins the notion of regaining control, but this contravenes well-established and powerful views of addiction. The debate here is not necessarily about the veracity of the view that controlled use is possible, but rather it points to the importance of understanding strongly held views and theories of addiction and the difficulties involved in challenging those beliefs.

Arguably one of the most widely known developments in treating addiction and substance use disorders is Prochaska and DiClemente's (1983) wheel of change. While not directly attributed to cognitive theoretical influences, this model demonstrates the importance of engaging with how individuals think about themselves and their substance use. The basic premise of the wheel of change is that the individual must be facilitated to think about their behaviour. In the terminology of the model, the individual needs to move from not thinking (pre-contemplation) to contemplation of their behaviour and the consequences of that behaviour in order to come to a decision about substance use and engage in a change plan.

In many ways more influential than behavioural or cognitive theory has been the associated developments of the combined cognitive behavioural–based treatment responses to substance misuse and addiction. Miller and Rollick's (2013) motivational interviewing approach to working with substance users (see Chapter 21), lauded as one with a strong evidence base while acknowledging the influence of Rogers's person-centred approach (see Chapter 3), has components that draw on both behaviour and cognitive theories. Motivation is viewed as a commitment to change behaviours, and the model of interview builds on developing a relationship between the motivational interviewer and the individual to facilitate thinking about behaviour, consequences and goals. Miller and Rollnick (2013) emphasize the importance of motivation in managing substance use problems. Motivation is not tied to some personality trait but is an active ingredient to be supported and encouraged. Central to this activity is a focus on change talk and working with an individual to consider change and what might build motivation for such change. The change can have a cognitive dimension but ideally will have a behavioural outcome.

Systems and social construction theories

Allen (2014, pp. 30–31), in reviewing why people use substances, makes the case that the single perspective theories, such as those outlined earlier, fail to meet the test of providing an explanation for all aspects of substance use. In support of this, he starts his consideration of theories of substance use by focusing on social and sociological perspectives. These perspectives facilitate developing our understanding of the links between substance use and social norms, gender, power, disadvantage (both economic and social), education, culture and subculture. The social lens provides for a more comprehensive analysis of why people use drugs, taking account not just of any individual propensity to use, but also allows for further consideration of family dynamics and family systems and draws attention to other systems such as communities, service providers, health and criminal justice systems and economic and political systems. Vakharia (2014, p. 695), considering the importance of systems in training social workers to work in substance use, states that the

> . . . systems perspective provides an ideal frame though which to view the current opioid overdose crisis because it can help students to view seemingly individual phenomenon as one that is actually dynamically impacting (and impacted by) interpersonal and family systems, health care delivery systems, human services agencies, criminal justice systems, the pharmaceutical industry, local/national policy and local/national public health policy.

More traditional approaches to substance use do attempt to include the family but do not encompass the mutuality and interactive dynamics demanded by systems thinking. Explaining these relationships with such concepts as co-dependency or adult children of 'alcoholics' results in pathologizing family members without capturing the resilience and coping strategies employed within families. Nor do they attempt to look beyond the individual or even the family to the broader systems within which the substance use problems are played out.

Behavioural theory has influenced some of the developments in working with families. O'Farrell and Fals-Stewart (2000) explored family-based interventions and identified family theory in relation to disease-oriented behavioural as well as family systems approaches to treatment. Some of the behavioural ideas are evident in the community reinforcement approach (Meyers & Miller, 2001). While these interventions acknowledge the impact of addiction on family and community, they focus on their potential role in challenging negative behaviours and supporting positive change, thus reflecting the reinforcement concepts of behavioural theory.

Attempts to understand substance use and family dynamics are not new. More traditional theories such as the disease concept underpin Al-Anon as a family support response. However, the complex interactions suggested in systems theories have not been developed and so have not gained the same influence as biological and psychological theories, despite the evidence that such interactions play an important part in dealing with the problems of substance use. Miller et al. (2011, p. 199) contend that 'newly found sobriety can require a redistribution of power and roles within a relationship'. Ideas such as power, roles and the function of the behaviour emerge from systems thinking. Miller et al. (2011, p. 200) also found that 'addressing both addiction and family functioning, outcomes for both can be significantly improved'. Social work education includes development of knowledge and skills regarding such relationship and family functioning, and so social workers should be in a strong position to apply these concepts to substance use within these systems.

Social construction theory (see Chapter 5) provides yet another challenge to traditional thinking about substance use. It provides a framework for understanding substance use as formulated by social context. It highlights discrepancies between the potential harmfulness of specific substances and the way a society views those substances. The controversial study by Nutt, King, and Phillips (2010) found that alcohol was the most damaging drug and that the current drug classification system has little relationship to evidence of harm. This construction of what is a dangerous drug then underpins the stigmatization, marginalization and criminalization of those who use those substances. It is further exasperated by the established links between substance use problems and social disadvantage (Loughran & McCann, 2006). There is much work to be done to shift the focus of intervention from an individual to a societal focus. Efforts such as community reinforcement models are attempting to engage with this but are limited by their behavioural underpinnings. Real engagement with these broader issues demands consideration of the challenges embedded in systems and social construction views of substance.

Concluding comments

Social workers have learned that adopting a deficit approach is usually unhelpful, as captured in both strengths perspectives and solution-focused work (Saleebey 2006; Ratner, George, & Iveson, 2012; see Chapters 22 and 23). Yet the profession is at risk of applying this same deficit analysis to its own involvement in substance use work. In the same way that a deficit model can underestimate service users, this approach underestimates the contribution of social work to substance use work. Social workers have a values system, knowledge base and skills set appropriate and applicable for substance use work. Butler (1996, p. 3), in discussing the social work ethos, comments that:

> . . . it must be regarded as an achievement that social workers have consistently articulated the validity and importance of the person-in-environment perspective as an alternative to the more technical vision of medicine or the militaristic dream of achieving a drug-free society as a result of victory in the 'war on drugs'. The importance of adopting a communal, as opposed to an individualistic, policy approach is now being advocated by a number of community groups.

Others, like Vakharia (2014), in discussing social work training, point out that evidence-based individual and group interventions are frequently part of social work training. These can include basic counselling skills, person-centred work, family work, motivational interviewing, solution-focused work, crisis intervention and cognitive behavioural work and are appropriate skills for working with substance use. As frontline and primary care workers, social workers need to be able to identify and assess substance use not just in the more severe level of addiction or dependency but across all levels of engagement with substance use. As child welfare and protection workers, they also need to be able to assess levels of risk to individuals and their children which are associated with substance use. Social workers are well grounded in assessment skills (National Institute of Health and Care Excellence, 2017; Department of Education, 2015), which, while focusing on child-centred practice, encompass issues related to parental capacity, a core aspect of assessing parents who use drugs. They are trained to develop relationships and engage service users. These skills are now recognized as core to any successful substance use intervention.

What is perhaps less evident is that the commitment to social justice and social inclusion is the foundation of social work practice. This can be seen in the radical and critical perspective which supports the transformational politicized dimensions of social work (Payne, 2005; see Chapter 30). Social work can bring additional value to substance use work by not just engaging with the biopsychosocial theories that can inform practice but by also highlighting the socio-political and economic understanding of substance use problems.

Research into clinical practices has assisted in identifying aspects of treatment responses that are more helpful than others. Miller et al. (2011) refer to brief interventions, motivational interviewing, community reinforcement and family-based work as evidence-based options. Yet, ironically, research is still somewhat equivocal. In reviewing evidence of successful outcomes in treatment, Orford (2008) suggests that we have been asking the wrong questions. Perhaps as a result, the focus of research has begun to shift and interest have developed in the quality of the relationship between service users and worker, and even more specifically on the role of empathy, as predictors of successful outcomes (Moyers & Miller, 2012). What is not ambiguous is that social, economic and political interventions can be effective, as can the shift in policy to harm reduction facilitated by the adoption of a public health approach to supplement, if not replace, the criminal, public order orientation (Butler, Elmeland, Thom, & Nicholls, 2017).

A comprehensive understanding of addiction or substance use must be inclusive; that means drawing on the bio-psycho-socio-economic-political perspectives in informing both policies and practice. Social workers are ideally placed to mediate this with their competence base professional standards in terms of values, knowledge base and skills and with their fundamental commitment to viewing service users' experiences from a social context and not from an individual deficit perspective.

Further reading

Allen, G. (2014). *Working with substance users: A guide to effective interventions.* Basingstoke: Palgrave Macmillan.

Galvani, S. (2015). *Alcohol and other drugs: The roles and capabilities of social workers.* Manchester: Manchester Metropolitan University.

Loughran, H., & Livingston, W. (Eds.). (2014). Substance abuse in social work education and training (Special ed.). *Social Work Education, 33*(5).

References

Allen, G. (2014). *Working with substance users: A guide to effective interventions.* Basingstoke: Palgrave Macmillan.

American Psychiatric Association. (2013). *Diagnostic and statistical manual of mental disorders* (5th ed.). Washington, DC: Author.

Butler, S. (1996). Substance misuse and the social work ethos. *Journal of Substance Misuse, 1*(3), 149–154.

Butler, S., Elmeland, K., Thom, B., & Nicholls, J. (2017). *Alcohol, power and public health: A comparative study of alcohol policy.* London: Routledge.

Carter, A., & Hall, W. (2013). Addiction neuroethics: Ethical and social implications of genetic and neuro science research on addiction. In P. Miller (Ed.), *Biological research on addiction: Comprehensive addictive behaviours and disorders* (vol. 2., pp. 541–549). Amsterdam: Elsevier Science.

Department of Education. (2015). *Working together to safeguard children: A guide to inter-agency working to safeguard and promote the welfare of children.* London: HM Government.

Department of Health and National Treatment Agency. (2006). *Models of care for alcohol misusers.* London: National Treatment Agency. Retrieved from https://webarchive.nationalarchives.gov.uk/201301240 73233/http://www.dh.gov.uk/prod_consum_dh/groups/dh_digitalassets/@dh/@en/documents/digitalasset/dh_4136809.pdf

Galvani, S., & Forrester, D. (2011). How well prepared are newly qualified social workers for working with substance use issues? Findings from a national survey in England. *Social Work Education, 30*(4), 422–439.

Jellinek, E. M. (1952). Phases of alcohol addiction. *Quarterly Journal of Studies on Alcohol, 13*(4), 673–684.

Jellinek, E. M. (1960). *The disease concept of alcoholism.* New Brunswick: Hillhouse Press.

Kim Berg, I., & Reuss, N. (1998). *Solutions step by step: A substance abuse treatment manual.* New York: Norton.

Loughran, H. (2002). *A study of alcohol problems and marriage from a treatment perspective.* (Unpublished PhD thesis). University College Dublin.

Loughran, H. (2010). *Understanding crisis therapies: An integrative approach to crisis intervention and post-traumatic stress.* London: Jessica Kingsley.

Loughran, H., Hohman, M., & Finnegan, D. (2010). Predictors of role legitimacy and role adequacy of social workers working with substance using clients. *British Journal of Social Work, 40*, 239–256.

Loughran, H., & Livingston, W. (Eds.). (2016). *Substance use in social work education and training: preparing for and supporting crisis.* Abingdon: Routledge.

Loughran, H., & McCann, M. E. (2006). *A community drugs study: Developing community indicators for problem drug use.* Dublin: NACD.

Meyers, R. J., & Miller, W. (Eds.). (2001). *A community reinforcement approach to the treatment of addiction.* Cambridge, UK: Cambridge University Press.

McCrady, B., & Epstein, E. (1999). *Addictions: A comprehensive guidebook.* New York: Oxford University Press.

Miller, W., Forcehimes, A., & Zweben, A. (2011). *Treating addiction: A guide for professionals.* New York: Guilford.

Miller, W. R., & Rollnick, S. (2013). *Motivational interviewing: Helping people change* (3rd ed.). New York: Guilford.

Morgen, K. (2017). *Substance use disorders and addictions.* London: Sage.

Moyers, T., & Miller, W. (2012). Is low therapist empathy toxic? *Psychology of Addictive Behavior, 27*(3), 878–884.

National Institute for Health and Care Excellence. (2017). *Child abuse and neglect* (Guideline NG76). Retrieved from www.nice.org.uk/guidance/ng76/resources/child-abuse-and-neglect-pdf-1837637587141

Nutt, D., King, L., & Phillips, L. (2010). Drug harms in the UK: A multi-criteria decision analysis. *The Lancet, 376*(9752), 1558–1565.

O'Farrell, T., & Fals-Stewart, W. (2000). Behavioral couples therapy for alcoholism and drug abuse. *Journal of Substance Abuse Treatment, 18*, 51–54.

Orford, J. (2008). Asking the right questions in the right way: The need for a shift in research on psychological treatments for addiction. *Addiction, 103*(6), 875–885.

Payne, M. (2005). *Modern social work theory* (3rd ed.). Basingstoke: Palgrave Macmillan.

Prochaska, J. O., & DiClemente, C. C. (1983). Stages and processes of self-change of smoking: Toward an integrative model of change. *Journal of Consulting and Clinical Psychology, 51*(3), 390–395.

Ratner, H., George, E., & Iveson, C. (2012). *Solution focused brief therapy: 100 key points and technique*. Abingdon: Routledge.

Saladin, M., & Santa Ana, E. (2004). Controlled drinking: More than just a controversy. *Current Opinion Psychiatry, 17*(3), 175–187.

Saleebey, D. (2006). *The strengths perspective in social work practice* (4th ed.). Boston: Pearson/Allyn & Bacon.

Smith, M., Whitaker, T., & Weismiller, T. (2006). Social workers in substance abuse treatment field: A snapshot of service activities. *Health and Social Work, 31*(2), 109–115.

Vakharia, S. (2014). Incorporating substance use content into social work curricula: Opioid overdose as a micro, mezzo and macro problem. *Social Work Education, 33*(5), 692–698.

Valentine, P. (1998). The etiology of addiction. In C. McNeece & D. DiNitto (Eds.), *Chemical dependency: A systems approach* (2nd ed., pp. 23–33). Boston: Allyn & Bacon.

White, W. (2000). The history of recovered people as wounded healers: II. The era of professionalization and specialization. *Alcoholism Treatment Quarterly, 18*(2), 1–25.

World Health Organization. (1992). *International classification of diseases: Classification scheme for mental and behavioural disorders* (10th ed.). Geneva: WHO. Retrieved from www.who.int/substance_abuse/terminology/definition1/en/

World Health Organisation. (2017a). *Management of substance abuse: Harmful use*. Retrieved from: https://www.who.int/substance_abuse/terminology/definition2/en/

World Health Organisation. (2017b). *Management of substance abuse: Hazardous use*. Retrieved from: https://www.who.int/substance_abuse/terminology/definition3/en/

38

Disability theory and social work practice

Stephen J. Macdonald and Lesley Deacon

Introduction

This chapter presents a summary of disability theory with reference to social work practice. We consider five models of disability, of which we advocate that three are essential for social work practice to support disabled service users. We discuss two medical models and three versions of the social model with reference to their theoretical origins. The chapter will suggest that the biomedical models employ an essentialist perspective to disability and impairment (see Chapter 6), whereas the social models draw on historical materialism, critical realism and post-structuralism philosophies. We use examples from our research to illustrate how these theoretical lenses emerge and can be applied in different situational professional spaces.

We argue that social work practitioners should not be constrained by one theoretical perspective. Rather, an eclectic toolkit should be utilized to facilitate inclusive and anti-discriminatory practices (Deacon & Macdonald, 2017). A post-positivist perspective is employed to bring together the different models by using a mixed-method approach in our research, which is presented in this chapter. Thus, we exemplify our theoretical, qualitative and quantitative research to progress a social scientific approach in disability studies to inform social work practice. As Williams (2003) suggests, a post-positivist position has now been embraced: i.e. that both a positivist *and* an interpretivist position can be occupied. This pragmatic approach therefore acknowledges that some 'realities' can be counted and measured and some cannot (Patton, 2002). The chapter aims to give clear direction for social work practitioners to understand different models of disability to develop a critical practice to move away from the current medicalized healthcare approach that dominates contemporary social work.

Medical models of disability and impairment

In the UK, social work emerged from 19th-century philanthropy, which had a significant influence on the lives of disabled people, particularly individuals living in poverty (Bamford, 2015). Although historical definitions of disability are usually affiliated with the rise of clinical medicine through normative measurement of the body, charitable organizations also allied themselves to medicine. The rise of modern medicine led firstly to the categorization of human physiology through the notion of 'normal' and 'abnormal' biological function and secondly to an attempt to develop successful interventions to 'cure' these biological abnormalities (Barnes, 2010; Barnes & Mercer, 2010). By the late 19th century, these normative measurements were extended beyond the physical body to pathologically categorize 'abnormal' behaviours (i.e. mental health issues) and 'abnormal' intellect (i.e. learning or intellectual impairments) (Barnes 2010, 2012; see Chapter 39). It is these early clinical definitions that led to the formation of the biomedical model in the 20th century. Charitable organizations in the late 19th and early 20th centuries, rather than rejecting biomedical movements such as eugenics, actively engaged with these practices (Simmons, 1978; O'Brien, 2011). With the emergence of medical social work in the early 20th century, the biomedical model became enshrined within social work practice concerning disability (Oliver, 1983).

The biomedical model of disability

In social science, the biomedical model can be characterized as an essentialist theoretical perspective. This model uses positivist methodological techniques to collect statistical measurements of human pathologies through the notions of 'function' and 'dysfunction'. From this essentialist perspective, the impairment impacts 'normal' behaviours, restricting interaction and social participation resulting in disability. Hence, impairment is directly linked to disability due to a physiological or neurological 'dysfunction'. With reference to professional practice, this model was defined by WHO's 'International Classification of Impairments, Disabilities and Handicaps' in the 1980s as:

Impairment: any loss or abnormality of psychological, physiological or anatomical structure or function.

- A deviation from a statistical 'norm' in an individual's biomedical status
- Includes loss/defect of tissue-mechanism-system-function
- Temporary or permanent

Disability: any restriction or lack (resulting from impairment) of the ability to perform an activity in the manner or within the range considered normal for a human being.

- Functional limitation expresses itself as a reality in everyday life
- Tasks, skills and behaviour
- Temporary or permanent

(adapted from Semple, Smyth, Burns, Darjee, & McInrosh, 2013, p. 90)

Although WHO has now replaced this classification, it still appears in prominent contemporary clinical medical texts (see *Oxford Handbooks of Psychiatry* and *Clinical Medicine*; *Oxford Concise Medicine Dictionary*). The model conceptualizes disability through a disease approach, where the role of professional practice is to 'cure' or to 'normalize' the physiological or psychological defects of a condition. Although the role of the social worker does not directly engage in the concept of 'cure', practitioners often work alongside healthcare to facilitate treatment. For example, social workers may support a service user into an NHS residential care home or ensure that a person is complying with their prescribed psycho-pharmaceutical medications. This would be justified, as conditions like schizophrenia are conceptualized as health conditions which need medical treatments. As Maynard, Boutwell, and Vaughn (2016, p. 5) suggest:

While schizophrenia is now understood as a disorder of brain function . . . research examining the contributions of biological and social factors has also led to a better understanding of the role and interaction of socio-environmental factors in the course of schizophrenia.... Thus, while understanding the biological factors is important, turning our attention to include biological factors in social work . . . does not presume a biological intervention. Indeed, it can lead to the identification and refinement of psycho-social interventions that affect or mitigate biological factors.

Applying a biomedical approach within social work practice employs a rehabilitative perspective which normalizes the disabling factors experienced by service users. In allying themselves to medicine to reduce a person's impairment effect, social workers assist in the rehabilitation process and support medical interventions. For some service users, rehabilitation *may* lead to 'cure', which is the desirable outcome. Yet for most disabled people, impairment is permanent, and 'cure' is not possible as their bodies have permanently changed or are physiologically different.

The biopsychosocial model of illness, impairment and disability

Within the UK, and globally, the biopsychosocial model has become the dominant approach when theoretically conceptualizing disability, both in healthcare and in social work practice (Barnes, Green, & Hopton, 2007; Berzoff & Drisko, 2015; Shakespeare, Watson, & Abu Alghaib, 2016). This model developed from the work of George Engel, a psychiatrist who viewed the biomedical model and social constructionist approaches as reductionist in nature. For Engel, the biomedical model reduced disease entirely to the molecular level and left no possibility for social factors to be incorporated within professional practice (Engel, 1977). Engel also rejected the anti-psychiatry movement of the time, which dismissed entirely any biological causation of mental illness (see Szasz, 1974). In a 1977 article entitled 'The need for a new medical model', he suggested that illness is affected by social environments and biochemical changes within the body, which have a psychological impact on a person's wellbeing. Engel proposed a need to develop an updated biomedical model which incorporated the biological, psychological and social.

The biopsychosocial model is still founded within an essentialist theoretical perspective since it does not reject the concept that it is a person's biological 'function' or 'dysfunction' which disables. However, this model advocates that the onset of illness, impairment and disability is complex and is affected by multiple different sociological and psychological factors. Conditions like schizophrenia cannot be entirely reduced to a biochemical deviation experienced by an individual. From the biopsychosocial perspective, the onset of schizophrenia *will* have occurred due to biological conditions: i.e. biochemical genetic properties. However, harmful behaviour may also have triggered the condition: i.e. experience of abuse or substance misuse. Certain social situations may also leave particular groups at greater risk of experiencing these harmful behaviours. As White (2005) illustrates, the biopsychosocial approach is holistic and examines the causal links between the biological, psychological and social to comprehend the onset of disease, illness and impairment. An example of this can be viewed in the work of Garland and Howard (2010):

> The social work profession's historical emphasis on the social environment as the context for individual wellbeing is supported by research over the past decade. Neuroplasticity and psychosocial genomic research indicate that socioenvironmental forces have the potency to alter human wellbeing through their effects on neurobiology.... Indeed, Engel's biopsychosocial paradigm is rooted in the philosophical principle of complementarity . . . instead of the 'either/or' mentality of dualistic reductionism, biopsychosocial research should

embrace a 'both/and' logic, where reports of subjective experience garnered through validated instruments and qualitative interviews are correlated ... [This] can add value to Social Work as a primary mental health and allied-health profession.

(Garland & Howard, 2010, pp. 8–9)

As with the biomedical approach, social work practitioners work alongside health professionals, this time to employ a holistic approach to support service users. Healthcare professionals provide appropriate medical treatment which is supplemented with a care package. The role of the social worker enables appropriate care packages to support a service user's biological (medical), psychological (psychiatric, also medical) and social (social care) needs. Garland and Howard (2010) argue that this model targets the complex and multiple needs of disabled service users to develop an appropriate and effective care model.

Yet the key criticism of this approach is that it individualizes disability and cultivates care packages designed around a person's impairment type. Therefore, a service user who has recently experienced a permanent severe spinal fracture may receive pain relief through medical services; get access to assistive technology, such as a wheelchair; require environmental changes within the home and receive some social care home support. If the person is struggling emotionally to deal with the loss of mobility, they *may* also get access to psychiatric services. Although biopsychosocial practice does provide individualized support, it does not deal with the structural inequalities that, for example, a wheelchair user will face within the wider social context. Thus, the biopsychosocial model *still* medicalizes the experiences of disabled people.

Social models of disability and impairment

The social model of disability has become a significant model within social work practice since Oliver (1983) first defined this approach in his book *Social Work with Disabled People*. Since its emergence in the 1980s and the formation of 'disability studies' as an academic field of inquiry, this approach has led to the rise of what is now defined as 'disability theory'. Since the turn of the 21st century, disability studies have witnessed the emergence of three significant theoretical approaches. These have transformed the social model of disability and led to the formation of alternative models (Barnes, 2012). The social model of disability was originally underpinned by a historical materialist perspective as disability was conceptualized as emerging from social and economic structural barriers which exclude disabled people. As the social model focused entirely on disability (i.e. structural disabling barriers), one of the key criticisms was its lack of attention to the effect that impairment has in a person's life (Shakespeare, 2013).

This criticism has led to the development of two further theoretical approaches underpinned by post-structural (Goodley, 2014) and critical realist theory (Shakespeare, 2015). Hence, the inclusion of impairment became a central concern within disability studies. From the post-structuralist perspective, not only is disability a social construct, but so is impairment. This draws on a linguistic interpretation of disability and impairment, suggesting that both concepts are cultural constructs of medicine based on dialectic binary notions of normative cultural constructions of the body (Goodley, 2014). Critical realism, in contrast, argues for incorporating the concept of biological impairment within a disabling barrier approach, developing an interactionist approach where disability and impairment interrelate (Shakespeare, 2013).

Within disability studies, there has been a significant amount of debate concerning the most effective theoretical approach when conceptualizing disability and impairment within theory and practice. Yet we suggest that social work practitioners are not constrained to one theoretical perspective and should employ an array of approaches to inform practice. The popularity of the biopsychosocial model in social work practice may give the impression of a holistic approach, but this perspective is dominated by a biomedical ideology of disability, and this results in the medicalization of people's abilities and inabilities through professional practice (Oliver & Sapey, 2006; Barnes & Mercer, 2010). We suggest that using different disability studies theories and models can offer social work practitioners different perspectives to embed the *social* rather than the *pathological* explanations of disability. A social worker should demonstrate sociological expertise aimed at understanding, intervention, support and inclusion for service users (Deacon, 2017).

In the following sections, we use examples of our own research, demonstrating how different models and theories of disability can be used to conceptualize the complex nature of support for disabled service users within society. We do not attempt to merge each model of disability but argue that each model is effective depending on the nature and circumstances of a specific service user group, due to the eclectic nature of social work practice (Deacon & Macdonald, 2017).

The social model of disability and historical materialism

The social model of disability initially developed from grassroots disability politics in response to the biomedical model which dominated health and social care in the 1970s and 1980s (Oliver, 2009). The early definition of the social model emerged from an activist group founded by Paul Hunt and Vic Finkelstein called the Union of the Physically Impaired against Segregation (UPIAS). Finkelstein and Hunt suggested that medicine offered them no solutions for overcoming problems associated with their impairments. Both men were wheelchair users and proposed that the problems they experienced were not due to their 'dysfunctional' bodies but rather due to environmental issues that excluded and oppressed them and other disabled people in society.

Oliver (1983) used UPIAS's definition of 'impairment' and 'disability' to identify the 'social model' for social work practitioners. His later work expresses a clear definition of the social model:

> Disability: a disadvantage or restriction of activity caused by a contemporary social organization which takes no or little account of people who have . . . impairments and thus excludes them from the mainstream of social activities.
>
> *(Oliver, 2009, p. 42)*

From this perspective, the problems that disabled people experience are due not to functional limitation but to environmental factors that prevent people with a range of impairments from fully participating in social life. The model was originally designed for people with physical impairments. By the 1990s, however, this expanded to people with sensory as well as intellectual impairments, followed later by individuals from the neuro-diversity and mental health communities. As Barton states:

> An extensive range of research findings has demonstrated the extent of the institutional discrimination which disabled people experience in our society. This involves access and opportunities in relation to work, housing, education, transport, leisure and support services. Thus, the issues go far beyond the notion that the problem is one of individual

disabilist attitudes. These are . . . structured by specific, historical, material conditions and social relations. Goodwill, charity and social services are insufficient to address . . . [these] factors.

(Barton, 1993, p. 242)

The social model led to the formation of disability studies, underpinned by a historical material-ist approach. A key element of this was to represent the voices and experiences of disabled peo-ple. This directly critiques the biomedical model as a system of social exclusion or oppression, which individualizes the social problems experienced by disabled people. An example of this can be seen in our research (Macdonald, 2009, 2012) on the impact that dyslexia has on adult-hood. What is significant is the intersectional relationship between disabling barriers and social class inequalities. The research illustrates how people from lower socio-economic backgrounds experience additional disabling barriers to their middle-class counterparts. This was particularly relevant for the group of participants who had engaged in criminality. Macdonald (2012) iden-tifies that the overrepresentation of service users with dyslexia in the criminal justice system is not due to a pathological link between dyslexia and criminality (Dåderman, Meurling, & Levander, 2012), but rather to structural inequalities. He suggests that more affluent participants had increased access to educational support and knowledge of assistive technologies, allowing them to confront many of the disabling barriers experienced in education and later in adult-hood. Macdonald and Clayton (2016) later further explored the relationship between disability, technology and socio-economic status. They found that disabled people had access to fewer technologies than the non-disabled population and therefore were unable to perceive them as helpful in addressing disabling barriers.

[F]rom an individual model perspective . . . the ability to use ICT depends on impairment (i.e. visual, hearing, motor and cognitive, etc.). Someone with no functional vision is more likely to experience difficulties using the Internet than someone with restricted lower body movement. . . . [A]lthough impairment impacts on how individuals use technology, the authors have presented evidence that there are structural barriers, such as poverty, skills/ knowledge and inaccessibility, which prevent disabled people in this study from using a range of digital technologies. . . . Therefore, if access to digital technologies is only for peo-ple who can afford them, then digital and assistive technologies, rather than benefit disabled people, will create a new level of social inequality reinforcing the digital divide within the United Kingdom. This study concludes by . . . claim[ing] that access to digital technology that helps remove barriers of exclusion for disabled people should be seen as a 'right' rather than a privilege for disabled people.

(Macdonald & Clayton, 2016, pp. 128–129)

Because social workers engage in practice at a micro level, they often miss the macro level (see Chapter 27). The social model enables them to understand what is needed (macro) rather than what is available (micro). These research examples illustrate the intersectional relation-ship between poverty and disability, and as Oliver (2009) suggests, if interventions are devel-oped based on impairment (biomedical), this leads to a one-size-fits-all approach. Our research highlights, however, that people with the same impairment experience very different disabling barriers, depending on their social and economic backgrounds. For example, a disabled person from an upper-middle-class background can afford to purchase additional assistive technologies while those from a lower-class background are subject to what is available through the NHS (Macdonald, 2009; Macdonald & Clayton, 2016). Therefore, their experience of disability is completely transformed by their social position. This requires social work practice to focus on disabling barriers rather than impairment type to take a truly service user perspective.

The social relational model of disability and critical realism

Within the UK, by the 21st century, the social model of disability had offered an alternative theoretical lens through which to conceptualize disability, which transformed research and social work practice (Macdonald, 2017). However, during this time the social model began to attract several criticisms. The first significant critique of the social model could be seen in the work of Liz Crow (1994), a disability activist. She acknowledged the importance of the social model in redefining disability and suggested that it had transformed her identity from a person with a dysfunctional pathology to an individual who belonged to an excluded minority group. She illustrated, however, that although the social model was directed at macro structural inequalities, it completely overlooked the concept of impairment.

> In fact, impairment, at its most basic level, is a purely objective concept which carries no intrinsic meaning. Impairment simply means that aspects of a person's body do not function or they function with difficulty. Frequently this has taken a stage further to imply that a person's body, and ultimately the person, is inferior. However, the first is fact; the second is an interpretation.
>
> *(Crow, 1994, p. 211)*

For Crow, impairment-related issues, such as pain or fatigue, had a significant impact on her experience of disability, so she argues for the necessity of incorporating impairment within the social model of disability. Shakespeare and Watson (2001) then described the social model as an 'outdated ideology'. They suggested that, to develop a theory of disability, one must incorporate both disability (as structural inequality) and impairment (as a physical limitation). Shakespeare and Watson (2001) argued for a dualist perspective; therefore, disability and impairment interact, resulting in disabling factors that impact on disabled people's lives.

> Experientially, impairment is salient to many. As disabled feminists have argued, impairment is part of our daily personal experience, and cannot be ignored in our social theory or our political strategy. Politically, if our analysis does not include impairment, disabled people may be reluctant to identify with the disability movement, and commentators may reject our arguments as being 'idealistic' and ungrounded. We are not just disabled people, we are also people with impairments, and to pretend otherwise is to ignore a major part of our biographies.
>
> *(Shakespeare & Watson, 2001, p. 11)*

Shakespeare (2013) later argues that pain is a significant disabling factor that impacts on people's lives. In his work we see the emergence of critical realism within disability studies. From this perspective, disability is constructed through structural barriers, and impairment relates to functional difficulties that impact on an individual's daily realities. Shakespeare draws on the work of Danermark (2001) and Bhaskar, Danermark, and Price (2017) suggesting that different levels of reality exist concerning disability and impairment. For others, the critical realist approach has been adopted as the 'social relational model of disability' (Ferrie & Watson, 2015). This was initially defined by Thomas (2007) to complement the social model by incorporating the emotional experiences of disability.

Examples of the social relational model can be viewed in our other studies. The impact of diagnosis and labelling is discussed with reference to dyslexia (Macdonald, 2010). In this research, a significant disabling barrier related to participants' lack of access to a diagnosis. Macdonald (2010) rejects the concept that dyslexia is merely a social construct and argues that the condition is both socially constructed and a biological reality. We argue that there are realities which formed the social experiences of participants within this study, and those realities are constructed by the effects of disability *and* impairment. Macdonald and Deacon (2015) extended this study to employ a quantitative approach, exploring the lives of homeless service users with dyslexia from a social relational model perspective. This study illustrates that service users with dyslexia are more prone to long-term addiction problems, are more likely to be processed through the criminal justice system and are at increased risk of self-harm and suicide attempts, when compared to the non-dyslexic homeless population. Yet there had been no attempt to comprehend the impact that dyslexia had on this group. Macdonald and Deacon (2015) argue that social workers must understand the impairment effect as this significantly impacts the specific disabling barriers experienced by homeless people with dyslexia. They illustrated that participants did not have access to specialized adult services relating specifically to their dyslexia; many service users had access to mental health and drug and alcohol support yet dyslexia went completely unnoticed in social work practice.

> [P]eople with dyslexia are overrepresented within the homeless population in the UK. As demonstrated, a number of statistically significant relationships have appeared within the data findings. These findings seem to suggest that for participants with dyslexia, once they become homeless, they have an increased risk of spiralling into the episodic and chronic homeless population. This study does not reject the importance of current support packages with reference to financial stability, drug and alcohol services and mental health support. . . . However, there also seems to be a need for specialist forms of support for dyslexia which is demonstrated in the findings; which requires further research.
>
> *(Macdonald & Deacon, 2015, p. 89)*

Macdonald and Deacon (2015) argue that participants with dyslexia experience significant disabling barriers in adulthood, but these barriers are impairment-related. A key problem for this service user group, therefore, is a lack of services that concentrated on impairment-specific barriers in adult life.

Although Shakespeare (2013) argues for the discontinuation of the social model, replacing it with a social theory, we argue that both models can be useful in different practice settings, taking the social work eclectic approach (Deacon & Macdonald, 2017). From this perspective, the social model of disability is effective when dealing with universal structural barriers, whereas the social relational model can be employed to conceptualize the disabled people's embodied experiences of disability and impairment.

Cultural disability studies and the affirmation model of disability

Further significant critiques of the social model of disability emerged from a cultural perspective, drawing on post-structuralism as a critical linguistic analysis of disability and impairment. From this perspective, impairment, along with disability, is socially constructed; this differs significantly from the critical realist perspective. Cultural disability studies have been considerably influenced by writers such as Davis (1995), Corker (1999) and Goodley (2011). Disability and impairment are conceptualized as linguistic constructs arising from social, economic and cultural ideas at a particular point in time. From a cultural disability studies perspective, medical diagnostic labels are attached to bodies and are medically referred to as impairment types. These labels are not universal or inevitable, but linguistic cultural constructs of a society that problematizes biological abilities according to their economic and cultural value. Medicine presents these diagnostic labels as scientific and objective, but cultural disability studies propose that these labels are produced within a sociocultural political landscape.

> This uneasy transhumanist dance between the binaries of disability/normalcy, deficiency/capacity, essentialism/freedom of choice demonstrates the ethically questionable ambitions of human enhancement when the erasure of disability is implicated. While disability studies recognises the disavowal of disabled people as rejected citizens of wider society, critical ableist studies questions transhumanist ambitions around human improvement and the negation of limited normal humanness.
>
> *(Goodley, 2014, p. 25)*

For Goodley (2014), disability is conceptualized through linguistic binary notions of 'normality' and 'abnormality', which are products of bourgeois moralities. This is justified through medical language which dissects disability into impairment categories and justifies those categories through discourses of universalism and science. Foucault's (2003) work is influential on this approach as medicine is an institution of power which manufactures discourses that categorize physical variations through normative biological measurements (Goodley, 2014). This 'medical gaze' exercises power over its cultural subjects as a system of social control. Therefore, impairment categories exist due to the political, cultural and economic need for particular labels at any given time.

This post-structuralist perspective offers the most radical interpretation of disability and impairment. It develops an oppositional discourse, thus rejecting terms like 'disability' and 'disablism' and replacing them with the concept of ableism. From Goodley's (2014) perspective, disability is now a construct of neo-liberalism, and so the cultural production of this discourse must be examined. Drawing on this perspective, we have applied this radical approach to the study of mental health within social work practice. Macdonald, Charnock, and Scutt (2018) explored the lived experiences of service users who had been diagnosed with a significant mental health problem. These service users had been engaging with services since the 1970s and 1980s, and the research explored how service user lives have changed after deinstitutionalization of care within the UK. The study discovered that discourses around care had changed, but the majority were still living within an institution (i.e. residential care), as well as taking a range of psycho-pharmaceutical medication.

> Although, contemporary psychiatry refers to the dismantling of mental hospitals through the process of deinstitutionalisation . . . there seems to be evidence in this study that there is still the reminiscent of the old hospitals in the current care system. In this study, the long term housing of economically deprived mental health patients is no longer delivered by the hospital, but now is provided by a privately run residential care system. Based on the majority of service user/survivor experiences, the marketisation of mental health services seems not to have led to the deinstitutionalisation of care, but has resulted in the process of trans-institutionalisation where service users/survivors have been moved from state owned to privately run care units.
>
> *(Macdonald et al., 2018, p. 27)*

In this study, service users' lives were significantly affected by institutional environments which controlled every aspect of their lives administratively. Although service users were free to leave their institutional care homes at any time of the day, few reported engaging in any activities outside the residential setting. Although the discourse of 'cure' was discussed, participants had been receiving medication as a form of therapy for 30 to 50 years. The key conclusion of this study was that although the large mental hospitals were closed during the period of deinstitutionalization, these were replaced by smaller residential care homes within the community. Therefore, the discourse of institutionalization has changed, but the practice has stayed the same. Macdonald et al. (2018) found that the discourse of 'cure' was used to justify the use of medication over a long period of time and in an institutional setting. Hence, the discourse of 'cure' has developed into a practice of social and political control.

Although cultural disability studies offer a radical perspective to question every aspect of medicalization, this approach can be associated with the development of the affirmation model of disability. Although it was initially defined by Swain and French (2010), Cameron (2011) provides a clear definition. For him, the construction of normality is a cultural performance which relates to a given set of societal norms. Within bourgeois culture, normality is celebrated where (dis)ability is commiserated. Drawing on a linguistic perspective, this model confronts negative connotations associated with (dis)ability as a tragedy in order to celebrate (dis)abled people through minority status.

> Disability [refers to] a personal and social role which simultaneously invalidates the subject position of people with impairments and validates the subject position of those identified as normal.
>
> *(Cameron, 2011, p. 20)*

From this perspective, the (dis)abled pathologies are constructed through the notion of abnormality, therefore validating the role of normality in society. Linguistic norms are produced in a historically specific cultural setting. So, for Cameron, if disability and impairment are culturally and historically constructed, then, in effect, this can be changed. He conceptualizes impairment through the notion of *difference* rather than as a personal and *social tragedy*.

From a social work perspective, cultural disability studies offer a radical critical discourse which questions all aspects of professional practice concerning disability. For the most part, this criticism has developed with reference to mental health services, particularly around medication and hospitalization (LeFrancois, Menzies, & Reaume, 2013; LeFrancois, 2017). Again, social work is viewed as an ally of medical practice and engages in dominant medical discourses which exercise disciplinary power to make service users engage with (pharmaceutical) treatment and place many disabled people in institutional settings (Macdonald et al., 2018). Not only does a cultural disability studies perspective offer social work a critical toolkit to interrogate concepts such as disability and impairment within professional practice, but it also gives us a model that can celebrate human and biological diversity within society. From this perspective, because culture constructs notions of disability and impairment, these meanings can be altered through radical ideas and practices.

Conclusion

The aim of this chapter is to present a range of perspectives which allow social work practitioners to understand and apply different theoretical lenses to support disabled service users and develop services. The chapter has outlined the dominant biopsychosocial approach which is employed globally within social work practice. We have suggested that this model is an extension of the traditional biomedical approach in contemporary practice. The biopsychosocial model, we argue, medicalizes service users' abilities and inabilities by conceptualizing disabilities through the notion of pathological dysfunction. This also allows an over-simplistic approach, which reinforces the current neoliberalization of social work practice, meaning that social work practitioners manage disability through services aimed at the biological (medicine), the psychological (psychiatric services) and the social (social care). From this position, the social work practitioner may perceive that they have successfully assessed and commissioned services based on a holistic approach to support the needs of a disabled service user. However, as medicine dominates, this applies a disease model in treatment and support of people with a range of impairments. We argue in this chapter that, although the biomedical has been renamed as the biopsychosocial model, this operates to individualize and medicalize social work practice.

Although we have illustrated the biomedical models, we do not advocate the use of these approaches for practice. Rather, we have presented examples of the authors' research which identifies alternative approaches to conceptualizing and supporting disabled people within the community, based on social models of disability. These models, which have emerged from disability studies, are often presented as opposing theoretical perspectives when defining disability. The authors argue, however, that these approaches can be complementary if used as part of the practitioner's eclectic toolkit. As Deacon (2017) suggests, social work theory consists of a range of possibilities, from neoliberal individualism to radical psychological and sociological constructionism. The aim of the social work practitioner is to devise and apply an eclectic toolkit to understand behaviours and facilitate effective and inclusive interventions, achieved through anti-discriminatory practice. Practice *must*, however, be facilitated by theoretical perspectives that are grounded within research (Deacon & Macdonald, 2017), as demonstrated in this chapter.

Shakespeare (2018) argues that disability studies have progressed in three waves. The first is the formation of the social model (in the work of, for example, Barnes, Finkelstein, Oliver); the second refers to debates around the impact of impairment (Shakespeare, Thomas, Watson) and the third refers to the cultural constructions of (dis)ability and impairment (Davis, Goodley). This chapter proposes a fourth wave to disability studies based on a post-positivist perspective, where theoretical and qualitative explorations, using disabled people's experiences, are quantified to progress representative evidence-based research to facilitate professional social work practice. Therefore, this study concludes by suggesting that the role of social work practitioners is not to be the silent partners of health professions, but rather to be social experts equipped to deal with complex social problems in everyday practice. What is unique about disability theory is that the theoretical knowledge which emerges from research has been produced in partnership with disabled people. The authors argue that rather than applying an updated biomedical model (i.e. the biopsychosocial model) to professional practice, social work practitioners can use a range of sociologically informed theoretical perspectives to facilitate inclusion and social change for disabled service users.

Further reading

Goodley, D. (2014). *Dis/ability studies: Theorising disablism and ableism*. Oxford: Routledge.

Oliver, M., Sapey, B. J., & Thomas, P. (2012). *Social work with disabled people* (4th ed.). London: Palgrave Macmillan.

Shakespeare, T. (2013). *Disability rights and wrongs revisited* (2nd ed.). Oxford: Routledge.

References

Bamford, T. (2015). *A contemporary history of social work: Learning from the past.* Bristol: Policy Press.

Barnes, C. (2010). A brief history of discrimination and disabled people. In L. J. Davis (Ed.), *The disability studies reader* (3rd ed., pp. 20–32). Oxford: Routledge.

Barnes, C. (2012). Understanding the social model of disability: Past, present and future. In N. Watson, A. Roulstone, & C. Thomas (Eds.), *Routledge handbook of disability studies* (pp. 12–29). London: Routledge.

Barnes, H., Green, L., & Hopton, J. (2007). Social work theory, research, policy and practice: Challenges and opportunities in health and social care integration in the UK. *Health and Social Care in the Community*, *15*(3), 191–194.

Barnes, C., & Mercer, G. (2010). *Exploring disability: A sociological introduction* (2nd ed.). Cambridge, UK: Polity Press.

Barton, L. (1993). The struggle for citizenship: The case of disabled people. *Disability, Handicap & Society*, *8*(3), 235–248.

Berzoff, J., & Drisko, J. (2015). What clinical social workers need to know: Bio-psycho-social knowledge and skills for the twenty first century. *Clinical Social Work Journal*, *43*, 263–273.

Bhaskar, R., Danermark, B., & Price, L. (2017). *Interdisciplinarity and wellbeing.* London: Routledge.

Cameron, C. (2011). Not our problem: Impairment as difference, disability as role. *Journal of Inclusive Practice in Further and Higher Education*, *3*(2), 10–25.

Corker, M. (1999). Differences, conflations and foundations: The limits to 'accurate' theoretical representation of disabled people's experience? *Disability and Society*, *14*(5), 627–642.

Crow, L. (1994). Including all of our lives: Renewing the social model of disability. In C. Barnes & G. Mercer (Eds.), *Exploring the divide* (pp. 55–72). Leeds: Disability Press.

Dåderman, A. M., Meurling, A. W., & Levander, S. (2012). 'Speedy action over goal orientation': Cognitive impulsivity in male forensic patients with dyslexia. *Dyslexia*, *18*(4), 226–235.

Danermark, B. (2001). Interdisciplinary research and critical realism: The example of disability research. *Interdisciplinary Research*, *4*, 56–64.

Davis, L. J. (1995). *Enforcing normalcy: Disability, deafness, and the body.* New York: Verso.

Deacon, L. (2017). Introduction to social work theory. In L. Deacon & S. J. Macdonald (Eds.), *Social work theory and practice* (pp. 5–10). London: Sage.

Deacon, L., & Macdonald, S. J. (2017). *Social work theory and practice.* London: Sage.

Engel, G. (1977). The need for a new medical model: A challenge to biomedicine. *Science*, *196*, 129–136.

Ferrie, J., & Watson, N. (2015). The psycho-social impact of impairments: The case of motor neurone disease. In T. Shakespeare (Ed.), *Disability research today: International perspectives* (pp. 185–203). Oxford: Routledge.

Foucault, M. (2003). *Abnormal: Lectures at the college de France 1974–1975.* London: Verso.

Garland, G., & Howard, M. O. (2010). Neuroplasticity, psychosocial genomics, and the biopsychosocial paradigm in the 21st century. *Health Social Work*, *34*(3), 191–199.

Goodley, D. (2011). *Disability studies: An interdisciplinary introduction.* London: Sage.

Goodley, D. (2014). *Dis/ability studies: Theorising disablism and ableism.* Oxford: Routledge.

LeFrancois, B. (2017). *Mad studies: Maddening social work.* New Brunswick: St Thomas University.

LeFrancois, B., Menzies, R., & Reaume, G. (2013). *Mad matters: A critical reader in Canadian mad studies.* Toronto: Canadian Scholars Press.

Macdonald, S. J. (2009). Windows of reflection from adults with dyslexia: Conceptualising dyslexia using the social model of disability. *Dyslexia*, *15*(4), 347–362.

Macdonald, S. J. (2010). Towards a social reality of dyslexia. *British Journal of Learning Disabilities*, *38*(1), 21–30.

Macdonald, S. J. (2012). Biographical pathways into criminality: Understanding the relationship between dyslexia and educational disengagement. *Disability and Society*, *27*(3), 427–440.

Macdonald, S. J. (2017). Five models of disability. In L. Deacon & S. J. Macdonald (Eds.), *Social work theory and practice* (pp. 174–186). London: Sage.

Macdonald, S. J., Charnock, A., & Scutt, J. (2018). Marketing 'madness': Conceptualising service user/survivors biographies in a period of deinstitutionalisation. *Disability and Society*.

Macdonald, S. J., & Clayton, J. (2016). Back to the future, disability and the digital divide. In A. Roulstone, A. Sheldon, & J. Harris (Eds.), *Disability and technology* (pp. 114–130). Oxford: Routledge.

Macdonald, S. J., & Deacon, L. (2015). 'No sanctuary': Missed opportunities in health and social services for homeless service users with dyslexia. *Social Work and Social Sciences Review*, *17*(2), 22–56.

Maynard, B. R., Boutwell, B. B., & Vaughn, M. G. (2016). Advancing the science of social work: The case for biosocial research. *British Journal of Social Work, 47*(5), 1572–1586.

O'Brien, G. V. (2011). Eugenics, genetics, and the minority group model of disabilities: Implications for social work advocacy. *Social Work, 56*(4), 347–354.

Oliver, M. (1983). *Social work with disabled people.* Basingstoke: Palgrave Macmillan.

Oliver, M. (2009). *Understanding disability: From theory to practice* (2nd ed.). Basingstoke: Palgrave Macmillan.

Oliver, M., & Sapey, B. J. (2006.). *Social work with disabled people* (3rd ed.). Basingstoke: Palgrave Macmillan.

Patton, M. (2002). *Qualitative research and evaluation methods* (3rd ed.). Thousand Oaks, CA: Sage.

Semple, D., Smyth, R., Burns, J., Darjee, R., & McInrosh, A. (2013). *Oxford handbook of psychiatry* (2nd ed.). Oxford: Oxford University Press.

Simmons, H. G. (1978). Explaining social policy: The English mental deficiency act of 1913. *Journal of Social History, 11*(3), 387–403.

Shakespeare, T. (2013). *Disability rights and wrongs revisited* (2nd ed.). Oxford: Routledge.

Shakespeare, T. (Ed.). (2015). *Disability research today: International perspectives.* Oxford: Routledge.

Shakespeare, T. (2018). *Disability: The basics.* Oxford: Routledge.

Shakespeare, T., & Watson, N. (2001). The social model of disability: An outdated ideology? In S. N. Barnartt & B. M. Altman (Eds.), *Exploring theories and expanding methodologies: Where we are and where we need to go* (pp. 9–28). London: Emerald.

Shakespeare, T., Watson, N., & Abu Alghaib, O. (2016). Blaming the victim, all over again: Waddell and Aylward's biopsychosocial (BPS) model of disability. *Critical Social Policy, 36*(4), 1–20.

Swain, J., & French, S. (2010). Towards an affirmation model of disability. *Disability and Society, 15*(4), 569–582.

Szasz, T. (1974). *The myth of mental illness: Foundations of a theory of personal conduct.* New York: HarperCollins.

Thomas, C. J. (2007). *Sociologies of disability and illness: Contested ideas in disability studies and medical sociology.* Basingstoke: Palgrave Macmillan.

White, P. (Ed.). (2005). *Biopsychosocial medicine.* Oxford: Oxford University Press.

Williams, M. (2003). *Making sense of social research.* London: Sage.

39

Accommodating cognitive differences

New ideas for social work with people with intellectual disabilities

Christine Bigby

People with intellectual disabilities are one of the most disadvantaged groups in Western societies with high rates of poverty, social exclusion and abuse (Bigby & Frawley, 2010). Mainstream service systems continue to fail them by not adjusting to their cognitive differences, and they are poorly positioned to benefit from the neoliberal changes to welfare states that offer self-direction over individualized services. More so than other groups, people with intellectual disabilities need trusting relationships and skilled support to claim resources, direct their own services and exercise rights as citizens to live good lives of their own choosing (Ellem, O'Connor, Wilson, & Williams, 2013; O'Connor, 2014). Social work, as the lead profession in human services, should play a key role in this by ensuring enabling individual support, challenging disabling social structures and securing the resources to redress social exclusion and other inequities. To achieve this, social workers must adapt their own direct practice and have the capacity to critically analyze social systems to identify levers for building the capacity of communities to be inclusive.

Despite the alignment of social work values and principles with rights-led disability policy, there is little social work–specific scholarship in this field (Bigby, 2013). The neglect of intellectual disability as a field of practice is compounded by the marginalization of people with intellectual disabilities in the disability rights movement and the emerging discipline of critical disability studies. Influential ideas, however, from this and other disciplines, are potentially applicable to issues of equity for people with intellectual disabilities and social work practice.

The social model of disability (Oliver, 1990; see Chapter 40), normalization (Brown & Smith, 1992) and deinstitutionalization (Mansell & Ericsson, 1996) were key influences during last decades of the 20th century. In the 21st century, they have been replaced by critical realist and relational models of disability (Shakespeare, 2014), theorizing about human rights (Carney, 2015) and new ideas about social inclusion from critical democratic theory and urban geography (Clifford Simplican, 2015). These new perspectives revolve around 'dilemmas of difference' (Stainton, 2002), which form a core theme of the chapter and pose questions such as:

> How to treat a person as an individual with equal rights and expectations of a quality of life similar to other citizens without disregarding their impairment or their need for

specific adaptations and support to attain equal outcomes. Yet in taking their impairment into account and drawing on knowledge about the category of 'intellectual disability' not marking the individual out as different from others or creating obstacles to their inclusion.

(Bigby & Frawley, 2010, p. 109)

A second interrelated theme of the chapter is that of 'dedifferentiation' – a recent trend of including people with intellectual disabilities as members of a broader undifferentiated group of people with disability and thus obscuring particular needs associated with cognitive impairment (Clegg & Bigby, 2017). Grappling with complex questions about if, when or how to respond to cognitive differences is not new in this field. Debates, however, are tainted with past failures, when too often recognition of difference had negative implications for people with intellectual disabilities, including exclusion from the class of rational people eligible for citizenship, removal of decision-making rights, incarceration in institutions, stigmatization and segregated second class services. The ideas discussed in this chapter provide more promising avenues for negotiating recognition and accommodations, as well as interacting across cognitive difference to realize the equal moral worth of people with intellectual disabilities. I explore these ideas and some of the limited empirical research they have spawned and consider implications for social work practice.

Putting impairment back in understandings of disability – critical realism

The social model reviewed in Chapter 40 was a blunt instrument for social work practice with people with intellectual disabilities. It exemplifies a dedifferentiated approach, theoretically including all people with a disability without attention to specific impairment groups. Yet most analyses implicitly only considered people without cognitive impairment. Goodley (2001) suggests that omission of people with intellectual disabilities from social model theorizing risks them being 'left in the realms of static, irreversible, individualized biology' (p. 212). For example, design of independent living schemes championed by social model theorists assumed the capacity of people with disability to hire and self-direct personal assistants through peer-led organizations. Very few social model scholars considered needs associated with independent living beyond personal care, such as support to express preferences, make decisions or form and negotiate relationships. Also largely ignored was overlaying complexity that cognitive impairment brings to self-directing support, so well described by Askheim (2003). Indeed, the limited research in this field suggests that social workers have felt ill equipped and reluctant to embrace individualized funding arrangements for people with intellectual disabilities (Sims & Gulyurtlu, 2014).

Little exploration has occurred of the subtle and less visible disabling barriers that more specifically affect people with intellectual disability, such as dominance of the written word to convey information, shift to multiskilling, loss of unskilled jobs and increasing reliance on inflexible technology to answer phones, pay bills or purchase tickets rather than direct or face-to-face encounters to transact public and private business. Notably, however, some research using a social model approach has drawn attention to the essentialist nature of impairment-saturated individualized models of disability that ignore intersections of class, race or gender. For example, the work of Llewellyn, Traustadottir, McConnell, and Signurjondsdottir (2010) on parents with intellectual disability identifies the way many of the problems they experience are sheeted back to intellectual impairment and poor mothering skills rather than the disabling impact of poverty, limited support and social networks.

More nuanced theoretical models of disability reviewed in Chapter 40 take greater account of the intertwining effects of impairment with socially constructed barriers to participation. Perhaps most important to the field of intellectual disability is the critical realist understanding of disability propelled to prominence by Shakespeare's (2006, p. 55) critique of the social model. Critical realism understands disability as 'an interaction between factors intrinsic to the individual, and extrinsic factors arising from the wider context'. Thus, people are disabled by both impairments and social arrangements that do not take account of impairments – the discriminatory structures and limiting social attitudes that compound the difficulties of low intellectual capacity, depriving people of rights, respect and dignity. This theory locates the causes of disability across multiple levels – the biological, social and cultural. It is similar to relational models of disability used by Scandinavian scholars (Gustavsson, 2004) and resembles in some respects the generic socio-ecological framework familiar to social workers.

Critical realism, like the social model of disability, takes a social justice perspective, seeking to explain phenomena in a way that leads to 'consideration of right conduct and the good life' (Houston, 2010, p. 74; see Chapter 11). It provides an important theoretical lens for social work practice with people with intellectual disabilities, holding together contrasting perspectives: consideration of real-world implications of individual limitations without locating the problem solely with the individual whilst also drawing out the disabling impact of social structures and the way society regards and interprets differences (Morgan, 2012).

Recognizing implications of cognitive impairment on life experiences and on how people learn, their capacity to understand ideas or language, make choices and judgements and manage social relationships and tasks of everyday living is important to all aspects of social work practice. It helps shape the types of private problems and public issues in interacting with social systems that people with intellectual disability experience. Such understanding gives insights into individual support or advocacy needs, as well as possibilities for community capacity building. O'Connor (2014), for example, illustrates the difficulties people with mild intellectual disability have in explaining their aspirations and needs during individualized planning or assessment processes. Partly, he suggests, this stems from limited experiences, limited understanding or communication difficulties, but also from a tendency to misrepresent their abilities in order to present well – something that is important for people with a history of failing and being looked down upon for non-achievement. As it becomes clearer that those with social capital benefit most from personalized service systems, O'Connor's reflections reinforce the significance of 'deep listening' to understand core messages about needs and the type of active approach to relationship and network building in practice with people with mild intellectual disabilities described by Ellem et al. (2013).

The finding that 37 percent of deaths of people with intellectual disability were avoidable, compared to 13 percent for the general population (Heslop et al., 2014) illustrates the imperatives of adjusting health systems to better accommodate their needs. While ways of embedding adjustments are found, individual support is critical to negotiate systems that assume patients are competent, self-managing consumers of services (Iacono & Bigby, 2016). The UK trial of named social workers is one example of a potential role of social work in adapting systems to accommodate people with intellectual disabilities, though the boundaries, practice skills and outcomes are yet to be explicated (James, Morgan, & Mitchell, 2017).

Craig's critical realist analysis of participation in community groups vividly illustrates the impact of social structures – durable, enduring patterns of behaviour, social rules and norms – on inclusion of people with intellectual disability (Craig, 2013; Craig & Bigby, 2015a, 2015b). Initially, she describes the visible processes at play, such as a differentiated response by group leaders who treated people with intellectual disability differently from any other new member, voicing concerns about the person fitting in or being manageable for the group; the imposition of conditions for attendance, such as being accompanied by a support worker and group processes of discernment about the viability of a person's participation that were influenced by factors such as members' expectations about whether this was the right place for a person with intellectual disability to be, where responsibility for their inclusion lay, and their familiarity with intellectual disability, as well as the skills and characteristics of the person themselves. For example, volunteers in a charity shop selling secondhand goods felt the shop was not the right place for a person with intellectual disability to be; rather, he should attend the 'special places built with the funds raised by the shop'. In this setting, too, the kindness of volunteers precluded giving direct feedback to the person about expected behaviour, hindering his capacity to change it. A second layer of analysis identified invisible generative and more structural mechanisms at various levels that underpinned entry pathways to groups and discernment processes. These are illustrated in Table 39.1.

Classification, protectionism and role differentiation worked against active participation of people with intellectual disabilities while meaningful contact, authority support, empathy and perspective taking promoted it. This analysis uncovered some of the deeply embedded structural obstacles to participation that must be tackled to bring about social change. It provides tools for analyzing potential inclusiveness of groups and suggests points of leverage for enabling individual participation, such provision of expert knowledge to assist group members deal with uncertainties about interactions and the key function of integrating activities in facilitating meaningful contact (Craig & Bigby, 2015a). This study demonstrates the analytical and professional skills required to support inclusion of people with intellectual disability in mainstream groups and possibilities for social workers in leading this type of practice. Too often, simplistic approaches

Table 39.1 Summary of generative key mechanisms of inclusion operating in a community group context

Domain	Mechanism	Operation in group context	Outcomes within group context for people with intellectual disability
Domain of polity/ economy	Classification (competence level)	Expectations	Beliefs about right place or wrong place. Designation to lowest (disability-specific) group.
Domain of culture	Protectionism	Inaccuracy of feedback	Protected from truth about effects of behaviour. Unable to adjust to group norms.
Domain of social settings	Role differentiation Authority support	Taking responsibility Positive leadership response	Allocation of responsibility for support to designated role rather than whole group. Shaped positive attitudes towards them and their right to be part of the group. Supported norm of acceptance in group.
Domain of situated activity	Meaningful contact	Familiarity	Reduced anxiety and confidence in interactions with person. Being seen as an individual rather stereotyped.
Domain of the person	Empathy Perspective taking	Kindness	Experienced a quality of warmth and genuineness in interactions.

Source: adapted from Craig (2013)

to supporting participation rely on support workers as companions rather than facilitators and fail to build the capacity of organizations, leading to presence rather than participation of people with intellectual disabilities (Wiesel & Bigby, 2014).

Human rights and supported decision-making

Rights discourses have powerfully influenced thinking about the position of people with intellectual disabilities. The 1971 United Nations Declaration on the Rights of Mentally Retarded [sic] Persons articulated rights to a decent standard of living, typical lifestyles and legal protection from abuse (United Nations, 1971). Decades later, the 2006 United Nations Convention on the Rights of Persons with Disabilities (the Convention), ratified by 174 countries, has reinvigorated debate about rights. On one hand, the Convention illustrates the strength of a dedifferentiated approach by addressing the collective interests of people with disabilities. On the other, it has led to unprecedented attention to the right of people with intellectual disabilities to make decisions about their own lives. In particular, Article 12, which addresses equity before the law, has been a catalyst for theorizing about legal provisions for supported decision-making and its underpinning practices (Bach, 2017; Carney & Beaupert, 2013).

Article 12 of the Convention asserts that all people with disabilities have the right to equal recognition as persons before the law and should enjoy legal capacity on an equal basis with others and obligates states to provide access to the support required to exercise legal capacity as well as safeguards against coercion. Interpretations of Article 12 suggest it breaks a connection between mental capacity and legal capacity – asserting the 'right to have rights' and make decisions about one's life regardless of cognitive ability. This is a landmark proposition as philosophical and political theorists have traditionally constructed the prerequisites for legal capacity as possession of rational thought, self-determination, independence or autonomy (Stainton, 1994). Failure to meet linguistic and cognitive norms has justified the exclusion of people with intellectual disabilities from full citizenship and removal of decision-making rights through guardianship or other regimes of substitute decision-making. Bach (2017, p. 4) invokes the term 'cognitive foreigners' to illustrate the exclusion experienced by people with intellectual disabilities based on mental capacity, as a result of cognitive ableism.

Article 12 brings to the fore philosophical ideas about relational autonomy and interdependence and is associated with promoting the concept of supported decision-making first developed in Canada in the 1990s (Gordon, 2000). Supported decision-making is founded on propositions that everyone has the right to self-determination and to exercise legal capacity and can express choices with the support in trusting relationships. The roles of supporters are to explain issues, explore options and support the expression of preferences (Carney & Beaupert, 2013). For people with more severe intellectual disabilities, this may involve interpreting signs and preferences, ascribing agency to a person's actions or co-constructing preferences (Series, 2015). Bach (2017, p. 11) summarizes supported decision-making as 'support needed to complement unique decision making abilities sufficient to exercise power over our lives and legal relationships . . . an interdependent way to exercise legal capacity with the communicative and interpretative assistance of trusted others'.

An example of a formal supported decision-making scheme is Representation Agreements found in British Columbia, Canada (Stainton, 2016). The flexible definition of mental capacity in this scheme enables people more commonly considered by the law to be incapable of entering into contracts to appoint a representative to assist them to make decisions and, if necessary, make decisions on their behalf. Such agreements give formal recognition to supporters and decision-making as a shared process.

Supported decision-making challenges the individual nature of decision-making and the idea that autonomy can only be exercised independently. It draws out the significance of enabling environments and personal relationships for people with intellectual disabilities (Wong, Clare, Holland, Watson, & Gunn, 2000), reflecting feminist conceptions of relational agency and autonomy that contend 'beliefs, values and decisions that inform autonomous acts are constituted within social relations of interdependence' (Mackenzie & Stoljar, 2000). Silvers and Francis (2009, p. 485) use the term 'prosthetic rationality' to draw an analogy between the support of a prosthetic limb and supporting a person to make decisions or express preferences. They explain that 'a trustee's reasoning and communicating can execute part or all of subject's own thinking processes without substituting the trustee's own ideas as if they were subject's own'.

Supported decision-making schemes have not yet replaced provisions for substitute decision-making in most jurisdiction. Reasons for this include issues of risk – fears about the vulnerability of people with cognitive impairment to coercion and abuse and the absence of empirical evidence about practice. Nevertheless, it has influenced ways of thinking about decision support which occurs in many contexts. These include intentionally established groups such as circles of support or micro boards or the preexisting individual formal or informal support relationships between people with intellectual disability and their families, friends or professionals. Expectations are clearly shifting towards a more rights-based approach to all decision support, placing a greater onus on supporters to acknowledge and respect the will, preference and rights of the person with cognitive impairment. This is illustrated, for example, by the principles and resources developed by law reform commissions and human service systems to guide decision support and better hold supporters to account (Australian Law Reform Commission, 2014; Department of Health, 2007)

Various schemes in Australia and elsewhere have trialled capacity-building programmes for formal and informal decision supporters of people with intellectual disabilities (Bigby et al., 2017). Positive outcomes have been reported for both supporters and decision makers and much has been learned about the viability, but resource-intense nature, of recruiting volunteer supporters and the value of access to advice for supporters. Research about the processes of decision-making support is beginning to identify key elements of good practice (Douglas, Bigby, Knox, & Browning, 2015), which are captured in the iterative framework of steps, principles and strategies developed by Bigby and Douglas (2016) illustrated in Figure 39.1.

Research, however, suggests a significant gap between theory and practice. Support for decision-making too often remains infused with paternalism, undue influence and risk avoidance, which override good intentions about respect for rights, will and preferences. Shifting decision support practices from outdated paradigms of best interests is a major task confronting the field. The principles of supported decision-making and knowledge about what constitutes good support for decision-making practice are important tools for social workers to contribute to this change.

Some aspects of supported decision-making, such as person-centredness and co-creation of preferences with trusted supporters, are already familiar to social workers as they resemble aspects of person-centred planning, user-led assessment and constructivist social work (Parton & O'Byrne, 2000). What supported decision-making offers, however, is a framework for practice more specific to people with intellectual disabilities, many of whom cannot easily articulate their feelings or preferences in a spoken dialogue and do not have strong networks of informal supporters to help them do so. Importantly, too, supported decision-making offers social workers a point of reference for judging the quality of decision support available to their clients with intellectual disabilities and alerting them to issues of coercion or undue influence or, indeed, the absence of needed support. This rights framework coalesces with the profession's code of ethics. It serves as another reminder, considering the multiple abuses uncovered by scandals and enquiries in recent years, that social work must rebuild its reputation as a 'trustworthy profession', and

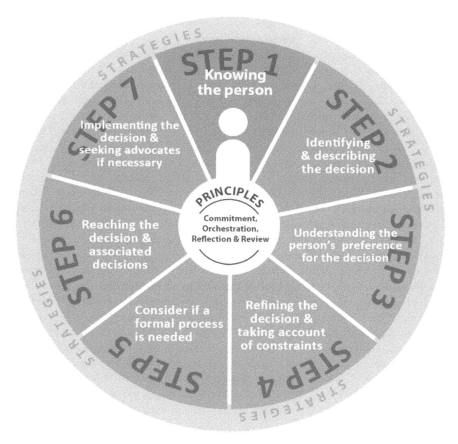

Figure 39.1   Support for decision-making: iterative steps, strategies and principles

every member must be 'courageous in speaking out about abuses of power that impact on the lives of people who use our services' (Healy, 2017, p. 7). The educational resources developed around supported decision-making which incorporate strategies for enabling risk will also assist social workers who occupy safeguarding roles and in building the capacity of supporters as well as holding them to account (Douglas & Bigby, 2018; http://www.enablingriskresource.com. au/; http://www.supportfordecisionmakingresource.com.au/).

Not just fitting in – disruptive ideas about social inclusion

Inclusion in the mainstream has been a policy ambition for people with intellectual disability since the 1970s. Initially driven by normalization and subsequently social role valorization theory, social inclusion was conceptualized as having 'an ordinary life in the community' – occupying valued social roles, relationships with community members and being part of the mainstream. These theories have been heavily critiqued for devaluing diversity and expecting people with intellectual disabilities to fit into existing social patterns (Brown & Smith, 1992).

Interpretations of inclusion have proliferated in the last two decades, turning it into a more ambiguous concept, hard to measure or design strategies to achieve. Nevertheless, there are enduring, and some would argue flawed, assumptions about the types of communities in which people with intellectual disabilities should be included and the underlying purposes of inclusion as creating a sense of value and belonging for individuals (Clifford Simplican, 2015). Critiques from political philosophy and urban geography are exposing assumptions and proposing new, more diverse ways of thinking about inclusion.

Clifford Simplican (2015) argues a communitarian ethos has dominated the meaning of inclusion through an emphasis on belonging to 'the community', where expectation of shared values and norms pervades self-identities of individuals. Privileging belonging to the mainstream and relationships with people without disabilities, communitarianism stifles thinking about difference. Effectively, it overlooks the interests of minority groups and, in the case of people with intellectual disabilities, the existence and significance of relationships with peers and the hurtfulness of the rejection they often experience and leaves little room for choice or voice about inclusion. These shortcomings are clearly captured in the paper aptly titled 'Whose "ordinary life" is it anyway?' (Brown & Smith, 1989).

Clifford Simplican (2015) uses radical democratic theory and its concern with the plurality of communities and centrality of difference, power and conflict to social life to offer non-normative understandings of inclusion. As she explains, central to her argument is 'how the creation of an "us" always implies a "them". The democratic paradox between abstract universal equality and [reality of] an exclusionary democratic community – is inescapable, and yet productive; the commitment to universal liberal equality enables citizens to challenge exclusion' (p. 722). Rather than people with intellectual disabilities being excluded from 'the community', her analysis sees inclusion as more fluid, opening up possibilities of belonging to multiple communities, based on self-identity, interest and preference as occurs for other minority groups. She draws attention to the procedural mechanisms put in place to challenge exclusion, such as monitoring processes for the Convention. Paradoxically, this and similar mechanisms, such as self-advocacy groups and employment of people with intellectual disabilities as advisors and representatives on reference groups, may also open competing forms of self-identification by strengthening participants' sense of belonging to alternative communities of excluded groups.

Inclusion, understood as being part of communities based on self-identity as a person with intellectual disability, or being excluded resemble the notion of counter publics in radical democratic theory. Here, 'a sense of belonging emerges against a backdrop of exclusion' (Clifford Simplican & Leader, 2015, p. 724). A similar perspective has emerged from social geographers who suggest, for people with intellectual disability, the most important part of community participation is the 'experiences of being there'. In response to their findings about the predominantly discriminatory and exclusionary experiences in the mainstream community echoed in many other studies, Milner and Kelly (2009, p. 59) suggest that people with intellectual disabilities will find community 'within self-authored segregated spaces and activities that celebrate the culturally distinctive mores of people with disabilities or harness their collective agency'. Indeed, empirical research is beginning to illustrate how segregated groups, based around activities such as drama, sports or self-advocacy, may be places of community for people with intellectual disability where, through participation, they gain a sense of identity and belonging. Reflecting Mouffe's paradox of democracy, while participation in a community of peers is important, the sense of belonging or identity derived as an artist, athlete or advocate also facilitates participation in other, perhaps more mainstream communities, through activities such as advocacy, exhibitions or sports carnivals (Bigby, Anderson, & Cameron, 2018). Anderson and Bigby (2018), for example, highlight the subtle radicalism that activities as a self-advocate bring about in community perceptions of the capabilities of people with intellectual disabilities.

However, such non-normative understandings of inclusion bring conundrums; they rely on choice and self-identification as a person with intellectual disability. The stigma associated with intellectual disability means some people with mild impairments reject being labelled in this way. For them, membership in anything other than the mainstream may not be acceptable. Notably, in Anderson's study, although members of self-advocacy groups, participants did not embrace an identity as people with intellectual disability but rather a mix of alternative excluded and mainstream identities – self-advocate, independent person, expert and businesslike person. Choice is pivotal; without it, there is the risk of reinventing the ghettoization of people with intellectual disabilities on the basis of externally assigned category.

Rather different new ideas about inclusion come from urban geography building on the proposal that fluid social networks now characterize modern cities, replacing place-based conceptions of communities with deep social ties (Wiesel & Bigby, 2016). The concept of 'convivial encounters' breaks the binary created by normalization between community presence (being in the mainstream) and community participation (having lasting relationships with other community members). Convivial encounters are neither free mingling in public places nor social

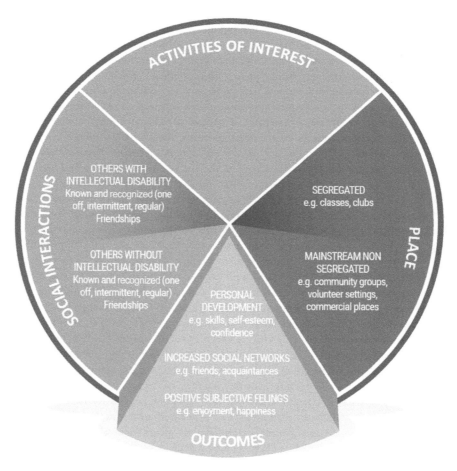

Figure 39.2   Heuristic of components and outcomes of community participation

interactions based on long-term relationships, but moments of pleasantness and warmth when people come together with a transitory shared identity or participate in a shared activity (Wiesel & Bigby, 2016). They can be fleeting and singular, such as an exchange in the supermarket queue; intermittent, such as recognition and greeting by the proprietor or other patrons at a local shop or longer and episodic, such as regular exchanges with other participants in a yoga class. Encounters for people with intellectual disability are important in themselves, signalling their recognition and being known as people with the right to be in mainstream places, but also hold potential for them to develop into lasting or deeper relationships. Research on how convivial encounters are supported or obstructed by supporters and difficult moments of social uncertainty negotiated provide important insights into skills necessary for practice (Bigby & Wiesel, 2015).

New ideas about inclusion take far greater account of cognitive difference and potential for inclusion in multiple and different communities. They suggest diverse combinations of places, activities and social interactions that constitute inclusion, which are illustrated in Figure 39.2.

These ideas suggest the importance of self-identity and choice to realizing inclusion, reinforcing the significance to practice of supported decision-making and trusted supporters who know a person well. From a collective perspective, they signal the need for representation and the voice of people with intellectual disabilities in debates about inclusion, monitoring, questioning progress and developing strategies. Hearing both collective and individual voices of people with intellectual disability will fundamentally challenge social workers in whatever role they occupy as expectations rise about user-led design of individualized support and co-production of programs, policies, education and research through participatory methods. In all of these endeavours, skilled accommodations are needed to enable communication across cognitive differences. Inevitably, the voices of people with mild impairments are easier to hear, and it behoves social workers to avoid common tendencies to use this group as a proxy for everyone by finding ways to amplify the voices of people with more severe and profound intellectual disabilities. Their collective and distinct needs must also inform policy, and their individual preferences must be recognized and respected to enable inclusion in their preferred communities.

Concluding comments

Supported decision-making is integral to ensuring the rights of people with intellectual disabilities to exercise choice and control over their own lives, which is so central in personalized consumer-driven welfare systems and to their citizenship. The profession has much to learn in this respect as even those who champion a rights approach to social work pay scant attention to people with intellectual disability (Ife, 2012). The new theoretical perspectives for understanding disability, developing practice around supported decision-making and disruptive ideas about inclusion discussed in this chapter can inform better social work practice with people with intellectual disabilities, particularly in the realms of user-led assessment and planning and enabling support for inclusion in the communities chosen by people themselves.

This chapter provides only a glimpse of ideas influencing social work practice with adults with intellectual disabilities. Other takes might have included new thinking about causes of challenging behaviour and the growing attention to people with intellectual disabilities as emotional beings understood through theories of attachment (see Chapter 14) rather than behaviourism (see Chapter 17), the influence of the feminist theorizing about the ethics of care (see Chapter 33) or family perspectives on including children with intellectual disability. Nevertheless, in whatever context social workers encounter people with intellectual disabilities and their families, they must first and foremost regard them as citizens with equal human rights. One of the biggest challenges will be seeing the person through multiple lenses often simultaneously and deciding if and how to take their cognitive differences into account to ensure equity of outcomes.

The framework below offers a general guide to practice with people with intellectual disabilities, which should

- Be person-centred (individualized and person directed).
- Start from people's visions about their own lives.
- Focus on a person's strengths and those of their social environment.
- Take a positive optimistic stance, whilst seeking to understand and make adjustments for personal and environmental obstacles.
- Adopt an open, shared process of engagement based on principles of supported decision-making, drawing on trusting and respectful relationship with the person and dialogue and collaboration with informal and professional others who know them well.
- Use multiple modes of communication which are adapted to a person's cognitive capacity.
- Use the power of competing interpretations drawn from different theoretical perspectives.
- Design individualized flexible support to enable preferred options here and now.
- Foster independence and skills development as well as building interdependence and relationships.
- Protect human rights and ensure any legally sanctioned incursion is the least restrictive as is possible.
- Build capacity for inclusion in chosen communities.
- Draw on combined resources of formal and informal worlds.
- Use transparent, ethical decision-making processes.

(adapted from Bigby & Frawley, 2010)

Further reading

Bigby, C., & Frawley, P. (2010). *Social work and intellectual disability: Working for change.* Basingstoke: Palgrave MacMillan.
Clifford Simplican, S. (2015). *The capacity contract: Intellectual disability and the question of citizenship.* Minneapolis: University of Minnesota Press.
Shakespeare, T. (2014). *Disability rights and wrongs revisited.* Abingdon: Routledge.

References

Anderson, S., & Bigby, C. (2018). Self-advocacy as a means to positive identities for people with intellectual disability: 'We just help them, be them really'. *Journal of Applied Research in Intellectual Disabilities, 13*(1), 109–120. Retrieved from https://doi.org/10.1111/jar.12223
Askheim, O. (2003). Personal assistance for people with intellectual impairments: Experiences and dilemmas. *Disability and Society, 18,* 325–339.
Australian Law Reform Commission. (2014). *Equality, capacity and disability in commonwealth laws: Final report.* Sydney: Australian Law Reform Commission.
Bach, M. (2017). Inclusive citizenship: Refusing the construction of 'cognitive foreigners' in neo-liberal times. *Research and Practice in Intellectual and Developmental Disabilities, 4*(1), 4–25.
Bigby, C. (2013). A national disability insurance scheme: Challenges for social work. *Australian Social Work, 66*(1), 1–6.
Bigby, C., Anderson, S., & Cameron, N. (2018). Uncovering conceptualisations and theories of change embedded in interventions to facilitate community participation for people with intellectual disability: A scoping review. *Journal of Applied Research in Intellectual and Developmental Disabilities, 31*(2), 165–180.
Bigby, C., & Douglas, J. (2016). *Support for decision-making: A practice framework.* Bundoora: Living with Disability Research Centre, La Trobe University. Retrieved from http://hdl.handle.net/1959.9/556875

Bigby, C., Douglas, J, Carney, T., Then, S, Wiesel, I., & Smith, E. (2017). Delivering decision-making support to people with cognitive disability: What has been learned from pilot programs in Australia from 2010–2015. *Australian Journal of Social Issues, 52*(3), 222–240.

Bigby, C., & Frawley, P. (2010). *Social work and intellectual disability: Working for change.* Basingstoke: Palgrave MacMillan.

Bigby, C., & Wiesel, I. (2015). Mediating community participation: Practice of support workers in initiating, facilitating or disrupting encounters between people with and without intellectual disability. *Journal of Applied Research in Intellectual Disability, 28*, 307–318.

Brown, H., & Smith, H. (Eds.). (1992). *Normalisation: A reader for the nineties.* London: Routledge.

Brown, H., & Smith, H. (1989). Whose 'ordinary life' is it anyway? *Disability, Handicap and Society, 4*, 105–119.

Carney, T. (2015). Supported decision-making for people with cognitive impairments: An Australian perspective? *Laws, 4*, 37–59.

Carney, T., & Beaupert, F. (2013). Public and private bricolage: Challenges balancing law, services & civil society in advancing CRPD supported decision-making. *UNSW Law Journal, 36*, 175–201.

Clegg, J., & Bigby, C. (2017). Debates about dedifferentiation: Twenty-first century thinking about people with intellectual disabilities as distinct members of the disability group. *Research and Practice in Intellectual and Developmental Disabilities, 4*(1), 80–97.

Clifford Simplican, S., & Leader, G. (2015). Counting inclusion with Chantal Mouffe: A radical democratic approach to intellectual disability research. *Disability & Society, 30*(5), 717–30.

Clifford Simplican, S., Leader, G., Kosciulek, J., & Leahy, M. (2015). Defining social inclusion of people with intellectual and developmental disabilities: An ecological model of social networks and community participation. *Research in Developmental Disabilities, 38*, 18–29.

Craig, D. (2013). *'She's been involved in everything as far as I can see': Supporting the active participation of people with intellectual disabilities in community groups.* (Unpublished PhD thesis). LaTrobe University Melbourne, Bundoora. Retrieved from http://hdl.handle.net/1959.9/536319

Craig, D., & Bigby, C. (2015a). 'She's been involved in everything as far as I can see': Supporting the active participation of people with intellectual disabilities in community groups. *Journal of Intellectual and Developmental Disability, 40*, 12–25.

Craig, D., & Bigby, C. (2015b). Critical realism in social work research: Examining participation of people with intellectual disability. *Australian Social Work, 68*, 309–323.

Department of Health. (2007). *Independence, choice and risk: A guide to best practice in supported decision-making.* London: Author.

Douglas, J., & Bigby, C. (2018). Development of an evidence-based practice framework to guide support for decision making. *Disability and Rehabilitation.* https://doi.org/10.1080/09638288.2018.1498546

Douglas, J., Bigby, C., Knox, L., & Browning, M. (2015). Factors that underpin the delivery of effective decision-making support for people with cognitive disability. *Research and Practice in Intellectual and Developmental Disabilities, 2*(1), 37–44.

Ellem, K., O'Connor, M., Wilson, J., & Williams, S. (2013). Social work with marginalised people who have a mild or borderline intellectual disability: Practicing gentleness and encouraging hope. *Australian Social Work, 66*, 56–71.

Goodley, D. (2001). 'Learning difficulties', the social model of disability and impairment: Challenging epistemologies. *Disability & Society, 16*, 207–231.

Gordon, R. M. (2000). The emergence of assisted (supported) decision-making in the Canadian law of adult guardianship and substitute decision-making. *International Journal of Law and Psychiatry, 23*(1), 61–77.

Gustavsson, A. (2004). The role of theory in disability research: Springboard or strait-jacket? *Scandinavian Journal of Disability Research, 6*, 55–70.

Healy, K. (2017). Becoming a trustworthy profession: Doing better than doing good. *Australian Social Work, 70*(Sup1), 7–16.

Heslop, P., Blair, P., Fleming, P., Hoghton, M., Marriott, A., & Russ, L. (2014). The confidential inquiry into premature deaths of people with intellectual disabilities in the UK: A population-based study. *The Lancet, 383*, 889–895.

Houston, S. (2010). Prising open the black box: Critical realism, action research and social work. *Qualitative Social Work, 9*, 73–91.

Iacono, T., & Bigby, C. (2016). The health inequalities of people with intellectual and developmental disabilities. In P. Liamputtong (Ed.), *Public health: Local and global perspectives* (pp. 294–312). Melbourne: Cambridge University Press.

Ife, J. (2012). *Rights and social work*. Melbourne: Cambridge University Press.

James, E., Morgan, H., & Mitchell, R. (2017). Named social workers: Better social work for learning disabled people? *Disability & Society, 32*(10), 1650–1655.

Llewellyn, G., Traustadóttir, R., McConnell, D., & Signurjóndsdóttir, H. (2010). *Parents with intellectual disabilities*. London: Wiley-Blackwell.

Mackenzie, C., & Stoljar, N. (2000). Autonomy refigured. In C. Mackenzie & N. Stoljar (Eds.), *Relational autonomy: Feminist perspectives on autonomy, agency, and the social self* (pp. 3–31). New York: Oxford University Press.

Mansell, J., & Ericsson, K. (1996). *Deinstitutionalisation and community living: Intellectual disability services in Britain, Scandinavia and United States*. London: Chapman & Hall.

Milner, P., & Kelly, B. (2009). Community participation and inclusion: People with disabilities defining their place. *Disability & Society, 24*, 47–62.

Morgan, H. (2012). The social model of disability as a threshold concept: Troublesome knowledge and liminal spaces in social work education. *Social Work Education, 31*, 215–226.

O'Connor, M. (2014). The national disability insurance scheme and people with mild intellectual disability: Potential pitfalls for consideration. *Research and Practice in Intellectual and Developmental Disabilities, 1*(1), 17–23.

Oliver, M. (1990). *The politics of disablement*. Basingstoke: Palgrave Macmillan.

Parton, N., & O'Byrne, P. (2000). *Constructive social work: Towards new practice*. Basingstoke: Palgrave Macmillan.

Series, L. (2015). Relationships, autonomy and legal capacity: Mental capacity and support paradigms. *International Journal of Law and Psychiatry, 40*, 80–91.

Shakespeare, T. (2006). *Disability rights and wrongs*. Abingdon: Routledge.

Shakespeare, T. (2014). *Disability rights and wrongs revisited*. Abingdon: Routledge.

Silvers, A., & Francis, L. (2009). Thinking about the good: Reconfiguring liberal metaphysics (or not) for people with cognitive disabilities. *Metaphilosophy, 40*(3–4), 475–498.

Sims, D., & Gulyurtlu, S. (2014). A scoping review of personalization in the UK: Approaches to social work and people with learning disabilities. *Health and Social Care in the Community, 22*, 13–21.

Stainton, T. (1994). *Autonomy and social policy: Rights, mental handicap and community care*. Aldershot: Avebury.

Stainton, T. (2002). Learning disability. In R. Adams, L. Dominelli, & M. Payne (Eds.), *Critical practice in social work* (pp. 190–198). London: Palgrave Macmillan.

Stainton, T. (2016). Supported decision-making in Canada: Principles, policy and practice. *Research and Practice in Intellectual and Developmental Disabilities, 3*, 1–11.

United Nations. (1971). *Declaration on the rights of mentally retarded persons*. General Assembly Resolution, 2857. Retrieved from https://www.ohchr.org/Documents/ProfessionalInterest/res2856.pdf

United Nations. (2006). *Convention on the rights of persons with disabilities*. Retrieved from www.un.org/disabilities/convention/conventionfull.shtml

Wiesel, I., & Bigby, C. (2014). Being recognised and becoming known: Encounters between people with and without intellectual disability in the public realm. *Environment and Planning A: Economy and Space, 46*(7). https://doi.org/10.1068/a46251

Wiesel, I., & Bigby, C. (2016). Mainstream, inclusionary and convivial places: Locating encounter between people with and without intellectual disability. *Geographic Review, 106*(2), 201–214.

Wong, J., Clare, I., Holland, A., Watson, P. C., & Gunn, M. (2000). The capacity of people with a 'mental disability' to make a health care decision. *Psychological Medicine, 30*, 295–306.

40

Social work theory and older people

Malcolm Payne

Much social work theorization about social work with older people concentrates on service provision and practical and emotional support of older people and their informal caregivers. This is sometimes detached from understanding about the changing political and social environment that affects the ageing process and the human lives of older people. Social attitudes, finance for services and the organization of service provision is often characterized by ageism: that is, prejudice and discrimination against a social group on grounds of age (Butler, 1969). But if social workers incorporate a co-production practice strategy favouring older people's positive engagement, sharing in planning and organizing care and support services, many barriers to a good quality of life and end of life for older people can be overcome. In these ways, social work can contest devaluing and oppressive views about ageing and older people.

Ageism and social work practice theory about older people

Ageist views suggest that older people's lives are coming to an end, they'll be dead soon, so all we need to do is make them comfortable, and then social workers can concentrate on children or mentally ill people who have a substantial lifetime available to be improved by our therapeutic and social change efforts. But the still-influential 19th century administrative convention sets the beginning of old age at 65. Even if this is rising in many countries to the mid to late 60s, older people on average live 20 or more years of life after this in most Western countries, well worth a concern for their needs and help for their family and other informal caregivers and applying critical analysis to their position in our postmodern, neoliberal societies.

Ayalon and Tesch-Römer (2018) identify several theories that might explain ageism. This range of theorization suggests that analysis of this social phenomenon is still unresolved. It provides, however, a context for considering approaches to ageing and practice with older people by pointing out that many social factors affect attitudes to ageing and influence policy and practice in service provision.

Ageism operates through group, organizational and social structures. Common examples of ageism arise in labour markets, where middle-aged or older people are thought to be too set in their ways to be employable or to be potentially challenging when subordinate to younger managers. Other examples are evolutionary assumptions, seeing younger people as important because they are 'the future', and age segregation, where older people are cut off from involvement in education organizations or community and family life. Intergroup threat and intergenerational conflict also provide theoretical explanations of ageism because some older people form a group with accumulated wealth – for example, owning housing or family resources– and younger generations are thwarted in economic and social progress by older people retaining control of resources (Willetts, 2010).

Modernization theory devalues older people by arguing that advances in technology and medicine have led older people to survive longer, placing a burden of frailty and disability on wider society. Thus, older people no longer represent an evolutionary 'survival of the fittest' but a burden of the weak. It also devalues older people's life experience in the face of rapid technological change. Increased focus on economic achievement and development, geographical mobility and secularization and embracing individualism reduces family links and supports that might value older people's participation in community, family and society. Instead, such trends enhance the value given to younger people's knowledge and skills. Intersectionality theory is also relevant to social work with older people because it makes clear that ageism is a lens through which other discrimination and oppression may be seen and that older people are a minority group that connects with the experience of other minority groups.

Ageism also operates through people's personal reactions to ageing and older people. Social identity theory proposes that people maintain a positive self-identity by valuing characteristics of youthfulness and distinguishing them from assumed negative characteristics of old age. Stereotype content theory argues that people classify others by perceived levels of warmth and competence. Physical slowing down in old age feeds an incompetence stereotype; emphasizing positive social roles such as grandparenting generates a warmth perception. Stereotype embodiment theory proposes that, as part of their social development, older people internalize a lifetime's experience of negative stereotypes of ageing. The life course and active ageing ideas that I discuss in this chapter implicitly accept these unhelpful stereotypes. They do this by emphasizing that ageing contrasts with youthfulness and promoting positive lifestyles that mimic youthful stereotypes rather than acknowledging the reality of physical and social difficulties in ageing. Because these ideas underlie common social and healthcare approaches in practice with older people, social work risks reproducing unhelpful stereotypes of ageing in its practice.

Also, at the interpersonal level, terror management theory claims that older people remind others of their mortality and vulnerability, stimulating them to an unconscious feeling of their own immortality (Greenberg, Solomon, & Pyszczynski, 1997). Separating and distinguishing themselves from older people allows them to preserve equanimity against fears of ageing. I think using the term 'terror' exaggerates the emotional content of an otherwise helpful analysis of ambivalences that many people have about the ageing process.

Social work practice with and social care services for older people must recognize and contest the social environment of ambivalence about ageing and devaluation of older people in personal relations and social structures. It is possible to do this through interventions at the macro level (see Chapters 26–29). This involves thinking critically about anti-oppressive and empowering practice within which older people, their informal caregivers and their communities can participate in and co-produce services and a social environment that promotes a quality of care that values both the humanity and participation of older people.

Approaches to ageing

Social and policy context

This critical social work practice with older people is affected by worldwide demographic changes; the proportion of older people in many populations is increasing as life expectancy extends due to social change and medical advance. Ageism leads policymakers in a neoliberal economic and political environment, consequently, to problematize older people as imposing a burden of dependence on the economy supported by the adult working population. It is this inappropriate claim of dependency burden that older people and social workers need to contest.

Rather than see the value of older people's contribution to and participation in society, therefore, much policy still focuses on the social and healthcare services required by dependence. This is reinforced by biomedical views of ageing, in themselves often supporting ageist views. The complexity of generating interlocking provision in housing, welfare and benefits, leisure and well-being, as well as social care to respond to older people's needs, means that the policy context of social work practice struggles to be creative in this field (National Audit Office, 2014, p. 6). The neoliberal political environment, prioritizing economic austerity, also restricts the development of a positive policy context in many countries. In this section, I explore some of the sources of policy for older people's care.

Biomedicine is the context of social interventions

Many approaches to ageing rely on biomedical thinking, raising issues discussed by Carey in Chapter 6 and by Deacon and Macdonald in Chapter 38. These are important for social workers because social work practice with older people intersects with healthcare services, and biomedicine is the taken-for-granted lens through which ageing is viewed by most people. Ageing is seen as a natural process, experienced by most animals. How evolutionary or genetic factors may influence this process is debated. So is the extent to which ageing is an accumulation of minor metabolic failures or injuries. Curative medicine focuses on reversing failures in metabolism in the major systems of the body: organs such as the heart, lungs or kidneys, which enable the body to function; process nutrition and perceive, react to and manage external events and pressures. Repairing these failures is an important objective of medicine, enabling people to return to independence from medical treatment, even if, post-treatment, they continue to be affected by some mental and physical impairments. Changes due to ageing may be slowed or sometimes avoided by lifestyle changes, including cosmetic and health and well-being actions such as improving fitness and avoiding risks of physical frailty such as falls.

Social gerontology as a source of theory

Gerontology studies the biological, cultural, social and psychological aspects of ageing. This is distinguished from geriatrics, medical practice with older people. Gerontological theories explore social responses to the physical changes of ageing and so are particularly relevant to social work practice. Social construction and critical theories have become important in social work. Developing within social work itself, ideas of citizenship incorporate concerns for social justice and inequality in practice with older people.

Social construction theories

Disengagement theory (Cumming & Henry, 1961) sees later life as a progressive disengagement from social relationships. This prepares people for the ultimate disengagement of advancing disease and death. Against this view, disengagement is not a universal process; people's preferences for social engagement vary throughout their lives (Rose, 1964). Older people and the people around them often do not see disengagement as desirable, and many continue to seek personal development and positive activity in social networks in later life. Also, any disengagement that appears to take place often derives from the social assumption that older people will step back from active engagement in the economy through retirement, taking up instead increased social provision, including retirement pensions and other social benefits. Thus, it is capitalist and neo-liberal society that disengages, rather than older people.

Ideas such as activity theory, continuity theory (Atchley, 1999) and successful ageing (Havighurst, 1961; Rowe & Kahn, 1987; Baltes & Baltes, 1990; Lupien & Wan, 2004) propose that we should emphasize maintaining and enhancing, into later life, positive activity and social engagement, downplaying age-related losses in mental and physical capacity. Continuity ideas stress a focus on maintaining what was valued during people's life course as a mark of successful ageing. These ideas lie behind political, health and social care services' efforts to promote arts and creativity, volunteering and social contributions such as grandparenting and other active social roles. Activity theory is criticized for imposing middle-class aspirations and family lifestyles on all older people (Katz, 2000). There is also little evidence to say what kinds of activity are useful and there is also criticism of pushing unremitting activity rather than a reflective, spiritual approach to later life. Activity theory is also problematic if it does not incorporate older people's needs and limitations (Versey, 2016).

'Successful ageing' perspectives are informed by life course theories which study continuity and change as people progress through life. Cohort studies explored the different directions children took as they developed through childhood into adulthood (Green, 2017), and sociological studies examined how individual biographies and social movements intersected with social structures (Elder, Johnson, & Crosnoe, 2003). These perspectives theorize that personal and social experiences and broader social change affect the physical, psychological and social development of individuals and the social networks of which they are a part. People go through a series of life stages, building the later on the previous stages. Erikson's (Erikson & Erickson, 1977) theory of life stages had an early influence in social work, although it is mainly concerned with childhood.

More recently, Robertson (2014) emphasized social transitions that occur in later life. These include retirement, downshifting from a family home into a home suitable for later life, becoming a grandparent, experiencing relationship breakdowns and establishing new intimate relationships, becoming an informal carer, bereavement, acquiring a long-term health condition, entering a care environment and preparing for the end of life. These transitions do not all happen to everyone, they occur over a lengthier period than traditionally defined old age (that is, post–65 years) and they are not necessarily associated with the ageing process. They are nevertheless typical social changes, and social workers need to be aware of how people adapt to ageing.

A significant recent influence is studies on health inequality, culminating in reports for the World Health Organization (WHO) and the British government (WHO, 2008; Marmot Review, 2010). They show that ill health in later life is significantly affected by 'social determinants of health'. There is a social gradient of health inequalities in which richer people, because they are more in control of their lives and work, are healthier for longer than poorer people. These draw attention to the concept of health capital, an aspect of Bourdieu's social capital (see Chapters 5 and 12). People have initial assets in their genetic make-up and build social assets through their lifetime, such as education, spiritual beliefs and support, social standing, control over their lives, cognitive capacity and emotional resilience such as humour. They also have biological assets in the capacity and fitness of their bodies. All these contribute human and social resources, enabling older people to respond to the challenges of ageing (Guimaraes, 2007). Social workers can usefully promote community, family and personal health and social capital as part of a strengths-based approach (see Chapter 18) to working with older people.

The social determinants approach thus contributes a preventive aspect to social work interventions by combating health inequalities and their impact in earlier phases of life. A useful policy (Marmot, 2010) is improving child development in the early years, education to improve people's social mobility and health understanding, organizing healthier work environments, reducing income inequalities and improving community support. Social work can make contributions in all these areas. Nevertheless, ageing brings with it increasing physical frailty and psychological stresses, which services must provide for.

Another social lens that has been influential sees ageing as being divided into third and fourth 'ages' (Laslett, 1996), distinguishing 'young-old' from 'old-old' people (Neugarten, 1974). The first two 'ages' (childhood and adulthood) are followed by a 'third-age' period. At this time, changes in middle age, such as children leaving home, stability in housing and income and career success give people a period of independence and agency. This increases their psychological and social control of the direction of their lives, aspirations for personal development and wider opportunities for new experiences. Although we might see this as benefiting only economically secure older people, even people with high support needs receiving considerable social and healthcare support value maintaining control of their lives and living a positive old age (Katz, Holland, Peace, & Taylor, 2011). 'Universities of the third age', where older people contribute education to their peers, is an example of the application of this idea. These are a potentially anti-oppressive intervention, enhancing community engagement and personal development, as in Jasiński's (2011) study of a Polish example.

Critical analysis of 'third age' ideas suggest that they push dependency and other problematic aspects of ageing into a 'fourth age', which people come to fear and see negatively. Moreover, as I suggested when considering ageism, all positive ageing ideas imply a negative view of dependency as a result of ageing, rather than focusing on the positives of interdependence within family and community.

Critical theory

A tradition of radical and critical accounts of social work practice theory builds on critical social policy ideas (Ray, Bernard, & Phillips, 2009; see Chapters 26–28). They emphasize ageism as a source of negative images of older people and, therefore, of general social discrimination against them. Older people's interests are disregarded by the current socio-economic system with its interest in economic growth and productivity. For example, economic policy sees greater value in economic outputs from the labour force, rather than artistic human achievements, personal and social satisfaction in relationships and enjoyment of leisure outside the workforce.

Feminist theory emphasizes how ageing accentuates gender divisions (see Chapter 31). Many psychosocial concerns about later life, for example, reflect a focus on men's interests. For example, retirement from the workforce is seen as problematic for men's well-being, rather than an opportunity for prioritizing reintegration into family and community life alongside and more equally with women.

Critical theory also questions common assumptions about services for older people, particularly medicalization and commodification. Medicalization sees the main issue with an ageing population as rising illness and disability, requiring care from social and health services. Commodification leads to policy for older people's services focusing on making society more efficient by reducing the cost of dependency on the working population which, in turn, supports socially divisive and negative austerity fiscal policies. Similarly, privatization and rationalization as important aims of services for older people focus on economic efficiency and reducing demands for needs to be met, rather than valuing support for older people's social contribution. Consequently, there is a perception that there is a systemic crisis in social provision for older people because increasing numbers of older people are dependent on smaller working populations, rather than valuing the economic and social contributions made by older people in their interdependency with community support and informal caregiving.

Citizenship approaches to incorporate social justice in care for older people

Citizenship is a legal and social identity and status denoting affiliation with a country. It is part of the structure of social order, connecting a population with the social and political structures that control a territory. Social and political citizenship incorporate civil rights to legal protection of freedoms and equality, political rights to participate in political processes and social rights to welfare and participation in social relationships with others.

Citizenship approaches in social work are professional strategies, reflecting humanistic theory (Payne, 2011a), to implement policies on people's opportunities to learn, grow and make decisions for themselves and on participation in interpersonal and social relationships and in political and social structures. Practice theory on citizen participation (Beresford & Croft, 1993) argues for facilitating social work client groups' participation in decision-making within institutions and services that affect them. Two theoretical accounts focus on older people.

One is Marshall and Tibbs's (2006, pp 16–18) distinction between medical, social and citizenship approaches to dementia. Medical models concentrate on managing the consequences of mental and physical decline in ageing. The social work contribution focuses on the social aspects of that decline. Social work helps families manage relationship changes that occur as older people need greater medical care, for example. The social approach to dementia connects with social models of disability (see Chapter 38). This sees older people as disadvantaged in pursuing their lives by the social and built environment, which fails to provide adequately for their needs. The social work contribution develops age-friendly environments, relevant services providing choice and flexibility, meeting care and other needs of older people. The citizenship model focuses on reciprocal relationships between older people and society. It sees older people as having the duty and right to participation in political and social relations within that society and society as having duties to engage with its citizens. The social work contribution is to facilitate older people's participation in social and political structures within society and to provide services that meet their needs.

My own account of citizenship social work with older people (Payne, 2011b, 2017) derives from more recent research viewing citizenship, rather than being a legal status or social right, as a process through which people gain or lose rights to participation in the community and society around them. This proposes that citizenship is developed. For example, children gain rights as they grow up, and migrants are accorded rights in a new homeland. Citizenship may also be lost, for example by social exclusion. I argue that social work practice should facilitate 'citizening', the process of building up rights relevant to a successful later life; should seek to prevent 'de-citizening', the process through which they lose existing rights and opportunities because of personal and social responses to ageing; and support 're-citizening', the process of building lost elements of later-life citizenship.

Citizenship ideas are important because they incorporate social justice arguments into the more conventional assumptions about our objectives in working with older people (see also Chapter 10).

Social work implications of policy on ageing

Current policy on services for older people has not yet escaped from historic patterns in family and intergenerational relationships. Many countries have not fully adapted to marked changes in social relations as more people survive into old age. In Germany, for example, life expectancy at birth early in the 20th century was 48 years (women) and 45 years (men). In the early 21st century, it was, respectively, 82 and 77 (Joint Academy Initiative on Aging, 2010). Labour force participation among older people, however, means that only 25 percent of Germans aged 60 to 65 years were employed in 2010 and only a few over that age. This trend has reversed as the official retirement age has been increased to 67 years. National and regional sources of statistics, such as, in the UK, the Office for National Statistics (www.ons.gov.uk) and, covering Europe, Eurostat (https://ec.europa.eu/eurostat) can inform service development and practice. Interpretation of statistics and social trends is available from national and international longevity centres (www.ilc-alliance.org).

An important policy debate is on financing the growing need for care services, and many countries have adapted funding models to increase funding so that people feel more secure in providing for long-term care (Elliott, Golds, Sissons, & Wilson, 2014). Curry, Castle-Clark, and Hemmings (2018) argue that a good feature of Japanese changes has been adoption of a 'whole system' model incorporating elements of public funding of care, private insurance, quality improvement and support of informal care.

Global policy on ageing is strongly influenced by WHO policy on ageing and health (WHO, 2015), which is influenced by and influences national agendas. It combines care, citizenship and social objectives, identifying six important policy areas creating an age-friendly world for older people to support their abilities to:

- meet basic needs for:

  - financial security
  - adequate housing
  - personal security

- learn, grow and make decisions
- be mobile
- build and maintain relationships
- contribute

Social workers can evaluate the services available in their country and area and their own practice against these objectives.

Service provision in healthcare focuses on:

- long-term health conditions (in particular, dementias)
- palliative care

The aim here is 'compression of morbidity' (Clarkson, 2012), to reduce the period at the end of life when serious conditions prevent older people from having a good quality of life. Another related strategy is to achieve 'dynamic equilibrium', where even though an older person has serious disabilities, other aspects of their health and well-being are managed to reduce the impact of the more serious conditions. Social work practice is interwoven with these important healthcare developments.

An increasingly important aspect of care provision for older people is to engage and support informal caregivers (see Chapter 7). This is crucial since most care is provided by family members and others in the local community.

Social work practice with older people

Social work practice with older people, called 'gerontological social work' in some European countries and the US, brings service provision and support activities together with therapeutic practice around personal change. The latter element is stronger in the US. Richardson and Barusch (2006), in an American text, for example, focus on individual psychological problems, such as depression, suicide and substance abuse, social psychological problems in family life and in end-of-life care, bereavement and responses to work and retirement. These are present worldwide and picked up by social workers in the context of service work.

UK texts, while covering some of these topics, particularly mental health issues, concentrate attention on planning care services, the major function of local government social workers, considered in the next section. Newer texts, for example, Hall and Scragg (2012), concentrate on responding to the diversity of older people. All these texts draw attention to the impact of dementia and long-term medical conditions on older people themselves and their families. Increasingly, they note that older people are approaching the end of life, and this aspect of people's life experience is important in care and because older people experience an accumulated burden of bereavement as friends and family die (Hayes et al., 2014; Payne, 2017; see Chapter 41). This is an important development because end-of-life care developed in the context of life-threatening illness, particularly cancer, in younger adults and its application of the age-group when most people die, older people, has been slow.

An international emphasis on autonomy, dignity, respect in professional relationships and developing feelings of well-being is also a strong element of practice in several professions, including social work (European Partnership for the Wellbeing and Dignity of Older People, 2012; see Chapters 8–9). UK literature strongly focuses on the legal and administrative role carried by local government social workers and others of safeguarding older people against abuse (Cooper & White, 2017).

Community and macro practice

Community and macro practice are important for social work with older people because efforts to sustain relationships across the life course into old age draw on connections within the locality. Both formal and informal community organizations provide volunteer labour and locations for older people's social provision. Social care services provided include opportunities for social interaction, day centres, meals services and arts and craft activities.

Policy objectives to create age-friendly environments and cities offer an international perspective on policy objectives that will best support older people (WHO, 2007). This includes work to develop outdoor spaces and buildings, transportation and housing that is adaptable for more frail and disabled older people. It also involves work to promote social participation, respect and social inclusion, civic participation and employment and good communication and information provision that will support citizening objectives.

Climate change has implications for older people (see Chapter 14). They are more vulnerable to the effects of serious adverse weather events. For example, older people's death rates are higher in heat waves, and they are more likely to be injured in earthquakes, floods or hurricanes (Hetherington & Boddy, 2013). Therefore, social work in climate and other disasters should make special provision for older people. Both older people and their families and local communities can consider what disasters might arise – for example, flooding, fires or weather damage – and make plans for keeping in touch with and supporting older people. People can keep an emergency kit available and have a chain of three people to contact in emergencies (American Psychological Association, 2018).

Elder abuse and safeguarding older people

As with children, preventing abuse of older people and safeguarding them from abuse is an important function of social work in most societies. There are two main types of abuse: first, intentional actions that cause harm or the risk of harm by caregivers or others who stand in a relationship of trust with an older person and second, neglect by both informal and paid caregivers failing to meet an older person's basic needs or protect them from harm (Lachs & Pillemer, 2004). Fallon's (2006) New Zealand study identifies four important elements of a safeguarding service:

- National policy development and coordination.
- Advisory group and support and local coordination for professionals and services engaged in safeguarding work.
- Professional health and social care interventions to help and protect individuals experiencing abuse and neglect and to investigate allegations of and concerns about abuse and neglect.
- Local services to support older people and respond to difficult and risky situations.

The main practice requirements are training to develop alertness among health and social care professionals and investigation of allegations and concerns expressed by older people and people in touch with them. This should lead to careful exploration and amelioration of relationship and behaviour difficulties. As with child protection (see Chapter 34), effective working together with other services and investigation resources, including the police, is an important strategy. Older people are particularly affected by financial abuse and scamming; social workers need to be alert both to keep older people well-informed and to secure against risks (Lee, Johnson, Fenge, & Brown, 2017).

Care management and person-centred, self-directed care

Case management, the original American term, or care management, the UK derivative, emerged in the 1980s as an important professional role in most adult social work provision and therefore in work with older people. It aims to integrate care services from different sources. A factor in its influence was the need to draw in resources, in service systems increasingly affected by neoliberal economic policies, from private and not-for-profit sectors of the economy as well as public provision. Adapting a conventional model of social work, it proposed a cycle of interventions starting with population screening to identify social needs, often now degraded in practice, to focus on prioritizing needs to facilitate service rationing in a constrained economic environment. The main phases of care management move on to assessment, followed by care planning, in which a 'package of services' is tailored to the identified needs of the older person. The package is implemented. Subsequently, it is monitored to ensure the delivery of the planned package and then reviewed periodically as the older person's needs change (Payne, 1995). This approach was implemented in the UK, primarily to facilitate the adoption of a quasi-market of multiple sectors of the economy, without much attention to its practice implications (Lewis & Glennerster, 1996).

Two common forms of care (case) management are identified. In administrative case management, the social worker carries out assessments, arranging services without a continuing relationship with client and carers. In clinical case management, the case manager provides a continuing supportive relationship as the services are used. This makes it possible to adapt them to the particular needs of clients and carers (Challis, 1994). Administrative case management was adopted in UK local authority social care and other public care systems internationally, primarily to facilitate managerial and budgetary control. It failed because there were insufficient resources to provide flexibly for care needs, so care managers became gatekeepers for scarce resources. Also, the separation of commissioner and provider roles in a quasi-market, separation from National Health Service funding sources and provision and the need for financial accountability in a large local authority service led to administrative rigidity and complexity.

This led to the development of current models of self-directed care (Pearson, Ridley, & Hunter, 2017), which aim to facilitate greater client influence over the care provision and its management. An international policy movement towards 'cash for care', rather than professionals organizing combinations of services for individuals, encourages direct payments to clients or caregivers who organize their own support (Ungerson & Yeandle, 2007). Formal services include care homes, nursing homes (care homes with nursing) and care services in clients' homes to assist with activities of daily living. Professional social work services include advice, information and social work for older people themselves and for informal caregivers and advocacy and brokerage with providers of care services and other local provision needed by older people. The process used varies across the world, but the crucial elements are co-production of care plans to establish a budget involving social workers, informal caregivers and clients. These can then be used to devise personalized service provision appropriate for each client and caregiver.

Examples of practice theory applied to work with older people

In addition to service development ideas about case management and self-directed care, some theories of social work practice have been specifically applied to work with older people. I summarize two examples here, which reflect some contemporary theoretical developments in humanistic and narrative practice (see Chapters 21–22).

Lantz and Walsh (2007) describe re-collection as a humanistic, existentialist technique in working with older people. They describe it as a process of 'honouring suppressed meaning potentials' (p. 59). Existential therapy focuses on how finding meaning in life experiences enhances people's capacity to overcome the vacuum that exists in their lives. The theoretical model emphasizes that older people, in their long lives, possess a stock of experiences that have at one time been important to them (e.g. what was valued in relationships with children, parents and former and present romantic partners). These have been suppressed and overlaid by later experiences. The aim of the technique is to collect again ('re-collect') and organize these meanings so that they may be valued again and made important in their present life. Practitioners discuss life experiences, helping clients 'actualize' the meaning of these past experiences by connecting them with present experiences and future 'potentials' (pp. 60–61). Artistic work, using photography, poetry or creative writing, helps to solidify these experiences. For example, a man was lent a camera to record important locations in his home area. He wrote captions explaining their importance in his life: e.g. the dance hall where he met his wife. Discussing the results brought together in a photo book with his grandchildren improved his relationships with later generations in the family and improved his grandchildren's acceptance of his living in their home.

One comprehensive attempt to apply a well-established social work practice theory, task-centred practice, to social work with older people is Naleppa and Reid's (2003) text on task-centred practice with older people.

Conclusion

In this chapter, I have drawn together elements of social work practice theory from other chapters in this book with policy directions and service development trends in work with older people. I have argued that, as with other client groups, the biomedical lens limits our view of appropriate responses to the needs of older people. Critical and social gerontological approaches offer alternative perspectives to inform social work thinking. There is the possibility of social work co-producing, together with older people and their informal caregivers, practice and services that increase the quality of life and well-being of all older people. This would enable social workers to build dignified and respectful provision for the real needs that a growing ageing population experiences, but also renew perceptions of the value older people bring to any society and combat the ageism present, sometimes hidden, in public perception and policy.

Further reading

Ayalon, L., & Tesch-Römer, C. (Eds.). (2018). *Contemporary perspectives on ageism*. Cham: Springer.
   A comprehensive analysis of sources and effects of ageism.
Hall, B., & Scragg, T. (Eds.). (2012). *Social work with older people: Approaches to person-centred practice*. Maidenhead: Open University Press.
   A useful up-to-date collection of articles, differentiating the needs of a range of groups of older people.
Ray, M., Bernard, M., & Phillips, J. (2009). *Critical issues in social work with older people*. Basingstoke: Palgrave Macmillan.
   The best account of critical practice with older people.

References

American Psychological Association [APA]. (2018). *Older adults and disasters how to be prepared and assist others*. New York: APA. Retrieved from www.apa.org/pi/aging/resources/older-adults-disasters.pdf
Atchley, R. C. (1999). *Continuity and adaptation in aging: Creating positive experiences*. Baltimore, MD: Johns Hopkins University Press.
Ayalon, L., & Tesch-Römer, C. (2018). Ageism: Concept and origins. In L. Ayalon & C. Tesch-Römer (Eds.), *Contemporary perspectives on ageism* (pp. 1–10). Cham: Springer.
Baltes, P. B., & Baltes, M. M. (Eds). (1990). *Successful aging: Perspectives form the social sciences*. Cambridge, UK: Cambridge University Press.
Beresford, P., & Croft, S. (1993). *Citizen involvement: A practical guide for change*. Basingstoke: Palgrave Macmillan.
Butler, R. N. (1969). Age-ism: Another form of bigotry. *Gerontologist*, *9*(4), 243–246.
Challis, D. (1994). *Care management: Factors influencing its development in the implementation of community care*. London: Department of Health.
Clarkson, P. (2012). What research tells social workers about their work with older people. In M. Davies (Ed.), *Social work with adults* (pp. 300–314). Basingstoke: Palgrave Macmillan.
Cooper, A., & White, E. (Eds.). (2017). *Safeguarding adults under the care act 2014: Understanding god practice*. London: Jessica Kingsley.
Cumming, E., & Henry, W. H. (1961). *Growing old: The process of disengagement*. New York: Basic Books.
Curry, N., Castle-Clarke, S., & Hemmings, N. (2018). *What can England learn from the long-term care system in Japan?* London: Nuffield Trust.
Elder, G. H., Johnson, M. K., & Crosnoe, R. (2003). The emergence and development of life course theory. In J. T. Mortimer & M. J. Shanahan (Eds.), *Handbook of the life course* (pp. 3–19). New York: Kluwer.

Elliott, S., Golds, S., Sissons, I., & Wilson, H. (2014). *Long-term care: A review of global funding models*. Edinburgh: Institute and Faculty of Actuaries.

Erikson, E., & Erikson, J. (1997). *The life cycle completed: Extended version*. New York: Norton.

European Partnership for the Wellbeing and Dignity of Older People. (2012). *European quality framework for long-term care services: Principles and guidelines for the wellbeing and dignity of older people in need of care and assistance*. Brussels: Age Platform Europe.

Fallon, P. (2006). *Elder abuse and/or neglect: Literature review*. Wellington: Centre for Social Research and Evaluation. Ministry of Social Development.

Green, L. (2017). *Understanding the life course: Sociological and psychological perspectives* (2nd ed.). Cambridge, UK: Polity Press.

Greenberg, J., Solomon, S., & Pyszczynski, T. (1997). Terror management theory of self-esteem and cultural worldviews: Empirical assessments and conceptual refinements. *Advances in Experimental Social Psychology, 29*, 61–139.

Guimaraes, R. M. (2007). Health capital, life course and ageing. *Gerontology, 53*(2), 96–101.

Hall, B., & Scragg, T. (Eds.). (2012). *Social work with older people: Approaches to person-centred practice*. Maidenhead: Open University Press.

Havighurst, R. J. (1961). Successful aging. *Gerontologist, 1*(1), 8–13.

Hayes, A., Henry, C., Holloway, M., Lindsay, K., Sherwen, E., & Smith, T. (2014). *Pathways through care at the end of life: A guide to person-centred care*. London: Jessica Kingsley.

Hetherington, T., & Boddy, J. (2013). Ecosocial work with marginalised populations: Time for action on climate change. In M. Gray, J. Coates, & T. Hetherington (Eds.), *Environmental social work* (pp. 46–61). Abingdon: Routledge.

Jasiński, Z. (2011). University of the third age as a form of social work. In J. Brągiel, I. Dąbrowska-Jabłońska, & M. Payne (Eds.), *Social work in adult services in the European Union: Selected issues and experiences* (pp. 188–199). London: College Publications.

Joint Academy Initiative on Aging. (2010). *More years, more life*. Stuttgart: Deutsche Akademie der Naturforscher Leopoldina.

Katz, J., Holland, C., Peace, S., & Taylor, E. (2011). *A better life: What older people with high support needs value*. New York: Joseph Rowntree Memorial Trust.

Katz, S. (2000). Busy bodies: Activity, aging and the management of everyday life. *Journal of Aging Studies, 14*(2), 135–152.

Lachs, M. S., & Pillemer, K. (2004). Elder abuse. *Lancet, 364*, 1263–1672.

Lantz, J., & Walsh, J. (2007). *Short-term existential intervention in clinical practice*. Chicago: Lyceum.

Laslett, P. (1996). *A fresh map of life: The emergence of the third age* (2nd ed.). Basingstoke: Palgrave Macmillan.

Lee, S., Johnson, R., Fenge, L-A., & Brown, K. (2017). Safeguarding adults at risk of financial scamming. In A. Cooper & E. White (Eds.), *Safeguarding adults under the care act 2014: Understanding good practice* (pp. 240–255). London: Jessica Kingsley.

Lewis, J., & Glennerster, H. (1996). *Implementing the new community care*. Buckingham: Open University Press.

Lupien, S. J., & Wan, N. (2004). Successful ageing: From cell to self. *Philosophical Transactions of the Royal Society of London, 359*, 1413–1426.

Marmot Review. (2010). *Fair society, healthy lives: Strategic review of health inequalities in England post-2010*. London: Marmot Review.

Marshall, M., & Tibbs, M-A. (2006). *Social work and people with dementia: Partnerships, practice and persistence* (2nd ed.). Bristol: Policy Press.

Naleppa, M. J., & Reid, W. J. (2003). *Gerontological social work: A task-centered approach*. New York: Columbia University Press.

National Audit Office. (2014). *Adult social care in England: Overview*. London: National Audit Office.

Neugarten, B. L. (1974). Age groups in American society and the rise of the young-old. *Annals of the American Academy of Political and Social Science, 415*(1), 187–198.

Payne, M. (1995). *Social work and community care*. Basingstoke: Palgrave Macmillan.

Payne, M. (2011a). *Humanistic social work: Core principles in practice*. Chicago: Lyceum.

Payne, M. (2011b). *Citizenship social work with older people*. Chicago: Lyceum.

Payne, M. (2017). *Older citizens and end-of-life care: Social work practice strategies for adults in later life*. London: Routledge.

Pearson, C., Ridley, J., & Hunter, S. (2017). *Self-directed support: Personalisation, choice and control*. Edinburgh: Dunedin.

Ray, M., Bernard, M., & Phillips, J. (2009). *Critical issues in social work with older people*. Basingstoke: Palgrave Macmillan.

Richardson, V., & Barusch, A. (2006). *Gerontological practice for the twenty-first century: A social work perspective*. New York: Columbia University Press.

Robertson, G. K. (2014). Transitions in later life: A review of the challenge and opportunities for policy development. *Working with Older People, 18*(4), 186–196.

Rose, A. M. (1964). A current sociological issue in social gerontology. *Gerontologist, 4*(1), 46–50.

Rowe, J. W., & Kahn, R. L. (1987). Human aging: Usual and successful. *Science, 237*, 143–149.

Ungerson, C., & Yeandle, S. (Eds.). (2007). *Cash for care in developed welfare states*. Basingstoke: Palgrave Macmillan.

Versey, H. S. (2016). Activity theory. In S. K. Whitbourne (Ed.), *Encyclopedia of adulthood and aging* (vol. 1., pp. 10–16). Chichester: Wiley.

Willetts, D. (2010). *The pinch: How the baby boomers took their children's future – And how they can give it back*. London: Atlantic.

World Health Organization. (2007). *Global age-friendly cities: A guide*. Geneva: WHO.

World Health Organization. (2008). *Closing the gap in a generation: Health equity through action on the social determinants of health*. Geneva: WHO.

World Health Organization. (2015). *World report on ageing and health*. Geneva: World Health Organization.

41

Holistic end-of-life care in social work

Cecilia L. W. Chan, Candy H. C. Fong and Y. L. Fung

Introduction

End-of-life social work interventions often focus on grief, anxiety, fear of death, pain and symptoms associated with the end of life, pathological adjustment to loss, problem behaviours, and subsequent co-morbidity and mortality (Christ, Messner, & Behar, 2015; Altilio & Otis-Green, 2011). Medical models are often taken as a core theoretical framework where sickness, discomforts and death are described as maladjustments or functional pathogenesis or seen as failures of medical intervention. Likewise, palliative care social work is heavily influenced by social work practice in hospital settings under the leadership of medical specialists in oncology, cardiology, nephrology, rheumatology, geriatrics and paediatrics. When patients are given an end-stage diagnosis, critical issues of physical care in the home, family adjustment to caring tasks, sudden loss of income and increases in health spending, anticipatory death anxiety and grief and shattered dreams and hopes can put the extended network of family and close friends into chaos. Dying is not an individual matter; it is a family and collective issue, which can be framed by a public health framework (Kellehear, 2005). Family members suffer from high emotional and practical distress but are often neglected by service providers. With high levels of unmet needs, especially on the psychosocial and spiritual aspects, there is a call for collective actions in curriculum design, training and standard setting in palliative and end-of-life social work and transdisciplinary teams (Otis-Green et al., 2009).

The first author has worked with advanced cancer patients for the past 30 years. She has witnessed many exceptional survivors who lived much longer than predicted by their oncologists. Many of these exceptional survivors could not afford traditional Chinese medicine, alternative treatment or expensive gene therapy. However, they could still survive by practising *qigong* exercises, going to church and serving as volunteers. Many of them rediscovered new meaning in life despite living with a deadly diagnosis. A more holistic approach is therefore worth considering in addition to the conventional pathological and symptom-management direction in end-of-life care (Chan & Dickens, 2015).

There are recent publications on theories related to the study of death, dying and bereavement from philosophical, sociological, psychological and community perspectives (Stillion & Attig, 2015). This chapter proposes a holistic framework to the understanding of end-of-life care for individuals, families and communities. The latest social work theories on end of life and challenges in theory development will be discussed.

Understanding end-of-life care from an individual perspective

Issues of practical needs in maintaining a daily routine, financial stress, emotional frustrations, family conflicts, fear of abandonment and the imminent death, uncertainties and witnessing loss of roles can be overwhelming to individuals and families. Loss of physical strength, frailty and inability to walk will make self-care, especially toileting, difficult and thus can rob individuals of their pride and sense of integrity. The loss of autonomy and dignity due to physical or cognitive frailty can be frustrating and demoralizing. Inability to handle practical chores and share thoughts on death will give rise to conflicts and disputes among patients and family members.

Ambiguous loss

'Ambiguous loss' can be a relevant theory to describe the situation of family members and patients at the end of their lives (Boss, 2002). Elizabeth Kübler-Ross used five simple words – denial, anger, bargaining, depression and acceptance – to describe the complex realities of death and dying for patients and family members (Smaldone & Uzzo, 2013). Her model is used widely in the palliative care community. Kübler-Ross's process model can be supplemented by Pauline Boss's theory on ambiguous loss (Boss, Roos, & Harris, 2011). Boss uses integrated role theory, symbolic interactionism with family boundary and system theories to explain the fluid and dynamic interaction of families in distress. When tackling death and end-of-life issues, members of the family and social network may tend to jump into the situation trying to rescue, but often in vain. They may intrude across each other's boundaries, causing frustrations and conflicts among members of the family. Loss of the past, present and future are also ambiguous. Patients and family members are usually caught in a tsunami of fear, uncertainty, demoralization, helplessness and hopelessness. As living with dying and anticipatory loss is ambiguous, inability to articulate the sense of loss of meaning can often lead to immense suffering and pain. Patients with physical and mental complications, such as those admitted to an intensive care unit or older adults with dementia, may experience greater ambiguity in the face of multiple losses (Kean, 2010).

A holistic model of bio-psycho-social-spiritual care

After being given an end-stage diagnosis, there is an urgency that all patients' core needs plus those of their loved ones be tackled as soon as possible. New social work theories are moving away from the pathology framework into contemporary approaches of holistic East-West well-being (Chan et al., 2014), transformation (Chan, Chan, & Ng, 2006), strengths-focused (Saleebey, 2012; see Chapter 18), meaning-driven (Neimeyer, 2000), holistic and integrative (Lee, Chan, Chan, Ng, & Leung, 2018) care through brief interventions. Along a similar line of thought, many research studies have provided evidence on the connectedness of mind-body research through positive psychology, meditation, guided imagery, hypnosis, mindfulness, diet, relaxation, *qigong*, chanting, cognitive behavioural therapy, psychotherapy, quantum touch and energy healing (Morone & Greco, 2007).

While the needs of persons at the end of their lives are often complex, there is a strong voice in search of an integrative bio-psycho-social-spiritual model. Dyer (2011) explained that this new model does not equal a summation of the 'bio', 'psycho', 'social' and 'spiritual' factors. Instead, it should be 'a harmonious integration of all the elements of healing realises and respects their complexity . . . ambiguity of the inevitable dimension of human existence' (Dyer, 2011, p. 297). The integrative body-mind-spirit social work framework was developed based on this long-outstanding quest for a holistic model (see Chapter 11).

An integrative body-mind-spirit social work framework

Key concepts of Chinese medicine, exercise, meridian (energy pathways in the body), dynamic balancing, mind-body connection and spirituality are all relevant to building a theoretical foundation for a holistic body-mind-spirit well-being (Lee et al., 2018). The Eastern framework of balance and harmony believes in a dynamic process of yin-yang elements within individual, family and community systems. A healthy flow of energy in the systems make regeneration and rejuvenation possible. If the energy is stuck, the health of the entity will be at risk (Ng, Chan, Ho, Wong, & Ho, 2006).

In recent years, research into integrative body-mind-spirit social work interventions found they were able to enhance the immune system, enhance anti-ageing protective enzymes and reduce stress hormones (Ho et al., 2017). Other research on mindfulness, yoga, breathing, qigong and neuroscience has provided empirical evidence on the improvement of the well-being of individuals before and after intervention. Connecting the deterioration of bodily functions with emotional and spiritual transcendence has yielded amazing stories of transformation. Through deep reflection from suffering and pain, individuals found new discoveries in their journeys through life.

The holistic body-mind-spirit model is based on a strengths-focused approach, emphasizing empowering patients and family carers to maintain hopes and dreams. Social support, assessment and enhancement of spiritual capital can contribute to building the patient's strengths (Wan, Leung, & Fong, 2014). By adopting a capacity-building framework, palliative care social workers will focus on social, emotional, intellectual, financial, artistic and communication strengths of patients and family carers (see Chapter 18).

Echoing anticipatory and ambiguous loss at the end of life, the existential crisis of loss of meaning in the midst of helplessness, hopelessness and total loss of control or dignity among patients and family members calls for spiritual intervention in sense making and meaning reconstruction. Spiritual issues are regarded as an important aspect of palliative care (Puchalski, Ferrell, & O'Donnell, 2011). Maugans (1996) suggests an assessment approach of spirituality at the end of life by asking questions on SPIRIT – spiritual belief, personal values, integration with the spiritual community, ritualized practices and restrictions, implications for clinical practice and terminal event planning.

Spirituality is relatively difficult to calibrate. There are increasing trends towards expressive arts, exercise, *qigong*, dance and alternative methods in serving cancer patients (Ho, Fong, Cheung, Yip, & Luk, 2016). Resilience and spiritual strengths can be enhanced with faith, hope, prayer, music, meditation and religious rituals. The search for spiritual meaning, a sense of comfort and peace and connection with God or a higher being are common among patients when lifespan is limited (Luskin, 2004). In recent decades, Eastern philosophies such as Buddhist and Daoist teachings have received increasing attention in supporting patients and families spiritually. Normalizing human suffering as part of life, with an emphasis on not knowing, non-attachment to life and death, respect for the law of nature, trust in the cause and effect in Dharma and being truthful, compassionate, kind and generous for the common good can help patients and families to cope with challenges in end-of-life care (Sik & Wu, 2015).

Hope originates from meaning, but it is also the biggest challenge for patients at the end of their lives. Existentialism, spirituality and meaning reconstruction theories are recognized as pivotal in end-of-life situations when individuals experience a strong craving for existential meaning (Villagomeza, 2005). Recent advances in logotherapy, sense-making processes, the study of suffering and growth through pain and the transformation of experiences of loss into personal capacity to embrace adversities have provided concrete frameworks for meaning making and reconstruction. Neimeyer (2000) developed elaborate techniques for helping patients and family members in retelling their stories, realigning their life priorities and developing a meaningful narrative in integrating new meanings to their lies and deaths. The constructivist psychotherapy approach in meaning making is still a major contemporary technique used by the professions in end-of-life care.

Resilience

A foundation of end-of-life care under the holistic model is facilitating the willingness of individuals to 'let go'. To be able to 'die in peace' requires high levels of emotional and spiritual intelligence. Some people can create a mess or chaos in family relationships and make life difficult for everyone before they die. These are 'dysfunctional' and 'high-conflict' families that tend to turn their anticipatory grief into hostile outbursts, creating hurts and opening up past wounds. Such interactions can create distance between the family members, resulting in detachment and disengagement.

The capacity for individuals and families to cope with adversity and not be immobilized by traumatic and ambiguous losses are regarded as resilient strengths. Resilience involves flexibility in coping; maintaining optimism, faith and hope despite physical decline; hardiness during constant frustrations and bad news; the ability to find meaning in suffering and the capacity to connect to a higher power or God at the end of life. These resilient capacities can be cultivated amid hurdles and difficulties in hostile environments. Patterson (2002) integrated family resilience and family stress theory into concepts explaining how resilience can provide strength in coping with relationship distress. Resilience is widely adopted in family adjustment to adversity and is also being adopted in palliative and end-of-life care (Walsh, 2012). Family intervention should focus on empowering family systems, enhancing family resources and facilitating family communication processes.

Adopting ecological, systems and family life-cycle developmental perspectives, resilience entails components of connectedness, nurturance, an enhanced sense of coherence, continuity, social and economic security, manageability and predictability in times of uncertainty, vulnerability and devastation. Mindfulness training for couples was found to be helpful (Hsiao et al., 2016) as it promotes an innate awareness of body sensation, thoughts, feelings, and experience without judgement, accepting and observing the experience moment by moment. This capacity to pay attention with deep listening and full presence can enable families to examine their fear of death and the importance of life. In the process of total and unconditional acceptance of self and others, loving kindness towards self and others will emerge.

Various interventions to enhance resilience focus on consolidating legacies of the past; making meaning of adversity as platform for growth and transcendence; affirming family strength and shared spirituality; developing a sense of purpose and meaning beyond apparent problems and finding strengths, comfort and guidance of loss through reconnection to values, rituals, and communal ceremonies and celebrations. Clinical trials found that palliative care can enhance resilience and perceived social support among family members (Somasundaram & Devamani, 2016). Many families become readier to express their positive emotions towards each other when a member is at the end of their life.

Understanding end-of-life care from a family perspective

The needs of family members of patients at the end of their lives cannot be ignored. The anxiety of family caregivers and patients is linked, and emotional distress among family carers can be higher than that of the patients (Chan et al., 2014). Caregiving chores are physically demanding, and family members of patients normally experience emotional dejection, anxiety and frustration (Mosher, Bakas, & Champion, 2013). Anticipatory grief, uncertainty and loss of control are also common for caregivers. Disrupted daily schedules, strained relationships, isolation and financial hardship can easily lead to burnout among the caregivers (Sanders, Bantum, Owen, Thorton, & Stanton, 2010).

Family interactions are often coloured by love, joy, intimacy, hate, alienation and disgust at different stages of family development. Unfortunately, intimate family relationships can also be violent, abusive and difficult at times, resulting in different patterns of family interaction that may be alienating, aggressive or high conflict. When it comes to the end of life, it is easy for families to become closer to each other or grow even further apart. Kissane and Hempton (2017) strongly advocate for more resources and training in facilitating family-centred palliative care. Palliative care family meetings are particularly relevant for high-conflict, disengaged, uninvolved and low-communication families and families with special needs and vulnerabilities. They deserve more attention and support from the care and support systems to facilitate communication, resolve conflicts, and tackle practical concerns. A family-centred palliative care approach can improve quality of death and reduce risks of prolonged bereavement.

Palliative care social workers need to support the family as a unit. Their role includes addressing caregiving stress and burdens, emotional distress and the sense of loss and grief in the caregiving and bereavement process. They should also be competent to handle relational issues within the family, including newly emerging or long-standing issues unveiled by end-stage illness. Social workers may also have a role in facilitating family communication on care planning and decision-making, ensuring that patients' values and preferences are being respected in the process and mediating possible family conflicts. Another core issue would be to help patients and family members achieve relational completion by facilitating the expression of love and forgiveness, passing on legacies and life wisdom, saying goodbyes and granting family members permission to live well after their departure.

Understanding end-of-life care from a community perspective

The purpose of social work intervention is to preserve the personhood of individuals who are confronted by imminent death. Most people fear the end of life and death as it may mean excruciating pain and severe disablement, as well as total loss of self-care abilities, pride and sense of meaning and purpose in life. Isolation, demoralization, destitution and poor quality of life during their last days of existence are also important issues. Yet the general death anxiety among community members creates extra barriers for dying persons to living with dignity in their own neighbourhoods. Community isolation, exclusion, meaninglessness, stigmatization and discrimination are common fears among families confronting death. Thus, active community engagement and collective participation to create a supportive and compassionate environment becomes crucial (Stillion & Attig, 2015; see Chapters 24 and 25).

Building compassionate communities: a health-promoting palliative care approach

Kellehear (2005) proposed a health-promoting palliative care approach for making large-scale, international efforts to incorporate principles of health promotion in end-of-life care. A series of social efforts by communities, governments, state institutions and social or medical care organizations would aim to create compassionate cities for improving health and well-being in the face of life-limiting illnesses (Sallnow, Richardson, Murray, & Kellehear, 2016). Since then, numerous regional and national guidelines and blueprints have been published and put into practice with several core principles identified (Gomez-Batiste & Connor, 2017):

1   Normalization of death: death and dying are perceived to be natural processes in life, and the dying process should not be over-medicalized and professionalized.
2   Integrative end-of-life care: The complex needs of patients and families should be addressed with a health promotion approach that promotes integrative well-being and fosters optimal functioning and living life to the full.
3   Continuum of end-of-life care: End-of-life care should start as early as possible in advanced age, with the diagnosis of an advanced chronic conditions or life-limiting illnesses, and extend beyond death into bereavement.
4   Community engagement: engage the entire community, policy and service leaders, health and social care professionals and advocates as active agents in changing the life experiences of patients and families.
5   Respecting the values and preferences of individuals: patients and families should be actively involved as partners in care planning and coordination so that patients' values and preferences are adequately addressed, and their sense of dignity preserved.

'Palliative care for all' approach

WHO pioneered a public health strategy, providing specific advice and detailed guidelines on how to integrate palliative care into existing healthcare systems. The model was further developed as a four-level approach, including the introduction of palliative care in all settings of care in the community; primary care and outpatient units; palliative specialist services and mixed palliative care specialists for specific health conditions such as dementia, cancer and AIDS (Gomez-Batiste & Connor, 2017).

One single step toward compassionate communities

While these ideas highlight the critical contribution of community, the question of how to engage the community in end-of-life care remains. The systematic review by Sallnow et al. (2016) summarizes four strategies from existing community engagement projects in end-of-life care:

1   Mobilization of community resources.
2   Influencing perceptions and reactions to death and dying.
3   Focus on the awareness and competence of the public.
4   Advocating policy reform.

Understanding the public perceptions of death and dying forms the essential basis for awareness campaigns, education programmes and training activities. When a society develops an open and positive attitude towards death and dying, it becomes more possible to mobilize community resources to support families and patients with life-limiting illnesses and to empower the community to advocate for policies favouring improvement in end-of-life care, which eventually contributes to building a compassionate community.

As an initial step to engage the community, there are extensive national and regional efforts on public engagement in European countries, the UK, the US, Canada and Asia (where death is often a taboo). They are effective means to understand public knowledge and attitudes towards issues in end of life as well as to guide service development and policy advocacy.

Public campaigns, such as the 'Death Café', which can be found in over 50 countries, enable people to discuss death and dying issues in a relaxed environment. 'Before I Die' walls have been created in 76 countries to provide a space in the community for people to re-examine life through thinking about death. There are projects such as 'Death Talks', 'Dying Matters', and the 'Conversation Project' to encourage people to initiate dialogues on end-of-life and death-related issues. Sharing by members of a community often becomes important collective action for social movements and policy advocacy.

Community-level palliative care social workers are resource persons who have a role in navigating through multiple systems for the best care of patients and families. They can take on the role of social change agent to facilitate communication across systems. This may empower patients and families as active agents and equal partners in care planning and decision-making, allowing their voices to be heard, their values and preferences respected and dignity conserved. It also helps other health and social care professionals communicate effectively with patients and families. Social workers can contribute to professional and community capacity building by organizing training for frontline clinical staff working in community settings, educational activities for the general public to increase community awareness and engagement in end-of-life issues, as well as recruiting, training and supervising volunteers.

The development of social work competency frameworks

The unique roles of social workers in end-of-life care for patients and families point towards an imperative need for continuous education in the field. Gomez-Batiste and Connor (2017) reviewed existing training and education programmes for health and social care professionals and summarized them into three aspects: professional specialization, complexity of intervention level and disciplinary approach. These three aspects are important to developing competency frameworks in end-of-life care as they help specify the aims, targets, levels and methods of training and education programmes. There are a few competency frameworks developed for the social work profession describing comprehensive curricula on knowledge, skills and practice values and attitude (Gwyther et al., 2005; Bosma et al., 2010). In line with the public health approach to palliative care, it is suggested that the aims, content and method of training be tailor made in accordance with social workers' positions, the nature of their work and their level of involvement in end-of-life care.

Challenges in theoretical development in end-of-life care

With increasing sophistication in technology and artificial intelligence in communication and caring, internet medicine, robotic care, multidisciplinary teams and holistic and energy healing, theorizing in end-of-life care may involve more fuzzy logic, computer language and blue-sky thinking (see Chapter 15). With patients and families becoming more educated, traditional professional end-of-life care will have to move towards active patient engagement and empowerment, treating patients as equal partners to prepare for their dying process. The new discoveries in medical treatment will create hope among patients with advanced diagnoses and may also distract them from dealing with end-of-life issues and defer relevant decisions. Risk-screening tools are effective in identifying persons in need of special interventions yet generic and basic needs of persons and families may be ignored. Focus on treatment compliance, advance directives and end-of-life pathways may build barriers for patients in accessing holistic psychosocial and spiritual care. Domiciliary palliative care as an integrative part of health and social care should be available to everyone in need because people spent most of their time at home in their last months of life. Measurement of the extent to which a good death is achieved, the capacity to let go and being able to be at peace with death is still in the process of development. More outcome measurements need to be developed to measure subtle states of affliction and equanimity (Chan et al., 2014). In situations of infectious diseases and behaviourally linked contagion such as AIDS, the issues of stigma and discrimination need to be tackled as well (Yu, Zhang, & Chan, 2016).

Further reading

Altilio, Y., & Otis-Green, S. (Eds.). (2011). *Oxford handbook of palliative social work*. New York: Oxford University Press.
This is a practical handbook on palliative social work with authors from all over the world contributing to guide practitioners on serving patients at the end of their lives.

Christ, G., Messner, C., & Behar, L. (Eds.). (2015). *Handbook of oncology social work: Psychosocial care for people with cancer*. New York: Oxford University Press.
This is a comprehensive handbook on oncology social work. Palliative care and symptom control are important aspects of oncology care.

Lee, M. Y., Chan, C. H. Y., Chan, C. L. W., Ng, S. M., & Leung, P. P. Y. (2018). *Integrative body-mind-spirit social work: An empirically based approach to assessment and treatment* (2nd ed.). New York: Oxford University Press.
This is a systematic guide to holistic and integrative body-mind-spirit social work. The second edition contains research and practice with online illustrations of intervention skills.

References

Bosma, H., Johnston, M., Cadell, S., Wainwright, W., Abernethy, N., Feron, A., . . . Nelson, F. (2010). Creating social work competencies for practice in hospice palliative care. *Palliative Medicine, 24*(1), 79–87.
Boss, P. (2002). *Loss, trauma, and resilience: Therapeutic work with ambiguous loss*. New York: Norton.
Boss, P., Roos, S., & Harris, D. L. (2011). *Grief in the midst of ambiguity and uncertainty: An exploration of ambiguous loss and chronic sorrow*. New York: Routledge.
Chan, C. H. Y., Chan, T. H. Y., Leung, P. P. Y., Brenner, M. J., Wong, V. P. Y., Leung, E. K. T., . . . Chan, C. L. W. (2014). Rethinking well-being in terms of affliction and equanimity: Development of a holistic well-being scale. *Journal of Ethnic Cultural Diversity in Social Work, 23*(3–4), 289–308.
Chan, C. L., & Dickens, R. R. (2015). Oncology social work practice in integrative medicine. In *Handbook of oncology social work: Psychosocial care for people with cancer* (p. 371). New York: Oxford University Press.
Chan, C. L. W., Chan, T. H. Y., & Ng, S. M. (2006). The strength-focused and meaning-oriented approach to resilience and transformation (SMART): A body-mind-spirit approach to trauma management. In G. Rosenberg & A. Weissman (Eds.), *International social health care policy, programs, and* studies (pp. 9–36). New York: Haworth.
Dyer, A. (2011). The need for a new 'new medical model': A bio-psychosocial-spiritual model. *Southern Medical Journal, 104*(4), 297–298.
Gomez-Batiste, X., & Connor, S. (Eds.). (2017). *Building integrated palliative care programs and services*. Retrieved from http://kehpca.org/wp-content/uploads/Go%CC%81mez-Batiste-X-Connor-S-Eds.-Building-Integrated-Palliative-Care-Programs-and-Services.-2017-b.pdf
Gwyther, L. P., Altilio, T., Blacker, S., Christ, G., Csikai, E. L., Hooyman, N., . . . Howe, J. (2005). Social work competencies in palliative and end-of-life care. *Journal of Social Work in End-of-Life & Palliative Care, 1*(1), 87–120.
Ho, R. T. H., Fong, T. C. T., Cheung, I. K. M., Yip, P. S. F., & Luk, M. Y. (2016). Effects of a short-term dance movement therapy program on symptoms and stress in breast cancer patients undergoing radiotherapy: A randomized controlled trial. *Journal of Pain and Symptom Management, 51*, 824–831.
Ho, R. T. H., Fong, T. C. T., Lo, P. H. Y., Ho, S. M. Y., Lee, P. W. H., Leung, P. P. Y., . . . Chan, C. L. W. (2017). Randomized controlled trial of supportive-expressive group therapy and body-mind-spirit intervention for Chinese non-metastatic breast cancer patients. *Supportive Care in Cancer, 24*(12), 4929–4937.

Hsiao, F. H., Jow, G. M., Kuo, W. H., Yang, P. S., Lam, H. B., Chang, K. J., . . . Chang, C. H. (2016). The long-term effects of mindfulness added to family resilience-oriented couples support group on psychological well-being and cortisol responses in breast cancer survivors and their partners. *Mindfulness, 7*, 1365–1376.

Kean, S. (2010). The experience of ambiguous loss in families of brain injured ICU patients. *Nursing in Critical Care*, 66–75.

Kellehear, A. (2005). *Compassionate cities: Public health and end-of-life care*. London: Routledge.

Kissane, D. W., & Hempton, C. (2017). Conducting a family meeting. In D. W. Kissane, B. Bultz, P. N. Butow, C. L. Byland, S. Noble & S. Wilkinson (Eds.), *Oxford textbook of communication in oncology and palliative care* (2nd ed., pp. 109–117). Oxford: Oxford University Press.

Luskin, F. (2004). Transformative practices for integrating mind-body-spirit. *Journal of Alternative and Complementary Medicine, 10*(1), S15–S23.

Maugans, T. A. (1996). The SPIRITual history. *Archives of Family Medicine, 5*, 11–16.

Morone, N. E., & Greco, C. M. (2007). Mind-body interventions for chronic pain in older adults: A structured review. *Pain Medicine, 8*(4), 359–275.

Mosher, C. E., Bakas, T., & Champion, V. L. (2013). Physical health, mental health, and life changes among family caregivers of patients with lung cancer. *Oncological Nursing Forum, 40*, 53–61.

Neimeyer, R. A. (2000). *Lessons of loss: A guide to coping*. Memphis, TN: Center for the Study of Loss and Transition, University of Memphis.

Ng, S. M., Chan, C. L. W., Ho, D. Y. F., Wong, Y. Y., & Ho, R. T. H. (2006). Stagnation as a distinct clinical syndrome: Comparing 'yu' (stagnation) in traditional Chinese medicine with depression. *British Journal of Social Work, 36,* 467–484.

Otis-Green, S., Ferrell, B., Spolum, M., Uman, G., Mullan, P., Baird, R. P., & Grant, M. (2009). An overview of the ACE Project – Advocating for clinical excellence: Transdisciplinary palliative care education. *Journal of Cancer Education, 2009, 24*(2), 120–126.

Patterson, J. M. (2002). Integrating family resilience and family stress theory. *Journal of Marriage and Family, 64*(2), 349–360.

Puchalski, C. M., Ferrell, B., & O'Donnell, E. (2011). Spiritual issues in palliative care. In E. Bruera & S. Yennurajalingam (Eds.), *Oxford American handbook of hospice and palliative medicine* (pp. 253–268). New York: Oxford University Press.

Saleebey, D. (Ed.). (2012). *The strengths perspective in social work practice* (6th ed.). Boston: Allyn & Bacon.

Sallnow, L., Richardson, H., Murray, S. A., & Kellehear, A. (2016). The impact of a new public health approach to end-of-life care: A systematic review. *Palliative Medicine, 30*(3), 200–211.

Sanders, S. L., Bantum, E. O., Owen, J. E., Thorton, A. A., & Stanton, A. L. (2010). Supportive care needs in patients with lung cancer. *Psychooncology, 19*, 480–489.

Sik, H. H., & Wu, B. W. Y. (2015). The importance of the Buddhist teaching on three kinds of knowing: In a school-based contemplative education program. In K. L. Dhammajoti (Ed.), *Buddhist meditative praxis: Traditional teachings and modern applications*. Hong Kong: Centre of Buddhist Studies, University of Hong Kong.

Smaldone, M. C., & Uzzo, R. G. (2013). The Kubler-Ross model, physician distress, and performance reporting. *Nature Reviews Urology*, 10, 425–428.

Somasundaram, R. O., & Devamani, K. A. (2016). A comparative study on resilience, perceived social support and hopelessness among cancer patients treated with curative and palliative care. *Indian Journal of Palliative Care, 22*(2), 135.

Stillion, J. M., & Attig, T. (Eds.). (2015). *Death, dying, and bereavement: Contemporary perspectives, institutions, and practices*. New York: Springer.

Villagomeza, L. R. (2005). Spiritual distress in adult cancer patients toward conceptual clarity. *Holistic Nursing Practice, 19*, 285–294.

Walsh, F. (2012). Family resilience: Strengths forged through adversity. In F. Walsh (Ed.), *Normal family processes* (pp. 399–427). New York: Guilford.

Wan, A. H. Y., Leung, P. P. Y., & Fong, C. H. C. (2014). Social support as spiritual capital of Chinese with cancer: Towards a holistic approach. In S. Chen (Ed.), *Social support and health: Theory, research, and practice with diverse populations* (pp. 193–208). New York: Nova.

Yu, N. X., Zhang, J. X., & Chan, C. L. W. (2016). Healthcare neglect, perceived discrimination, and dignity-related distress among Chinese patients with HIV. *AIDS Education and Prevention, 28*(1), 90–102.

Index

Note: numbers in *italic* indicate a figure & numbers in **bold** indicate a table.

Index

Milton Keynes UK
Ingram Content Group UK Ltd.
UKHW051852071024
449327UK00025B/1915